KU-733-489

LIBRARY
Learning
Resource Centre

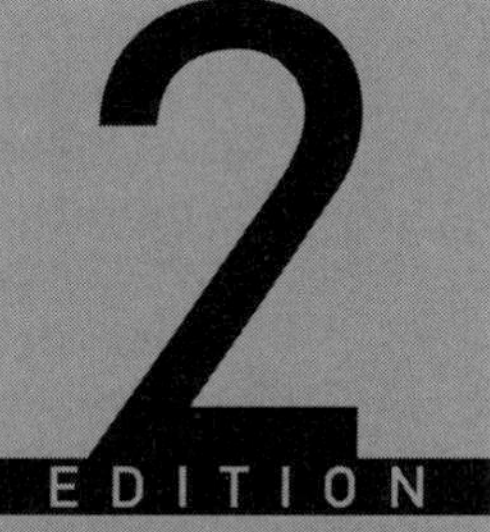

Handbook of Theories of Aging

Vern L. Bengtson, PhD, is research professor of gerontology and Professor Emeritus of Sociology at the University of Southern California. He has a PhD from the University of Chicago and is past president of the Gerontological Society of America. He has coauthored *How Families Still Matter: A Longitudinal Study of Two Generations* and coedited the *Cambridge Handbook of Age and Ageing*, the *Sourcebook of Family Theory and Research*, and *Aging in East and West: Families, States, and the Elderly*. His research articles have appeared in the *Journals of Gerontology*, *American Sociological Review*, *American Journal of Sociology*, and *Research on Aging*.

Merril Silverstein, PhD, is a professor in the Davis School of Gerontology and the Department of Sociology at the University of Southern California. He holds a doctorate degree in sociology from Columbia University. He was previously research assistant professor at Brown University and before that an NIA postdoctoral scholar in aging research at the University of Southern California. He has authored over 100 published works, including two edited volumes: *Intergenerational Relations Across Time and Place* and *From Generation to Generation: Continuity and Discontinuity in Aging Families*. He is a fellow of the Gerontological Society of America, the Brookdale National Fellowship Program, and the Fulbright International Senior Scholars Program.

Norella M. Putney, PhD, is a research assistant professor in the Department of Sociology at the University of Southern California and currently serves as project director of the Transmission of Religion Across Generations study, an investigation of religion and families, supported by a grant from the John Templeton Foundation. She holds a doctoral degree in sociology from the University of Southern California and has published on such topics as theories of aging, intergenerational relations, aging and the life course, and women's changing lives. She has coauthored chapters in several volumes, including the *Cambridge Handbook of Age and Ageing*, and the *Handbook of the Life Course*.

Daphna Gans, PhD, is a postdoctoral fellow in the study of aging at the Department of Labor and Population at RAND and a recipient of the National Institute on Aging Ruth L. Kirschstein National Research Service Award of Postdoctoral Training. She is a part-time lecturer at the Leonard Davis School of Gerontology at the University of Southern California. She earned her doctoral degree in gerontology from the University of Southern California and holds a master's degree in family studies from Michigan State University. She coauthored articles that were published in several professional journals, including *Journal of Marriage and Family* and *Journal of Family Issues*. During her studies at the University of Southern California, she served as data coordinator for a 4-year binational study on intergenerational support to the aged in Israel and the United States.

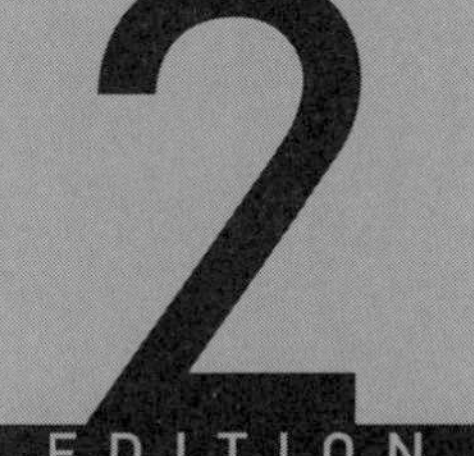

Handbook of Theories of Aging

Editors
Vern L. Bengtson, PhD
Merril Silverstein, PhD
Norella M. Putney, PhD
Daphna Gans, PhD

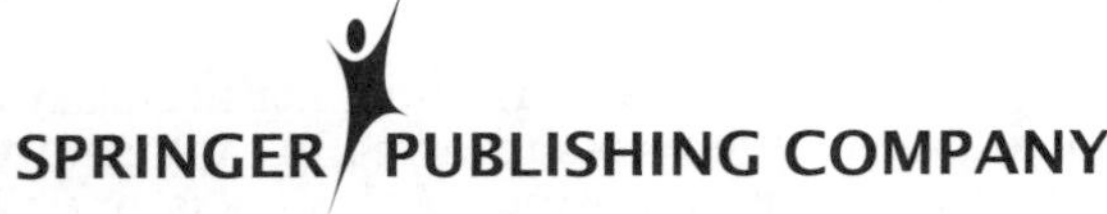

New York

Springer Publishing Company, LLC
11 West 42nd Street
New York, NY 10036
www.springerpub.com

Acquisitions Editor: Sheri W. Sussman
Production Editor: Julia Rosen
Cover design: Mimi Flow
Composition: Apex CoVantage

08 09 10 11 12/ 5 4 3 2 1

Library of Congress Cataloging-in-Publication Data
Handbook of theories of aging / [edited by] Vern Bengtson . . . [et al.].—2nd ed.
p. ; cm.
Includes bibliographical references and index.
ISBN 978-0-8261-6251-9 (alk. paper)
1. Aging—Research. 2. Gerontology—Research. I. Bengtson, Vern L.
[DNLM: 1. Aging—physiology. 2. Aging—psychology. 3. Geriatrics.
4. Models, Biological. WT 104 H236 2009]
HQ1061.H3366 2009
305.2601—dc22 2008033650

Printed in the United States of America by Hamilton Printing.

Dedication

Dedicated to,

James E. Birren, PhD, Dean Emeritus, USC Davis School of Gerontology

One of the founders of the field of gerontology
and originator of the first scientific theories in the psychology of aging
on his 90th birthday.

Contents

List of Figures and Tables

Chapter 27

Chapter 29

Chapter 32

Chapter 35

Chapter 39

Contributors

W. Andrew Achenbaum, PhD
Professor of History and Social Work at the University of Houston
Houston, TX

Katherine R. Allen, PhD
Professor of Human Development
Virginia Polytechnic Institute and State University
Blacksburg, VA

Hiroko Akiyama, PhD
Research Associate Professor, Survey Research Center, Institute for Social Research
University of Michigan
Ann Arbor, MI

Toni C. Antonucci, PhD
Associate Dean for Academic Programs and Interdisciplinary Studies
Ellizabeth M. Douvan Collegiate Professor of Psychology, Senior Research Scientist and Program Director of the Life Course Development Program in the Institute for Social Research
University of Michigan
Ann Arbor, MI

Steven N. Austad, PhD
Professor of Cellular and Structural Biology and the Barshop Institute for Longevity and Aging Studies
University of Texas Health Science Center
San Antonio, TX

Jan Baars, PhD
Professor of Interpretive Gerontology The Netherlands University for Humanistics
Professor of Philosophy of the Social Sciences and the Humanities, University of Tilburg
Utrecht, The Netherlands

Scott A. Bass, PhD
Provost and Professor of Public Affairs
American University
Washington, DC

Kira S. Birditt, PhD
Elizabeth Douvan Research Fellow, Institute for Social Research
University of Michigan
Ann Arbor, MI

Fredda Blanchard-Fields, PhD
Professor and Chair of the School of Psychology
Georgia Institute of Technology
Atlanta, GA

Toni Calasanti, PhD
Professor of Sociology
Virginia Polytechnic Institute and State University
Blacksburg, VA

Sara Carmel, MPH, PhD
Professor of Medical Sociology and Gerontology
Ben-Gurion University of the Negev
Beer-Sheva, Israel

Monique D. Cohen, MPH
Department of Health Policy and Administration
University of North Carolina Chapel Hill
Chapel Hill, NC

Eileen M. Crimmins, PhD
Associate Dean of the Davis School of Gerontology
Edna M. Jones Chair in Gerontology and Professor of Gerontology and Sociology
University of Southern California
Los Angeles, CA

Dale Dannefer, PhD
Selah Chamberlain Professor and Chair of the Department of Sociology
Case Western Reserve University
Cleveland, OH

Kelvin J. A. Davies, PhD, DSc
James E. Birren Professor of Gerontology and Professor of Molecular and Computational Biology
University of Southern California
Los Angeles, CA

Peggye Dilworth-Anderson, PhD
Professor of Health Policy and Administration
School of Public Health
Associate Director of Aging and Diversity
Institute on Aging
University of North Carolina Chapel Hill
Chapel Hill, NC

Israel Doron, PhD
Law Professor and Senior Lecturer in the Department of Gerontology
University of Haifa
Haifa, Israel

Rita B. Effros, PhD
Professor of Pathology and Laboratory Medicine
David Geffen School of Medicine
University of California
Los Angeles, CA

Kenneth F. Ferraro, PhD
Professor of Sociology and Director of the Center on Aging and the Life Course
Purdue University
West Lafayette, IN

Michael R. Foy, PhD
Professor of Psychology
Loyola Marymount University
Los Angeles, CA

Christine L. Fry, PhD
Professor of Anthropology Emerita
Loyola University
Chicago, IL

Stavros Gonidakis, BA
Doctoral Student
Integrative and Evolutionary Biology
University of Southern California
Los Angeles, CA

Michael Gurven, PhD
Associate Professor of Anthropology
University of California Santa Barbara
Santa Barbara, CA

Laurie Russell Hatch, PhD
Professor of Sociology and Director of the Center for Teaching and Learning at
Ohio University
Athens, OH

Jon Hendricks, PhD
Professor and former Dean
Oregon State University
Corvallis, OR

Robert B. Hudson, PhD
Professor and Chair, Department of Social Policy
Boston University School of Social Work
Boston, MA

Malcolm L. Johnson, PhD
Visiting Professor of Gerontology and End of Life Care
University of Bath
Emeritus Professor of Health and Social Policy
University of Bristol
Bristol, UK

Ben Lennox Kail, MS
Doctoral Student in Department of Sociology
Florida State University
Tallahassee, FL

Antje Kalinauskas, PhD
Postdoctoral Fellow, Blanchard-Fields' Adult Development Lab
Georgia Institute of Technology
Atlanta, GA

Hillard Kaplan, PhD
Professor of Anthropology
University of New Mexico
Albuquerque, NM

Jennifer Reid Keene, PhD
Associate Professor of Sociology
University of Nevada Las Vegas
Las Vegas, NV

Jessica A. Kelley-Moore, PhD
Associate Professor of Sociology
Case Western Reserve University
Cleveland, OH

Bob G. Knight, PhD
Merle H. Bensinger Professor of Gerontology and Professor of Psychology
Andrus Gerontology Center
University of Southern California
Los Angeles, CA

Neal Krause, PhD
Professor in the Department of Health Behavior and Health Education
School of Public Health
University of Michigan
Ann Arbor, MI

Nichole Kryla-Lighthall, BA
Doctoral Student in the Davis School of Gerontology
University of Southern California
Los Angeles, CA

Gisela Labouvie-Vief, PhD
Professor of Social-Emotional Development
Department of Psychology
University of Geneva
Geneva, Switzerland

Ken Laidlaw, PhD
Senior Lecturer in Clinical Psychology
Section of Clinical and Health Psychology
University of Edinburgh
Edinburgh, UK

Charles F. Longino Jr., PhD
Washington M. Wingate Professor of Sociology
Director of the Reynolda Gerontology Program
Wake Forest University
Winston Salem, NC

Valter D. Longo, PhD
Associate Professor of Biogerontology and Biological Sciences
Davis School of Gerontology
University of Southern California
Los Angeles, CA

Ariela Lowenstein, PhD
Professor of Aging Studies
University of Haifa
Haifa, Israel

Victor W. Marshall, PhD
Director, University of North Carolina Institute on Aging
Professor of Sociology, and Adjunct Professor of Health Behavior and Health Education
University of North Carolina Chapel Hill
Chapel Hill, NC

George M. Martin, PhD
Professor of Pathology Emeritus
University of Washington
Seattle, WA

Mike Martin, PhD
Professor of Gerontopsychology
Director of the Center of Gerontology
University of Zurich
Zurich, Switzerland

Mara Mather, PhD
Associate Professor of Gerontology and Psychology
University of Southern California
Los Angeles, CA

Chris Phillipson, PhD
Professor of Applied Social Studies and Social Gerontology
Keele University
Staffordshire, UK

Jason L. Powell, PhD
Senior Lecturer
School of Sociology and Social Policy
University of Liverpool
Liverpool, UK

Jill Quadagno, PhD
Professor of Sociology
Mildred and Claude Pepper Eminent Scholar Chair in Social Gerontology
Florida State University
Tallahassee, FL

Carol D. Ryff, PhD
Director of the Institute on Aging and Professor of Psychology
University of Wisconsin–Madison
Madison, WI

Markus H. Schafer
Doctoral Student in Sociology
Purdue University
West Lafayette, IN

K. Warner Schaie, PhD, ScD (hon.), DrPhil (hon.)
Evan Pugh Professor Emeritus of Human Development and Psychology
Pennsylvania State University
University Park, PA

Richard A. Settersten Jr., PhD
Professor of Human Development and Family Sciences
College of Health and Human Sciences
Oregon State University
Corvallis, OR

Tetyana Pylypiv Shippee
Doctoral Candidate in the dual-title PhD Program in Sociology and Gerontology
Purdue University
West Lafayette, IN

Reshma Shringarpure, PhD
Clinical Scientist in the Department of Clinical Research at Amylin Pharmaceuticals, Inc.
San Diego, CA

Burton Singer, PhD
Charles and Marie Robertson Professor of Public and International Affairs
Princeton University
Senior Research Scientist
University of Wisconsin–Madison
Madison, WI

Richard F. Thompson, PhD
Keck Professor of Psychology and Biological Sciences
University of Southern California
Los Angeles, CA

Mats Thorslund, PhD
Professor in Social Gerontology
Aging Research Center, Karolinska Institute/Stockholm University
Research Director at the Stockholm Gerontology Research Center
Stockholm, Sweden

Molly E. Trauten, MGS
Doctoral Student in the Department of Human Development and Family Sciences
Oregon State University
Corvallis, OR

Sarinnapha Vasunilashorn, MS
Doctoral Candidate and NIA Predoctoral Fellow
USC Davis School of Gerontology
University of Southern California
Los Angeles, CA

Alexis J. Walker, PhD
Petersen Chair in Gerontology and Family Studies
Professor of Human Development and Family Sciences
Oregon State University
Corvallis, OR

Alan Walker, PhD
Professor
Department of Sociological Studies
University of Sheffield
Sheffield, UK

Sherry L. Willis, PhD
Professor of Human Development
Pennsylvania State University
University Park, PA

Jeffrey Winking, PhD
Assistant Professor of Anthropology
Texas A&M University
College Station, TX

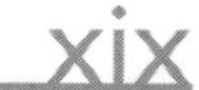

Diana S. Woodruff-Pak, PhD
Professor of Psychology, Neurology, and Radiology
Director of the Neuroscience Program
Temple University
Philadelphia, PA

Steven H. Zarit, PhD
Professor of Human Development and
Head, Department of Human Development and Family Studies
Pennsylvania State University
University Park, PA

Preface

Theory appears to be growing in importance in gerontology today. By theory, we mean "attempts to explain," and frequently in the past it was noted that "the field of gerontology is data-rich but theory-poor" (see the previous edition of this handbook). Recently, however, there seems to be an increase in "attempts to explain," going beyond descriptive data to propose mechanisms and processes underlying them. Perhaps nowhere is this more visible than in the growth of cross-disciplinary studies concerning the mechanism of aging, which is one of the underlying themes of this volume.

The purpose of this handbook is to advance the development and applications of theories of aging. Its intended audience is researchers who wish to build theory in order to better understand their findings about processes of aging. Another audience is the next generation of researchers in gerontology: graduate students, postdoctoral fellows, and junior investigators—those who will be leading the course of knowledge construction in aging in the 21st century.

As noted in the first edition, many of these future leaders in gerontological research were learning the tools of their trade in an intellectual and scientific context that seemed, at the end of the 20th century, increasingly dismissive of the importance of theory. Technological sophistication in statistical modeling—but not theoretically based explanations—were demanded by journal reviewers. Applications of research findings to specific problems—but not basic research to advance theoretical development—seemed to be the priority of National Institutes of Health study sections reviewing grants. At the same time, some critics were saying that we are at *The End of Science* (Horgan, 1996), while some postmodernists suggested that the very enterprise of theoretical explanation was little more than intellectual nonsense.

Since the first edition was published in 1999, however, there has been a renewed interest in encouraging theory-based research among editors of several distinguished journals, including the *Journals of Gerontology: Social Sciences* and, most recently, the *Journals of Gerontology: Psychological Sciences.* Editorial policy in these journals, among others, has changed to explicitly encourage the inclusion of manuscripts that report theory-based research findings as well as those presenting research findings that can contribute to theory.

The stated goal in the first edition of this handbook was to reestablish the importance of theory in discourse about problems of aging. Throughout the 25 chapters of the first edition of this handbook, authors addressed the primacy of explanation in the vastly expanding scientific literature reporting empirical findings about aging. The handbook was highly lauded and sold very well;

apparently, a host of readers were looking for attempts to explain, not just describe, phenomena of aging, and the chapter authors were eminently successful in doing so. The scope of the first edition of the handbook was multidisciplinary, reflecting the many scientific and applied disciplines engaged in gerontological research and interventions, encompassing the biology of aging, the psychology and sociology of aging, and social policy and practice concerning problems of aging. While the first edition was multidisciplinary—presenting an array of disciplinary theories of aging—the current edition aims at crossing disciplinary boundaries.

In this second edition of the handbook, the authors continue this tradition of developing explanations. But there is a new emphasis: cross-disciplinary or interdisciplinary explanations. In just the past few years, a number of investigators have reached out beyond traditional disciplinary boundaries to partner with researchers in adjacent fields in studying aging and age-related phenomena. Our goal in this book was to discuss, develop, and promote such interdisciplinary work. The chapters in this volume were commissioned from scholars whose research in aging has achieved international recognition and who we believe have something new to say about the advancement of cross-disciplinary theorizing in our field. In our letter of invitation to the contributors of this handbook, we included a specific request to discuss the interdisciplinary aspects of gerontological theory in their topic.

This edition of the handbook consists of 40 chapters written by 67 experts in the field of aging. It is organized in eight parts, reflecting major theoretical developments in gerontology since 1999.

1. *The context of theories of aging:* The three chapters in this part examine the role and dimensions of theories in gerontology, problems and prospects for multidisciplinary theories in aging, the history of theories of aging, and an evolutionary, anthropological perspective on aging and the human life span.
2. *Theorizing aging across disciplines:* Chapters in this part focus on biodemography, an example of gerontological inquiry across disciplines; a philosophical inquiry into the nature of time, age, and aging; meaning in life as a forum for interdisciplinary theory; and a biopsychosocial theory of healthy aging.
3. *Biological theories of aging:* Topics here include an overview of biological theories of aging; revisiting the immunological theory of aging; gene action and classical evolutionary theory of aging; neuroscientific theories of learning, memory, and aging; programmed longevity and aging theories; and free radicals and oxidative stress theories in aging.
4. *Psychological theories of aging:* These five chapters cover the convoys over the life course theory; building theories of social context, cognition, and aging; dynamic integration theory of emotion, cognition, and equilibrium in later life; a theory of cognitive plasticity; and a cognitive control theory of aging and emotional well-being.
5. *Social science perspectives on theories of aging:* Chapters in this part present an integrative theory of social gerontology; phenomenological theories and aging; life course theory and aging; cumulative inequality theory; theorizing lifestyle, agency, and structure in the life course; theories in feminist gerontology and sexuality; theorizing across cultures; anthropological theories and the experiences of aging; and theorizing about families and aging.

6. *Society, public policy, and theories of aging:* The six chapters in this part look at theoretical accounts of aging policy development in the United States, the political economy theory of aging, theory informing public policy with the life course perspective as a policy tool, theorizing the social in social policy and aging, the impact of globalization on aging, and aging policy in the welfare state.
7. *Translating theories of aging:* In this part, the issues discussed include theorizing the relationship between law and aging; spirituality, finitude, and theories of the life span; theories of a "good old age," mental health, and aging; translational theory and interventions to enhance well-being in later life; and the construction of knowledge in gerontological education.
8. *The future of theories of aging:* In a concluding chapter, the editors review some of the major themes and developments reflected in this volume. On the basis of these, they offer some predictions about the future of theory development in aging and some suggestions for the next generation of theory builders in gerontology.

The authors represent the United Kingdom, Switzerland, the Netherlands, Sweden, Israel, and the United States. Each has taken part in some cross-disciplinary research or writing in gerontology. All have labored long and hard to meet the demands of creating explanations for aging phenomena; one author said, "I feel like I've just taken my second doctoral oral." Theory building is hard work because it requires thinking.

This handbook includes a remarkable array of contributions that present state-of-the-art innovative inter- and intradisciplinary theorizing in the study of aging. It represents the current status of theoretical development in the study of aging. In the near future, we can expect a plethora of research articles presenting findings from innovative multidisciplinary and interdisciplinary collaborations in the study of aging. We hope that the authors of these publications will address the theoretical implications of their findings and pursue explanations that go beyond specific empirical findings. While theorizing—and especially theorizing across disciplines—is a challenging task, it is of crucial importance to the cumulative construction of knowledge.

Vern L. Bengtson
Merril Silverstein
Norella M. Putney
Daphna Gans
May 2008

Reference

Horgan, J. (1996). *The end of science: Facing the limits of science in the twilight of the scientific age.* New York: Broadway Books.

Acknowledgments

We wish to dedicate this volume to James E. Birren on his 90th birthday. He is one of the founders of scientific gerontology and one of the first presidents of the Gerontological Society of America. In his years at the National Institutes of Health, he fostered an amazing increase in research on aging, and in his decades at the University of Southern California's Andrus Gerontology Center, he mentored scores of students and younger scholars to careers in aging. Throughout his career, he has always been searching for explanations—and that is why we think he is truly the master of theory in our field.

In addition, we wish to acknowledge the contributions to this volume by Linda Hall, program manager at the University of Southern California. Linda has been involved in every stage of this project, from discussing the invitation for chapter authors to sending off the manuscript to the publisher (finally). In between, she edited chapters as they were sent in for correct style and sent gentle reminders to delinquent authors. This is the 15th book that Linda has shepherded into publication, and we are amazed by her skill. Thank you, Linda.

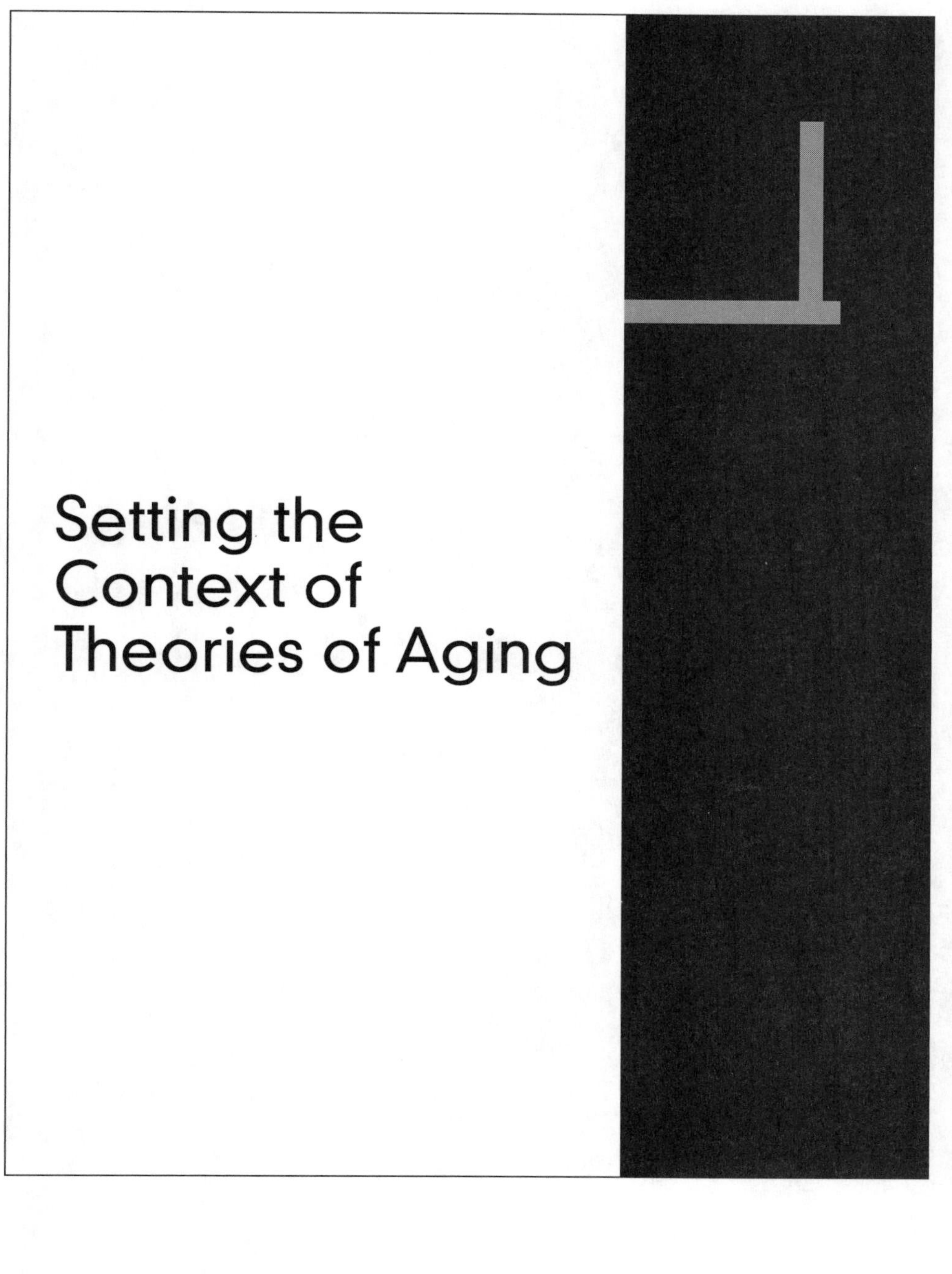

Setting the Context of Theories of Aging

1 Theories About Age and Aging

Vern L. Bengtson
Daphna Gans
Norella M. Putney
Merril Silverstein

Some humans are active and vital at age 90, while others are frail at age 60. Why? What causes aging? Why is there so much variation in aging among members of the same species? (see chapters 4, 5, 10, and 12)

Some older individuals perform as well as younger people on cognitive tasks, while others show significant deficits in cognitive functioning. Why? Is there a secret to avoiding memory loss, such as "keeping active"? (see chapters 15 and 17)

Some social contexts and societies provide significant care for their aged, while others leave it to the individual and his or her resources. Why? Why is there so much variation in public policy about aging? (see chapters 29, 31, and 34)

Some older adults appear to have emotionally gratifying lives despite experiencing significant losses. How do they manage this? (see chapters 18 and 37)

These are only a few examples of the many puzzles that gerontological researchers are addressing in their investigations. The answers to such "why" and "how" questions require theory, which is *an attempt to explain.*

The scientific study of aging is only three-quarters of a century old. But over the past three-quarters of a century, our field has accumulated a wealth of data about aging. We have come to know a great deal about cellular and molecular aging and changes in memory with age as well as the variation across societies in age-related health behaviors. At the same time, we do not know as much as we would like about *why* or *how* these aging phenomena and their consequences occur or about why and how there is so much variation in aging.

In this chapter, we attempt to present an overview of the multiple perspectives evident today concerning the nature and place of theorizing in our multidisciplinary field. We address three questions, three issues that we hope will guide tomorrow's researchers as they plan their investigations:

1. What is theory? How is it useful in research on aging?
2. What are the latest developments in theory from perspectives of biology, psychology, sociology, and social policy applied to aging?
3. What is interdisciplinary theorizing? Why is it the wave of the future in research on aging?

What Is Theory? Theorizing in Aging Research

Theorizing is a *process of developing ideas that allow us to understand and explain empirical observations.* The term *theory* is used in many ways to describe interpretations of ideas or observations—from theory as a conjecture or guess to what physicists define as a "coherent group of general propositions used as principles of explanation for a class of phenomena" (Webster, 2003). Even within a given field of knowledge such as gerontology, perspectives on theory change over time (as can be seen from the previous edition of this *Handbook of Theories of Aging* [Bengtson & Schaie, 1999]). But there are some features of theory that remain constant over time.

Theory as Explanation

"An attempt to explain" is the simplest and most direct way to define theory. Theorizing is the attempt to solve some puzzle we have encountered in our experience as scholars. Whether in the laboratory, in field studies, or in surveys—or indeed in everyday life—humans seek explanations and meanings for *what* they observe or experience. And that leads to their questioning the *why* and the *how* beyond their immediate observations. This is theorizing—the search for explanation.

Theories are like lenses. Look at an object through one kind of lens, and the viewer will see one thing; look at it through another lens, and the viewer will be able to see something different. For example, the field of aging and the social sciences is a multiple-paradigm arena, with several different theoretical perspectives or paradigms (e.g., critical theory and science-based theory) operating and changing all at the same time. It should be obvious that several lenses are required to see the complexity and diversity of aging processes.

Theory is crucial for useful research about aging. Lack of theory leads to one-shot, limited application of research findings that do not lead to building cumulative knowledge about an issue. Researchers—whether students or professors, whether using qualitative or quantitative methods—cannot design adequate studies without ideas about *what* it is they want to find out and *why* that is important. Making these explicit is crucial to a successful study design. And at the end of the process, when researchers select the most important results or findings to write about, they are theorizing—highlighting ideas that are important to share with others.

Theorizing as a Process

It may be helpful to refer to *theorizing* rather than use more passive terminology such as *using theory, applying theory, or developing theory.* The focus is on *theorizing,* the verb, rather than on *theory* as a noun or modifier. Theory should be viewed more as a *process* than as an end product. Too often "theory" is associated with some abstract set of ideas, disconnected from the process that led up to those ideas. Or it is associated with the memorization of the ideas and names of people long dead. As a graduate student said, "Theory is some arcane body of reasoning associated with a name that you have to memorize in order to appear knowledgeable in this class."

That is not the point of theory. We theorize, whether we are aware of it or not, in attempting to understand our observations and experiences. It is natural to go beyond describing the *what* of the data we have collected (whether from brain slices to census reports or in-depth qualitative interviews) to attempt to explain the *why* and *how* of the biological, social, or psychological processes underlying them. This is theorizing.

Theorizing Should Be Explicit

We submit that researchers should be *explicit* in theorizing. We should be aware that the data on aging we collect or statistically manipulate are not just "facts." They also constitute the essential raw materials of our reasoning and theorizing about our findings. Too frequently, theorizing is covert or implicit; this can lead to problems in research. In developing research, the investigators' "implicit theory" and underlying assumptions about the nature of the phenomena to be studied inevitably guide the selection of research questions as well as the concepts and variables to be measured. If the investigators do not recognize or acknowledge these implicit assumptions, this can bias or distort their interpretation of their findings.

Interdisciplinary Theories of Aging

Probably the most striking theoretical trend since the publication of the last edition of the *Handbook of Theories of Aging* 10 years ago has been the development of interdisciplinary theories of aging. Despite the difficulties in bridging traditional disciplinary boundaries and despite the challenges of working with different research paradigms and technologies, there have been significant breakthroughs in explanations of aging phenomena that take approaches from several disciplinary perspectives and blend them together into a unified theory.

The Foundations of Theories of Aging

Achenbaum (chapter 2) reminds us that theories of aging have a very long tradition in human thought, dating back at least to the epic of Gilgamesh in Babylonia about A.D. 3000. Hebrew and Christian Scriptures offered insights about the wisdom and suffering associated with gray hairs. Aristotle may have been the first to codify theories of age; he ascribed humors to four stages of life, with youth being hot and moist and old age cold and dry. Current theories about successful aging can be traced back to the texts of past masters; Coronaro in 1557 offered a regimen to promote healthful aging that consisted of exercise, diet, and temperance—eerily similar to that prescribed in Rowe and Kahn's (1998) bestseller four centuries later. That we "stand on the shoulders of giants" is unmistakably true of developing theories of aging. It is unfortunate that so many gerontological researchers appear not to be aware of this.

Certainly the growing body of evidence from evolutionary biology represents a foundation for current theories about the aging process. Kaplan, Gurven, and Winking (chapter 3) provide a useful review of such findings applied to species-typical aging. They note that an understanding of how the aging process and age-specific mortality respond to novel environmental variation requires a theory of how natural selection has acted on human biology over the course of human evolution. Their chapter presents such a theory, suggesting that the adaptive niche occupied by our species has selected for a coevolved suite of characteristics, what they call the *human adaptive complex.* They then present a theory about why the ability to live at least to age 65 has played such an important role in human adaptation, without which many other human characteristics could not have evolved.

Philosophical foundations are also crucial in attempts to understand aging, although researchers seem much less aware of these than the historical and evolutionary foundations. Baars (chapter 5) examines some epistemological attributes of the three central constructs in gerontology: *age, aged,* and *aging.* These are applications of the much larger concept of *time,* and the even broader concept of *change.* Theories of aging, then, are attempts to answer the question of how specific changes can be explained as part of processes of aging. Baars distinguishes between two kinds of time that are useful in gerontological research: *chronological time,* a causal representation, and *intrinsic time,* the personal and collective meanings given to past, present, and future. It is the latter that Baars suggests is the most useful perspective from which to examine human aging; it is too rich, he says, to be reduced to chronological age, life expectancy, or mortality rates.

Biodemography and Explaining Aging

The biodemography of aging, as summarized by Vasunilashorn and Crimmins (chapter 4), investigates questions relating to the variability in the rate of aging in populations. It attempts to understand how generalizable the current human condition is by examining different species or human populations in different settings. Researchers in the biodemography of aging are developing two types of theories. First are the "why" theories—why do animals and humans age? Why do some species, subpopulations, or societies age faster than others? Theories of programmed aging suggest that a biological clock drives the process of human development and aging process. Proposed explanations of these temporal molecular pathways include cellular aging and related genetics. Recent work has produced evidence that there are cross-species similarities in the patterning of life spans and also that within species life spans are considerably influenced by environment—for example, deviations in fertility and survival schedules in response to changing environmental conditions.

Second are the "who" theories—which populations age more quickly than others, and which individuals die sooner than others? Biopsychosocial theories attempt to explain how environmental, medical, and technological changes experienced by populations change the rate of aging. They attempt to determine which individuals within a population are most vulnerable to adverse health and age-associated conditions. The stress theory of health and aging has been proposed to explain such differences. This suggests that excess strains, because of greater exposure to chronic and acute strains, lead to increased risk for disease and disability. This theory is linked to the theory of cumulative disadvantage employed by sociologists (see Ferraro, Shippee, & Schafer, chapter 22). Most of these studies are motivated by the fundamental biodemographic question: how important is the role of environment on an individual's health and survival at later ages?

Multidisciplinary Theories of Meaning in Late Life

The search for a meaningful life has been a concern of philosophy and religion since humankind's earliest recorded history. But as Krause (chapter 6) points out, this is not merely an academic curiosity. Research on meaning in life is important because it speaks directly to key issues that face an aging population. A growing number of studies suggest that people who have found a sense of meaning in life tend to enjoy better physical health and tend to experience fewer symptoms of depression than individuals who have not been able to derive a sense that their lives have meaning. In addition, people with a stronger sense of meaning also tend to be happier and report higher levels of satisfaction with their lives.

Krause notes that meaning in life is a complex, multidimensional construct comprising four factors or dimensions: (a) having a clear set of values, (b) a sense of purpose, (c) goals for which to strive, and (d) the ability to reconcile things that have happened in the past. We can develop the theory by starting with a few key linkages: (a) personality traits shape the nature of social relationships that are formed by older adults; (b) relationships with significant others, in turn, help determine an older person's sense of meaning in life; (c) the social process of meaning making is influenced by the language that actors use at they jointly create a sense of meaning in life; and (d) once a sense of meaning has been negotiated and is firmly in place, findings from research in biology and physiology help show how it may affect health in late life. Scholars such as Frankl, Jung, Berger, and Maslow have argued that the ability to derive a sense of meaning in life represents the high-water mark of human development. If they are correct, then many of the biological, psychological, and sociological processes that researchers study should somehow contribute to the attainment of this ultimate goal.

Biopsychosocial Understanding of Healthy Aging

Almost everyone today would agree that there is no single fundamental cause of healthy aging but rather a multiplicity of factors working together to facilitate optimal functioning well into later life. But trying to understand the interplay among these multiple influences is a key challenge in formulating theory and executing empirical studies. Ryff and Singer (chapter 7) provide some innovative suggestions for making sense of these issues. First, they provide two definitions of "healthy aging" corresponding to biological and behavioral/medical orientations: (a) fending off cellular and molecular damage for the longest possible period of the life course and (b) the maximal delay of illness, disease, disability, and hence mortality—factors that keep the organism functioning optimally for the longest period of time. Second, they delineate an integrative approach to the task of understanding the causes, processes, and pathways of healthy aging, given the growing evidence that factors at multiple levels of influence are involved.

Healthy aging is fundamentally a biopsychosocial process involving three broad contributing factors: (a) social structural influences (gender, socioeconomic status, race, age, and cultural context), (b) individual influences (psychosocial and behavioral), and (c) biological influences (inflammatory and oxidative damage, damage to irreplaceable molecules and cells, and blood metabolic hormones). By integrating a huge body of literature concerning these processes, Ryff and Singer develop several propositions that are key to their biopsychosocial theory of healthy aging. For example, one proposition is about health promotion: positive psychosocial factors predict better biological regulation. Another is about resilience: positive psychosocial factors protect against the damaging effects of external adversity. A third concerns recovery and repair processes: positive psychosocial factors facilitate the regaining of functional and biological capacities. In each of these, we see the value of interdisciplinary investigation, which vaults us beyond traditional disciplinary boundaries and limitations.

Biological Theories and Aging

Part 3 of this handbook, on theories of the biology of aging, represents a set of chapters that, taken together, are inclusive of the major theoretical explanations for why aging occurs in living organisms. While the biological mechanisms responsible for aging are exceedingly numerous, the major theoretical paradigms guiding research in the field can be condensed into two general orientations:

stochastic processes (such as random genetic mutation and oxidative stress) and *programmed senescence* (structured genetic expressions in old age). This parsimonious rendering of biological theories of aging highlights both a growing degree of consensus about the role that evolution and natural selection play in the development of senescence and longevity and a sharpening contentiousness between competing perspectives about *how* this process might have occurred.

Generally, each chapter in this part favors one perspective while paying homage to the alternative perspective, and several chapters are formally integrative in their approach. Effros (chapter 9) reviews the role of the adaptive immune system in senescent aging and mortality. The immunological theory of aging posits that the very system that served a crucial protective function early in life becomes a liability in old age when it works less effectively because of replicative senescence of T cells—an explanation for aging generally known as *antagonistic pleiotropy*. The body is capable of forming a staggeringly large number of possible responses to fight the almost infinite number of foreign antigens that interfere with normal functioning. However, this fine-turned response system breaks down with aging, impairing the body's ability to resist these invaders. Dysregulated immune response has been linked to cardiovascular disease, inflammation, Alzheimer's disease, and cancer. Although direct causal relationships have not been established for all these detrimental outcomes, the immune system has been at least indirectly implicated. Effros points out that an immunological explanation for aging is not inconsistent with other wear-and-tear theories, such as oxidative stress—that may impair immune response or be exacerbated by it—as well as programmed aging, as deteriorated immune response appears to be related to shorter telomere length.

Martin (chapter 10) takes us on a grand tour of the main currents of thought in the biology of aging, taking the perspective of a classical evolutionary theorist. In the traditional evolutionary formulation, maladaptive genes responsible for the declines associated with aging have escaped the force of natural selection either because they are expressed only after reproduction or because they are expressed early in life with positive functions, only to have deleterious effects later in life. Martin is particularly concerned with species-specific variations in the life span that are related to environmental exposures. The particular genes that are selected for improved resistance or robustness in each species depends on the types of challenges presented by its unique environment. Thus, he uses universal principles of evolutionary theory to explain particularistic disease and life span outcomes within a species. In pointing out phenotypic differences between identical twins in later life, Martin suggests that stochastic processes in genes *and* exposures to random elements in the environment are inseparable in evolutionary theory, thereby bridging major camps in the biology of aging.

Woodruff-Pak, Foy, and Thompson (chapter 11) use a mouse model system to test hypotheses about mechanisms related to learning and memory. Using classical conditioning techniques related to eyeblinks (aural stimulus that is coupled with a puff of air), the authors are able to demonstrate variation in learning and age-related memory losses. They further find that estrogen appears to protect the hippocampus against the negative effects in adult and aged groups of mice. Their work suggests plasticity in neural brain structures and their consequent behavioral outcomes. In linking physiological and psychological processes, the authors add to our understanding of the malleable nature of aging.

Gonidakis and Longo (chapter 12) take a strong stand that aging is genetically programmed as an adaptive response to changing environmental conditions—a perspective that stands at odds with stochastic perspectives on aging. Key to their formulation is the notion that expression of genes is programmed to variously extend life or trigger senescence depending on the nutritional environment to which the organism is exposed. The authors seek to reconcile the apparent contradiction between findings that caloric restriction leads to life span extension (by directing energy toward maintenance rather than reproduction) and findings that programmed altruistic death improves the fitness of a population at the expense of individual fitness. Using a well-studied strain of yeast, the authors' experiments show that yeast cells senesce in order to provide nutrients for enhancing survival of better-adapted mutant cells that then repopulate the strain—a form of altruistic suicide by the older, less adapted yeast cells. The model proposes that programmed longevity and programmed aging are not contradictory but unique reactions to changing nutritional conditions.

The chapter by Shringarpure and Davies (chapter 13) provides a comprehensive review of the free radical theory of aging, the most prominent of the theories proposing that wear and tear is the root cause of senescence. When oxygen is metabolized, unpartnered electrons are discarded, causing damage to cells, DNA, and eventually body systems. Paradoxically, the very processes necessary for life—respiration and metabolizing nutrients—are oxidative. The authors propose that the accumulation of oxidative stress results in disease and death. While molecules in the body can absorb these free radicals and systems are adept at repairing such damage, the defense systems of the body are not completely effective and also weaken with age. The cumulative damage caused by free radicals over a lifetime and the weakened effectiveness of repair systems with aging putatively may cause a threat to survival. However, the authors point out that there is little direct evidence that increased oxidative stress accelerates aging and shortens the length of life. While oxidative stress remains a compelling theory of cellular aging, more research is needed before it can conclusively be viewed as a theory of human aging.

Austad (chapter 8) is the most sanguine that empirical evidence now points to a single theory for why all living organisms decline and die. In coming to this conclusion, he first takes up the question of what constitutes a theory. Resting his argument on the notion that theories are capable of explaining a wide variety of phenomena and (unlike hypotheses) are mutually exclusive, he argues that there are only three general theories of biological aging. He reviews the empirical support for rate-of-living (wear-and-tear), programmed aging, and evolutionary senescence theories of aging. Austad judges which of the theories is most consistent with the extant findings. He finds weak evidence for rate-of-living theories—among them, oxidative stress—noting that energy expenditure, speed of metabolism, and oxidative damage bear little relationship to overt markers of aging and longevity. He notes that while programmed aging (such as altruistic suicide) has merit in limited instances, it has been found too infrequently in nature to serve as an explanation for a phenomenon as ubiquitous as aging. Austad concludes that evolutionary senescence theory finds the greatest empirical support in the literature. This theory proposes that genes with deleterious effects in later life accumulate because they have escaped the force of natural selection. In Austad's view, empirical findings to date are most consistent with this explanation of senescent aging, thereby meeting his criterion that a successful theory is one that casts the widest net.

The chapters in this part reveal the enormously fertile state of theorizing in the biology of aging. Collectively, they reflect exciting intellectual enterprises to make sense of the wealth of data available and to fit them to the dominant theoretical orientations in the field. Much of what is presented points to a consolidation of knowledge and a growing parsimony in theory construction. As Austad points out, the more than 300 theories of aging identified by a review of the literature can be effectively reduced to three—a remarkable condensation but one that accurately describes theoretical paradigms and their scholarly camps. Each chapter in this part of the volume makes an effort to link to an "opposing" camp, but as of yet there is no unified theory on the horizon in the biology of aging. Taken as a whole, the chapters point to remaining fissures between theoretical orientations as well as irreconcilable differences between explanatory theories, making finding an integrative paradigm, however worthwhile, an elusive goal. Paradigmatic integration will require additional cross-level, cross-system, and cross-species research to gain further insight into the multiplex reasons for aging.

Psychological Theories and Aging

The chapters in part 4 are guided by the life span developmental perspective and the theory of selective optimization with compensation (Baltes & Baltes, 1990). Three chapters (Blanchard-Fields and Stange, chapter 15; Willis, Schaie, and Martin, chapter 17; Kryla-Lighthall and Mather, chapter 18) also extend socioemotional selectivity theory. Antonucci, Birditt, and Akiyama (chapter 14) offer the convoy model of social relations.

Contributors converge on such concepts as complexities and dynamic processes, the need to situate microprocesses in larger social and historical contexts, and the interplay between levels of analysis and reciprocal influences (e.g., chapter 17 emphasizes the reciprocal influences of neural structures, behaviors, and the sociocultural). The importance given the stress process brings together biological, psychological, sociological factors and signals the necessity of crossing disciplinary boundaries. Noteworthy in these chapters is the strong emphasis on articulating mechanisms: the *how.*

Contributors convey optimism about growing old and being old, focusing less on decline and more on the positive. Indeed, the leading concepts—adaptation, optimization and compensation, and plasticity—are revealing. On the other hand, there are thematic differences evident in the theories, fundamental some would say: change (reflected in the concepts of plasticity) versus stability (emotional regulation and equilibrium).

In chapter 14, Antonucci, Birditt, and Akiyama expand the theoretical scope and complexity of the convoy model of social relations. Based on life span development principles, the theory conceptualizes and explains individual development nested within social relations as they move across the life span and the abiding influence of social relations on health and well-being. A basic assumption of the model is that people need social relations. The major components of the social relations model include social networks, social support, and satisfaction with support. A dynamic feature of the model pertains to feedback provided by consociates, such as family members and friends, as an individual matures and grows old. The convoy metaphor acknowledges that individual lives are shaped by personal, situational, and support relations. A dimension of the latter category, social networks are the structures that provide the foundation from which subjective aspects of relations emerge. In addition to the objective characteristics of social networks or members of the convoy who provide tangible or emotional support of some type, the model incorporates an interpretative aspect of social relations, that is, the individual's personal evaluation of their relations.

Understanding the social relations of an individual's social convoy across time is extraordinarily important because of their far-reaching effects on health and well-being. Recent empirical and theoretical work has extended the model to include (a) stress and the role of social relations as a buffer, expanding its cross-disciplinary reach, and (b) development of a social relations/self-efficacy model to investigate mechanisms through which social relations affect well-being over time. A strength of the convoy model of social relations has been its widespread applicability in cross-national settings.

Guided by the theories of selective optimization with compensation and socioemotional selectivity, Blanchard-Fields and Stange (chapter 15) develop a model specifying the role that socioemotional context plays as it interacts with cognitive decline to moderate or compensate effects of decline on well-being. The authors are interested in the functional dynamics of everyday cognitive behavior beyond the laboratory. Their aim is to examine effects of contextual factors on social judgments by identifying developmental mechanisms and social contexts that determine when older adults' social judgment is adaptive and when it is not. As with the other contributions to theory in this part, the central issue in this model concerns adaptation; the outcomes of interest are life satisfaction, quality of life, and health.

The authors argue that past research on cognitive loss and aging is incomplete and that a very different picture emerges when socioemotional context is taken into account. Emotional processing, social expertise, and emotional regulation can remain intact in the face of cognitive decline. The authors show that cognitive resource limitations may operate in conjunction with other social or personal correlates, such as social expertise, or, when personal beliefs are violated, to produce a reliance on dispositional inferences instead of situational adjusted inferences. If social expertise is present, snap judgment (dispositional inference) could result in an adaptive outcome. Outcomes of social judgments can include health and quality-of-life issues in old age, so it is important to include social judgments in models of cognitive loss and aging. The task is to assess when a social judgment such as a dispositional inference is biased or contextually adaptive. As noted in chapter 17, the age–period–cohort problem can challenge interpretation of findings in life span developmental research. Referencing related research on causal attribution biases, Blanchard-Fields and Stange found that differences in social beliefs and values accounted for age differences in causal attribution biases. But on closer examination, they determined that those age differences were in fact generational or cohort differences in beliefs that subjects perceived were violated, causing social judgment bias.

Labouvie-Vief (chapter 16) advances a theory of dynamic integration, drawing from life span development and the work of Piaget. This psychological theory of aging focuses on mechanisms for maintaining emotional regulation at older ages. Labouvie-Vief observes that there have been two views of the developmental course of emotions in adulthood and aging. One is that in aging, an increase in emotional well-being is the result of general improvement in emotion regulation. The alternative view states that older adults' ability to process affective information is frequently compromised. Dynamic integration theory (DIT) integrates these two views. This theory articulates a dynamic interaction of developmental, situational, and individual difference-related mechanisms that result in more and less effective ways of regulating equilibrium. Emotion regulation is seen as a dynamic response to challenges. The question is how older people, in the face of decline, manage to maintain good self-concepts and well-being.

The theory predicts that highly activating situations create escalating levels of emotional arousal in older adults more easily than in younger ones. Studies indicate that older individuals may have difficulty inhibiting high emotional arousal. The theory predicts that with advancing age, the capacity to integrate a sense of well-being and high levels of complexity will be impaired. In addition to older age, increased vulnerability is more likely under conditions of resource limitations, high levels of activation (arousal), or low levels of socioemotional resources. Labouvie-Vief is skeptical of socioemotional selectivity theory's focus on changes and adjustments, seeing them as higher-level intentional processes assessed by inference.

Using a life span developmental perspective, Willis, Schaie, and Martin (chapter 17) extend the theory of selective optimization with compensation by presenting a theory of cognitive plasticity in adulthood. The theory is predicated on the idea that development is a process of lifelong adaptation and as such is modifiable or plastic at all phases of development. The research agenda integrates the contributions of developmental psychology, concerned with cognitive plasticity, and neuropsychology, concerned with cognitive reserve. A central focus is interindividual and intraindividual variability, and what needs to be specified is why there are interindividual differences in intraindividual adaptation and plasticity.

The authors discuss five issues that must be addressed in developing a comprehensive theory of cognitive plasticity: (a) the levels where adaptivity and compensation can be observed: neural, behavioral, and sociocultural (research must take account of the reciprocal influence between the brain, experience, and behavior); (b) different time scales, short term and long term; (c) the processes and mechanisms associated with plasticity; (d) developmental issues, such as sensitive or critical periods associated with learning and cognition and periods associated with reductions in plasticity or reductions in neural patterns of functional connectivity; and (e) methodological issues in the study of plasticity.

Willis, Schaie, and Martin give attention to positive aspects of aging that follows from the notion of adaptability and provide some ideas how better understanding of cognitive plasticity might be applied to improve the lives of older people. For example, they observe how cognitive potential can remain even when neural structure has been compromised. Neurogenesis can occur even in older humans and animals as a result of cognitively stimulating activities at the behavioral level. Efficient acquisition of new cognitive skills and behaviors in later life depends on reconfiguration and customization of cortical networks in the brain, represented as critical mechanisms for brain plasticity.

More recently, the study of cognitive plasticity has given attention to sociocultural influences. Here researchers are using cohort-sequential designs to try to distinguish age effects from cohort effects (increased education and exposure to technology). A bioconstructionist perspective suggests that there are reciprocal influences between individual and cultural plasticity. It indicates that increasing cultural resources are required for cognitive plasticity with age but that utilization of these cultural resources becomes less efficient with age.

In chapter 18, Kryla-Lighthall and Mather present a cognitive control theory of emotional well-being. Their research is in concert with the emphasis on positive aging now prevalent in gerontological research, which contrasts with a view of aging as inevitable decline. The chapter attempts to explain "the surprising robustness of emotional well-being" among older people. Building on socioemotional selective theory, the authors propose a theoretical framework that integrates findings from cognition, emotion, and neuroscience research. Socioemotional selective theory posits that the perception of time is a major determinant of human motivation. In contrast to younger people, who are motivated to invest in the future by focusing on knowledge acquisition goals, older people, who are more cognizant of time limitations, shift their attention to emotional regulation goals. A key proposition is that with advancing age, cognitive control resources are increasingly allocated for enhancing emotional well-being.

Older adults use control strategies, such as inhibiting negative information, refreshing goal-relevant information, and selectively rehearing positive memories, to achieve their emotional goals. For example, a key strategy is the "positivity effect," whereby older adults devote more attention and processing time to positive stimuli and less to negative stimuli. Kryla-Lighthall and Mather indicate that because memory recollection is affected by internal goals, older people will selectively distort their memories in order to promote emotional well-being. Another strategy used to reach emotion regulation goals is selective attention, allowing older people to focus on more positive information. Kryla-Lighthall and Mather note that age-related changes to cognitive control structures appear to negatively affect emotional regulation. But despite these declines, regulation of emotion and frontal lobe–controlled social behavior functions well in old age. The authors point to recent imaging research showing that older adults spontaneously recruit additional cognitive resources to meet their processing needs and in so doing enhance their emotional well-being. This corresponds to the selective optimization with compensation model and the plasticity of cognitive function discussed by Willis, Schaie, and Martin (chapter 17).

Social Science Theories and Aging

In contrast to theory development in the biological and behavior sciences, theoretical progress has been more challenging in social gerontology. In part this is because social phenomena over the course of life are extraordinarily complex and fluid but also because researchers approach their topics with different epistemologies.

What Is Meant by Theory?

Earlier in this chapter, we examined what is meant by theory and how it is used. In a majority of the 10 chapters in part 5, on social science theories of aging, the authors define theory as an explanation and are in alignment with the scientific perspective on knowledge development. Phenomenology, as presented by Longino and Powell (chapter 20), uses an interpretive approach to knowledge and focuses on understanding rather than explanation. Those writing from a feminist perspective, as evidenced by Calasanti (chapter 25), Dilworth-Anderson and Cohen (chapter 26), and Allen and Walker (chapter 28), often combine interpretive and critical theory approaches, depending on the topic of interest. We point out that a chapter topic and how it is addressed theoretically and epistemologically in this part of the handbook may not necessarily reflect the author or authors' preferred perspective. An author may elect a critical approach toward a topic in one theoretical essay or project, combine interpretive and critical approaches in addressing another topic, and use a scientific approach toward still another. Some authors see virtue in being eclectic in their theorizing.

Inequality and Cumulative Disadvantage

Inequality is a major theoretical focus among the contributors to the social science perspectives on theories of aging. Many of the chapters demonstrate a convergence of thought on the theoretical and substantive significance of *cumulative advantage or disadvantage* across the life course. For example, Ferraro, Shippee, and Schafer (chapter 22) develop the ideas of cumulative advantage and disadvantage and present a middle-range formal theory of cumulative inequality. The authors point out that while social advantage and disadvantage are often seen as outcomes for individuals, they use the term *inequality* to emphasize the importance of systemic properties in how individuals become stratified. The authors selected cumulative inequality as a more concise phrase than cumulative advantage/disadvantage. The theory incorporates elements of macro- and microsociological content and takes account of the way that social systems generate inequality on multiple levels. Cumulative inequality theory gives explicit attention to *perceptions* of disadvantage rather than just the objective conditions of their situations, which has been the dominant approach in previous studies of accumulating disadvantage. In addition, their cumulative inequality theory gives explicit attention to the intergenerational nature of inequality, which is not systematically covered in cumulative advantage/disadvantage theory.

Theoretical concern with cumulative advantage and disadvantage is also evident in the chapters by Hendricks and Hatch (chapter 23) and Settersten and Trauten (chapter 24) in terms of their focus on *social class as an explanatory mechanism.* Settersten and Trauten predict that social class will almost certainly become the most powerful factor in determining life course patterns and outcomes and will continue to create even greater disparities within societies.

In her discussion of anthropological perspectives on aging, Fry (chapter 27) highlights cultural diversity—a constituent element in the cumulative advantage/disadvantage framework. A theoretical interest in inequality can be inferred when Fry observes how modernization as an explanatory concept in anthropology has been replaced by globalization.

Feminist theorists are also centrally concerned with inequality. Allen and Walker (chapter 28) observe that feminist thought shares the common assumption that the various power/privilege asymmetries of gender, race, class, age, and sexual orientation are major and intersecting, not competing, inequalities, and that they make up systems of influences on people's everyday lives. "Intersectionality" is advanced as a key concept in feminist theorizing. Calasanti (chapter 25) argues that a focus on intersecting inequalities is critical to understanding those experiences of aging and that feminist gerontology is uniquely able to offer scholars a lens through which to view these intersections.

It is perhaps not surprising that scholarly concurrence on the need for theorizing inequality should emerge now, as evidenced in so many of these chapters, at a time when wealth disparities are increasing in all societies. The authors of chapters in part 6 theorize why this has occurred.

Life Course and Social Forces

A focus on the life course perspective represents another important theme among the chapters in this part. Certainly those concerned with cumulative advantage and disadvantage are using a life course perspective. Hendricks and Hatch (chapter 23) present a theory of lifestyles within a life course perspective. The authors articulate how lifestyles, through their connection to life choices and life changes, can link agency and structure, a major theoretical goal in social gerontology. Lifestyles can be conceptualized as a central mechanism within the life course framework and more generally as a linkage between the micro and macro in developing theories of aging. Moreover, lifestyles can be empirically grounded.

Dannefer and Kelley-Moore (chapter 21) contend that while the life course perspective has become increasingly useful and widely applied, a sociological theory that explains how social forces shape the life course is still needed. The authors dissect life course theorizing to show an overemphasis on agency and "personalogic" explanations and a neglect of "sociologic" explanations. They also assert that there has been a neglect of within-cohort variability. They extend their model of life course *explanans* and *expalanadas* by adding a cultural component—perhaps with a nod to Dilworth-Anderson and Cohen (chapter 26) and Fry (chapter 27). They define this as a "symbolic apparatus of age-related meanings, values, and norms."

Also reflecting the life course focus, Settersten and Trauten (chapter 24) consider the implications for how societies might function when age-based norms vanish—a consequence of the deinstitutionalization of the life course—and suggest that these implications pose new challenges for theorizing aging and the life course in postindustrial societies. Dramatic reductions in mortality, morbidity, and fertility over the past several decades have so shaken up the organization of the life course and the nature of educational, work, family, and leisure experiences that it is now possible for individuals to become old in new ways. The configurations and content of other life stages are being altered as well, especially for women. In consequence, theories of age and aging will need to be reconceptualized.

Toward Interdisciplinarity

The chapter by Bass (chapter 19) is illustrative of efforts to cross disciplinary and epistemological boundaries in theorizing. Bass argues that social gerontology is becoming an integrative discipline in its own right. But in contrast to the rapid evolution of interdisciplinary work in the natural sciences and engineering, Bass suggests that social gerontology—and the social sciences more generally—has not kept pace. Despite the benefits that would come from cross-fertilization of knowledge bases, disciplines in the social sciences have not produced widely shared methodologies or theories. Nevertheless, Bass observes that social gerontology is maturing. A small but growing group of scholars in social gerontology have advanced theoretical thinking in the past two decades, bringing fresh ideas and insights. Bass suggests that out of this theoretical ferment, at least two "schools of thought" have emerged in social gerontology: critical gerontology and postmodern gerontology. He contrasts these two theoretical perspectives, their epistemological grounding and assumptions and topics of concern. A central focus is how to theorize the aging individual within a larger historical, political, social, cultural, and economic environment, one characterized by increasing risk where social responsibilities are shifting from the state to individuals and families.

Bass takes up the interdisciplinarity challenge by proposing an integrative theory of social gerontology. This theory blends a macroperspective, examining the larger social, economic, environmental, cultural, and political contexts that influence human behavior and health, with the micro-individual, and family perspectives. Critical to this framework is how these macrostructures differentially allocate resources and support an aging population and, as a result, how individuals respond to their own aging and others aging around them.

A Phenomenological Approach

Phenomenology, an established theoretical tradition in the social sciences, provides an epistemological underpinning for several theoretical approaches in social gerontology (feminist theories, critical theories, and postmodernist perspectives). In their chapter, Longino and Powell (chapter 20) extend theoretical understanding by presenting the theory of phenomenology and its application in the study of aging. The focus of phenomenology is on illuminating the human meanings of social life. By using phenomenology through its in-depth qualitative gathering of intimate human feelings and meanings, the approach emphasizes how individuals understand the means by which phenomena, originating in human consciousness, come to be experienced as features of the social world.

In our previous review of theories in social gerontology (Bengtson, Burgess, & Parrott, 1997; Bengtson, Putney, & Johnson, 2005), social constructivism was described as one of the most frequently used microlevel perspectives for understanding the experiences of older people and their families and the subjective meanings of age and aging. In fact, social constructivism is a constituent element of the phenomenology approach to knowledge. Researchers using feminist theories such as Allen and Walker (chapter 28) and Calasanti (chapter 25) are guided by social constructivist ideas and methods. Longino and Powell provide us with a greater understanding of social constructivism within the theory of phenomenology and in so doing extend its range of application in social gerontological theorizing.

Dilworth-Anderson and Cohen (chapter 26) draw conceptual guidance from social constructivism and phenomenology to explore the meanings and understandings of a group of elderly caregivers from diverse ethnic backgrounds caring for an older relative with dementia. They describe the importance of values in studying culturally diverse groups and how it challenges researchers to uncover what culture means to those being studied. In their research, they combined social constructivism with a sociocultural perspective that recognizes that meaningful experiences are interpreted within one's own culture (see also Fry, chapter 27). The authors note how "the very fabric of social order is determined by the meanings assigned by its members as well as the interpretations that they make in legitimizing what they have created." The authors describe how they used a grounded theory approach that lends itself to social constructivism and the search for meanings.

Society, Public Policy, and Theories of Aging

Part 6 addresses theories of aging as they explain the complex interrelationships among societal process at the macrolevel, the formation of public policy, and the welfare of the aged population. The chapters in this part demonstrate how social processes can shape old-age policy and in turn shape the experience of the aged population or even construct old age (see chapter 29 for the United States and chapter 34 for Sweden), how the interactions between social processes and old-age policy can have differential effects on different subgroups within the aged population (chapters 30 and 33), how larger social forces such as globalization affect the aged population (chapter 33), and how individuals themselves can shape the very social structures (that in turn shape their social context) by exercising agency (chapter 32). This process of interdependence between individuals, or the principle of "linked lives," as well as the understanding that agency is embedded within social structure, is supported by both critical theories (chapter 32) and the life course perspective (chapter 31).

Hudson (chapter 29) takes readers on a fascinating journey of the development of American old-age policy. The journey is guided by an integrative discussion of three clusters of theoretical explanations of aging policy formation. The first cluster addresses economic theories and discusses how emerging industrial economies conditioned welfare state development. The second cluster introduces society-centered approaches and focuses on values, behaviors, and actions of individuals and groups and their interactions with policy formation. The third cluster is state centered, discussing both the state itself and the policy outcomes. Hudson's discussion illuminates how old-age policy has transformed the status of the aged in the United States from a vulnerable population defined by needs to an increasingly well-organized and well-off population. In concluding this theoretically driven analysis of old-age policy formation, Hudson reminds us that aging policy constructs old age by providing an answer to the question of "*who is old?*" Following this line of thought, Hudson claims that the current debate over raising the age of eligibility to Social Security benefits is more than just a practical matter. Raising age eligibility may, in his words, carry significant consequences, as it may undo the achievements of old-age policy and transform the aged from the institutionalized population that they are today back to a vulnerable group, a process he calls "reresidualizing the aged."

While Hudson focuses on old-age policy in the United States, Thorslund and Silverstein (chapter 34) provide a stimulating discussion of the development of the welfare state in Sweden. An important aspect of Swedish policy is the recognition that there is a third party affecting social welfare in addition to the individual and the state. This third party includes traditional community organizations such as civic or religious groups that provide services to those in need. A reduction in state involvement in caring for the aged population may result in a renewed increased involvement of such organizations in supporting the aged population. While Thorslund and Silverstein discuss this as a possible way to maintain the well-being of the aged population even in an era of budget cuts, such a solution is indeed based on viewing the aged as a "needy" group, perhaps leading to exactly what Hudson (chapter 29) discusses as "reresidualizing the aged."

Phillipson (chapter 33) goes beyond national contexts and discusses the effects of globalization on the aged and the aging experience. He suggests that globalization produced a "distinctive stage in the history of aging" where the distinctions between domestic or national and international are blurry and less well defined. In such a climate, tensions arise between state-based policies and those formulated by global institutions. While globalization affects aging directly through its effects on the economy, Phillipson claims that its most central effect is in "redefining the social"—creating deregulation of the social order. Again, this takes place in a much less predictable and regulated environment. Thorslund and Silverstein (chapter 34) suggest that national values regarding the welfare state in terms of the target population and the preferences for care are mediating factors between the effects of macrolevel factors such as globalization and the microlevel aging experience. However, Phillipson observes that globalization may very well shape and redefine the very national norms that once were so important to national old-age policy formation.

Walker (chapter 32) takes the reader through the captivating process of theory formation that explains the social. The social is defined as "the outcome of constantly changing processes through which people, to a greater or lesser extent, realize themselves as interacting social beings." This self-realization process is interdependent with the creation of collective identities. As individuals interact with one another, they often have to compromise and sometimes face constraints. In such an approach, therefore, agency or choice is viewed as embedded within structure. The role of the welfare state is to enable choice and "to empower people to negotiate their way through the rapidly changing life course." Welfare state policies and rational or individual choice should be seen not as competitors but rather as compensatory.

While Walker uses critical gerontology to emphasize that agency is embedded within structure, Marshall (chapter 31) reaches a similar conclusion from a completely different theoretical direction—the life course perspective. In an innovative chapter, Marshall discusses the life course perspective, often used to explain individual developmental changes over the life course, as a useful analytical approach to inform public policy formation. Using the case of an innovative Canadian policy initiative, Marshall discusses the tenets of the life course perspective and its strength in guiding policy formation. Marshall pays special attention to the importance of considering interdependence among individuals—the life course principle of "linked lives" over time. The life course perspective allows policymakers to view individuals as nested within families and broader social institutions that present opportunities and constraints. It further emphasizes the importance of historical analysis and the understanding that cohorts differ in the way they experience aging.

While the aged population on average may be better off financially when compared to other age-groups (see chapters 29 and 34), the proponents of critical gerontology (see chapters 32 and 33) argue that the interaction between the state and the economy in the social construction of old age creates inequalities in the experience of growing old. Kail, Quadagno, and Keene (chapter 30) theorize economic disparities among the aged population. They present a unique integrative theoretical approach to explain how economic inequalities accumulate over the life course of individuals and even further as they are transmitted across generations. Driven by the political economy of aging theory, the chapter presents a unique integration among several other theories—the cumulative disadvantage approach, feminist theories, and the concept of moral economy. Their approach leads to the proposition that economic disparities among the aged population are a result of systematic inequalities based on gender, race, ethnicity, minority status, and marital status across the life course. Moreover, even the policies that are designed to support the aged population—old-age policies—are socially constructed within a generational debate of the young versus the old, leading to a probable reduction of current distributional policies.

Taken together, these chapters provide a unique view of the various complexities of the continually changing interdependent relationships between individuals as they exercise agency and construct their own aging experience, the social institutions that provide constraining context to such individual choice, the state that facilitates and shapes these interactions, and larger social forces such as globalization, that affect all these factors.

Translating Theories of Aging

In part 7, authors discuss theories in four distinct applications of gerontology: application of theories to elder law (chapter 35); critique of the relationship between spirituality, finitude, and theories of the life span (chapter 36); applications of theories of aging to psychological interventions to enhance well-being in old age (chapters 37 and 38); and a proposal of a new interdisciplinary gerontological education framework that strives at blending research and practice (chapter 39).

Doron (chapter 35) presents a multidimensional approach to the study of elder law. Despite the implied importance of aging theories in the formation of elder law, Doron claims that elder law has received little attention in the gerontological literature. He calls the attention of gerontologists to the theoretical basis of elder law and terms this area of study "jurisprudential gerontology." His multidimensional approach goes beyond consideration of the core legal principles of human and civil rights protection to other dimensions, including, for example, the familial and informal supportive dimension, discussing the role of the state in forming a legal environment that supports those caring for the aged. Using his model, he encourages researchers to think in terms of several dualisms that underlie the field of elder law: paternalism versus autonomy and individual versus society. By discussing elder law within the framework of these underlying values, Doron connects the field of elder law to the policy arena as discussed by others (see chapters 32, 33, and 34).

In chapter 36, Johnson presents a unique perspective on theories of aging and specifically the life span or life course theories. Johnson criticizes these theories for neglecting to give adequate attention to a uniquely important aspect of the life course—death and dying. Johnson suggests that while some attention was given to the topics of finitude—the "awareness of the imminence" of one's death—and to spirituality, which encompasses "transcendental, religious, and self-explorations," these areas of research have been isolated from the traditional research on the life course. Johnson makes a passionate plea to integrate these topics in the study of the life course, suggesting that it is mortality that creates the very culture we live in, or, as he says, "without death, there would be no culture."

Chapters 37 and 38 present two approaches to understand well-being in old age and to design interventions that aim to promote personal growth toward enhancing one's individual aging experience. In chapter 37, Zarit opens with a paradox. While late life is typically accompanied by losses and challenges, older adults as a group seem to fare better in terms of their mental health compared to other age-groups. With the exception of dementia, most mental illnesses are less prevalent in old age, and Zarit therefore raises the question. With all the losses and challenges, why are older people happy? He utilizes several psychological theories of aging to explain this paradox, including Rowe and Kahn's successful aging; Baltes's selection, optimization, and compensation model; Carstensen's socioemotional selectivity theory; various dimensions of emotional control; and the concept of wisdom. Finally, drawing on Erikson's theory, Zarit discusses the need to find a sense of integrity in old age and examines life review as a method of achieving such sense. Zarit concludes that a good old age is certainly possible and that individuals can make their added years meaningful and productive. While he recognizes and acknowledges the existence of disease and other hardships, Zarit proposes a theory-driven intervention plan at the primary prevention level that may allow individuals to overcome challenges and compensate for losses, allowing them to be meaningfully involved in a good old age. These set of skills include good health habits, skills for managing chronic illness, good social skills, skills for managing emotions, good cognitive skills, leisure skills, good economic skills, and, finally, development of a sense of self-efficacy for the ability to change one's life.

Knight and Laidlaw (chapter 38) provide a fascinating description of theory formation that is a product of a fruitful collaboration between two applied researchers. By merging their two individually developed parallel models, Knight and Laidlaw illustrate the role of good theory in promoting knowledge and progressing the field of the study of aging. Advocating a broad and inclusive pantheoretical approach, Knight developed a contextual, cohort-based maturity/specific challenge model for psychotherapy with older people. More recently, Knight developed the contextual adult life span theory for adapting psychotherapy (CALTAP). At the same time, Laidlaw and colleagues developed a comprehensive conceptualization framework (CCF) that was designed to adapt cognitive-behavioral therapy. While these approaches differ in emphasis, both the CALTAP and the CCF model share many similarities that are also emphasized by the life course perspective, including an emphasis on cohort membership and social context.

In this chapter, Knight and Laidlaw merge their theories and create a new theory that benefits from both of their individual theories and adds a unique component—an emphasis on the achievement of wisdom, or, as they define it, "knowing how." Like Zarit (chapter 37), Knight and Laidlaw recognize the possible barriers to wisdom attainment in the form of disease as well as societal barriers. However, much like Zarit, they believe that individual change through psychological intervention may prove to be an effective mechanism enhancing well-being in old age. Their theory-based intervention model provides a useful illustration for putting theories of aging into action.

Lowenstein and Carmel (chapter 39) discuss the need to find a systematic venue to create a more harmonious collaboration between researchers and practitioners as well as a closer integration between research and practice in educating future gerontologists. Lowenstein and Carmel view the educational system and, more specifically, graduate and undergraduate gerontology programs as the natural agents of such creation. They propose an interdisciplinary gerontological education paradigm that aims at enhancing theory-driven study and research at the graduate level, leading to the production of highly trained gerontologists who are equipped in relevant applicable knowledge. In order to be successful, such an educational framework should address the complex needs of the heterogeneous and diverse aging populations. The programs should present with a flexible modular geared to the individual training needs of the students, depending on the specific subgroup they will be serving, including specific ethnic groups, immigrants, or the chronically disabled. The programs should be interdisciplinary and draw on collaborations with other school and departments.

Conclusion

As will be seen in the remainder of this volume, there has been a resurgence in the explicit use of theory to develop explanations and understandings of the aging process. More and more, investigators are choosing to grapple with the *why* and *how* questions of aging rather than simply describe the *what*. Among the most promising developments recently is the noticeable increase in efforts to advance interdisciplinary theories of aging and a greater willingness to intersect traditional disciplines of biology, psychology, and the social and policy sciences. This trend has opened up avenues for more inclusive explanations of why and how health, mortality, and quality of life change with aging. In particular, attempts to bridge micro- and macro-environments of aging have yielded more comprehensive understandings of senescence and the aging process. From the widest analytic focus on population dynamics to the tightest focus on molecular biology, seemingly disparate and disciplinary-specific theories of aging are increasingly juxtaposed, linked, and, sometimes, integrated, in spite of institutional structures (in the academy and the research community) that tend to keep them apart.

There has also been a rise in attempts to incorporate social and physical environments in theories of aging, reflecting awareness that differing contexts can explain variation in the aging process across human groups and species. Recognition that aging includes internal and external processes that interact with each other has enriched theories of aging and inspired the use of multilevel approaches. There is growing awareness that agency (individual interpretations and actions), social constraints (class, race, gender, and culture), and societal institutions (health care and state pension systems) must be acknowledged in any analysis of the causes and consequences of aging. Further, humans are purposeful, reflexive actors who accommodate or reduce the impact of aging by personally modifying their behaviors and collectively modifying the policy environments that determine the resources available for older adults.

Rapid expansion of aging research over the last several decades has made theory more, not less, important. An inductive approach of sifting through voluminous amounts of data is useful for unearthing patterns and making important serendipitous discoveries, but it is no substitute for the rigorous refinement and synthesis of theory, without which scientific explanations and epistemological understandings of aging cannot be readily achieved. The future of aging research, as we discuss in chapter 40, will likely see even greater attention to theory, particularly interdisciplinary theories. Although difficult to orchestrate and expensive to develop, theory-driven interdisciplinary investigations of aging are nevertheless the wave of the future.

References

Baltes, P. B., & Baltes, M. M. (1990). Psychological perspectives on successful aging: The model of selective optimization with compensation. In P. B. Baltes & M. M. Baltes (Eds.), *Successful aging: Perspectives from the behavioral sciences* (pp. 1–34). New York: Cambridge University Press.

Bengtson, V. L., Burgess, E. O., & Parrott, T. M. (1997). Theory, explanation, and a third generation of theoretical development in social gerontology. *Journal of Gerontology: Social Sciences, 52,* S72–S88.

Bengtson, V. L., Putney, N. M., & Johnson, M. (2005). Are theories of aging necessary? In M. Johnson, V. L. Bengtson, P. Coleman, & T. Kirkwood (Eds.), *The Cambridge handbook of age and ageing* (pp. 3–20). Cambridge: Cambridge University Press.

Bengtson, V. L., & Schaie, K. W. (Eds.). (1999). *Handbook of theories of aging.* New York: Springer Publishing.

Rowe, J. W., & Kahn, R. L. (1998). *Successful aging.* New York: Pantheon.

Webster, N. (2003). *Webster's new American dictionary.* New York: HarperCollins.

A Metahistorical Perspective on Theories of Aging

2

W. Andrew Achenbaum

Originally published in 1966, Gerald Gruman's (2003) *A History of Ideas About the Prolongation of Life,* still the definitive guide to the subject, posits that the earliest recorded theories of aging were enmeshed in representations of death, late life, and futile quests for immortality. Notions about aging originated respectively in the epic of Gilgamesh, which traces back to Babylonia around 3000 B.C.E.; in the myths of Prometheus and Pandora as recounted by Hesiod, who lived roughly 22 centuries later; and in the legend of Tithonos, dating from the seventh or eighth century B.C.E. Aristotle (384–322 B.C.E.), Gruman claims, was the first person in the West to codify and modify theories of age. Aristotle ascribed humors to four stages of life (youth was hot and moist, old age cold and dry), based on theories of the body and nature set forth by physicians who subscribed to the teachings of Hippocrates (460–377 B.C.E.). Theories about aging also circulated in the East during this era: Taoists melded alchemy and philosophy in their writings about longevity (Gruman, 2003).

Prevailing theories of aging thereafter built on precedents transmitted from generation to generation. To wit, scientists such as William Harvey (1578–1657) and philosopher René Descartes (1596–1650) reworked the writings of Galen (129–199), who had incorporated Greco-Roman ideas. Hebrew and Christian Scriptures offered insights about the wisdom and suffering associated with gray hairs. Physicians and alchemists in the Far East and in Arabia borrowed from Western sources as they formulated their own empirical observations. Teachings of Jabir (721–815) pervaded Islamic views of physical and spiritual aging for centuries. Popular art complemented scientific theory building in the Middle Ages. Artisans' depictions of the Journey of Life allegorized the human life, blending moral and religious casuistry with physical and biological causality. This pattern of accretion continues to the present day. Current metaphors and theories about successful aging can be traced back to the texts of past masters. To cite one example, Luigi Cornaro's *Discorsi della vita sobria* (1557) offered a regimen to promote healthful aging, consisting of temperance, diet, and exercise. Cornaro framed his discourses with references to age-old maxims illustrating how to avoid premature death (Cole, 1992).

Historical works have grounded theory building in the United States since the founding of the Republic, as even the following cursory overview indicates. Benjamin Rush invoked Cicero's *De Senectute* (44 B.C.E.) and Cornaro, among others, to bolster his observations about how the American climate and environment improved the health status of those who lived past the age of 80. Even in their dying days, Rush believed, the survivors of the Revolution were valuable mentors to rising generations. Similarly, an 1881 English translation of Jean-Martin Charcot's *Lecons cliniques sur les maladies des vieillards and les maladies chroniques* influenced American biologists and medical researchers who were technologically and scientifically receptive to physiological and pathological models of senescence then in vogue in France and Germany. Charcot cited the scientific principles of 17th-century British physician Francis Bacon to corroborate his analysis of lesions in late life (Achenbaum, 1978). Harvard comparative anatomist Charles Sedgwick Minot was a contrarian: he invoked the past mainly to discount its relevance to "modern" science. In *The Problem of Age, Growth and Death,* Minot (1908) disparaged previous ideas about aging in order to celebrate the theories and methods of "modern" biomedical science.

Edmund Vincent Cowdry's (1939) publication of *Problems of Ageing: Biological and Medical Aspects* marked the emergence of gerontology as a scientific field of inquiry in the United States. Cowdry recruited 25 top-flight contributors largely from the Union of American Biological Societies. Nobel laureates led Cowdry's roster, which included anatomists, biochemists, clinicians, dermatologists, pathologists, and physiologists. With support from the Josiah Macy Jr. Foundation and the National Research Council, authors reviewed the current state of theories and knowledge about aging in their scientific area. Cowdry also encouraged the specialists to critique each other's work in order to define the scope and parameters of research on aging. As John Dewey noted in his introduction to *Problems of Ageing,* theory building depended on the creativity of seasoned, reflexive scholars. Cowdry's collaborators not only re-presented theories of aging that had survived the test of time, but they also embraced cross-disciplinary ways of conceptualizing problems and collecting and analyzing data (Achenbaum, 1995).

The subtitle of Cowdry's volume stressed biological and medical aspects of aging, as had theoretical and clinical work in the field during the first 150 years of U.S. history. (The predominance of biomedical approaches until 1800 is evident in Gruman's monograph. Americans conformed to a larger gerontological pattern of historical theory building.) Some social scientists and social workers generated theories on aging prior to World War II. G. Stanley Hall (1922) traced to aging theory building from ancient times in *Senescence*. So did Simone de Beauvoir (1972) in *The Coming of Age*.

With the creation of professional organizations devoted to research and teaching on aspects of aging—notably the founding of the American Geriatrics Society in 1942 and of the Gerontological Society of America three years later—the number of competing theories about senescence, explicating continuities and changes from the cellular to the societal levels, has mushroomed. Social and behavioral scientists have been as prolific in theory building as members of the biomedical community. Gerontologists' capacity for constructing theories lagged behind their data collecting. In *Emergent Theories of Aging*, James Birren and Vern Bengtson (1988) urged "researchers to begin to address the data-rich but theory-poor state of current research on aging, and to encourage cross-disciplinary interchange that focuses on theory development in aging" (p. ix). Advances in gerontology, the pair contended, required bridging "islands of knowledge" via "basic theoretical principles" at several levels of complexity.

Historical perspectives facilitate the present process of theory building on aging by charting a comparative, temporal baseline of conceptual progress and setbacks. The second edition of Robert Binstock and Ethel Shanas's *Handbook of Aging and the Social Sciences* (1985), for instance, devoted two chapters to reconstructing the foundations of gerontology's theoretical scope and methods (Achenbaum, 1985; Maddox & Campbell, 1985). Bengtson has been remarkably trenchant and prolific (see especially Bengtson, Parrott, & Burgess, 1996; Bengtson, Rice, & Johnson, 1999; Bengtson & Schaie, 1999) in arguing that robust theories are a prerequisite to advance gerontology. Historical commentaries by Scott Bass (2006; see also Bass & Ferraro, 2000), Jon Hendricks (Hendricks & Achenbaum, 1999), and Victor Marshall (1995, 1999) merit scrutiny. H. R. Moody (1988) advocated "critical gerontology" as a window on U.S. theory building; scholars from Canada (Katz, 1996) and Britain (Biggs, Lowenstein, & Hendricks, 2003; Phillipson, 1998) as well as U.S. scholars such as Carroll Estes, Martha Holstein, and Meredith Minkler have challenged mainstream thinking. They offer alternative theories that borrow heavily from other disciplines.

Some historically grounded constructs offer a narrow focus, not an overview. For example, scholars evaluate how disengagement theory stirred the gerontological imagination while provoking spirited debates (Achenbaum & Bengtson, 1994). Other case studies revisit "how structural functionalism informed disengagement, modernization, and age stratification theories; symbolic interactionism influenced activity and subculture theories; social constructivist theories of aging built on phenomenology and ethnomethodology; and life course studies combined macro-micro perspectives in the social sciences" (Katz, 2003, p. 17).

Emphasizing theoretical breakthroughs in the social sciences and humanities does not mean that there has been a lack of interest in the history of biomedical theories. In *Prolongevity*, Albert Rosenfeld (1976), a science editor for *Life*, critiqued the historical origins of and the cross-disciplinary links between successive wear-and-tear, immunological, and hormonal theories. "Each sortie into the frontier areas of aging research provides a reminder of how totally in flux those frontiers are" (p. vii). In *Maximum Life Span*, Roy Walford (1983) put the "theories of aging I love best" in historical context. Lewis Lipsitz (Lipsitz & Goldberger, 1992, 1995) invoked Cowdry's *Problems of Ageing* and chaos theory to explain people's vulnerability to cardiovascular disease as they aged.

Given the available resources, there is little reason to add to the treasure trove yet another historiography of theories of aging. Instead, I intend to look for dominant patterns of defining and categorizing issues found in historical perspectives on theories of aging. Hayden White (1973) calls this mode of classifying and explicating motifs in historical documents *metahistory*. The historical text itself becomes contextualized:

> *One of the ways that a scholarly field takes stock of itself is by considering its history. Yet it is difficult to get an objective history of a scholarly discipline, because if the historian is himself a practitioner of it, he is likely to be a devotee of one or another of its sects and hence biased; and if he is not a practitioner, he is unlikely to have the expertise necessary to distinguish between the significant and the insignificant events of the field's development. . . . Metahistory seeks to [address] itself to such questions as, What is the structure of a particular* historical *consciousness? What is the epistemological status of historical* explanations. . . . *What are the possible* forms *of historical representation and what are their bases? (White, 1978, p. 81)*

After establishing the significance of "dualisms" in theory building across intellectual domains, I investigate the positive and negative effects of dualistic thinking among researchers on aging. I then propose an alternative way of using dualisms to create dialectical approaches to generating theories in gerontology.

The Significance of Dualisms in Theory Building

Juxtaposing two irreducible, heterogeneous principles—sometimes complementary, sometimes in conflict—to analyze the process of knowing or to explain the nature of reality dates back to ancient civilizations. Rather than delve into the history of dualistic thought across disciplines and professions, it suffices for our purposes to ascertain how theoreticians identified the bipolar dimensions of a problem and used dualisms to describe and explain events in nature and human relations. Dualisms historically have been a common way of organizing reality in theoretical terms.

Ancient Greek mythologies abound in dualisms. Sages and ordinary people distinguished gods from mortals. Among the divinities, Greeks differentiated celestial from terrestrial gods and identified monsters antagonistic to gods who protected households or the heavens. Plato, in *Phaedo*, articulated a doctrine of Forms that became the ontological prototype for making phenomena intelligible. Aristotle rejected Plato's contention that Forms existed independently, but he did not challenge dualistic conceptualizations of reality. In the East, dualistic ways of thinking also took root. Hindu philosophers emphasized the eternal tension between an ultimate reality and the illusory nature of phenomena. Taoists in China postulated that the overarching notion of yin and yang embraced all pathways to knowledge.

Mind–body dualisms animated various schools of philosophy over the centuries. The strategy gave rise to the Cartesian dualism, which remains the basis for subsequent scientific inquiry. Descartes (1641) stressed causal interactions between the immaterial mind and the material body. His ideation was challenged by Leibniz (among others) who stressed parallels rather than interactions in dualities. Many modern scientists, ranging from those who study lobes of the brain or changes in the environment, contend that dualisms are obsolescent. Yet dualisms persist in contemporary research paradigms: the distinction between "gender" and "sex" and essentialism and sexism lace contemporary feminist theories of science ("Dualism, Philosophy of Mind," 2007).

Similar mind–behavior dualisms have existed in the behavioral sciences. Psychologists today seek internal and external causes to describe and explicate events or emotions under scrutiny. Basic researchers often pursue different questions from applied practitioners. Different modes of experimental and nonexperimental methods are utilized in both camps ("Aspects of Psychology," 1996).

Theologians invoke moral dualisms as they probe the nature of good and evil, the sacred and the profane. Dualisms help scholars accentuate the presence (or lack) of universality in particularity. Despite Paul's claim that "there is no longer Jew nor Greek; there is no longer slave nor free; there is no longer male and female" (Galatians 3:28), such theory drives theological distinctions between "insiders" and "outsiders." Still, ecumenicists deploy dualisms to respect differences in appeals to unity (Gunnes, 2003).

This survey sets the stage for what follows. Dualisms have been central to organizing knowledge since the dawn of civilization. Theoreticians in disparate fields of inquiry invoke dualisms. I deliberately eschewed how dualisms affect biomedical researchers because in the next section we will see that dualisms have been integral to the gerontological enterprise.

Dualisms, Past and Present, in Theories of Aging

Researchers historically have constructed theories of aging that were (and in some instances remain) framed by at least one of the following eight dualisms.

1. Aging as a Disease/Aging as a Normal Process

The origins of this dualism can be traced back to classical Rome. Seneca (4 B.C.E.–65 C.E.) emphasized quality over the length of life. In *De Brevitate Vitam,* he claimed that a short life could abound in meaning if lived productively. Conversely, that the aphorism "*senectus morbidus est*" ("old age is a disease") is attributed to Seneca indicates his fear of living so long as to be diminished socially and physically. Cicero (106–43 B.C.E.), in contrast, proclaimed in *De Senectute* that one of the glories of late life was that it freed persons from the follies of youth. Old age, like earlier stages of life, had distinctive advantages. Insofar as "old men retain their mental faculties, provided their interest and application continue," Cicero observed, "such strength as a man has he should use, and whatever he does should be done in proportion to his strength" (quoted in Falconer, 2001, pp. 31, 37).

The contrast between the theories of aging enunciated by Seneca and Cicero should not be overdrawn. "Life is a voyage, in the process of which, we are perpetually changing our scenes," wrote Seneca. "We first leave childhood behind us, then youth, then the years of ripened manhood, then the more pleasing part of old age" (quoted in Cole, 1992, p. 120). Late life, in Seneca's construct, was not entirely a disease-ridden stage devoid of compensations. Similarly, Cicero's *De Senectute* is not an unalloyed paean to old age: he acknowledged physical decline as well as losses of pleasures and esteem. Nonetheless, pathological and "normal" models of aging competed in the minds of alchemists, physicians, scientists, philosophers, and other commentators.

The contrast was especially evident in the United States at the beginning of the 20th century. Nobel laureate Elie Metchnikoff emphasized the pathological features of old age. "The theory of old age and the hypotheses which are connected with it may be summarized in a few words: the senile degeneration of our organism is entirely similar to the lesions induced by certain maladies of a microbic origin," Metchnikoff (1904) postulated. "Old age, then, is an infectious chronic disease which is manifested by degeneration, or an enfeebling of the noble elements, and by the excessive activities of the macrophages" (p. 548).

A decade later, I. L. Nascher, emphasizing cumulative changes in cells and tissues with maturation, questioned whether old age per se was a malady. Nascher called for a new cadre of specialists to care for the elderly, analogous to creation in 1881 of pediatrics as a specialty for those who attended to the diseases and conditions of childhood. In *Geriatrics,* Nascher (1914) described old age as a normal, distinct physiological stage of life beset by a "pathological process in a normally degenerating body" (pp. 47–48).

Once again, it is tempting to accentuate the theoretical differences between Metchnikoff and Nascher. Metchnikoff (1908) held fast to his notion that old age was a disease, but he was no nihilist. "It is useful to prolong life," he declared in *Prolongation of Life: Optimistic Studies* (p. 135), confident that scientific theories and techniques someday would prevent premature old age and precocious deaths. Nascher, on the other hand, consistently differentiated "senility" from "senile pathology." He devoted most of *Geriatrics* to discussing 37 primary senile diseases, 21 secondary diseases, 33 "preferential" diseases, 27 diseases that presented symptoms differently in late life, and 56 diseases unlikely to strike in advanced years. The points of convergence in the men's models did not vitiate fundamental differences in their respective characterizations of late life.

Pathological and physiological models of aging compete in gerontology's biomedical circles today. Disease-driven theories enable pathologists, surgeons, and bench scientists to solve problems; it may fuel ageism in the health care arena. The persistence of negative images of age accounts in part for the shortage of geriatric physicians, nurses, and social workers attending to the chronic maladies that multiply with advancing years.

2. Prolongevity/Natural Limits to Aging

Alchemists, philosophers, and healers long have sought a magical potion or miracle to bestow immortality on mortal beings. Thus far, the quest has been futile, though increases in life expectancy at birth and at age 40 during the past 150 years lead some investigators to predict even more dramatic future gains in the number of years that men and women can expect to live. Sometimes the gift of immortality has unintended consequences, as the torturous decrepitude suffered by Tithonos granted long life but not commensurate health. The quest for eternal vitality can be fatal: Seminoles killed Ponce de Leon when he found a Fountain of Youth (Olshansky & Carnes, 2003).

Hebrew Scripture is one of many ancient texts, in contrast, that posits a natural limit to the duration of life: "Their days shall be one hundred twenty years" (Genesis 6:3). Perhaps the verse should not be taken literally since the fifth chapter of Genesis portrays Patriarchs living between 500 and 1,000 years. Yet the 120-year figure is remarkably close to the 125-year maximum for human life that for several centuries has been an outside limit to the duration of mortal existence. Similarly, the message of Psalm 90:10—"The days of our life are seventy years, or perhaps eighty if we are strong; even then their span is only toil and trouble; they are soon gone, and we fly away"—presaged the distinction that Bernice Neugarten made between the young-old and old-old. Old age is not a homogeneous phase of human development.

Biologists have addressed the dualism at the cellular level. In 1912, Nobel laureate Alexis Carrel grew fibroblasts (bundles of connective tissues) from chicken's hearts in his laboratory at Rockefeller Institute. In an ideal environment, Carrel theorized, cells were inherently immortal. This hypothesis was accepted as paradigmatic until the 1960s, when Dr. Leonard Hayflick demonstrated that human fibroblasts could not divide more than 50 times. The discrepancy was traced to a faulty technique in Carrel's lab. Yet the dualism did not implode: Dr. Ana Aslan sold Gerovital premised on the presumably scientific rationale that cellular immortality was possible (Walford, 1983).

Indeed, the battle between those who foresee dramatic extensions in life and those who accept limits to growth continues today. The American Academy of Anti-Aging Medicine (A4M) claims more than 11,000 adherents, more than double the membership of the Gerontological Society of America. The A4M's leadership claims that pharmacological and technological interventions soon will make it possible to extend human life beyond 150 years (Binstock, 2003). Better yet, there will be an increase in the proportion of healthful years among the long lived. Future generations of elders will not befall Tithonos's fate with added years of life before them.

Proponents of "successful" and "productive" aging urge people to remain physically active and socially and economically engaged. Without necessarily endorsing the mantra of the American Association of Retired Persons that "60 is 30," the model stretches the attributes of middle age to those in the third quarter of life, thereby tacitly acknowledging limits to competency and activity somewhere along the life course before the onset of death.

3. Disengagement Theory/Activity Theory

Disengagement theory is one of the few theories of aging constructed for and by gerontologists. Its prime proponents, Elaine Cumming and William Henry (1961), stipulated that "aging is an inevitable, mutual withdrawal or disengagement, resulting in decreased interaction between the aging person and others in the social systems he belongs to" (p. 14). The formulation provoked immediate controversy because it described modalities as if they were innate, unidirectional, and universal. Disengagement, Cumming and Henry assumed, was immune to mediating circumstances or variations by race, ethnicity, gender, or class (Hochschild, 1975).

Activity theory arose in response to disengagement theory. Late-life satisfaction, asserted Bernice Neugarten (1964), among others, depended on the active maintenance of one's relationships and continuing involvement in meaningful pursuits. Prevailing theories of productive and successful aging, which arise from activity theory, have been challenged. Critics claim that activity theory and its offspring ignore health and economic disparities that may curtail or diminish the desire and opportunities for some older people to engage in familiar activities. Some elders do not wish to take on fresh challenges. Neither end of the dualism, in short, captures the range of potentials and pitfalls common to late life or the circumstances that affect widening and/or withdrawing social bonds and meaningful endeavors that people engage in as they grow older.

4. The Marginalized/The Self-Dependent

Most gerontologists acknowledge late-life diversity. Societal factors, ranging from gender and racial discrimination to the consequences of policy decisions, adversely affect the identities of aging men and women, marginalizing them in the workplace, the community, and other social institutions. In the United States, Carroll Estes (1979, 2001) and Meredith Minkler and Carroll Estes (1998) theorized that the elderly's disadvantageous position resulted from the political or moral economy of aging. British scholars such as Peter Townsend (1981), Chris Phillipson (1982), and Alan Walker (1986) formulated "dependency" theories that underscored the institutionalization of a construct of disadvantaged, marginalized old age.

Another school of thought stresses the elderly's growing sense and realization of empowerment. Recent cohorts of older people enjoy on average better health and have more resources, both financial and political, at their disposal, enabling them to assert their rights to better treatment or to choose to cut back on priorities. "Autonomy" was a buzzword in the United States especially in the 1980s. Bioethicists scrutinized nursing home practices that restrained residents' freedoms. The right to autonomy colored debates over euthanasia and, less dramatically, doctor–patient decisions about providing or withdrawing treatment (Minkler & Estes, 1998).

As with the other dualisms, many gerontologists framed the debate between "marginalization" and "autonomy" at one extreme or the other. They often failed to incorporate evidence that did not fit their model. This observation, in turn, leads us to four dualisms that inhere in the construction of gerontological theories themselves.

5. Reductionist/Holistic Approaches to Gerontologic Theory Building

Reducing problems to the lowest possible level of analysis is a standard modus operandi in biomedical circles. Since physicians and bench scientists dominated research on aging for most of the 20th century, their commitment to reductionism suffused theory building.

As gerontology emerged as a field of scientific inquiry, however, architects like Lawrence Frank (1956) urged a more holistic approach:

> *To develop a field theory, we must apparently give up the concept of special entities with rigidly defined boundaries, and recognize that we are dealing with a total field in which we can distinguish continually fluctuating components. . . . We are attempting to get away from fixed boundaries since they create a difficult problem of how to get across those boundaries. (pp. 354, 357)*

Gerontological theory building required multidisciplinary, cross-disciplinary, and, ideally, interdisciplinary collaborations in order to capture the dynamic dimensions of senescence. Disciplinary-specific reductionism has its place, but that approach is not enough to grow a field premised on limning the "big picture."

6. Continuity/Dialogic Theories of Aging

On the presuppositions of activity theory, Robert Atchley (1999), among others, proposed a theory of human development that accentuated continuities in adults' experiential learning. People learn to adapt to changes in their identities and environment. Despite empirical evidence that validated this strategy, critics felt that continuity theory minimized the significance of exogenous, societal factors. Donald Cowgill and Lowell Holmes (1972), building on social scientists' constructs of modernization theory, hypothesized that economic, social, and political factors disrupt life trajectories. Matilda White Riley and R. L. Kahn (1994) emphasized the salience of structural and cultural lags that altered the status quo, forcing older adults to cope with dysfunctions in the dynamics of societal trends.

7. Chronological/Age-Irrelevant Definitions of the Last Stage(s) of Life

Throughout U.S. history, 65, give or take 15 years, has signaled the onset of old age. Consistent with the age-graded transitions in childhood and youth, policymakers select 55, 60, 62, 66, or 72 to be neutral markers for establishing eligibility criteria and allocating resources. Yet most gerontologists recognize that chronological age is a poor predictor of any important dimension in late life. A certain ambivalence thus pervades the theoretical literature. Bernice Neugarten (1974) affixed age brackets in distinguishing between the "young-old" and "old-old," though she urged readers not to reify them. Yet in *Age or Need?*, Neugarten (1982) urges that "need" shape age-based policies.

8. Stereotypes/Varieties of Age

Negative images of old age abound in American history. Ageism, Robert Butler (1975) hypothesized, is "a systematic stereotyping of and discrimination against people because they are old, just as racism and sexism accomplish this with skin color and gender" (p. 12). Gerontologists often homogenize representations of late life, though most theories of old age account for the varieties of late-life meanings and experiences. A theoretical conundrum arises when analysts try to determine whether race, gender, ethnicity, class, or region are more influential than age per se in tracking continuities and changes over the life course.

Dialectical Approaches to Gerontological Theory Building

In framing conceptual issues and research problems in terms of dualisms, gerontologists conform to an age-old, ubiquitous mode of advancing knowledge. The strategy, however, has impeded their theoretical objectives. Investigators typically justify novel constructs as necessary antidotes to deficiencies in existing models. Ironically, by emphasizing a particular set of dimensions in the meanings and experiences of growing older that have been underplayed in prevailing theories, gerontologists too often fail to validate and incorporate strengths and insights in the constructs they wish to challenge.

To wit, the major flaw in disengagement theory was that it presumed that the process of withdrawing from the labor force and social networks, which *does* occur, was a universal, inevitable phenomenon of human aging. This is not the case. Proponents of activity theory rightly sought to correct this flaw in disengagement theory by offering empirical evidence that those older people who wish(ed) to stay engaged and maintain contacts increased their life satisfaction. Yet this alternative representation failed to take sufficient account of subsets of the elderly population who physically and mentally were incapable of working. Activity theorists rarely addressed structural barriers older people faced because of age, race, gender, or ethnicity. Thus, both disengagement theory and activity theory eventually gave way to different ways of thinking about late life.

To the extent that theories of aging, viewed along a historical continuum, tend to swing from one extreme version of a dualism to another, gerontologists thus far have not succeeded in formulating theories of aging that sustain the test of time. This lesson from the past too often is lost on rising cohorts of researchers on aging. Look at the indexes of both editions of this handbook: scholars across disciplines once cited the work of Bernice Neugarten; now her theoretical and policy-relevant insights are rarely read or mentioned by those who mimic her ideas without even knowing they are doing so. And in this lost legacy—the continuing relevance of a past master's ideas—lies a final metahistorical perspective on theories of aging: we already have within our reach a way to transcend dualistic fallacies.

A dialectical approach to theory building in gerontology can rest on the dualisms to be found in our historical treasure trove. According to Brian Fay (1996),

> *In a* dialectical *approach, differences are not conceived as absolute, and consequently the relation between them is not one of utter antagonism. Indeed, on a dialectical view, alternatives, while genuinely competing, only appear to be completely "other" to each other. They are in fact deeply interconnected, and the confrontation between them can be comprehended and transcended. . . . Competing alternatives originally thought to have exhausted the possibilities*

can then be replaced with a wider viewpoint which recognizes the worth in the original positions but which goes beyond them. (p. 224)

Dialectical orientations that build on gerontological insights and borrow from other disciplines and professions shape current theories of aging. Let me cite four examples:

- George Engel, M.D., in the 1950s formulated a "biopsychosocial model" to serve as a general theory for searching the causes of illness and for seeking preventive factors in healing. Engel drew inspiration from the mechanistic conceptions of Jacques Loeb, a contributor to Cowdry's *Problems of Ageing* (Brown, 2000). His paradigm helped to unify medical and behavioral sciences, dissolving the classical mind–body dualism. Engel's model fell out of favor in psychiatry when neuroscientists, who began to dominate the specialty in the 1990s, opted for different approaches (Dowling, 2005). By then, however, geriatricians had designed holistic paradigms that paralleled Engel's biopsychosocial approach in the clinic, laboratory, and classroom.
- Research on aging has benefited from a healthy infusion of feminist theory, which has transformed constructs in the humanities and social sciences and, to a lesser degree, the biomedical sciences. Along with others, the critiques of Martha Holstein (1999) challenge androcentric perspectives in gerontology and demand that researchers on aging take seriously the often marginalized voices of women. Feminist theories have enriched applied research as well as basic research. Feminist standpoint theory as well as ecofeminism informs social work research on aging (Besthorn & McMillen, 2002; Swigonski, 1994).
- As previously noted, "critical gerontology" has multidisciplinary roots in the humanities (especially philosophy) and the social sciences (notably in theories about dependency as well as political and moral economy). Practitioners challenge and reconceptualize basic definitional terms, epistemological issues, and interpretations of data. Critical gerontology has entered the gerontological mainstream without losing its edge.
- Narrative discourse builds on Robert Butler's insistence on the value that older individuals derive from engaging in life review and on models of late-life human development conceived by Joan and Erik Erikson, among others. Practitioners are less interested in capturing every autobiographical detail than in probing the meanings that inhere in key moments of a person's sense of self. Insofar as narrative discourse seeks to empower the inner voice of aging, it has natural affinities with branches of psychology and clinical practices (Kenyon, Ruth, & Mader, 1999).

What links these four dialectical approaches is their common effort to construct models and methods appropriate for gerontology's multidisciplinary orientation. They resemble the imaginative work unifying Cowdry's (1939) *Problems of Ageing*. Theories, as E. O. Wilson (1998) declared, are critical: "Nothing in science—nothing in life for that matter—makes sense without theory. . . . Scientific theories are a product of imagination—*informed* imagination" (pp. 56–57). A metahistorical perspective on gerontology attests to the fundamental importance of solid, cogent theory building as a guide to shaping imaginative inquiries into the nature, dynamics, and mysteries of human lives as they mature over time.

References

Achenbaum, W. A. (1978). *Old age in the new land: The American experience since 1790.* Baltimore: Johns Hopkins University Press.

Achenbaum, W. A. (1985). Societal perceptions of aging and the aged. In R. H. Binstock & E. Shanas (Eds.), *Handbook of aging and the social sciences* (2nd ed., pp. 129–148). New York: Van Nostrand Reinhold.

Achenbaum, W. A. (1995). *Crossing frontiers.* New York: Cambridge University Press.

Achenbaum, W. A., & Bengtson, V. L. (1994). Re-engaging the disengagement theory of aging: On the history and assessment of theory development in gerontology. *The Gerontologist, 34,* 756–763.

Aspects of psychology. (1996). Retrieved November 7, 2007, from http://www.personal.psu.edu/faculty/j/5/j5j/psy002/P00s-96/dualis8.htm

Atchley, R. C. (1999). *Continuity and adaptation in old age.* Baltimore: Johns Hopkins University Press.

Bass, S. (2006). Gerontological theory: The search for the Holy Grail. *The Gerontologist, 46,* 139–144.

Bass, S., & Ferraro, K. (2000). Gerontological education in transition: Considering disciplinary and paradigmatic evolution. *The Gerontologist, 40,* 97–106.

Bengtson, V. L., Parrott, T. M., & Burgess, E. O. (1996). Progress and pitfalls in gerontological theorizing. *The Gerontologist, 36,* 768–772.

Bengtson, V. L., Rice, C. J., & Johnson, M. L. (1999). Are theories of aging important? Models and explanations in gerontology at the turn of the century. In V. L. Bengtson & K. W. Schaie (Eds.), *Handbook of theories of aging* (pp. 3–20). New York: Springer Publishing.

Bengtson, V. L., & Schaie, K. W. (Eds.). (1999). *Handbook of theories of aging.* New York: Springer Publishing.

Besthorn, F. H., & McMillen, D. P. (2002). The oppression of women and nature: Ecofeminism as a framework for an expanded ecological social work. *Families in Society, 83,* 221–232.

Biggs, S., Lowenstein, A., & Hendricks, J. (2003). *The need for theory: Critical approaches to social gerontology.* Amityville, NY: Baywood Publishing.

Binstock, R. H. (2003). The war on "anti-aging medicine." *The Gerontologist, 43,* 4–14.

Binstock, R. H., & Shanas, E. R. (1985). *Handbook of aging and the social sciences.* New York: Academic Press.

Birren, J. E., & Bengtson, V. L. (Eds.). (1988). *Emergent theories of aging.* New York: Springer Publishing.

Brown, T. M. (2000). *The growth of George Engel's biopsychosocial model.* Retrieved December 7, 2007, from http://human-nature.com/free-associations/engel1.html

Butler, R. N. (1975). *Why survive? Growing old in American society.* New York: Putnam.

Cole, T. R. (1992). *The journey of life: A cultural history of aging in America.* New York: Cambridge University Press.

Cowdry, E. V. (Ed.). (1939). *Problems of ageing: Biological and medical aspects.* Baltimore: Williams and Wilkins.

Cowgill, D. O., & Holmes, L. D. (Eds.). (1972). *Aging and modernization.* New York: Appleton-Century-Crofts.

Cumming, E., & Henry, W. E. (1961). *Growing old.* New York: Basic Books.

de Beauvoir, S. (1972). *The coming of age.* New York: Putnam's Sons.

Dowling, A. S. (2005). George Engel, M.D. (1913–1999). *American Journal of Psychiatry, 162,* 2039.

Dualism, philosophy of mind. (2007). Retrieved November 11, 2007, from http://en.wikipedia.org/wiki/Cartesian_dualism

Estes, C. (1979). *The aging enterprise.* San Francisco: Jossey-Bass.

Estes, C. (2001). *Social policy & aging.* Thousand Oaks, CA: Sage.

Falconer, W. A. (Trans.). (2001). *Cicero, De Senectute.* Cambridge, MA: Harvard University Press.
Fay, B. (1996). *Contemporary philosophy of social science.* Malden, MA: Blackwell.
Frank, L. K. (1956). Analysis of various types of behavior. In R. R. Grinker (Ed.), *Toward a unified theory of human behavior* (pp. 251–269). New York: Basic Books.
Gruman, G. J. (2003). *A history of ideas about the prolongation of life.* New York: Springer Publishing. (Original work published 1966)
Gunnes, G. (2003). In defense of dualisms. *Mozaik, 27,* 10–12.
Hall, G. S. (1922). *Senescence: The last half of life.* New York: D. Appleton & Sons.
Hendricks, J., & Achenbaum, W. A. (1999). Historical development of theories of aging. In V. L. Bengtson & K. W. Schaie (Eds.), *Handbook of theories of aging* (pp. 21–39). New York: Springer Publishing.
Hochschild, A. R. (1975). Disengagement theory: A critique and proposal. *American Sociological Review, 40,* 553–569.
Holstein, M. (1999). Women and productive aging: Troubling implications. In M. Minkler & C. L. Estes (Eds.), *Critical gerontology: Perspectives from political and moral economy* (pp. 37–49). Amityville, NY: Baywood Publishing.
Katz, S. (1996). *Disciplining old age: The formation of gerontological knowledge.* Charlottesville: University Press of Virginia.
Katz, S. (2003). Critical gerontological theory. In S. Biggs, A. Lowenstein, & J. Hendricks (Eds.), *The need for theory* (pp. 15–31). Amityville, NY: Baywood Publishing.
Kenyon, G. M., Ruth, J.-E., & Mader, W. (1999). Elements of a narrative gerontology. In V. L. Bengtson & K. W. Schaie (Eds.), *Handbook of theories of aging* (pp. 40–58). New York: Springer Publishing.
Lipsitz, L. A., & Goldberger, A. L. (1992). Loss of "complexity" and aging. *Journal of the American Medical Association, 267,* 1806–1809.
Lipsitz, L. A., & Goldberger, A. L. (1995). Age-related changes in the "complexity" of cardiovascular dynamics. *Chaos, 5,* 102–109.
Maddox, G. L., & Campbell, R. T. (1985). Scope, concepts, and methods in the study of aging. In R. H. Binstock & E. Shanas (Eds.), *Handbook of aging and the social sciences* (2nd ed., pp. 203–222). New York: Van Nostrand Reinhold.
Marshall, V. L. (1995). Social models of aging. *Canadian Journal of Aging, 14,* 12–34.
Marshall, V. L. (1999). Analyzing social theories of aging. In V. L. Bengtson & K. W. Schaie (Eds.), *Handbook of theories of aging* (pp. 434–455). New York: Springer Publishing.
Metchnikoff, E. (1904). Old age. In *Annual Report of the Smithsonian Institution for the Year Ending June 30, 1904* (pp. 45–64). Washington, DC.
Metchnikoff, E. (1908). *The prolongation of life: Optimistic studies.* New York: G. P. Putnam's Sons.
Minkler, M., & Estes, C. (1998). *Critical gerontology.* Amityville, NY: Baywood Publishing.
Minot, C. S. (1908). *The problem of age, growth, and death: A study of cytomorphosis.* New York: G. P. Putnam's Sons.
Moody, H. R. (1988). Toward a critical gerontology: The contribution of humanities theories of aging. In J. E. Birren & V. L. Bengtson (Eds.), *Emergent theories of aging* (pp. 19–40). New York: Springer Publishing.
Nascher, H. (1914). *Geriatrics.* New York: Scribners.
Neugarten, B. L. (1964). *Personality in middle and late life.* New York: Atherton Press.
Neugarten, B. L. (1974). Age groups in American society and the rise of the young-old. *Annals of the American Academy of Political and Social Science, 415,* 187–198.
Neugarten, B. L. (1982). *Age or need? Public policies for older people.* Beverly Hills, CA: Sage.
Olshansky, S. J., & Carnes, B. A. (2003). *The quest for immortality: Science at the frontiers of aging.* New York: Diane Publishers.
Phillipson, C. (1982). *Capitalism & the construction of old age.* London: Macmillan.
Phillipson, C. (1998). *Reconstructing old age: New agendas in social theory and practice.* London: Sage.
Riley, M. W., & Kahn, R. L. (Eds.). (1994). *Age and structural lag.* New York: Wiley.
Rosenfeld, A. (1976). *Prolongevity.* New York: Avon.
Swigonski, M. E. (1994). The logic of feminist theory in social work research. *Social Work, 39*(4), 387–393.

Townsend, P. (1981). Structured dependency of the elderly. *Ageing & Society, 1,* 5–28.
Walford, R. L. (1983). *Maximum life span.* New York: Norton.
Walker, A. (1986). Pensions and the production of policy in old age. In C. Phillipson & A. Walker (Eds.), *Aging and social policy* (pp. 86–99). Aldershot: Gower.
White, H. (1973). *Metahistory.* Baltimore: Johns Hopkins University Press.
White, H. (1978). *Tropics of discourse.* Baltimore: Johns Hopkins University Press.
Wilson, E. O. (1998). *The new frontiers of science.* New York: HarperCollins.

An Evolutionary Theory of Human Life Span: Embodied Capital and the Human Adaptive Complex

3

Hillard Kaplan
Michael Gurven
Jeffrey Winking

The future of human longevity remains an open question and is the subject of a vigorous debate among population scientists. There are scientists who propose that human life expectancy is not likely to exceed 85 years (Fries, 1989; Hayflick, 2007). Others suggest that life expectancy may reach 100 years in the 21st century (e.g., Vaupel, 1997). The difference between these two positions stems from beliefs about the relative importance of environmental and genetic variance in determining life expectancy. Those who expect limited future gains in life expectancy believe that most of the existing gains came from improvements in preadult survivorship and that there is an innate program of physiological decay. On the other hand, those who expect greater improvements base their views on evidence suggesting that secular trends in life expectancy due to improvements in the environment (broadly conceived in terms of public health, social services, and so on) show no signs of deceleration to date. At the same time, even as medical science is advancing, there are trends toward increasing obesity, diabetes, and hypertension in both developed and developing nations (Crimmins et al., 2005; Hossain, Kawar, & El Nahas, 2007; Seidell, 2000), causing concern that those environmental improvements may be offset by food abundance and greater ensuing risk for those diseases.

An understanding of how age-specific mortality, the aging process, and behavior respond to novel environmental variation requires a theory of how natural selection has acted on our biology over the course of human evolution. This chapter presents such a theory and attempts to make sense of those two opposing views, suggesting that both are partially correct and partially incorrect. We argue that in the environments in which humans spent the majority of their evolutionary history, natural selection has resulted in a species-typical human life span of about seven decades, as part of a larger adaptive complex. We also argue that the human response to the novel environments of today grows out of our evolutionary history and, to a large extent, is predictable.

The chapter begins with a general framework for understanding gene–environment interactions affecting age-specific mortality and longevity and the role of natural selection in determining the evolution of population gene distributions over time. We then present an extension of standard life history theory, which we term the "embodied capital theory of life history evolution." These ideas are then applied to an understanding of the human case, and we argue that the adaptive niche occupied by our species selected for a coevolved suite of characteristics, or the *human adaptive complex*. We then present the theory about why the ability to live at least to age 65 has played an important role in the human adaptation, without which many other human characteristics could not have evolved. Together with a long life span, these characteristics form an adaptive peak that is unique to humans, with other species being at other peaks in the adaptive landscape. The chapter concludes with a discussion of the present and future that derives from this theory.

A General Framework

Figure 3.1 depicts graphically a conceptual framework for analyzing the factors underlying the evolutionary process relevant to aging and its demographic and physiological outcomes. The two boxes to the left represent the gene–environment interactions that determine diet, work effort, and state of cell and organ tissue by age. Beginning with the upper box, human populations, over evolutionary time, experienced distributions of environmental assaults, including viral and bacterial disease, parasitism, predation, accidents, and trauma. While those assaults undoubtedly varied over time and geography, there was likely a characteristic range of variation to which evolving humans were exposed during the 2 million years our species lived as nomadic foragers.

With respect to pathogen burden, it is likely that evolving hominids were exposed to an array of pathogens, many common to other wild primate species (Nunn et al., 2004). A general assumption is that virgin-soil epidemics were mostly nonexistent in isolated populations prior to modernization and the advent of agriculture and large-scale settlement (Fiennes, 1978; McNeil, 1989).

3.1

Effects of natural selection on organ condition and age schedules of mortality and reproduction.

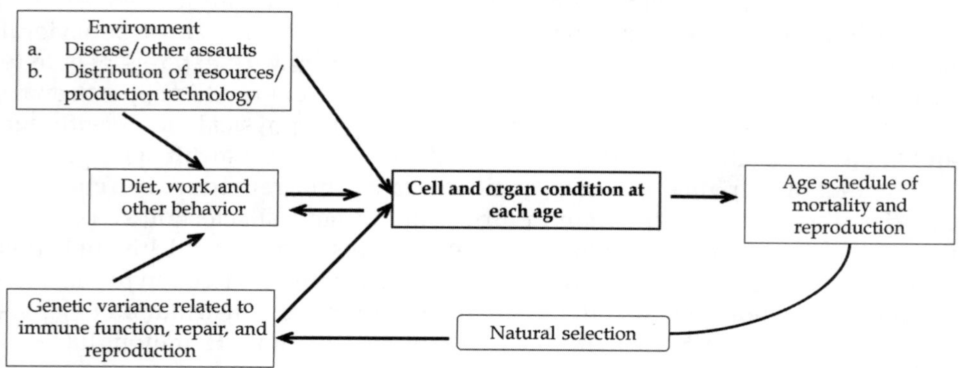

While there is a great deal of uncertainty regarding disease exposure during our evolutionary past, recent work suggests that common infections that have been traditionally associated with high population density, such as tuberculosis (Buikstra, 1981; Clark, Kelley, Grange, & Hill, 1987) and trypanosomiasis (Coimbra, 1988), were present in pre-Columbian South America. The presence of antibodies to viral infections, such as herpes, Epstein-Barr, and varicella, has been documented in relatively isolated Amazonian groups (Black, Woodall, Evans, Liebhaber, & Henle, 1970; Salzano & Callegari-Jacques, 1988). There is strong evidence that cytomegalovirus, Epstein-Barr virus, pneumonias, intestinal geohelminths, herpes, hepatitis B, and arboviruses have long coexisted among precontact Amazonian populations (Black, 1975). More important, recent phylogenetic evidence for a variety of pathogens that were previously assumed to postdate the advent of agriculture and animal domestication also strongly suggests an earlier evolutionary history of exposure to many common pathogens, including smallpox, falciparal malaria, and tuberculosis (see review in Pearce-Duvet, 2006). Sexually transmitted diseases also likely have a long evolutionary history among humans (Donovan, 2000). While virulence of some pathogens may have changed with dense reservoirs of human and animal hosts, ancestral humans were likely exposed to a wide diversity of viruses, bacteria, protozoa, and parasites (Finch & Stanford, 2004).

At the same time as evolving humans faced a distribution of environmental assaults, they also lived in environments with characteristic distributions of food resources and characteristic technologies that changed over evolutionary time. It appears that humans, at least over the past several hundred thousand years, have eaten an omnivorous diet based on both hunting and gathering, with much higher amounts of meat than other primates (Kaplan, Hill, Lancaster, & Hurtado, 2000). This, along with advents in cooking technology (Wrangham, Jones, Laden, Pilbeam, & Conklin-Brittain, 1999), allowed them to do much less physiological processing, such as bacterial fermentation of leaves, in order to have adequate amounts of fat and protein in their diet.

Genes (depicted in the lower left of Figure 3.1) that control defenses against pathogens, repair of cell damage, and reproduction interact with those environmental assaults to determine population distributions of individuals of different ages and their associated physical states at the cellular and organ levels. Genes also interact with environmental conditions (including distributions of energy in the environment and production technologies) and with physical state to determine diet, work, energy budget, and reproductive behavior. Those behavioral patterns have feedback effects on physical state since work exposes people to risks of injury and physical stress but also provides energy to support repair, immune defenses, and reproduction. Both changing physical states with age and behavior result in mortality and reproductive schedules with age.

Population variance in age-specific mortality and reproductive schedules associated with genetic variation in turn result in natural selection since some genotypes are associated with lower or higher fitness than others. Ultimately, this process of natural selection feeds back on the distribution of genotypes in subsequent generations. Presumably, this process produces a distribution of genotypes that tends to maximize fitness over generational time (Hamilton, 1966).

Embodied Capital, Development, and Aging

Two fundamental trade-offs determine the action of natural selection on reproductive schedules and mortality rates. The first trade-off is between current and future reproduction. By growing, an organism can increase its energy capture rates in the future and thus increase its future fertility. For this reason, organisms typically have a juvenile phase in which fertility is zero until they reach a size at which some allocation to reproduction increases lifetime fitness more than continued growth. Similarly, among organisms that engage in repeated bouts of reproduction (humans included), some energy during the reproductive phase is diverted away from reproduction and allocated to maintenance so that they can live to reproduce again. Natural selection is expected to optimize the allocation of energy to current reproduction and to future reproduction (via investments in growth and maintenance) at each point in the life course so that genetic descendants are maximized (Gadgil & Bossert, 1970). Variation across taxa and across conditions in optimal energy allocations is shaped by ecological factors, such as food supply, disease, and predation rates.

A second fundamental life history trade-off is between offspring number (quantity) and offspring fitness (quality). This trade-off occurs because parents have limited resources to invest in offspring and each additional offspring produced necessarily reduces average investment per offspring. Most biological models (Lack, 1954; Lloyd, 1987; Smith & Fretwell, 1974) operationalize this trade-off as number versus survival of offspring. However, parental investment may affect not only survival to adulthood but also the adult productivity and fertility of offspring. This is especially true of humans. Thus, natural selection is expected to shape investment per offspring and offspring number so as to maximize the product of offspring number and average per-offspring lifetime fitness.

The embodied capital theory integrates life history theory with capital investment theory in economics (Becker, 1975; Mincer, 1974) by treating the processes of growth, development, and maintenance as investments in stocks of somatic or embodied capital. In a physical sense, embodied capital is organized somatic tissue—muscles, digestive organs, brains, and so on. In a functional sense, embodied capital includes strength, speed, immune function, skill, knowledge, and other abilities. Since such stocks tend to depreciate with time, allocations to maintenance can also be seen as investments in embodied capital. Thus, the present–future reproductive trade-off becomes a trade-off between investments in own embodied capital and reproduction, and the quantity–quality trade-off becomes a trade-off between the embodied capital of offspring and their number.

The embodied capital theory allows us to treat problems that have not been addressed with standard life history models. For example, physical growth is only one form of investment. The brain is another form of embodied capital, with special qualities. On the one hand, neural tissue monitors the organism's internal and external environment and induces physiological and behavioral responses to stimuli (Jerison, 1973, 1976). On the other hand, the brain has the capacity to transform present experiences into future performance. This is particularly true of the cerebral cortex, which specializes in the storage, retrieval, and processing of experiences. The expansion of the cerebral cortex among higher primates represents an increased investment in this capacity (Armstrong, 1982; Fleagle, 1999; Parker & McKinney, 1999). Among humans, the brain supports learning and knowledge acquisition during both the juvenile and the adult period, well after the brain has reached its adult mass. This growth in the stock of knowledge and functional abilities is another form of investment.

The action of natural selection on the neural tissue involved in learning, memory, and the processing of stored information depends on the costs and benefits realized over the organism's lifetime. There are substantial energetic costs of growing the brain early in life and of maintaining neural tissue throughout life. Among humans, for example, it has been estimated that about 65% of all resting energetic expenditure is used to support the maintenance and growth of the brain in the first year of life (Holliday, 1978). Another potential cost of the brain may be decreased performance early in life. The ability to learn may entail reductions in "preprogrammed" behavioral routines and thus decrease early performance. The incompetence of human infants—and even children—in many motor tasks is an example.

Taking these costs into account, the net benefits from the brain tissue involved in learning are then fully realized only as the organism ages. In a niche where there is little to learn, a large brain might have higher costs early in life and a relatively small impact on productivity late in life. Natural selection may then tend to favor the small brain. In a more challenging niche, however, although a small brain might be slightly better early in life, because of its lower cost, it would be much worse later, and the large brain might be favored instead.

The brain is not the only system that learns and becomes more functional through time. Another example is the immune system, which requires exposure to antigens in order to become fully functional. Indeed, the maturation of the immune system is a primary factor in the decrease in mortality with age from birth until the end of the juvenile period.

A positive relationship between brain size and life span (controlling for body size) is found in empirical studies of mammals (Sacher, 1959) and primates

(Allman, McLaughlin, & Hakeem, 1993; Hakeem, Sandoval, Jones, & Allman, 1996; Judge & Carey, 2000). Such considerations led us to propose that brain size and longevity coevolve for the following reasons. Since the returns to a large brain lie in the future, ecological conditions favoring large brains also favor greater expenditure on survival. Conversely, exogenous ecological conditions that lower mortality favor increased expenditure on survival and hence also much greater investment in brain capital (Abrams, 1993; Carey, 2001; Williams, 1957).

This logic suggested an alternative approach to standard evolutionary treatments. Standard treatments generally define two types of mortality: (a) extrinsic, which is imposed by the environment and is outside the control of the organisms (e.g., predation or weather), and (b) intrinsic, over which the organism can exert some control over the short run or which is subject to selective control over longer periods. In most models of growth and development, mortality is treated as extrinsic and therefore not subject to selection (Charnov & Berrigan, 1993; Kozlowski & Wiegert, 1986). Models of aging and senescence (Promislow, 1991; Shanley & Kirkwood, 2000) frequently treat aging as affecting intrinsic mortality, with extrinsic mortality, in turn, selecting for rates of aging. For example, in the Makeham-Gomperz mortality function, where the mortality rate, μ, equals $A + Be^{ux}$ (with A, B, and μ being parameters and x referring to age), this entails treating the first term on the right-hand side of the equation, A, as the extrinsic component and the second term as the intrinsic component.

In our view, this distinction between types of mortality is misleading and generates confusion. Organisms can exert control over virtually all causes of mortality in the short or long run. Susceptibility to predation can be affected by vigilance, choice of foraging zones, travel patterns, and anatomical adaptations, such as shells, cryptic coloration, and muscles facilitating flight. Each of those behavioral and anatomical adaptations has energetic costs that reduce energy available for growth and reproduction. Similar observations can be made regarding endogenous responses to disease and temperature. The extrinsic mortality concept has been convenient because it provided a reason for other life history traits, such as age of first reproduction and rates of aging. However, this has prevented the examination of how mortality rates themselves evolve by natural selection.

Since all mortality is, to some extent, intrinsic or "endogenous," a more useful approach is to examine the functional relationship between mortality and effort allocated to reducing it. Exogenous variation can be thought of in terms of varying "assault" types and varying "assault" rates of mortality hazards. For example, warm, humid climates favor the evolution of disease organisms and therefore increase the assault rate and diversity of diseases affecting organisms living in those climates. Exogenous variation also may affect the functional relationship between mortality hazards and endogenous effort allocated to reducing them.

The recognition that all mortality is partially endogenous and therefore subject to selection complicates analysis because it requires multivariate models, but it also generates insights about evolutionary coadaptation or coevolution among life history traits. One of the benefits of modeling life history evolution formally in terms of capital investments is that their analysis is well developed in economics with many well-established results. The next section summarizes some formal results of applying capital investment theory to life history evolution with informal graphical illustrations.

Capital Investments and Endogenous Mortality

As a first step, it is useful to think of capital generally as the bundle of functional abilities of the soma. Organisms generally receive some energy from their parents represented as an initial stock of capital, say, K_0. Net energy acquired from the environment, F, at each point in time, t, is a positive function of the capital stock, with diminishing returns to capital. This energy can be used in three ways that are endogenous and subject to selection. It can be reinvested in increasing the capital stock, that is, in growth. Define $\nu(t)$ as flow of investment at time t, so that dK/dt equals $\nu(t)$. Since growth and development take time, it is useful to impose a maximal investment rate, $\bar{\nu}$. Some energy, s, may also be allocated to reducing mortality, μ, for example, via increased immune function. The probability of reaching any age, $p(t)$, is then a function of mortality rates at each earlier age, so that $p(t) = e^{-\int_0^t \mu(t)dt}$. Finally, energy can also be used for reproduction, which is the net excess energy available after allocations to capital investments and mortality reduction, y; thus, $y(t) = F(K) - \nu(t) - s(t)$.

The dynamic optimization program is to find the largest solution r of $\int_0^\infty p(t)y(t)e^{-rt}dt = C_0$, where C_0 is the cost of producing a newborn. This equation is an economic extension of the continuous-time Euler-Lotka equation for the long run growth rate in a species without parental investment after birth. Under most conditions (e.g., for most of human evolutionary history), the average r must be close to zero. It can then be shown that an optimal life history would choose capital investment and mortality reduction so as to maximize total expected surplus energy over the life course. The results of the analysis have been presented and proven formally (Kaplan & Robson, 2002). At each point in time, the marginal gain from investments in capital and the marginal gain from increased expenditure on survival must equal their marginal costs. During the capital investment period, where v is greater than zero, the value of life, J, which is equal to total expected future net energy, is increasing with age since productivity is growing with increased capital. The optimal value of s also then increases. At some age, a steady state is reached when capital is at its optimum level, and both capital and mortality rates remain constant.

Two important comparative results emerge from this analysis. An environmental change that increases the productivity of capital has two reinforcing effects: it increases the optimal level of capital investment (and hence the length of the investment period) and decreases mortality through increases in s because it increases the value of life. A reduction in mortality rates has two similar effects. It increases the optimal capital stock and produces a reinforcing increase in s. Overall, these two effects would tend to increase the expected life span.

It is interesting to note that the model does not result in senescence, as defined by increasing mortality rates with age. Even if capital were to depreciate over time—say, if $dK/dt = (1 - \lambda)K(t) + \nu(t)$, with λ being the proportional depreciation rate—a steady state still would be achieved where depreciation would be exactly offset by investment (Arrow & Kurz, 1970; Intriligator, 1971).

In a recent paper, Kaplan and Robson (n.d.) provide a model of senescence by disaggregating embodied capital into its two dimensions of *quantity* and *quality*. The quantity of embodied capital can be defined in terms of the number of cells in the soma, and cell quality, interpreted as functional efficiency in our model, is endogenous. Its deterioration can always be slowed or reversed by investment in repair. Without such investment, cell quality depreciates over time because of the buildup of deleterious by-products of cell metabolism. For example, somatic capital can be disaggregated into its two components, the quantity and quality of tissue, where optimal levels of quality decline with age, even when quantity grows and then remains stable.

A key result from these analyses is that key life history variables under selection, such as time spent growing (i.e., the capital investment period), mortality rates, and reproductive rates, jointly respond to ecological parameters and therefore coevolve. The settings of different ecological parameters, such as the productivity of somatic capital and the costs of mortality reduction, jointly determine the *complex* of life history characteristics exhibited by a species. In the next section, we illustrate the components of an adaptive complex for the human case.

Life Span and the Human Adaptive Complex

Our proposal is that natural selection impacting immune function, DNA repair, energy metabolism, growth, and behavior produced a specific life history pattern in the environmental context in which humans evolved. In particular, we hypothesize that the ecological niche that our ancestors occupied in the majority of the world's environments consisted of a coadapted set of traits, including (a) the life history of development, aging, and longevity; (b) diet and dietary physiology; (c) energetics of reproduction; (d) social relationships among men and women; (e) intergenerational resource transfers; and (f) cooperation among related and unrelated individuals (Gurven & Kaplan, 2006; Gurven, Kaplan, & Gutierrez, 2006; Gurven & Walker, 2006; Kaplan, 1997; Kaplan & Gurven, 2005; Kaplan, Hill, Lancaster, & Hurtado, 2001; Kaplan, Mueller, Gangestad, & Lancaster, 2003; Kaplan & Robson, 2002; Kaplan et al., 2000; Robson & Kaplan, 2003). We refer to this set of traits as the *human adaptive complex* (HAC).

According to the theory, the HAC is a very specialized niche, characterized by (a) the highest-quality, most nutrient-dense, largest-package-size food resources; (b) learning-intensive, sometimes technology-intensive, and often cooperative food acquisition techniques; (c) a large brain to learn and store a great deal of context-dependent environmental information and to develop creative food acquisition techniques; (d) a long period of juvenile dependence to support brain development and learning; (e) low juvenile and even lower adult mortality rates, generating a long productive life span and population age structure with a high ratio of adult producers to juvenile dependents; (f) a three-generational system of downward resource flows from grandparents to parents to children; (g) biparental investment with men specializing in energetic support and women combining energetic support with direct care of children; (h) marriage and long-term reproductive unions; and (i) cooperative arrangements among kin and unrelated individuals to reduce variance in food availability through sharing and to more effectively acquire resources in group pursuits. Following is a review of some evidence supporting this view.

Diet, Net Food Production Over the Life Course, and Intergenerational Transfers

There is now mounting evidence from various sources, including digestive anatomy, digestive biochemistry, bone isotope ratios, archaeological assemblages, and observational data on hunter-gatherers, that humans are specialized toward the consumption of calorie-dense, low-fiber foods that are rich in protein and fat. Contrary to early generalizations based on incomplete analysis and limited evidence (Dunn, 1968), more than half the calories in hunter-gatherer diets are derived from animal meat. There are 10 foraging societies and five chimpanzee communities for which caloric production or time spent feeding were monitored systematically (Kaplan et al., 2000). Modern foragers all differ considerably in diet from chimpanzees. Measured in calories, the major component of forager diets is vertebrate meat. This ranges from about 30% to around 80% of the diet in the sampled societies with most diets consisting of more than 50% vertebrate meat (equally weighted mean = 60%), whereas chimpanzees obtain about 2% of their food energy from hunted foods. Similarly, using all 229 hunter-gatherer societies described in the Ethnographic Atlas (Murdock, 1967) and Murdock's estimates based on qualitative ethnographies, Cordain et al. (2000) found median dependence on animal foods of 66% to 75%.

The next most important food category in the 10-society sample is extracted resources, such as roots, nuts, seeds, most invertebrate products, and difficult-to-extract plant parts, such as palm fiber or growing shoots. They may be defined as nonmobile resources that are embedded in a protective context such as underground or in hard shells or bearing toxins that must be removed before they can be consumed. In the 10-forager sample, extracted foods accounted for about 32% of the diet, as opposed to 3% among chimpanzees.

In contrast to hunted and extracted resources, which are difficult to acquire, collected resources form the bulk of the chimpanzee diet. Collected resources, such as fruits, leaves, flowers, and other easily accessible plant parts, are simply gathered and consumed. They account for 95% of the chimpanzee diet, on average, and only 8% of the human forager diet. The data suggest that humans specialize in rare but nutrient-dense resource packages or patches (meat, roots, and nuts), whereas chimpanzees specialize in ripe fruit and low-nutrient-density plant parts.

Although the data are still relatively thin, it appears that this dietary shift can be traced to the origins of the genus *Homo* about 2 million years ago. Compared to chimpanzees and australopithecines, early *Homo* appears to have a reduced gut (Aiello & Wheeler, 1995), and radio-isotope data from fossils also suggest a transition from a more plant-based diet to greater reliance on meat (Schoeninger, Bunn, Murray, Pickering, & Moore, 2001). There is significant archaeological evidence of meat eating by *Homo* in the early Pleistocene (Bunn, 2001), and radio-isotope evidence from Neanderthal specimens (Richards & Hedges, 2000) and anatomically modern humans in Europe (Richards & Hedges, 2000) during the late Pleistocene show levels that are indistinguishable from carnivores. It is interesting that this dietary transition occurs at about the same time as the hominid brain expanded beyond the size of the ape brain around

2 million years ago (Aiello & Wheeler, 1995). The next section discusses the comparative evidence on brain development and its psychological correlates.

Figure 3.2 compares human and chimpanzees in terms of age profiles of net production (food produced minus food consumed) and mortality rates. Seen on the right vertical axis, the chimpanzee net production curve shows three distinct phases. The first phase, lasting to about age 5, is the period of complete and then partial dependence on mother's milk. Net production during this phase is negative. The second phase during which net production is zero is independent juvenile growth, lasting until adulthood, about age 13 for females. The third phase is reproductive, during which females but not males produce a surplus of calories that they allocate to nursing.

Humans, in contrast, produce less than they consume for close to 20 years. Net production becomes increasing negative until about age 14 (with growth in consumption due to increased body size outstripping growth in production) and then begins to climb. Net production in adulthood among humans is much higher than among chimpanzees and peaks at a much older age. Peak net production among humans reflects the payoffs to the long dependency period. It is about 1,750 calories per day, but it is not reached until about age 45. Among chimpanzee females, peak net production is only about 250 calories per day, and since fertility decreases with age, net productivity probably decreases during the adult period.

This delay in productivity and then the great increase during adulthood is due to the difficulty involved in acquiring foods. In most environments, fruits are the easiest resources that people acquire. Daily production data among Ache foragers show that both males and females reach their peak daily fruit production by their mid- to late teens. Some fruits that are simply picked from the ground are collected by 2- to 3-year-olds at 30% of the adult maximum rate. Ache children acquire five times as many calories per day during the fruit season as during other seasons of the year (Kaplan, 1997). Similarly, among the Hadza, teen girls acquired 1,650 calories per day during the wet season when fruits were available and only 610 calories per day during the dry season when fruits were not. If we weight the wet- and dry-season data equally, Hadza teen

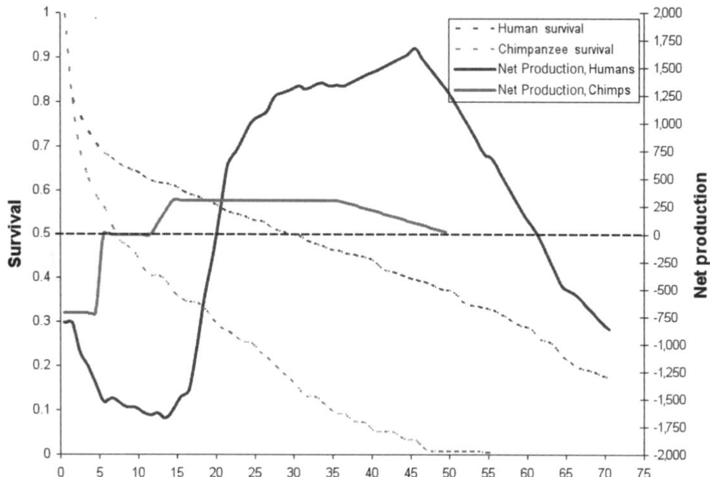

3.2

Net food production and survival: Human foragers and chimpanzees.

Adapted from Kaplan et al. (2000).

girls acquire 53% of their calories from fruits, compared to 37% and 19% for reproductive-aged and postreproductive women, respectively (Blurton Jones, Hawkes, & O'Connell, 1989).

In contrast to fruits, the acquisition rate of extracted resources often increases through early adulthood as foragers acquire necessary skills. Data on Hiwi women show that root acquisition rates do not asymptote until about age 35 to 45, and the rate of 10-year-old girls is only 15% of the adult maximum. Hadza women appear to obtain maximum root digging rates by early adulthood (Blurton Jones et al., 1989). Hiwi honey extraction rates by males peak at about age 25. Again the extraction rate of 10-year-olds is less than 10% of the adult maximum (Kaplan et al., 2000). Experiments done with Ache women and girls clearly show that young adult girls are not capable of extracting palm products at the rate obtained by older Ache women (Kaplan et al., 2000). Ache women do not reach peak return rates until their early 20s. !Kung (Ju/'hoansi) children crack mongongo nuts at a much slower rate than adults (Blurton Jones, Hawkes, & Draper, 1994), and Bock (1995) has shown that nut-cracking rates among the neighboring Hambukushu do not peak until about age 35. Finally, chimpanzee juveniles also focus on more easily acquired resources than adult chimpanzees. Difficult-to-extract activities, such as termite and ant fishing or nut cracking, are practiced less by chimpanzee juveniles than adults (Boesch & Boesch, 1999; Hiraiwa-Hasegawa, 1990; Silk, 1978).

The skill-intensive nature of human hunting and the long learning process involved are demonstrated dramatically by data on hunting return rates by age (for details regarding why hunting is so cognitively demanding, see Kaplan et al., 2001). Hunting return rates among the Hiwi do not peak until age 30 to 35 with the acquisition rate of 10-year-old and 20-year-old boys reaching only 16% and 50% of the adult maximum, respectively. The hourly return rate for Ache men peaks in the mid-30s. The return rate of 10-year-old boys is about 1% of the adult maximum, and the return rate of 20-year-old juvenile males is still only 25% of the adult maximum (Walker et al., 2002). Marlowe (unpublished data) obtains similar results for the Hadza. In addition, boys switch from easier tasks, such as fruit collection, shallow tuber extraction, and baobab processing, to honey extraction and hunting in their mid- to late teens among the Hadza, Ache, and Hiwi (Blurton Jones et al., 1989; Blurton Jones, Hawkes, & O'Connell, 1997; Kaplan et al., 2000). Even among chimpanzees, hunting is strictly an adult or subadult activity (Boesch & Boesch, 1999; Stanford, 1998; Teleki, 1973).

A complex web of intra- and interfamilial food flows and other services supports this age profile of energy production. First, there is the sexual division of labor. Men and women, however, specialize in different forms of skill acquisition with correspondingly different foraging niches and activity budgets and then share the fruits of their labor. The specialization generates two forms of complementarity. Hunted foods acquired by men complement gathered foods acquired by women because protein, fat, and carbohydrates complement one another with respect to their nutritional functions (Hill, 1988) and because most gathered foods, such as roots, palm fiber, and fruits, are low in fat and protein (nuts are an exception). The fact that male specialization in hunting produces high delivery rates of large, shareable packages of food leads to another form of complementarity. The meat inputs of men shift the optimal mix of activities for women, increasing time spent in child care and decreasing time spent in food acquisition. They also shift women's time to foraging and productive activities that are compatible with child care and away from activities that are dangerous to them and their children (Brown, 1970; Hurtado, 1992).

On average among adults in the 10-group sample, men acquired 68% of the calories and almost 88% of the protein; women acquired the remaining 32% of calories and 12% of protein. Given that, on average, these calories are distributed to support adult female consumption (31%), adult male consumption (39%), and offspring (31%), respectively, women supply 3% of the calories to offspring, and men provide the remaining 97%. Men supply not only all the protein and fat to offspring but also the bulk of the protein and fat consumed by women. This contrasts sharply with most mammalian species (>97%), where the female supports all the energetic needs of the offspring until it begins eating solid foods (Clutton-Brock, 1991) and males provide little or no investment. It is the high productivity of men that has probably allowed for the evolution of physiological adaptations among women, such as fat storage at puberty and again during pregnancy, which is not found in apes.

Strikingly, the survival curves in Figure 3.2 depicted with dashed lines and scaled on the left vertical axis show that only about 30% of chimpanzees ever born reach 20, the age when humans produce as much as they consume, and that less than 5% ever born reach 45, when human net production peaks. The relationship between survival rates and age profiles of production is made even clearer in Figure 3.3. This panel plots net expected cumulative productivity by age, multiplying the probability of being alive at each age times the net productivity at that age and then cumulating over all ages up to the present age. The thin and bold lines show cumulative productivity by age for chimpanzees and humans, respectively. The long human training period is evident when the troughs in the human and chimpanzee curves are compared. The dashed line is a hypothetical cross of human production profiles with chimpanzee survival rates. It shows that the human production profile would not be viable with

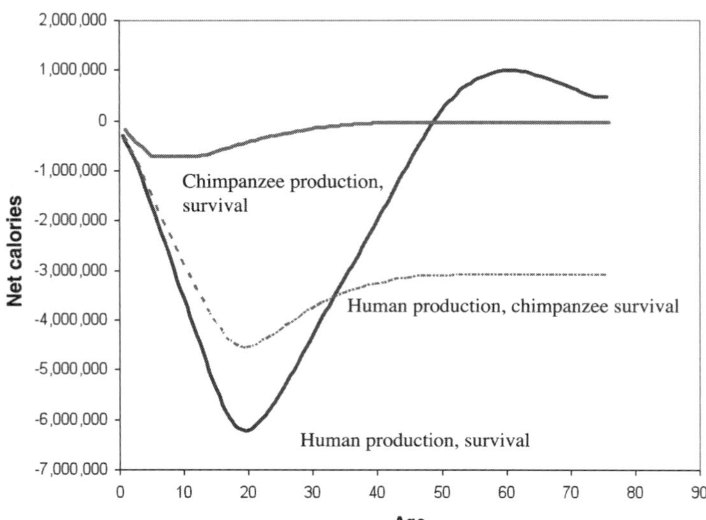

3.3 Cumulative expected net caloric production by age: Humans and chimpanzees.

Adapted from Kaplan et al. (2000).

chimpanzee survival rates because expected lifetime net production would be negative. The next section examines human longevity in greater detail.

Traditional Human Life History and Demography

Figure 3.4 shows expected future years of life remaining (e_x), conditional on living to each age for the human groups with the most reliable data and for wild and captive chimpanzees. While there is significant variation across groups in life expectancy at early ages, there is significant convergence after about age 30. With the exception of the Hiwi, who show more than 10 years less remaining during early ages and more than 5 years less remaining during adulthood, and of the Hadza, whose life expectancy at each age is about 2 years longer than the rest at most adult ages, all other groups, including 18th-century Sweden, are hardly distinguishable. This figure also shows that at age 40, the expected age at death is about 63 to 66 (i.e., 23 to 26 additional expected years of life), whereas by age 65, expected age at death is only about 70 to 76 years of age. By that age, death rates become very high.

In contrast, chimpanzees show a very different life course, with higher mortality and lower age-specific survival, especially during adulthood. Even placing chimpanzees in protected environments and modern medical care, which greatly reduces juvenile mortality, does not achieve the longevity experienced by traditional humans without medical care. Captivity raises infant and juvenile survival greatly, from 37% surviving to age 15 to 64%, similar to the human averages. However, while the probability of reaching 45 increases 10-fold from 3% in the wild to 20% with captivity, it is still just half as high as humans living in premodern conditions. The difference between chimpanzees and humans after age 45 is even greater, with an expected future life span of chimpanzees in captivity of only 7 years, about a third of the human expectation. It appears

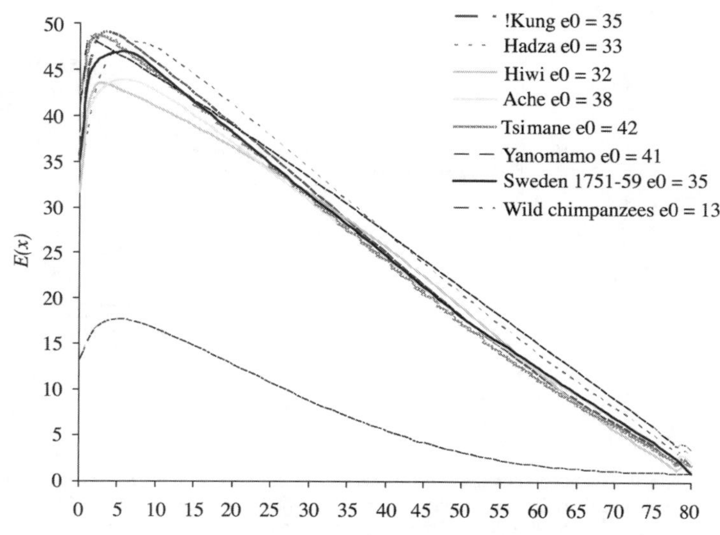

3.4

Age-specific life expectancy among foragers and chimpanzees.

Expected number of years remaining for six sample populations with sufficient data quality and Sweden, 1751–1759. Curves are based on life table estimates using the Siler model. Adapted from Gurven and Kaplan (2007).

that chimpanzees simply age much faster than humans and die earlier, even in protected environments.

Human adult mortality rates in traditional groups also do not rise at a constant proportional rate. Senescence is usually defined as an increase in the endogenous rate of mortality (Finch, Pike, & Whitten, 1990; Rose, 1991). It has been reported that in many populations, mortality reaches its minimum at reproductive maturity and then increases thereafter at a constant proportional (Gompertz) rate, although noticeable decreases in vital functions do not occur until at least age 30 (Shock, 1981; Weale, 2004).

For most traditional human groups, however, we find strong evidence of departure from linearity. The slope of mortality increase is greater after age 40 than before age 40 (Gurven & Kaplan, 2007). From age 15 until about 35, we see virtually no change in mortality rates with age. This is a period of prime adulthood. However, after age 40, mortality rates rise steadily with age. This delay in senescent decline may play an important role in the greater longevity of our species.

The effective end of the human life span under traditional conditions seems to be just after 70 years of age. Following the lead of Kannisto (2001) and Lexis (1878), we examine the modal ages of "normal" adult death and the variance around these modes to examine the extent of stability in adult life spans among and within our study populations (see Figure 3.5 and Table 3.1).

3.5

Modal ages of adult death. Adapted from Gurven and Kaplan (2007).

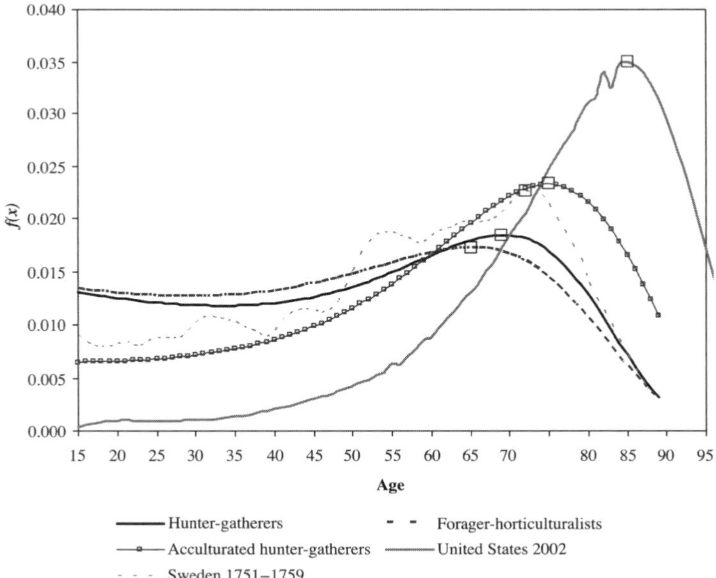

Frequency distribution of ages at death $f(x)$ for individuals over age 15 show strong peaks for hunter-gatherers, forager-horticulturalists, and acculturated hunter-gatherers, Sweden 1751–1759, and the United States, 2002. All curves except for the United States are smoothed by using Siler estimates. Adapted from Gurven and Kaplan (2007).

3.1 Modal Ages of Adult Death[a]

Population	Modal age at death	Standard deviation	% of adult deaths at mode	% adult deaths at and above mode
Hadza	76	6.0	2.5	24.1
Hiwi	68	3.3	3.3	17.9
Ache	71	7.7	2.1	24.5
Yanomamo Xilixana	75	7.3	1.9	22.8
Tsimane	78	5.9	3.0	30.5
!Kung, 1963–1974	74	7.8	2.7	35.4
Ache reservation	78	5.9	3.0	30.5
Aborigines	74	7.8	2.7	35.4
Wild chimpanzees	15	16.8	4.6	100.0
Captive chimpanzees	42	7.5	2.6	38.5
Sweden, 1751–1759	72	7.4	2.3	24.3
United States, 2002	85	1.7	3.5	35.3

[a] The extent of variation around the mode is usually defined as four standard deviation units around the mode (Cheung et al., 2005). Adapted from Gurven and Kaplan (2007).

Figure 3.5 shows the frequency distribution, $f(x)$, of deaths at age x, conditional on surviving to age 15, for our composite categories of hunter-gatherer, forager-horticulturalists, and acculturated hunter-gatherer samples using all populations with high data quality and age specificity. All curves (except Sweden and the United States) are based on the Siler models. Data from early-eighteenth-century Sweden and the modern United States are shown for comparative purposes. This sample of premodern populations shows an average modal adult life span of about 72 years of age (range: 68 to 78; Table 3.1).

While modal age at death is not the same as the effective end of the life span because it refers to a peak in the population distribution of adult deaths, it may reflect an important stage in physiological decline. While there is significant individual variation in rates of aging, the modal age at death may be the age at which most people experience sufficient decline that if they do not die from one cause, they are soon to die from another. This is consistent with our anecdotal impressions of frailty and work in foraging societies. While many individuals remain healthy and vigorous workers through their 60s, few are in good health and capable of significant work in their 70s, and it is the rare individual who survives to age 80.

The Evolved Human Life Span

A fundamental conclusion to be drawn from this analysis is that extensive longevity appears to be a novel feature of *Homo sapiens*. The demographic data derived from foragers and forager-horticulturalists allow us to assess how those benefits can change with age. The two panels in Figure 3.6, derived from data on Tsimane forager-horticulturalists, compare age-specific numbers of dependent descendants with mortality rates. The top panel shows the weighted sum of children and one-half the number of grandchildren by age (since grandchildren share, on average, a quarter of their genes with grandparents, whereas parents share half with their own children). The bottom panel shows age-specific mortality rates. Even though a woman still has descendants who could benefit from assistance, the number of offspring and grandoffspring, especially dependents less than 18 years old, drops considerably after about 65 years. This is the point when mortality begins to rise precipitously. The late age decline in dependents is similar to the modal age at death from Figure 3.4. We have tabulated actual flows of food and observed that men and women invest in children and grandchildren after reproduction has ceased, with a shifting emphasis from mostly children to mostly grandchildren as they age.

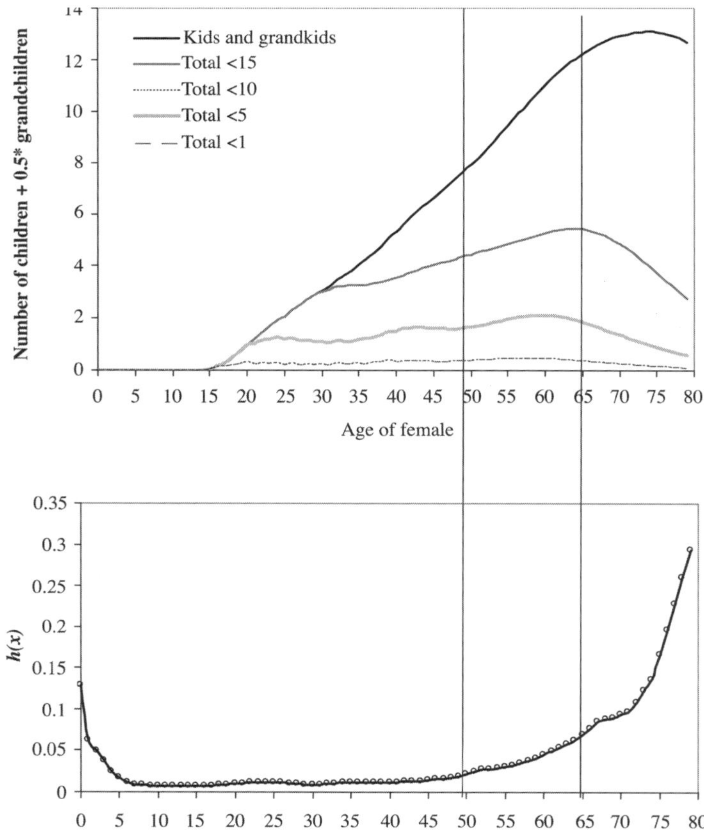

3.6

Age-specific dependency and adult mortality.

Number of children and one-half the number of grandchildren by age of a Tsimane woman (top panel) compared against age-specific mortality rate for Tsimane (bottom panel). Adapted from Gurven and Kaplan (2007).

As the number of closely related dependent kin eligible to receive investment decreases after age 65, the fitness benefits of longer life decrease, and there is less evolutionary incentive to pay increasing maintenance and repair costs to remain alive and functional beyond this period. Similar results are obtained when the same exercise is done with other populations. Data on males would also show a similar pattern, except that the male peak is 3 to 5 years later because of their later age at marriage. This is potentially why few people lived beyond the seventh decade of life.

Conclusions: The Present and the Future

In response to modern conditions, the same genome results in a different life history profile. We began this chapter by considering the debate on the future of human longevity. While average life expectancy has changed significantly over recent history, it is an open question whether gains will continue linearly and whether maximum life span itself will still increase (Vaupel, 1997; Wilmoth, 1997). The model we propose in Figure 3.1 can be expanded to shed light on this issue. In Figure 3.7, we add changed features to human environments to the model.

If we imagine the environments in which our ancestors evolved, environmental assaults and access to energy to combat those assaults are likely to have varied across time and locale. Such variation is likely to select for some phenotypic plasticity in allocations to defense and repair. At the same time, the hunting-and-gathering adaptation practiced by evolving humans was built on a complex of long-term child dependence during which learning trumps productivity and the extremely high productivity of adults, especially in middle age. Together, the costs of slowing senescence and mortality prevention and the benefits of extended investment in descendants produced selection for a

3.7

Modernization effects on life span.

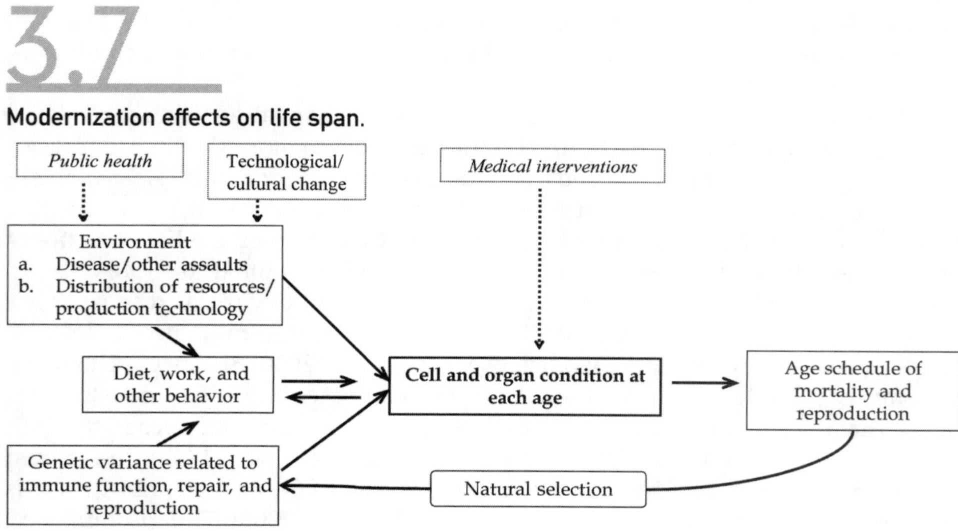

characteristic human life span, with some variance around the central tendency. The comparison of the data from 18th-century Sweden to the hunting-and-gathering populations suggests that relatively similar age distributions of adult deaths occur under a relatively broad range of environmental conditions.

The reductions in infectious diseases and improvements in food supply dramatically lower the assault rate on people's bodies as modernization occurs. Aging individuals are increasingly insulated from assaults as well. The same set of defenses that evolved to be phenotypically plastic (at least to some degree) in relation to ancestral environmental variation produces a very different distribution of deaths under modern conditions. In that sense, when one considers the evolved human life span, it is perhaps best conceived as a population-level distribution of deaths that corresponds to the characteristic range of environments in which our ancestors lived.

In this light, it is likely that neither of the two extreme views (a fixed upper limit to human life span or unlimited flexibility in relation to environmental change) is correct. However, we suspect that environmental change will ultimately have decelerating effects on life expectancy improvement. With relatively constant selection over much of human history, the different somatic subsystems of an organism should tend toward a shared rate of senescence (i.e., stochastically at the population level). In response to a radically changed environment, however, such coordination is not necessarily to be expected, and there may be much carryover from the selective environment, thereby limiting life span extension. The chimpanzee–human comparison also suggests that species differences tend to overwhelm differences in environmental conditions in determining mortality hazards as individuals age. This implies that some differences in our respective genomes have resulted in basic differences in rates of repair and tissue maintenance that manifest themselves in physiological deterioration at older ages.

On the other hand, we differ from those who expect few gains in life expectancy because our view suggests that a reduction in the assault rate, coupled with medical interventions and increases in energy balance, should increase longevity (Abrams, 1993). In addition to lowered assault rates slowing physiological damage, we can expect on theoretical grounds that the evolved human repair and defense system will respond to improved environmental conditions, leading to greater longevity.

We do not yet understand the mechanisms underlying the effects of modernization. Do members of industrialized countries senesce more slowly, in a physiological sense, than people exposed to higher assault environments? Alternatively, are most of the mortality improvements due to reductions in cause-specific mortality at specific ages through prevention of assaults or medical treatment of illnesses? Is a 50-year-old Hadza as robust and functional as a 50-year-old American? It has been argued that aging and the onset of chronic disease is accelerated in response to poor nutrition, infectious disease, and chronic inflammatory processes in general (Bengtsson & Lindstrom, 2000; Blackwell, Hayward, & Crimmins, 2001; Elo & Preston, 1992). For example, there is increasing evidence that chronic diseases, such as diabetes, occurred at earlier ages in the 19th century in the United States than occur today (Fogel & Costa, 1997). In contrast to the United States, the Tsimane show higher levels of C-reactive protein across all ages (Gurven, Kaplan, Crimmins, Finch, & Winking, 2008). This protein is an acute-phase marker that promotes inflammation and among Tsimane associates with disease load and presence of parasites. There is also increasing evidence that malnutrition and health insults during fetal and perinatal development produce a set of cascading effects leading to a greater risk of coronary heart disease later in life (Barker & Osmond, 1986; Cameron & Demerath, 2002). Together, these results suggest that aging and old-age mortality are modulated through energy allocation decisions made early in life in a particular disease ecology. Nevertheless, definitive answers to these questions await further research.

References

Abrams, P. A. (1993). Does increased mortality favor the evolution of more rapid senescence? *Evolution, 47,* 877–887.

Aiello, L., & Wheeler, P. (1995). The expensive-tissue hypothesis: The brain and the digestive system in human and primate evolution. *Current Anthropology, 36,* 199–221.

Allman, J., McLaughlin, T., & Hakeem, A. (1993). Brain weight and life-span in primate species. *Proceedings of the National Academy of Sciences of the United States of America, 90*(1), 118–122.

Armstrong, E. (1982). A look at relative brain size in mammals. *Neuroscience Letters, 34,* 101–104.

Arrow, K. J., & Kurz, M. (1970). *Public investment, the rate of return, and optimal fiscal policy.* Baltimore: Johns Hopkins University Press.

Barker, D. J. P., & Osmond, C. (1986). Infant mortality, childhood nutrition, and ischaemic heart disease in England and Wales 1986. *Lancet, 1,* 1077–1081.

Becker, G. S. (1975). *Human capital.* New York: Columbia University Press.

Bengtsson, T., & Lindstrom, M. (2000). Childhood misery and disease in later life: The effects on mortality in old age of hazards experienced in early life, southern Sweden, 1760–1894. *Population Studies, 54,* 263–277.

Black, F. L. (1975). Infectious disease in primitive societies. *Science, 187,* 515–518.

Black, F. L., Woodall, J. P., Evans, A. S., Liebhaber, H., & Henle, G. (1970). Prevalence of antibody against viruses in the Tiriyo, an isolated Amazonian tribe. *American Journal of Epidemiology, 91,* 430–438.

Blackwell, D. L., Hayward, M. D., & Crimmins, E. M. (2001). Does childhood health affect chronic morbidity in later life? *Social Science & Medicine, 52,* 1269–1284.

Blurton Jones, N. G., Hawkes, K., & Draper, P. (1994). Differences between Hadza and !Kung children's work: Original affluence or practical reason? In E. S. Burch & L. Ellana (Eds.), *Key issues in hunter gatherer research* (pp. 189–215). Oxford: Berg.

Blurton Jones, N. G., Hawkes, K., & O'Connell, J. (1989). Modeling and measuring the costs of children in two foraging societies. In V. Standen & R. A. Foley (Eds.), *Comparative socioecology of humans and other mammals* (pp. 367–390). London: Basil Blackwell.

Blurton Jones, N. G., Hawkes, K., & O'Connell, J. (1997). Why do Hadza children forage? In N. L. Segal, G. E. Weisfeld, & C. C. Weisfield (Eds.), *Uniting psychology and biology: Integrative perspectives on human development* (pp. 297–331). New York: American Psychological Association.

Bock, J. (1995). *The determinants of variation in children's activities in a Southern African community.* Unpublished manuscript.

Boesch, C., & Boesch, H. (1999). *The chimpanzees of the Tai Forest: Behavioural ecology and evolution.* Oxford: Oxford University Press.

Buikstra, J. E. (Ed.). (1981). *Prehistoric tuberculosis in the Americas.* Evanston, IL: Northwestern University Archaeological Program.

Bunn, H. T. (2001). Hunting, power scavenging, and butchering by Hadza foragers and by Plio-Pleistocene *Homo*. In C. B. Stanford & H. T. Bunn (Eds.), *Meat-eating and human evolution* (pp. 199–218). Oxford: Oxford University Press.

Cameron, N., & Demerath, E. W. (2002). Critical periods in human growth and their relationship to diseases of aging. *American Journal of Physical Anthropology, 35*(Suppl.), 159–184.

Carey, J. R. (2001). Insect biodemography. *Annual Review of Entomology, 46,* 79–110.

Charnov, E., & Berrigan, D. (1993). Why do female primates have such long lifespans and so few babies? *Evolutionary Anthropology, 1,* 191–194.

Cheung, S. L. K., Robine, J.-M., Robine, J. M., Jow-Ching, E., & Caselli, G. (2005). Three dimensions of the survival curve: Horizontalization, verticalization and longevity extension. *Demography, 42,* 243–258.

Clark, G. A., Kelley, M. A., Grange, J. M., & Hill, M. C. (1987). The evolution of mycobacterial disease in human populations: A reevaluation. *Current Anthropology, 28,* 45–62.

Clutton-Brock, T. H. (1991). *The evolution of parental care*. Princeton, NJ: Princeton University Press.

Coimbra, C. E. A., Jr. (1988). Human settlements, demographic patter, and epidemiology in lowland Amazonia: The case of Chagas' disease. *American Anthropologist, 90,* 82–97.

Cordain, L., Brand Miller, J., Eaton, B., Mann, N., Holt, S. H. A., & Speth, J. D. (2000). Plant-animal subsistence ratios and macronutrient energy estimations in hunter-gatherer diets. *American Journal of Clinical Nutrition, 71,* 682–692.

Crimmins, E., Alley, D., Reynolds, S., Johnston, M., Karlamangla, A., & Seeman, T. (2005). Changes in biological markers of health: Older Americans in the 1990s. *Journal of Gerontology: Medical Sciences, 60,* 1409–1413.

Donovan, B. (2000). The repertoire of human efforts to avoid sexually transmissible diseases: Past and present. Part 1. Strategies used before or instead of sex. *Sexually Transmitted Infections, 76,* 88–93.

Dunn, F. L. (1968). Epidemiological factors: Health and disease in hunter-gatherers. In R. B. Lee & I. DeVore (Eds.), *Man the hunter* (pp. 221–228). Chicago: Aldine.

Elo, I. T., & Preston, S. H. (1992). Effects of early-life conditions on adult mortality: A Review. *Population Index, 58,* 186–212.

Fiennes, R. (1978). *Zoonoses and the origins and ecology of human disease.* London: Academic Press.

Finch, C. E., Pike, M. C., & Whitten, M. (1990). Slow mortality rate accelerations during aging in animals approximate that of humans. *Science, 249,* 902–905.

Finch, C., & Stanford, C. (2004). Meat-adaptive genes and the evolution of slower aging in humans. *Quarterly Review of Biology 79*, 3–50.

Fleagle, J. G. (1999). *Primate adaptation and evolution.* New York: Academic Press.

Fogel, R. W., & Costa, D. L. (1997). A theory of technophysio evolution, with some implications for forecasting population, health care costs and pension costs. *Demography, 34,* 49–66.

Fries, J. F. (1989). The compression of morbidity: Near or far? *Milbank Quarterly, 67,* 208–232.

Gadgil, M., & Bossert, W. H. (1970). Life historical consequences of natural selection. *American Naturalist, 104,* 1–24.

Gurven, M., & Kaplan, H. (2006). Determinants of time allocation to production across the lifespan among the Machiguenga and Piro Indians of Peru. *Human Nature, 17*(1), 1–49.

Gurven, M., & Kaplan, H. (2007). Longevity among hunter-gatherers: A cross-cultural comparison. *Population and Development Review, 33,* 321–365.

Gurven, M., Kaplan, H., Crimmins, E., Finch, C., & Winking, J. (2008). Lifetime inflammation in two epidemiological worlds: The Tsimane of Bolivia and the United States. *Journal of Gerontology: Biological Sciences, 63A*(2), 196–199.

Gurven, M., Kaplan, H., & Gutierrez, M. (2006). How long does it take to become a proficient hunter? Implications for the evolution of delayed growth. *Journal of Human Evolution, 51*, 454–470.

Gurven, M., & Walker, R. (2006). Energetic demand of multiple dependents and the evolution of slow human growth. *Proceedings of the Royal Society of London, Series B: Biological Sciences, 273,* 835–841.

Hakeem, A., Sandoval, G. R., Jones, M., & Allman, J. (1996). Brain and life span in primates. In R. P. Abeles, M. Catz, & T. T. Salthouse (Eds.), *Handbook of the psychology of aging* (pp. 78–104). San Diego: Academic Press.

Hamilton, W. D. (1966). The molding of senescence by natural selection. *Journal of Theoretical Biology, 12,* 12–45.

Hayflick, L. (2007). Biological aging is no longer an unsolved problem. *Annals of the New York Academy of Sciences, 1100,* 1–13.

Hill, K. (1988). Macronutrient modifications of optimal foraging theory: An approach using indifference curves applied to some modern foragers. *Human Ecology, 16,* 157–197.

Hiraiwa-Hasegawa, M. (1990). The role of food sharing between mother and infant in the ontogeny of feeding behavior. In T. Nishida (Ed.), *The chimpanzees of the Mahale Mountains: Sexual and life history strategies* (pp. 267–276).Tokyo: Tokyo University Press.

Holliday, M. A. (1978). Body composition and energy needs during growth. In F. Falker & J. M. Tanner (Eds.), *Human growth* (Vol. 2, pp. 117–139). New York: Plenum Press.

Hossain, P., Kawar, B., & El Nahas, M. (2007). Obesity and diabetes in the developing world—A growing challenge. *New England Journal of Medicine, 356,* 213–215.

Intriligator, M. D. (1971). *Mathematical optimization and economic theory.* Englewood Cliffs, NJ: Prentice Hall.

Jerison, H. (1973). *Evolution of the brain and intelligence.* New York: Academic Press.

Jerison, H. J. (1976). Paleoneurology and the evolution of mind. *Scientific American, 234,* 90–101.

Judge, D. S., & Carey, J. R. (2000). Postreproductive life predicted by primate patterns. *Journal of Gerontology: Biological Sciences, 55,* B201–B209.

Kannisto, V. (2001). Mode and dispersion of the length of life. *Population: An English Selection, 13,* 159–171.

Kaplan, H. (1997). The evolution of the human life course. In K. Wachter & C. Finch (Eds.), *Between Zeus and Salmon: The biodemography of aging* (pp. 175–211). Washington, DC: National Academies Press.

Kaplan, H., Gurven, M., & Hurtado, A. M. (2005). The natural history of human food sharing and cooperation: A review and a new multi-individual approach to the negotiation of norms. In H. Gintis, S. Bowles, R. Boyd, & E. Fehr (Eds.), *Moral sentiments and material interests: The foundations of cooperation in economic life* (pp. 75–113). Cambridge, MA: MIT Press.

Kaplan, H., Hill, K., Lancaster, J., & Hurtado, A. M. (2000). A theory of human life history evolution: Diet, intelligence, and longevity. *Evolutionary Anthropology, 9,* 156–185.

Kaplan, H., Hill, K. R., Lancaster, J. B., & Hurtado, A. M. (2001). The embodied capital theory of human evolution. In P. T. Ellison (Ed), *Reproductive ecology and human evolution* (pp. 293–317). Hawthorne, NY: Aldine de Gruyter.

Kaplan, H., Mueller, T., Gangestad, S., & Lancaster, J. (2003). Neural capital and lifespan evolution among primates and humans. In C. E. Finch, J.-M. Robine, & Y. Christen (Eds.), *The brain and longevity* (pp. 69–98). Berlin: Springer Verlag.

Kaplan, H. S., & Robson, A. (2002). The emergence of humans: The coevolution of intelligence and longevity with intergenerational transfers. *Proceedings of the National Academy of Sciences of the United States of America, 99,* 10221–10226.

Kaplan, H., & Robson, A. (n.d.). *Why aging is optimal: Senescence and size-dependent costs of somatic repair.* Unpublished manuscript. Department of Anthropology, University of New Mexico.

Kozlowski, J., & Wiegert, R. G. (1986). Optimal allocation to growth and reproduction. *Theoretical Population, 29,* 16–37.

Lack, D. (1954). *The natural regulation of animal numbers.* Oxford: Oxford University Press.

Lexis, W. (1878). Sur la Durée Normale de la Vie Humaineet sur la Théorie de la Stabilité des Rapports Statistiques. *Annales de Démographie Internationale, 2,* 447–460.

Lloyd, D. G. (1987). Selection of offspring size at independence and other size-versus-number strategies. *American Naturalist, 129,* 800–817.

McNeil, W. H. (1989). *Plagues and peoples* (2nd ed.). New York: Anchor Books.

Mincer, J. (1974). *Schooling, experience, and earnings.* Chicago: National Bureau of Economic Research.

Murdock, G. P. (1967). Ethnographic Atlas: A summary. *Ethnology, 6,* 109–236.

Nunn, C. L., Altizer, S., Sechrester, W., Jones, K., Barton, R., & Gittleman, J. (2004). Parasites and the evolutionary diversity of primate clades. *American Naturalist, 164*(Suppl.), S90–S103.

Parker, S. T., & McKinney, M. L. (1999). *Origins of intelligence: The evolution of cognitive development in monkeys, apes and humans.* Baltimore: Johns Hopkins University Press.

Pearce-Duvet, J. M. C. (2006). The origin of human pathogens: Evaluating the role of agriculture and domestic animals in the evolution of human disease. *Biological Reviews, 81,* 369–382.

Promislow, D. E. L. (1991). Senescence in natural populations of mammals: A comparative study. *Evolution, 45,* 1869–1887.

Richards, M. P., & Hedges, R. M. (2000). Focus: Gough's Cave and Sun Hole Cave human stable isotope values indicated a high animal protein diet in the British Upper Paleolithic. *Journal of Archeological Science, 27,* 1–3.

Robson, A., & Kaplan, H. (2003). The evolution of human life expectancy and intelligence in hunter-gatherer economies. *American Economic Review, 93*(1), 150–169.

Rose, M. R. (1991). *Evolutionary biology of aging.* New York: Oxford University Press.

Sacher, G. A. (1959). Relation of lifespan to brain weight and body weight in mammals. In G. E. W. Wolstenhome & M. O'Connor (Eds.), *Ciba Foundation Colloquia on Ageing* (pp. 115–133). London: Churchill.

Salzano, F. M., & Callegari-Jacques, S. (1988). *South American Indians: A case study in evolution.* (*Research monographs on human population biology,* No. 6.). Oxford: Oxford University Press.

Schoeninger, M., Bunn, H. T., Murray, S., Pickering, T., & Moore, J. (2001). Meat-eating by the fourth African ape. In C. B. Stanford & H. T. Bunn (Eds.), *Meat-eating and human evolution* (pp. 179–195). Oxford: Oxford University Press.

Seidell, J. C. (2000). Obesity, insulin resistance and diabetes—A worldwide epidemic. *British Journal of Nutrition, 83*(Suppl. 1), S5–S8.

Shanley, D. P., & Kirkwood, T. B. L. (2000). Calorie restriction and aging: A life-history analysis. *Evolution, 54,* 740–750.

Shock, N. W. (1981). Indices of functional age. In D. Danon, N. W. Shock, & M. Marois (Eds.), *Aging: A challenge to science and society* (pp. 302–319). Oxford: Oxford University Press.

Silk, J. B. (1978). Patterns of food-sharing among mother and infant chimpanzees at Gombe National Park, Tanzania. *Folia Primatologica, 29,* 129–141.

Smith, C. C., & Fretwell, S. D. (1974). The optimal balance between size and number of offspring. *American Naturalist, 108,* 499–506.

Stanford, C. B. (1998). *Chimpanzee and red colobus: The ecology of predator and prey.* Cambridge, MA: Harvard University Press.

Teleki, G. (1973). *The predatory behavior of wild chimpanzees.* Lewisburg, PA: Bucknell University Press.

Vaupel, J. W. (1997). The remarkable improvements in survival at older ages. *Philosophical Transactions of the Royal Society of London. Series B, Biological Sciences,* 1799–1804.

Weale, R. A. (2004). Biorepair mechanisms and longevity. *Journal of Gerontology: Biological Sciences, 59,* 449–454.

Wilmoth, J. (1997). In search of limit. In K. Wachter and C. Finch (Eds.), *Between Zeus and Salmon: The biodemography of longevity* (pp. 38–64). Washington, DC: National Academy Press.

Wrangham, R. W., Jones, J. H., Laden, G., Pilbeam, D., & Conklin-Brittain, N. (1999). The raw and the stolen. *Current Anthropology, 40,* 567–594.

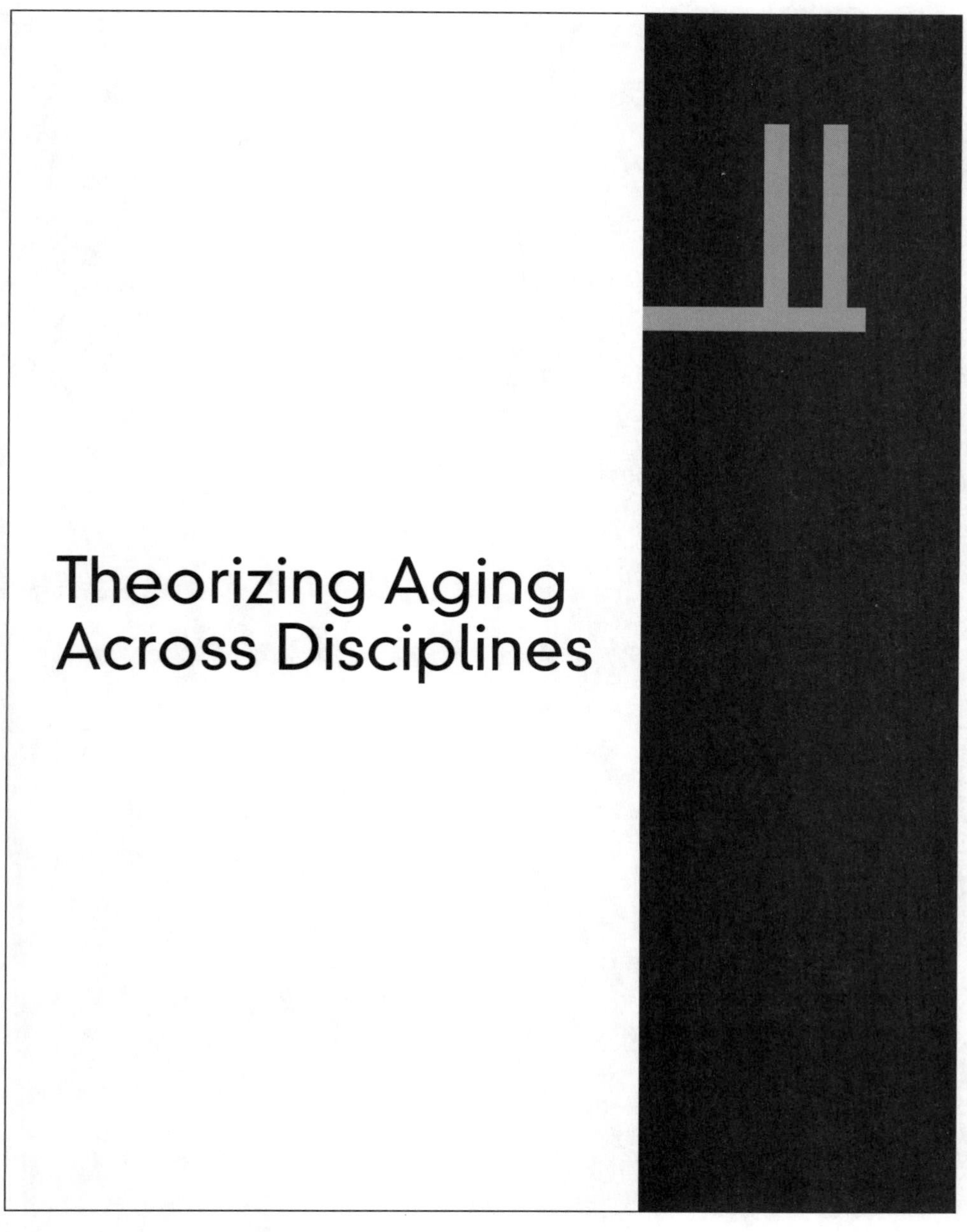

II

Theorizing Aging Across Disciplines

Biodemography: Integrating Disciplines to Explain Aging

4

Sarinnapha Vasunilashorn
Eileen M. Crimmins

Biodemography, a new subfield of demography, incorporates biological theory and measurement with traditional demographic approaches to better understand variation in health and mortality across populations and among individuals within those populations. Traditionally, demographers studied a limited number of life transitions: births, marriages, deaths, and migration; over time, however, demography has incorporated a wider range of life events and statuses, including changes in labor force participation and educational attainment, family structure, living arrangements, intergenerational resource transfers, and health.

With the rapid aging of populations and declines in mortality that occurred in recent years, a number of questions have become central to studies in the demography of aging. These include the following: What is the limit to human life span for individuals? What is the maximum average life expectancy for populations? Are people living longer healthy lives as well as longer lives? and How do you explain the variability in the aging process across individuals and groups? In other words, the focus of work in the demography of aging has changed from descriptions of population aging to understanding how and why aging occurs and the plasticity of human aging to environmental, social, behavioral, and technological changes. Hence, biodemography, which became a natural outgrowth of past demographic research on health and mortality, focused on these questions because social scientists were limited in their ability to provide answers without considering biological and medical theory and information.

Biodemography has two subfields: (a) biomedical demography with a focus on variability in human health and links to epidemiology and medicine and (b) biological demography with links to population and evolutionary biology (Carey & Vaupel, 2007). Demographic focus on population characteristics and processes affecting population change are central to both aspects of biodemography. Generally, the biodemography of aging investigates questions relating to variability in the rate of aging across or within populations and attempts to understand how generalizable the current human condition is by comparing humans to other species or comparing human populations across time and place. *Between Zeus and the Salmon* (Wachter & Finch, 1997), the first book on biodemography, reflects these interests using theory and empirical evidence reflecting biological demography. Zeus is an immortal Greek god who lives forever; in contrast, salmon have preprogrammed life spans, dying shortly after reproduction, and the focus is where humans fall on this continuum. The second book in this National Research Council series of books on biodemography, *Cells and Surveys* (Finch, Vaupel, & Kinsella, 2002; Olshansky, 1998), reflects the interest in the more biomedical approach to understanding population health and addresses how biomedical information can inform demographic understanding of health and mortality. The third book in the series, *Biosocial Surveys* (Weinstein, Vaupel, & Wachter, 2008), clarifies how rapidly the biomedical aspect of biodemography has grown by showing results from the incorporation of biological indicators in many population surveys as well as the wealth of biological information being incorporated into population studies now and in the near future.

While researchers have attempted to determine a general theory of aging and longevity (Gavrilov & Gavrilova, 2003), there is no one theory that drives the study of biodemography. There are, however, two major types of biological theories that have fostered its development: programmed theories and biopsychosocial theories of aging. Programmed theories of aging, synonymous with "why" theories, underline the driving forces that cause aging to occur. In contrast, the "who" theories of aging, of which the biopsychosocial approach is often used, examine why some individuals or populations age earlier than others.

History of the Biodemography of Aging

While biodemography of aging is a relatively young discipline (Carnes & Olshansky, 1993; Olshansky & Carnes, 1994; Wachter & Finch, 1997), its foundations originated in the 18th century with zoologist Georges Buffon, who suggested that "physical laws" and not lifestyle behaviors or diet regulate life span across multiple species (Buffon, 1812). Here, physical laws link the biological clock guiding growth and development to the biological clock determining life span. For instance, Buffon concluded that the time between birth and reproductive maturity remained relatively constant for a given species: about 30 days for rabbits, 56 days for cats, 60 days for guinea pigs, 64 days for dogs, and 14 years for humans. If other biological processes, including aging, followed the same fixed laws as those that maintained the timing of sexual maturity, then Buffon hypothesized that life span must also be fixed: a fixed amount of time for gestation, a fixed time for growth, and ultimately a fixed time for the duration of life (i.e., life span).

In examining the life span characteristics of several species, Buffon suggested that the average life span of individuals, also known as life expectancy at birth, is proportional to the amount of time dedicated to growth and development. More specifically, he noted that life expectancy was about six to seven times the duration from birth to sexual maturity. Assuming that in humans, for example, the age at puberty is 14 years, this would predict a life expectancy of between 85 and 100 years.

The first mathematical support for Buffon's study was provided by Benjamin Gompertz, who showed that after maturity the risk of death increases exponentially with age (Gompertz, 1825). Gompertz empirically demonstrated this pattern and regularity in death rates as evidenced in what is now called "the Gompertz curve" (Windsor, 1932), which has been the source of a number of hypotheses tested recently using the biodemographic approach.

While Gompertz's law was well known by demographers, there was little emphasis on mortality at older ages until the last quarter of the 20th century. After mortality at young ages and after infectious diseases were largely eliminated in much of the world by the 1960s, mortality became concentrated among the old and was attributable largely to a small number of chronic diseases. With these changes, the demographic focus moved to the end of the life span. It is also true that at this time, mortality at the end of the life span began to fall sharply (Crimmins, 1993).

Biodemography of Aging Theories

With rapid declines in old age mortality occurring in the 1970s and 1980s in much of the world, researchers in the demography of aging became interested in whether life expectancy was approaching a predetermined limit and whether future predictions of population size and life expectancy should be built on such assumptions. In addition, questions arose as to whether healthy life expectancy, as well as total life expectancy, was increasing. A focus on the quality of life as well as the quantity of life developed both in international agencies and among policymakers in a number of countries.

In the 1980s, increasing interest in the biodemography of aging was spurred with the publication of James Fries's well-known article "Compression of Morbidity," which linked these two questions (Fries, 1980; Vaupel, 2004). In this article, Fries described two types of death: premature and senescent. Premature deaths are a result of accidental events and conditions that shorten an individual's life. On the other hand, senescent deaths occur as a natural consequence of approaching one's maximum possible life span.

Fries thought that while potential life span could not be altered by medical, environmental, or behavioral changes, the likelihood that persons in a given population will approach and live to their maximum potential life span can be changed. In other words, while we cannot extend our maximum potential years of life, we can increase the number of years that members of the population will potentially live and the proportion that will achieve this maximal life span.

Fries's concept of death has parallels to Aristotle's depiction of mortality, in which he symbolizes death by the flames of a fire. In his analogy, premature death resembles a flame that is extinguished by water, while senescent death resembles a fire that gradually ceases to burn on its own (Vaupel, 2004). Similar to Fries's assertion that humans have a fixed maximum life span, Aristotle also states that all individuals have a given amount of "fuel," akin to a fixed supply of wood available to maintain the flames of a fire. Ultimately, Fries's greatest contribution stemmed from his ability to distinctly pinpoint specific aspects of Aristotle's description of mortality and to provide an empirical illustration of maximum life spans. As life expectancy at even the oldest ages has increased, there has been little empirical evidence pointing to a maximum value at which life expectancy is fixed (Robine & Michel, 2004); however, while there is obviously more plasticity in population life expectancy than Fries thought, no one has lived longer than Jean Calment's 122 years.

The introduction of the idea of the "Compression of Morbidity" has resulted in biodemographers investigating morbidity as well as mortality. Mortality is now considered the end of a process of health change captured in the disablement process (Vebrugge & Jette, 1994). Studying morbidity as well as mortality has generally led to the conclusion that the length of healthy life has increased along with the total length of life (Crimmins, Saito, & Ingegneri, 1997). In addition, demographers have shown how mortality and morbidity are often not closely related in that many causes of morbidity and disability are not necessarily causes of mortality. Demographic modeling has also shown how the direction of change in population health can be opposite to the change in length of life in a population (Crimmins, Hayward, & Saito, 1994; Preston, 1987).

Joining of the Social and Biological Sciences

In the 1950s and 1960s, evolutionary biologists began formulating a theory of aging rooted in the Darwinian view of evolution and survival of the fittest. Essentially, this theory states that the fittest animals or individuals in a given population will reproduce more and be more likely to pass on of their genes than less fit individuals. Hence, those fit enough to survive to reproductive maturity and fit enough to reproduce will ensure that their genes remain in the next generation's gene pool.

This concept of evolutionary drive is linked to the aging process because detrimental mutations that affect individuals in postreproductive ages will not be "weeded out" and will be passed on to later generations. Mutations that lower mortality or increase fertility during younger ages, even if deleterious in later years, will be selected for. This concept, known as antagonistic pleiotrophy, attempts to explain why certain mutations that are detrimental in later years remain in the gene pool across generations (Williams, 1957). While they are costly in late life, their beneficial effects during earlier years assert their maintenance over time. This may be one explanation for the increase in age-related health change and adverse health outcomes occurring with age.

In the early 1990s, researchers in the biodemography of aging began investigating common biological influences contributing to similarities in age patterns of death across human and animal species (Finch & Pike, 1996; Vaupel et al., 1998). During this time, the field of biodemography continued to incorporate both biological and social science theories, with its theoretical basis derived largely from evolutionary biology (Hamilton, 1966; Kirkwood, 1977; Medawar, 1951; Williams, 1957).

"Why" Theories

Based on an evolutionary perspective, the "why" theories (Ricklefs & Finch, 1995) attempt to understand why animals and humans age. Generally, these theories use cross-species comparisons (Longo & Finch, 2003), or cross-time comparisons of human populations (Crimmins & Finch, 2006; Finch & Crimmins, 2004), to suggest explanations as to why some species, subpopulations, or societies age faster than others (Finch & Austad, 2001). These theories also underscore common aspects of the aging process across species.

Theories of programmed aging suggest that a biological clock drives the process of human development and aging processes. Proposed explanations of these conserved molecular pathways (e.g., the glucose or insulin-like growth factor [IGF]-1 pathways) include cellular aging and related genetics. The programmed aging view (Cristofalo, Tresini, Francis, & Volker, 1999) is supported by the discovery of common pathways of aging among various animal models that exhibit similar life trajectories. For instance, the glucose or IGF-1 pathways are similar among yeast, worms, flies, mice, and humans (Longo & Finch, 2003). These pathways are vital to the livelihood of these species because they regulate energy and fat accumulation, ultimately affecting growth, aging, and mortality.

Akin to Aristotle's and Fries's theories of fixed resources over one's lifetime, cellular aging is also rooted in the discovery that most cellular tissues can divide only a finite number of times. On average, human cells from embryonic tissues stop dividing after 50 cumulative population doublings (CPDs). This phenomenon, introduced by Leonard Hayflick and Paul Moorhead (1961), is known as Hayflick's limit or replicative senescence (RS) (for additional information, see Kirkwood, 1999).

Across species, there is an association between the number of CPDs and longevity. For instance, cells from a Galapagos tortoise, which can live more than 100 years, divide approximately 110 times, while cells from mice, which live less than 5 years, divide about 15 times. Moreover, cells from individuals with Werner syndrome (WS), a progeroid syndrome in which individuals undergo accelerated aging, have far fewer CPDs than cells from normal, non-WS individuals. However, exceptions to Hayflick's limit do exist, with some cells never reaching RS. These "immortal" cells include embryonic germ cells and cells from some tumors.

While the bulk of biodemographic studies investigate humans, a handful of studies have examined age patterns of fertility and mortality in other species to better understand aging and mortality from an evolutionary standpoint. Vaupel et al. (1998) compared death rates of humans, four strains of flies, yeast, and worms. While the trajectories of death varied across animal species, a common characteristic was found: the overall deceleration of mortality at the oldest ages. Other smaller-scale studies have reported equivalent findings in beetles, flies, and humans (Finch, 1990; Tatar, Carey, & Vaupel, 1993; Wilson, 1994).

Such cross-species studies have underscored three important biodemographic concepts: mortality correlation, induced demographic schedules, and heterogeneity in frailty (Vaupel et al., 1998). Mortality rates at various ages are correlated across populations and over time (Coale & Demeny, 1983; Crimmins & Finch, 2006; Lee & Carter, 1992). We see this from Buffon's initial hypothesis discussing the relationship between time of sexual maturity and time of death: multiply the time of sexual maturity by six or seven to determine the species' time of death. Moreover, in comparing mortality trajectories across species, we find evidence for a potential conservation of mortality deceleration and mortality correlation as basic characteristics of these complicated animal systems (Vaupel, 1997). Ultimately, utilizing this cross-species biodemographic approach allows researchers to better determine and understand the shared (and differential) biological pathways involved in aging processes and aging outcomes. In comparing links across age in human populations living in a variety of circumstances, we uncover mechanisms that link early-life experiences to late-life outcomes (Finch & Crimmins, 2004).

The induction of demographic schedules is based largely on the Lotka equation, which underscores an important concept in evolutionary theory. The Lotka equation indicates how population characteristics, such as the increasing prevalence of an advantageous mutation, are based on age-specific schedules of fertility and survival assuming that these fertility and survival schedules remain fixed over time (Lotka, 1939). This is often not the case for most species that are frequently required to adapt to fluctuating environmental conditions (Mangel & Clark, 1988; Orzack & Tuljapurkar, 1989), which induce or result in changing demographic schedules of survival and fertility. For example, medflies require protein, which is not always available, to reproduce. When fed protein, they are able to reproduce, and their age at mortality in turn decreases.

Thus, while we have evidence that there are cross-species similarities in the patterning of life span, we also have evidence that within-species life spans are affected by the environment. This has come from studies of opossums, guppies, and grasshoppers in different locations (Austad, 1993; Reznick, Shaw, Rodd, & Shaw, 1997; Tatar, Khazaeli, & Curtsinger, 1997). Among insects with social, hierarchical networks (e.g., bees), the same genome across the species can be programmed to result in short-lived worker bees or long-lived queen bees (Finch, 1990). Support for the heterogeneity-in-frailty hypothesis was also shown in cohorts of flies that were exposed to a stressor that killed the frail files and left only the nonfrail survivors. A comparison of mortality trajectories among the stressed cohorts and the nonstressed control cohorts revealed the remarkable extent of heterogeneity between the two groups (Curtsinger & Khazaeli, 1997; Vaupel, Yashin, & Manton, 1987). We also know that several species have evolved physiological modes or conditions allowing them to deal with uncertain external conditions. These physiological modes have been termed the stationary phase in yeast, hibernation in bears, dauer states in *Caenorhabditis elegans* (a worm), and diapause in some insects. Hence, across species, we find evidence for deviations in fertility and survival schedules in response to ever-changing environmental conditions.

Many model organisms have been used to examine the effect of genetic changes on longevity. With relatively small genetic modifications, the life spans of nematodes, yeast, and mice have been extended dramatically (Guarente & Kenyon, 2000; Longo & Kennedy, 2006; Tatar, Bartke, & Antebi, 2003). Results from some of this work are surprising for those who study humans. For instance, in studying longevity in nematodes, one can examine length of life in a population of genetically identical individuals who live in identical environments. A social scientist might expect to find no variability in longevity with no variability in genes or environment, but results indicate almost as much variability in length of life among these nematodes as would be found in a population of humans (Kirkwood & Finch, 2002). Even individuals with the same genetic makeup exhibit some degree of heterogeneity in phenotypic traits. For instance, some individuals become more frail than others because of environmental influences or random developmental events (Finch & Kirkwood, 2000). This has also been shown for human twins (Yashin & Iachine, 1995).

"Who" Theories

While aging is inevitable for all species, in humans, some populations "age" more quickly than others, and within populations some individuals "age" more quickly than others. Biopsychosocial theories attempt to explain how environmental, medical, and technological changes experienced by populations change the rate of aging. They also focus on determining which individuals within a population are most vulnerable to adverse health- and age-associated conditions. Over the past few decades, the scope of potential analyses relating demographic research to health outcomes has been expanded because of theoretical, methodological, and empirical developments (Crimmins, 1993; Hummer, 1996; Mosley & Chen, 1984; Preston & Taubman, 1994; Rogers, Hummer, & Nam, 2000).

Over time, demographers of aging who study human populations have enlarged their scope to study the entire disablement process, shifting their focus away from studying only mortality. The field quickly expanded from studies investigating solely mortality and life expectancy to focusing on conditions and diseases associated with aging, such as cognitive loss, heart disease, and declines in functioning and frailty. As indicated previously, the reasons for this included ongoing health changes and trends in the population, but it also relied on the availability of large-scale population-based longitudinal data sets that monitored the aging process over representative samples of individuals (Crimmins, 1993).

In order to better study health in large-scale population studies, biomarkers are often now included to better understand physiological processes that change with age, diseases with age-linked onset, and the aging process itself (Alley, 2007). Biomarkers are used to monitor and predict the health of the population, to identify individuals with particular resistance or susceptibility to health problems, and to evaluate therapeutic interventions. The utility of biomarkers rests on the notion that they represent early physiological change or provide information on existing diseases or loss of function. Health change in an aging population begins with the development of risk factors and continues at somewhat later ages to the onset of diseases and conditions, to functioning loss or loss of ability to perform certain physiological functions, and ultimately to the onset of disability (Vebrugge & Jette, 1994). Using biomarkers to investigate this first stage of deterioration in physiological status allows researchers to better identify individuals and populations at risk of developing diseases and adverse health conditions before manifestation of clinical symptoms.

At the other end of the health continuum is frailty, an emerging concept in the study of health outcomes specific to older age (Cohen, 2000; Fried et al., 2001; Morley, Perry, & Miller, 2002). It signifies a downward trajectory in health and the ability to perform daily tasks due to the accumulation of acute and chronic diseases as well as physiological decline and dysregulation that accompany the onset of diseases and advanced age (Cohen, 2000). A number of indicators of frailty have also been included in recent population-based health surveys. In this respect, biomarkers can be used to indicate the presence of health changes in any of the following aspects: risk, disease, functioning loss, disability, frailty, or imminent death.

Most of the important age-related health outcomes (including mortality, cancer, cardiovascular disease, and loss of physical and cognitive functioning ability) appear to be somewhat interrelated and to be associated with similar risk factors. In attempts to understand the mechanisms by which these conditions arise, the biodemographic approach considers the complex interplay among demographic, psychological, behavioral, and biological factors on these health outcomes. The broadening of the concept of health and the increasing knowledge of the links between dimensions of health and causal factors are key to the extension of biodemographic research into non–mortality-associated health and mortality outcomes across species (Vebrugge & Jette, 1994).

In order to more fully understand change and differentials in disease, disability, and the relative burden of mortality within a population, the biodemographic approach has incorporated explanations originating in sociological, psychological, behavioral, medical, and biological research. Figure 4.1, taken from Crimmins and Seeman (2004), details a heuristic model of several potentially interacting pathways of interest in understanding health outcomes linked to aging.

This model indicates that chronic health conditions and physiological change in old age stem from lifetime social, economic, behavioral, and psychological conditions. The links between lifecycle conditions and health can, of course, vary by the context in which they occur. Although these social, behavioral, and psychological mechanisms contribute to health in different ways, at some point all of them affect aging and health outcomes through some biologi-

4.1

Biopsychosocial model of health outcomes.

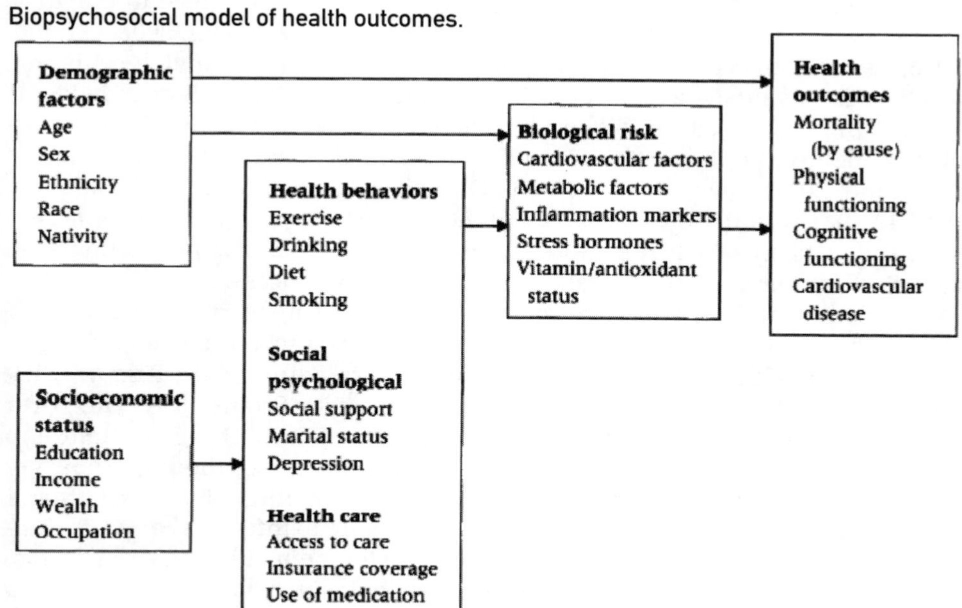

Note. From Crimmins and Seeman (2004).

cal mechanism, as there must be some way that social and psychological factors "get under the skin" to cause health problems.

One of the major concerns of biodemography has been explaining differentials in population health. A large body of research suggests that individuals with less education have a greater risk of disease onset, loss of physical functioning, impairments in cognition and physical function, and mortality compared to those with higher education, although demographers have clarified how selection processes change these differences with age (Adler et al., 1993; Crimmins, Hayward, & Seeman, 2004; Crimmins, Kim, & Seeman, in press; Hayward, Crimmins, Miles, & Yang, 2000; Smith 1999; Williams, 1990). Additionally, chronic conditions (including hypertension, heart disease, diabetes, disability, cognitive impairment, and loss of functioning) related to morbidity and mortality have been linked to low education levels (Albert et al., 1995; Crimmins, Hayward, & Seeman, 2004; Jones & Gallo, 2002; Seeman et al., 2005). Ethnic-minority populations and individuals with low socioeconomic status (SES) also exhibit both a higher level and earlier onset of age-related physiological deterioration and disease, including cardiovascular disease and diabetes (Brancati, Whelton, Kuller, & Klag, 1996; Crimmins, Kim, Alley, Karlamangla, & Seeman, 2007; Kaplan & Keil, 1993).

The stress theory of health and aging has been proposed as one explanation of these differences (Finch & Seeman, 1999). Stress theories of aging suggest that excess stress, due to greater exposure to chronic and acute strains, leads to increased risk for disease and disability. This theory is also linked to the ideas of cumulative disadvantage employed by sociologists (Dannefer, 2003; O'Rand, 1996). Empirical evidence has supported the idea that accumulated lifetime levels of disadvantage experienced by individuals with low SES or individuals undergoing prolonged periods of chronic stress have higher levels of physiological deterioration in later life and adverse health outcomes (Hamil-Luker & O'Rand, 2007; Hayward et al., 2000; O'Rand & Hamil-Luker, 2005; Singer & Ryff, 1999). These theories allow researchers to investigate the underlying reasons and mechanisms as to why health disparities exist within populations and contribute to our overall understanding of the aging process.

Biodemographers also have looked across contemporary populations for clues to how large-scale changes in environment and income are related to differences in health outcomes across countries (Crimmins, Soldo, Kim, & Alley, 2005; Palloni, Pinto-Aguirre, & Pelaez, 2002; Thomas & Strauss, 1997) and over time (Crimmins & Finch, 2006; Fogel & Costa, 1997). Most of these studies are motivated by the fundamental biodemographic question of the importance of the environment and behaviors on an individual's health and survival at later ages. In humans, for instance, nutrition and exposure to infections during gestation and childhood have been related to the development of biologic risk factors (e.g., high blood pressure and diabetes) associated with adverse cardiovascular health in middle to later years of life (Barker, 1992; Elo & Preston, 1992; Finch & Crimmins, 2004; Fogel & Costa, 1997). Such findings have given rise to numerous research questions and ignited exciting debates. This has pushed the initial boundaries of biodemography and shed light on the interplay between innate and acquired biological circumstances, as well as social and environmental conditions.

Introducing Biomarkers Into the Study of Population Health

Because incorporation of the study of biological factors in human populations has been such a large part of the recent expansion of biodemography, we discuss this more fully in this section. As indicated previously, many health outcomes connected to aging have similar risk factors. This is because physiological changes across systems in the body are often interrelated and because decline in one area may be related to declines in other areas. In addition, physiological changes interact so that a set of small changes across a number of systems may be more important to the health and functioning of the organism than a large change in one system. This is the idea behind the concept of allostatic load, which has provided important guidance in the development of many biodemography studies (Crimmins & Seeman, 2004; McEwen, 2004; Seeman, McEwen, Rowe, & Singer, 2001). For instance, stress has been associated with the disruption in regulation of several physiological systems, including the sympathetic nervous system, the immune system, the hypothalamic–pituitary–adrenal axis, inflammatory responses, and the cardiovascular system. Chronically high levels of stress can result from continued exposure to adverse environmental conditions (e.g., occupations that expose individuals to harmful ultraviolet rays) or psychological stressors (e.g., job stress, family stress, financial constraints, or being a caregiver for a family member).

Inclusion of biomarkers for health outcomes in population studies has benefited from the identification of risk factors and health states in large-scale community and population studies, including the Framingham Heart Study and the National Health and Nutrition Examination Survey. It has also been encouraged by changes in technology that have allowed the collection of biomarkers using less invasive methods as well as technological developments in laboratory methods (McDade, Williams, & Snodgrass, 2007). The MacArthur Study of Successful Aging was the first large-scale community-based study to collect an extensive array of biomarkers in a home-based setting. Because of increases in scientific knowledge of aging and improvements in technology for collection, a growing number of recent population studies have included biomarkers along with collection of social, economic, and psychological information (Weinstein, Vaupel, & Wachter, 2008).

The incorporation of biomarkers into studies of biodemography has contributed to our understanding of the potential mechanisms related to differentials in mortality within populations. Hence, biodemographers have used biomarkers to understand gender differences in mortality, as well as differences in health among individuals with different SES. Such studies have found gender and SES differences in a number of cardiovascular, metabolic, and inflammatory biomarkers in addition to markers of immunity and infection.

Using Biomarkers to Understand Differences Within Populations

Females have an average life expectancy of about 80 years, while males live to around 75 years (Hoyert et al., 2006). A large part of this difference in life expectancy is due to mortality after age 60 and to cardiovascular health (Waldron, 1995). In examining biomarkers related to cardiovascular and metabolic function, gender differences have been found. While the relationship varies across age groups, generally males have higher blood pressure (Goldman et al., 2004; Price & Fowkes, 1997), cholesterol (Goldman et al., 2004), triglycerides (Seidell et al., 1991), glycated hemoglobin (Crimmins, Kim, Alley, Karlamangla, & Seeman, 2006), and homocysteine (Brattstrom, Lindgren, Israelsson, Andersson, & Hultberg, 1994; Jacques et al., 1999) compared to females.

Differences in health outcomes among SES groups have also been related to levels of biological risk. Individuals with low SES, often defined as having less education and being at or near poverty, have greater disability (Crimmins, Hayward, & Seeman, 2004; Hayward, Crimmins, Miles, & Yang, 2000) and mortality (Rogot, Sorlie, Johnson, & Schmitt, 1992) compared to individuals with high SES. In fact, the occurrence of diseases and deaths have been estimated to be 5 to 10 years earlier for people with low SES (Crimmins, Hayward, & Seeman, 2004; Hayward, Crimmins, Miles, & Yang, 2000). Additionally, people with low SES have on average more biological risk factors (Seeman, McEwen, Rowe, & Singer, 2001; Seeman et al., 2008), including elevated blood pressure, pulse, total cholesterol, glycated hemoglobin, C-reactive protein (CRP), albumin, waist-to-hip ratio, and low levels of high-density lipoprotein.

In the following sections, we outline some of these biomarkers and others now frequently collected and analyzed in research on the health of older populations. We briefly describe the markers and why they are important in understanding aging, health, and mortality. This list represents a small selection from a significantly larger number of markers that could potentially be described. Our intent is to provide basic information on the most frequently used measures. For a more in-depth discussion of these and other biomarkers of aging, see Crimmins, Vasunilashorn, Kim, and Alley (2008).

Cardiovascular Biomarkers

Heart disease is the most important cause of death within the older adult population and is one of the most important causes of disability (Sahyoun, Lentzner, Hoyert, & Robinson, 2001), hence markers of the cardiovascular system are especially useful in determining health among older adults as well as differences in health among individuals. Systolic blood pressure (SBP) and diastolic blood pressure (DBP), the most commonly measured biomarkers and markers of cardiovascular health, have been strongly associated to cardiovascular disease (Franklin et al., 2001; Izzo, Levy, & Black, 2000). For instance, SBP strongly predicts coronary heart disease (CHD) and life expectancy at later ages (Stamler, Neaton, & Wentworth, 1989), while DBP has been inversely related to CHD risk among individuals aged 60 and over (Franklin et al., 2001). Since males and individuals with low SES tend to have higher levels of SBP and DBP (Lawlor, Ebrahim, & Davey Smith, 2001; Seeman et al., 2008), this may be one link as to why these individuals have higher risk of poor cardiovascular health and mortality.

Other markers of cardiovascular health typically studied in population surveys include pulse pressure and heart rate. Pulse pressure (PP), an indicator of the difference between the SBP and DBP, also predicts risk of CHD in old age as well as middle age (Benetos et al., 1997; Franklin et al., 2001). Heart rate, considered one of the four vital signs, is associated with increased risk of CHD in addition to cardiovascular, noncardiovascular, and all-cause mortality (Gann, Daviglus, Dyer, & Stamler, 1995; Gillum, Makuc, & Feldman, 1991; Seccareccia et al., 2001). High risk levels of heart rate are more common among people at the poverty level compared to individuals with incomes five times the poverty level (Seeman et al., 2008) and represent an increased risk of cardiovascular and noncardiovascular mortality.

Metabolic Biomarkers

Markers of the metabolic system have been associated with cardiovascular outcomes and have frequently been measured to evaluate an individual's risk for heart disease. The most commonly used metabolic markers include two components of total cholesterol: low-density lipoprotein (LDL) and high-density lipoprotein (HDL) cholesterol. High levels of LDL, often referred to as "bad" cholesterol, are correlated with CHD (Colpo, 2005). Generally, elevated LDL cholesterol levels have been found to contribute to the increased risk of mortality and heart disease (Reed, Yano, & Kagan, 1986). In contrast, high levels of HDL are protective for heart disease, while low levels of HDL have been associated with an increased risk of heart disease (Gordon et al., 1989). More individuals living in households with incomes below the poverty level have high risk levels of HDL and total cholesterol compared to people with incomes above the poverty level (Seeman et al., 2008).

High levels of triglycerides, another metabolic biomarker, have also been associated with adverse cardiovascular outcomes, including heart attacks (Gaziano, Hennekens, O'Donnell, Breslow, & Buring, 1997), CHD (Cullen, 2000), and coronary artery disease (Linton, Fazio, & NCEP-ATPIII, 2003).

As an alternative to fasting blood glucose, many researchers measure glycosylated hemoglobin (HbA1c) since it can be collected in a nonfasting sample (Rohlfing et al., 2000). High levels of HbA1c are indicative of prediabetes or controlled diabetes and have been linked to cardiovascular disease and mortality (Khaw et al., 2004), both of which are higher in males than females (Castelli, 1984; Jackson et al., 1997) and among individuals with low SES (Cooper, 2001; Rogot et al., 1992).

High risk levels of anthropometric measures related to adiposity, including body mass index (BMI, the ratio of weight to height squared [kg/m^2]) and waist-to-hip ratio, have been associated with a greater risk of heart disease, diabetes, stroke, and disability (Davison, Ford, Cogswell, & Dietz, 2002; Himes, 2000; Larsson et al., 1984; Must et al., 1999; Ohlson et al., 1985; Welin, Svardsudd, Wilhelmsen, Larsson, & Tibblin, 1987). Although differences in BMI by gender are not universal, in the U.S. women generally are more obese while men are more overweight (Crimmins, Kim, Alley, Karlamangla, & Seeman, 2006). Also, those who are poorer and of lower SES generally have higher levels of most indicators of weight and adiposity (Seeman et al., 2008).

Biomarkers of Inflammation, Immunity, and Infection

Age-related changes in inflammatory markers are complex and include a wide range of potential indicators. CRP, is often used as an indicator of an acute-phase response to infection and systemic level of inflammation. Levels of CRP may be elevated because of the presence of chronic conditions, including diabetes, asthma, rheumatoid arthritis, and heart disease (Amos, Constable, Crockson, Crockson, & McConkey, 1977; Danesh, Collins, Appleby, & Peto, 1998; Pradhan, Manson, Rifai, Buring, & Ridker, 2001; Ridker, Hennekens, Buring, & Rifai, 2000; Rifai & Ridker, 2001; Takemura et al., 2006). CRP has been shown to be predictive of mortality (Harris et al., 1999) as well as declines in physical and cognitive function (Reuben et al., 2002). Additionally, elevated levels of CRP have been related to lower SES (Alley et al., 2006), which is linked to higher cardiovascular disease and mortality (Cooper, 2001; Rogot, Sorlie, Johnson, & Schmitt, 1992).

Interleukin-6 (IL-6), one of a class of immune system regulators (or cytokines) that respond to acute illness or injury, is another more commonly measured inflammatory marker in population surveys. Levels of IL-6 increase with age and are related to a variety of chronic, age-associated conditions, including osteoporosis, arthritis, type 2 diabetes, certain cancers, and Alzheimer's disease, declines in cognition and physical functioning, and mortality (Ferrucci et al., 1999; Harris et al., 1999; Papanicolaou, Wilder, Manolagas, & Chrousos, 1998; Scholz, 1996; Reuben et al., 2002; Weaver et al., 2002). Similar to CRP, there is an inverse relationship between IL-6 and SES levels, indicating that SES is associated with inflammatory risk factors related to cardiovascular outcomes (Loucks et al., 2006).

Fibrinogen, a protein that assists in the blood clotting, has been strongly predictive of both mortality (Fried et al., 1998) and the onset of cardiovascular disease (Kannel, Wolf, Castelli, & D'Agostino, 1987; Tracy et al., 1995). In addition, the relationship between SES and fibrinogen levels has been suggested as another potential mechanism linking low social status and stress to cardiovascular disease (De Boever et al., 1995; Markowe et al., 1985; Wilson et al., 1993).

These biomarkers have contributed to our understanding of health and mortality, and they have underscored the complexity of the relationships of biomarkers to health outcomes across populations. For instance, high heart rate has been linked to increased mortality in older women but not men (Perk et al., 2003); however, high DBP seems to have a greater impact on CHD mortality in males compared to females. Further use of biomarkers will enable researchers to better understand these complex relationships.

Genetic Biomarkers

Genetic markers denote another category of indicators that are recently being included in a number of population studies. Use of genetic markers will allow for further consideration of additional, independent indicators of risk, as well as modifiers of risk for individuals with other behavioral, biological, or genetic characteristics. Ultimately, this will broaden the entire approach to the inclusion of biomarkers in understanding population health. Presently, only a few genetic indicators have been included in population studies, and several of these genetic indicators have not shown clear-cut relationships between health and longevity found in animal models (Christensen, Johnson, & Vaupel, 2006).

The most commonly examined genetic indicator and the marker with the greatest evidence of associations with several health outcomes is apolipoprotein E (APOE). Studies have found higher risk for late-onset Alzheimer's disease among people with the APOE-ε4 genetic allele (Corder et al., 1993; Poirier et al., 1993), as well as increased risk for cardiovascular diseases, such as heart attack, stroke, and coronary artery disease (Leon et al., 2004; Schmitz et al., 2001).

The inclusion of biologic markers and, to a lesser extent, genetic markers of health and aging have substantially contributed to our understanding of biological risk factors associated with several age-associated conditions. As both biologic and genetic markers become increasingly investigated in large-scale population studies in multiple societies, we will have better insight as to why such differences occur across cultures and within populations. These findings will help elucidate the paths toward understanding social, cultural and behavioral links to health and policies toward improving health and decreasing health disparities.

Importance of Biodemography

As stated throughout this chapter, aging of populations and changes in health in humans and across various animal models represents a composite outcome of complex processes replete with interconnections between the biological and social arenas. Since demographers often examine trends and changes in order to forecast future trends in health and survival, this requires knowledge of both fixed and modifiable biological factors. By merging the biological sciences with the social sciences, researchers will be better equipped to determine the causes of current trends, forecast future trends, and explain why the differences in subpopulations and across societies exist.

In the study of aging in humans, for example, it is apparent that some individuals age without becoming frail, while others are greatly disabled at much younger ages. It is also apparent that while some species have a life span of a few days (yeast), others may live to 100 years (humans). Even among humans, some subpopulations tend to live much longer than others. While we are just beginning to understand how genetic, biologic, and environmental circumstances contribute to these disparities, our understanding remains superficial. By including more biology into our research on aging populations, we have increased our potential to address some fundamental questions about the complexities of health and aging within a given society.

Strengths of Biodemography

The biodemographic approach has the potential to affect our understanding of some of the most important questions facing gerontology today, largely because it provides a biopsychosocial approach to understanding populations. As a special subfield, biodemography encompasses several strengths. First is the approach of demographic analyses, which use mathematical models and data from large representative population samples to clarify how processes of change affect population characteristics and individual life-cycles (Preston, 1987). This is a strength in that age-stratified processes can have unexpected consequences—for example, increasing healthy life and deteriorating population health (Crimmins, Hayward, & Saito, 1994).

Second, the versatility of its biodemographic approach in studying various areas related to health and aging is an additional strength. Its most commonly employed application uses this perspective to underscore the mechanisms by which the social and economic environment, behaviors, and medical interventions affect health outcomes. For example, biodemography is already widely used to investigate health disparities by determining ways in which sociodemographic characteristics, such as race and SES, "get under the skin" to affect later-life health (Taylor, Repetti, & Seeman, 1997). More specifically, measures of stress (as indicated by the hormone cortisol) and indicators of accelerated aging (marked by telomere length, which is a region of repetitive DNA at the end of chromosomes that has an inverse relationship with increasing age) are currently being collected in studies of caregiving and have already begun to elucidate the paths by which caregivers are at greater risk of disease and disability (de Vugt et al., 2005; Epel et al., 2004). The biodemographic approach is evident in clarifying how the length of life lived in various states of health, the years of life lost, and the life expectancy of subgroups is affected by socioeconomic status, physiological status, behaviors, and medical interventions (Crimmins, Kim, & Seeman, in press; Crimmins & Saito, 2001; Lievre, Alley, & Crimmins, 2008; Peeters et al., 2003).

Another application of biodemography examines the relationship between health and social outcomes. While this approach has received less attention, it depicts another interesting approach to integrative research studies. For instance, the relationship between the economic distribution of resources and social relationships has laid the foundation for understanding the importance of the postreproductive population (e.g., grandparents and great grandparents) within social and family structures. This has led to studies of both modern and anthropological societies examining inter- and intragenerational transfers from an evolutionary perspective (Kaplan & Robson, 2002).

Although it is a relatively new field of study, the biodemography of aging has quickly found its place in the research realm. From its initial inception, it was clear that an interdisciplinary approach and genuine communication between and within the social and life sciences was necessary (Wachter & Finch, 1997). This led to more concerted efforts toward collaborations across disciplines and marked a significant point in the convergence of the biological and social sciences. This "marriage" between these two disciplines has signified a joining and synthesis of microlevel analyses related to mortality (as examined by biologists) and macrolevel analyses of population-level research (as examined by demographers; Wachter, 1997). Research in biodemography of aging has already greatly contributed to our overall understanding of human health and longevity. The next few years hold great promise for the field, as researchers are beginning to delve further into the biologic, genetic, environmental, and social effects that conjointly contribute to health outcomes across the life span.

References

Adler, N. E., Boyce, T. W., Chesney, M. A., Cohen, S., Folkman, S., & Syme, L. S. (1993). Socioeconomic inequalities in health: No easy solution. *Journal of the American Medical Association, 269,* 3140–3145.

Albert, M. S., Jones, K., Savage, C. R., Berkman, L., Seeman, T., Blazer, B., et al. (1995). Predictors of cognitive change in older persons: MacArthur Studies of Successful Aging. *Psychology and Aging, 10,* 578–589.

Alley, D. E. (2007). Biomarkers of aging. In K. S. Markides (Ed.), *Encyclopedia of health and aging* (pp. 77–80). Thousand Oaks, CA: Sage.

Alley, D. E., Seeman, T. E., Kim, J. K., Karlamangla, A., Hu, P., & Crimmins, E. M. (2006). Socioeconomic status and C-reactive protein levels in the US population: NHANES IV. *Brain, Behavior, and Immunity, 20,* 498–504.

Amos, R. S., Constable, T. J., Crockson, R. A., Crockson, A. P., & McConkey, B. (1977). Rheumatoid arthritis: Relation of serum C-reactive protein and erythrocyte sedimentation rates to radiographic changes. *British Medical Journal, 1,* 195–197.

Austad, S. (1993). FRAR course on laboratory approaches to aging: The comparative perspective and choice of animal models in aging research. *Aging, 5,* 259–267.

Barker, D. J. (1992). The effect of nutrition of the fetus and neonate on cardiovascular disease in adult life. *Proceedings of the Nutrition Society, 51,* 135–144.

Benetos, A., Safar, M., Rudnichi, A., Smulyan, H., Richard, J. L., Ducimetiére, P., et al. (1997). Pulse pressure: A predictor of long-term cardiovascular mortality in a French male population. *Hypertension, 30,* 1410–1415.

Brancati, F. L., Whelton, P. K., Kuller, L. H., & Klag, M. J. (1996). Diabetes mellitus, race, and socioeconomic status: A population-based study. *Annals of Epidemiology, 6,* 67–73.

Brattstrom, L., Lindgren, A., Israelsson, B., Andersson, A., & Hultberg, B. (1994). Homocysteine and cysteine: Determinants of plasma levels in middle-aged and elderly subjects. *Journal of Internal Medicine, 6,* 633–641.

Buffon, G. L. L. (1812). *Natural history, general and particular* (W. Smellie, Trans.). London: T. Cadell and W. Davis. (Original work published 1747)

Carey, J. R., & Vaupel, J. W. (2007). Biodemography. In G. Ritzer (Ed.), *Encyclopedia of sociology* (pp. 283–287). Boston: Blackwell.

Carnes, B. A., & Olshansky, S. J. (1993). Evolutionary perspectives on human senescence. *Population and Development Review, 19,* 793–806.

Christensen, K., Johnson, T. E., & Vaupel, J. W. (2006). The quest for genetic determinants of human longevity: Challenges and insights. *Nature Reviews Genetics, 7,* 436–448.

Coale, A., & Demeny, P. (1983). *Regional model life tables and stable populations.* New York: Academic Press.

Cohen, H. J. (2000). In search of the underlying mechanisms of frailty. *Journal of Gerontology: Biological Sciences, 55,* 706–708.

Colpo, A. (2005). LDL cholesterol: "Bad" cholesterol, or bad science? *Journal of American Physicians & Surgeons, 10,* 83–89.

Corder, E. H., Saunders, A. M., Strittmatter, W. J., Schmechel, D. E., Gaskell, P. C., Small, G. W., et al. (1993). Gene dose of apolipoprotein E type 4 allele and the risk of Alzheimer's disease in late onset families. *Science, 261,* 921–923.

Crimmins, E. (1993). Demography: The past 30 years, the present, and the future. *Demography, 30,* 579–591.

Crimmins, E. M., & Finch, C. E. (2006). Infection, inflammation, height, and longevity. *Proceedings of the National Academy of Sciences of the United States of America, 103,* 498–503.

Crimmins, E., Hayward, M. D., & Saito, Y. (1994). Changing mortality and morbidity rates and the health status and life expectancy of the older U.S. population. *Demography, 31,* 159–175.

Crimmins, E. M., Hayward, M. D., & Seeman, T. (2004). Race/ethnicity, socioeconomic status, and health. In N. Anderson, R. Bulatao, & B. Cohen (Eds.), *Critical perspectives on race and ethnic differences in health in later life* (pp. 310–352). Washington, DC: National Academies Press.

Crimmins, E., Kim, J. K., Alley, D., Karlamangla, A., & Seeman, T. (2006). Recent changes in cardiovascular risk factors among women and men. *Journal of Women's Health, 15,* 734–746.

Crimmins, E. M, Kim, J. K., Alley, D. A., Karlamangla, A., & Seeman, T. (2007). Hispanic paradox in biological risk profiles. *American Journal of Public Health, 97,* 1305–1310.

Crimmins, E. M., Kim, J. K., & Seeman, T. E. (in press). Poverty and biological risk: The earlier "aging" of the poor. *Journal of Gerontology: Biological Sciences.* Forthcoming.

Crimmins, E., & Saito, Y. (2001). Trends in disability free life expectancy in the United States, 1970–1990: Gender, racial, and educational differences. *Social Science and Medicine, 52,* 1629–1641.

Crimmins, E. M., Saito, Y., & Ingegneri, D. (1997). Trends in disability-free life expectancy in the U.S.: 1970–1990. *Population and Development Review, 23,* 555–572.

Crimmins, E. M., & Seeman, T. E. (2004). Integrating biology into the study of health disparities. *Population & Development Review, 30,* 89–107.

Crimmins, E. M., Soldo, B. J., Kim, J. K., & Alley, D. E. (2005). Using anthropometric indicators for Mexicans in the United States and Mexico to understand the selection of migrants and the "Hispanic paradox." *Social Biology, 52,* 164–177.

Crimmins, E. M., Vasunilashorn, S., Kim, J. K., & Alley, D. E. (2008). Biomarkers related to aging in human populations. *Advances in Clinical Chemistry, 46,* 161–215.

Cristofalo, V. J., Tresini, M., Francis, M. K., & Volker, C. (1999). Biological theories of senescence. In V. L. Bengtson & K. W. Schaie (Eds.), *Handbook of theories of aging* (pp. 98–112). New York: Springer Publishing.

Cullen, P. (2000). Evidence that triglycerides are an independent coronary heart disease risk factor. *American Journal of Cardiology, 86,* 943–949.

Curtsinger, J. W., & Khazaeli, A. (1997). A reconsideration of stress experiments and population heterogeneity. *Experimental Gerontology, 32,* 727–729.

Danesh, J., Collins, R., Appleby, P., & Peto, R. (1998). Association of fibrinogen, C-reactive protein, albumin, or leukocyte count with coronary heart disease: Meta-analyses of prospective studies. *Journal of the American Medical Association, 279,* 1477–1482.

Dannefer, D. (2003). Cumulative advantage/disadvantage and the life course: Cross-fertilizing age and social science theory. *Journal of Gerontology: Social Sciences, 58,* 327–337.

Davison, K. K., Ford, E. S., Cogswell, M. E., & Dietz, W. H. (2002). Percentage of body fat and body mass index are associated with mobility limitations in people aged 70 and older from NHANES III. *Journal of the American Geriatric Society, 50,* 1802–1809.

De Boever, E., De Bacquer, D., Braeckman, L., Baele, G., Rosseneu, M., & De Backer, G. (1995). Relation of fibrinogen to lifestyles and to cardiovascular risk factors in a working population. *International Journal of Epidemiology, 24,* 915–921.

de Vugt, M. E., Nicolson, N. A., Aalten, P., Lousberg, R., Jolle, J., & Verhey, F. R. (2005). Behavioral problems in dementia patients and salivary cortisol patterns in caregivers. *Journal of Neuropsychiatry & Clinical Neuroscience, 17,* 201–207.

Elo, I. T., & Preston, S. H. (1992). Effects of early-life conditions on adult mortality: A review. *Population Index, 58,* 186–212.

Epel, E. S., Blackburn, E. H., Lin, J., Dhabhar, F. S., Adler, N. E., Morrow, J. D., et al. (2004). Accelerated telomere shortening in response to life stress. *Proceedings of the National Academy of Sciences of the United States of America, 101,* 17312–17315.

Ferrucci, L., Harris, T. B., Guralnik, J. M., Tracy, R. P., Corti, M. C., Cohen, H. J., et al. (1999). Serum IL-6 level and the development of disability in older persons. *Journal of the American Geriatrics Society, 47,* 639–646.

Finch, C. E., (1990). *Longevity, senescence, and the genome.* Chicago: University of Chicago Press.

Finch, C. E., & Austad, S. N. (2001). History and prospects: Symposium on organisms with slow aging. *Experimental Gerontology, 36,* 593–597.

Finch, C. E., & Crimmins, E. M. (2004). Inflammatory exposure and historical changes in human life-spans. *Science, 305,* 1736–1739.

Finch, C. E., & Kirkwood, T. B. L. (2000). *Chance, development, and aging.* Oxford: Oxford University Press.

Finch, C. E., & Pike, M. C. (1996). Maximum life span predictors from the Gompertz mortality model. *Journal of Gerontology: Biological Sciences, 51,* 183–194.

Finch, C. E., & Seeman, T. E. (1999). Stress theories of aging. In V. L. Bengtson & K. W. Schaie (Eds.), *Handbook of the theories of aging* (pp. 81–97). New York: Springer Publishing.

Finch, C. E., Vaupel, J. W., & Kinsella, K. G. (2002). *Cells and surveys: Should biological measures be included in social science research?* Washington, DC: National Academies Press.

Fogel, R. W., & Costa, D. L. (1997). A theory of technophysio evolution, with some implications for forecasting population, health care costs, and pension costs. *Demography, 34,* 49–66.

Franklin, S. S., Larson, M. G., Kahn, S. A., Wong, N. D., Leip, E. P., Kannel, W. B., et al. (2001). Does the relation of blood pressure to coronary heart disease risk change with aging?: The Framingham Heart Study. *Circulation, 103,* 1245–1249.

Fried, L. P., Kronmal, R. A., Newman, A. B., Bild, D. E., Mittlemark, M. B., Polak, J. F., et al. (1998). Risk factors for 5-year mortality in older adults: the Cardiovascular Health Study. *Journal of the American Medical Association, 279,* 585–592.

Fried, L. P., Tangen, C. M., Walston, J., Newman, A. B., Hirsch, C., Gottdiener, J., et al. (2001). Frailty in older adults: Evidence for a phenotype. *Journal of Gerontology: Biological Sciences, 56,* 146–156.

Fries, J. F. (1980). Aging, natural death, and the compression of morbidity. *New England Journal of Medicine, 202,* 130–135.

Gann, P. H., Daviglus, M. L., Dyer, A. R., & Stamler, J. (1995). Heart rate and prostate cancer mortality: Results of a prospective analysis. *Cancer Epidemiology Biomarkers & Prevention, 4,* 611–616.

Gavrilov, L. A., & Gavrilova, N. S. (2003). The guest for a general theory of aging and longevity. *Science of Aging Knowledge Environment, 28,* 1–10.

Gaziano, J. M., Hennekens, C. H., O'Donnell, C. J., Breslow, J. L., & Buring, J. E. (1997). Fasting triglycerides, high-density lipoprotein, and risk of myocardial infarction. *Circulation, 96,* 2520–2525.

Gillum, R. F., Makuc, D. M., & Feldman, J. J. (1991). Pulse rate, coronary heart disease, and death: The NHANES I Epidemiologic Follow-Up Study. *American Heart Journal, 121,* 172–177.

Goldman, N., Weinstein, M., Cornman, J., Singer, B., Seeman, T., & Chang, M. (2004). Sex differentials in biological risk factors for chronic disease: Estimates from population-based surveys. *Journal of Women's Health, 13,* 393–403.

Gompertz, B. (1825). On the nature of the function expressive of the law of human mortality and on a new mode of determining life contingencies. *Philosophical Transactions of the Royal Society of London, 115,* 513–585.

Gordon, D. J., Probstfield, J. L., Garrison, R. J., Neaton, J. D., Castelli, W. P., Knoke, J. D., et al. (1989). High-density lipoprotein cholesterol and cardiovascular disease: Four prospective American studies. *Circulation, 79,* 8–15.

Guarente, L., & Kenyon, C. (2000). Genetic pathways that regulate aging in model organisms. *Nature, 408,* 255–262.

Hamil-Luker, J., & O'Rand, A. M. (2007). Gender differences in the link between childhood socioeconomic conditions and heart attack risk in adulthood. *Demography, 44,* 137–158.

Hamilton, W. D. (1966). The moulding of senescence by natural selection. *Journal of Theoretical Biology, 12,* 12–45.

Harris, T. B., Ferrucci, L., Tracy, R. P., Corti, M. C., Wacholder, S., Ettinger, W. H., et al. (1999). Associations of elevated interleukin-6 and C-reactive protein levels with mortality in the elderly. *American Journal of Medicine, 106,* 506–512.

Hayflick, L., & Moorhead, P. (1961). The serial cultivation of human diploid cell strains. *Experimental Cell Research, 25,* 585–621.

Hayward, M., Crimmins, E. M., Miles, T., & Yang, Y. (2000). The significance of socio-economic status in explaining the race gap in chronic health conditions. *American Sociological Review, 65,* 910–930.

Himes, C. L. (2000). Obesity, disease, and functional limitation in later life. *Demography, 37,* 73–82.

Hoyert, D., Heron, M., Murphys, S., & Kung, H. (2006). *Deaths: Final data for 2003* (No. 54). Hyattsville, MD: National Center for Health Statistics.

Hummer, R. (1996). Black-white differences in health and mortality: A review ad conceptual model. *Sociological Quarterly, 37,* 105–125.

Izzo, J. L., Levy, D., & Black, H. R. (2000). Importance of systolic blood pressure in older Americans. *Hypertension, 35,* 1021–1024.

Jacques, P. F., Rosenberg, I. H., Rogers, G., Selhub, J., Bowman, B. A., Gunter, E. W., et al. (1999). Serum total homocysteine concentrations in adolescent and adult Americans: Results from the third National Health and Nutrition Examination Survey. *American Journal of Clinical Nutrition, 69,* 482–489.

Jones, R. N., & Gallo, J. J. (2002). Education and sex differences in the mini-mental state examination: Effects of differential item functioning. *Journal of Gerontology: Social Sciences, 57,* 548–558.

Kannel, W. B., Wolf, P. A., Castelli, W. P., & D'Agostino, R. B. (1987). Fibrinogen and risk of cardiovascular disease: The Framingham study. *Journal of the American Medical Association, 258,* 1183–1186.

Kaplan, G. A., & Keil, J. E. (1993). Socioeconomic factors and cardiovascular disease: A review of the literature. *Circulation, 88,* 1973–1998.

Kaplan, H. S., & Robson, A. J. (2002). The emergence of humans: The coevolution of intelligence and longevity with intergenerational transfers. *Proceedings of the National Academy of Sciences of the United States of America, 99,* 10221–10226.

Khaw, K. T., Wareham, N., Bingham, S., Luben, R., Welch A., & Day, N. (2004). Association of hemoglobin A1c with cardiovascular disease and mortality in adults: The European prospective investigation into cancer in Norfolk. *Annals of Internal Medicine, 141,* 413–420.

Kirkwood, T. B. L. (1977). Evolution of aging. *Nature, 270,* 301–304.

Kirkwood, T. B. L. (1999). *Time of our lives: The science of human aging.* Oxford: Oxford University Press.

Kirkwood, T. B. L., & Finch, C. E. (2002). Ageing: The old worm turns more slowly. *Nature, 419,* 794–795.

Larsson, B., Svardsudd, K., Welin, L., Wilhelmsen, L., Bjorntorp, P., & Tibblin, G. (1984). Abdominal adipose tissue distribution, obesity, and risk of cardiovascular disease and death: 13 year follow up of participants in the study of men born in 1913. *British Medical Journal, 288,* 1401–1404.

Lawlor, D. A., Ebrahim, S., & Davey Smith, G. (2001). Sex matters: Secular and geographical trends in sex differences in coronary heart disease mortality. *British Medical Journal, 323,* 541–545.

Lee, R. D., & Carter, L. R. (1992). Modeling and forecasting US mortality. *Journal of the American Statistical Association, 87,* 659–675.

Leon, A. S., Togashi, K., Rankinen, T., Després, J. P., Rao, D. C., Skinner, J. S., et al. (2004). Association of apolipoprotein E polymorphism with blood lipids and maximal oxygen uptake in the sedentary state and after exercise training in the HERITAGE family study. *Metabolism, 53,* 108–116.

Lievre, A., Alley, D., & Crimmins, E. (2008). Educational differentials in life expectancy with cognitive impairment among the elderly in the United States. *Journal of Aging and Health, 20,* 456–477.

Linton, M. F., Fazio, S., & National Cholesterol Education Program (NCEP)—the third Adult Treatment Panel (ATPIII). (2003). A practical approach to risk assessment to prevent coronary artery disease and its complications. *American Journal of Cardiology, 92,* 19–26.

Longo, V. D., & Finch, C. E. (2003). Evolutionary medicine: From dwarf model systems to healthy centenarians? *Science, 299,* 1342–1346.

Longo, V. D., & Kennedy, B. K. (2006). Sirtuins in aging and age-related disease. *Cell, 126,* 257–268.

Lotka, A. J. (1939). *Théorie Analytique des Associations Biologiques.* Paris: Hermann.

Loucks, E. B., Sullivan, L. M., Hayes, L. J., D'Agostino, R. B., Sr., Larson, M. G., Vasan, R. S., et al. (2006). Association of educational level with inflammatory markers in the Framingham Offspring Study. *American Journal of Epidemiology, 163,* 622–628.

Mangel, M., & Clark, C. W. (1988). *Dynamic modeling in behavioral ecology.* Princeton, NJ: Princeton University Press.

Markowe, H. L., Marmot, M. G., Shipley, M. J., Bulpitt, C. J., Meade, T. W., Stirling, Y., et al. (1985). Fibrinogen: A possible link between social class and coronary heart disease. *British Medical Journal, 291,* 1312–1314.

McDade, T. W., Williams, S., & Snodgrass, J. J. (2007). What a drop can do: Dried blood spots as a minimally invasive method for integrating biomarkers into population-based research. *Demography, 44,* 899–925.

McEwen, B. S. (2004). Protective and damaging effects of mediators of stress and adaptation: Allostasis and allostatic load. In J. Schulkin (Ed.), *Allostasis, homeostasis and the costs of physiological adaptation* (pp. 65–98). Cambridge: Cambridge University Press.

Medawar, P. B. (1951). *An unsolved problem in biology.* London: Lewis.

Morley, J. E., Perry, H. M., III, & Miller, D. K. (2002). Editorial: Something about frailty. *Journal of Gerontology: Biological Sciences, 57,* 698–704.

Mosley, W. H., & Chen, L. C. (1984). An analytical framework for the study of child survival in developing countries. *Population Development Review, 10,* 25–45.

Must, A., Spadano, J., Coakley, E. H., Field, A. E, Colditz, G., & Dietz, W. H. (1999). The disease burden associated with overweight and obesity. *Journal of the American Medical Association, 282,* 1523–1529.

Ohlson, L. O., Larsson, B., Svärdsudd, K., Welin, L., Eriksson, H., Wilhelmsen, L., et al. (1985). The influence of body fat distribution on the incidence of diabetes mellitus. 13.5 years of follow-up of the participants in the study of men born in 1913. *Diabetes, 34,* 1055–1058.

Olshansky, S. J. (1998). On the biodemography of aging: A review essay. *Population & Development Review, 24,* 381–393.

Olshansky, S. J., & Carnes, B. A. (1994). Demographic perspectives on human senescence. *Population & Development Review, 20,* 57–80.

O'Rand, A. M. (1996). The precious and the precocious: Understanding cumulative disadvantage and cumulative advantage over the life course. *The Gerontologist, 36,* 230–238.

O'Rand, A. M., & Hamil-Luker, J. (2005). Processes of cumulative adversity linking childhood disadvantage to increased risk of heart attack. *Journal of Gerontology: Social Sciences, 60,* 117–124.

Orzack, S., & Tuljapurkar, S. (1989). Population dynamics in variable environments. VII. Demography and evolution of iteropartiy. *American Naturalist, 133,* 901–923.

Palloni, A., Pinto-Aguirre, G., & Pelaez, M. (2002). Demographic and health conditions of ageing in Latin America and the Caribbean. *International Journal of Epidemiology, 31,* 762–771.

Papanicolaou, D. A., Wilder, R. L., Manolagas, S. C., & Chrousos, G. P. (1998). The pathophysiologic roles of interleukin-6 in human disease. *Annals of Internal Medicine, 128,* 127–137.

Peeters, A., Barendregt, J. J., Willekens, F., Mackenback, J. P., Mamun, A. A. L., & Bonneux, L. (2003). Obesity in adulthood and its consequences for life expectancy: A life-table analysis. *Annals of Internal Medicine, 138,* 24–32.

Perk, G., Stessman, J., Ginsberg, G., & Bursztyn, M. (2003). Sex differences in the effect of heart rate on mortality in the elderly. *Journal of the American Geriatric Society, 51,* 1260–1264.

Poirier, J., Davignon, J., Bouthillier, D., Kogan, S., Bertrand, P., & Gauthier, S. (1993). Apolipoprotein E polymorphism and Alzheimer's disease. *Lancet, 342,* 697–699.

Pradhan, A. D., Manson, J. E., Rifai, N., Buring, J. E., & Ridker, P. M. (2001). C-reactive protein, interleukin 6, and risk of developing type 2 diabetes mellitus. *Journal of the American Medical Association, 286,* 327–334.

Preston, S. H. (1987). Relations among standard epidemiologic measures in a population. *American Journal of Epidemiology, 126,* 336–345.

Preston, S., & Taubman, P. (1994). Socioeconomic differences in adult mortality and health status. In L. Martin & S. Preston (Eds.), *Demography of aging* (pp. 279–318). Washington, DC: National Academies Press.

Price, J., & Fowkes, F. (1997). Risk factors and the sex differential in coronary artery disease. *Epidemiology, 8,* 584–591.

Reed, D., Yano, K., & Kagan, A. (1986). Lipids and lipoproteins as predictors of coronary heart disease, stroke, and cancer in the Honolulu Heart Program. *American Journal of Medicine, 80,* 871–878.

Reuben, D. B., Cheh, A. I., Harris, T. B., Ferrucci, L., Rowe, J. W., Tracy, R. P., et al. (2002). Peripheral blood markers of inflammation predict mortality and functional decline in high-functioning community-dwelling older persons. *Journal of the American Geriatrics Society, 50,* 638–644.

Reznick, D. N., Shaw, F. H., Rodd, F. H., & Shaw, R. G. (1997). Evaluation of the rate of evolution in natural populations of guppies (*Poecilia reticulata*). *Science, 275,* 1934–1937.

Ricklefs, R. E., & Finch, C. E. (1995). *Aging: A natural history.* New York: Scientific American Library.

Ridker, P. M., Henne Kens, C. H., Buring, J. E., & Rifai, N. (2000). Creactive protein and other markers of inflammation in the prediction of cardiovascular disease in women. *New England Journal of Medicine, 342,* 836–843.

Rifai, N., & Ridker, P. M. (2001). High-sensitivity C-reactive protein: A novel and promising marker of coronary heart disease. *Clinical Chemistry, 47,* 403–411.

Robine, J. M., & Michel, J. P. (2004). Looking forward to a general theory on population aging. *Journal of Gerontology: Biological Sciences, 59,* 590–597.

Rogers, R., Hummer, R., & Nam, C. (2000). *Living and dying in the USA: Behavioral, health, and social differentials of adult mortality.* San Diego: Academic Press.

Rohlfing, C. L., Little, R. R., Wiedmeyer, H. M., England, J. D., Madsen, R., Harris, M. I., et al. (2000). Use of GHb (HbA1c) in screening for undiagnosed diabetes in the U.S. population. *Diabetes Care, 23,* 187–191.

Sahyoun, N. R., Lentzner, H., Hoyert, D., & Robinson, K. N. (2001). *Trends in causes of death among the elderly. Aging trends* (No. 1). Hyattsville, MD: National Center for Health Statistics.

Schmitz, K. H., Schreiner, P. J., Jacobs, D. R., Leon, A. S., Liu, K., Howard, B., et al. (2001). Independent and interactive effects of apolipoprotein E phenotype and cardiorespiratory fitness on plasma lipids. *Annals of Epidemiology, 11,* 94–103.

Scholz, W. (1996). Interleukin 6 in diseases: Cause or cure? *Immunopharmacology, 31,* 131–150.

Seccareccia, F., Pañoso, F., Dima, F., Minoprio, A., Menditto, A., Noce, C., et al. (2001). Heart rate as a predictor of mortality: The MATISS project. *American Journal of Public Health, 91,* 1258–1263.

Seeman, T. E., Huang, M. H., Bretsky, P., Crimmins, E., Launer, L., & Guralnik, J. M. (2005). Education and APOE-ε4 in longitudinal cognitive decline: MacArthur Studies of Successful Aging. *Journal of Gerontology: Social Sciences, 60,* 74–83.

Seeman, T. E., McEwen, B. S., Rowe, J. W., & Singer, B. H. (2001). Allostasis, homeostasis, and the cost of physiological adaptation. In J. Schulkin (Ed.), *Allostatic load: Operationalizing allostatic load* (pp. 113–149). Cambridge: Cambridge University Press.

Seeman, T. E., Merkin, S. S., Crimmins, E., Koretz, B., Charette, S., & Karlamangla, A. (2008). Education, income, and ethnic differences in cumulative biological risk profiles in a national sample of US adults: NHANES III (1988-1994). *Social Science & Medicine, 66,* 72–87.

Seidell, J. C., Cigolini, M., Charzewska, J., Ellsinger, B. M., Bjorntorp, P., Hautvast, J. G., et al. (1991). Fat distribution and gender differences in serum lipids in men and women from four European communities. *Atherosclerosis, 87,* 203–210.

Singer, B., & Ryff, C. D. (1999). Hierarchies of life histories and associated health risks. *Annals of the New York Academy of Sciences, 896,* 96–115.

Smith, J. (1999). Healthy bodies and thick wallets: The dual relation between health and economic status. *Journal of Economic Perspectives, 13,* 145–166.

Stamler, J., Neaton, J. D., & Wentworth, D. N. (1989). Blood pressure (systolic and diastolic) and risk of fatal coronary heart disease. *Hypertension, 13,* 2–12.

Takemura, M., Matsumoto, H., Niimi, A., Ueda, T., Matsuoka, H., Yamaguchi, M., et al. (2006). High sensitivity C-reactive protein in asthma. *European Respiratory Journal, 27,* 908–912.

Tatar, M., Bartke, A., & Antebi, A. (2003). The endocrine regulation of aging by insulin like signals. *Science, 299,* 1346–1351.

Tatar, M., Carey, J. R., & Vaupel, J. W. (1993). Long-term cost of reproduction with and without accelerated senescence in *Callosobruchus maculatus:* Analysis of age-specific mortality. *Evolution, 47,* 1302–1312.

Tatar, M., Khazaeli, A. A., & Curtsinger, J. W. (1997). Chaperoning extended life. *Nature, 390,* 30.

Taylor, S. E., Repetti, R. L., & Seeman, T. (1997). Health psychology: What is an unhealthy environment and how does it get under the skin? *Annual Review of Psychology, 48,* 411–447.

Thomas, D., & Strauss, J. (1997). Health and wages: Evidence on men and women in urban Brazil. *Journal of Economics, 77,* 159–185.

Tracy, R. P., Bovill, E. G., Yanez, D., Psaty, B. M., Fried, L. P., Heiss, G., et al. (1995). Fibrinogen and factor VIII, but not factor VII, are associated with measures of subclinical cardiovascular disease in the elderly: Results from the Cardiovascular Health Study. *Arteriosclerosis, Thrombosis, and Vascular Biology, 15,* 1269–1279.

Vaupel, J. W. (1997). Trajectories of mortality in advanced ages. In K. W. Wachter & C. E. Finch (Eds.), *Between Zeus and the salmon: The biodemography of longevity* (pp. 17–37). Washington, DC: National Academies Press.

Vaupel, J. W. (2004). The biodemography of aging. *Population and Development Review, 30,* 48–62.

Vaupel, J. W., Carey, J. R., Christensen, K., Johnson, T. E., Yashin, A. I., Holm, N. V., et al. (1998). Biodemographic trajectories of longevity. *Science, 280,* 855–860.

Vaupel, J. W., Yashin, A. I., & Manton, K. G. (1987). Debilitation's aftermath: Stochastic process models of mortality. *Mathematical Population Studies, 1,* 21–48.

Vebrugge, L., & Jette, A.M. (1994). The disablement process. *Social Science Medicine, 38,* 1–14.

Wachter, K. W. (1997). Between Zeus and the salmon: Introduction. In K. W. Wachter & C. E. Finch (Eds.), *Between Zeus and the salmon: The biodemography of longevity* (pp. 1–16). Washington, DC: National Academies Press.

Wachter, K. W., & Finch, C. E. (1997). *Between Zeus and the salmon: The biodemography of longevity.* Washington, DC: National Academies Press.

Waldron, I. (1995). Contribution of biological and behavioral factors to changing sex differences in ischemic heart disease mortality. In A. D. Lopez, G. Casselli, & T. Valkonen (Eds.), *Adult mortality in developed countries: from description to explanation* (pp. 161–178). Oxford, England: Clarendon Press.

Weaver, J. D., Huang, M. H., Albert, M., Harris, T., Rowe, J. W., & Seeman, T. E. (2002). Interleukin-6 and risk of cognitive decline: MacArthur Studies of Successful Aging. *Neurology, 59,* 371–378.

Weinstein, M., Vaupel, J. W., & Wachter, K. W. (2008). *Biosocial surveys.* Washington, DC: National Academies Press.

Welin, L., Svardsudd, K., Wilhelmsen, L., Larsson, B., & Tibblin, G. (1987). Analysis of risk factors for stroke in a cohort of men born in 1913. *New England Journal of Medicine, 317,* 521–526.

Williams, D. R. (1990). Socioeconomic differentials in health: A review and redirection. *Social Psychology Quarterly, 53,* 81–99.

Williams, G. C. (1957). Pleiotrophy, natural selection and the evolution of senescence. *Evolution, 11,* 398–411.

Wilson, D. L. (1994). The analysis of survival (mortality) data: Fitting Gompertz, Weibull, and logistic functions. *Mechanisms of Ageing and Development, 74,* 15–33.

Wilson, T. W., Kaplan, G. A., Kauhanen, J., Cohen, R. D., Wu, M., Salonen, R., et al. (1993). Association between plasma fibrinogen concentration and five socioeconomic indices in the Kuopio Ischemic Heart Disease Risk Factor Study. *American Journal of Epidemiology, 137,* 292–300.

Windsor, C. P. (1932). The Gompertz Curve as a growth curve. *Proceedings of the National Academy of Sciences of the United States of America, 18,* 1–8.

Yashin, A. I., & Iachine, I. A. (1995). Genetic analysis of durations: Correlated frailty model applied to survival of Danish twins. *Genetic Epidemiology, 12,* 529–538.

Problematic Foundations: Theorizing Time, Age, and Aging

5

Jan Baars

It may be one of the main gerontological paradoxes that all human beings *age*, but at a certain moment in their lives they are labeled as "aged" or "older" (older than whom?) and their living beyond that point as "aging." The expressions "aged" and "aging" are without any further explanation used as references to an abnormal group, although these expressions actually indicate a universal and continuous process of living in time. Persons are transformed into "aging," "aged," or "older" bodies at a particular chronological age without any evidence that important changes are taking place at that age apart from this sudden cultural relocation. Seen from the chronological framework of life expectancies, this may take place very early, at 40 or 50 years of age.

Concepts of time have something to do with understanding *changes*, and gerontology is supposed to answer the question of how specific changes can be explained as part or as consequences of the processes of aging. Arriving at such explanations and giving answers will be an arduous task, as many different processes and contexts play their roles. But this does not justify overly simplified ways of studying aging.

Gerontological studies usually begin by defining their populations in terms of chronological age and present their results in diagrams where the interrelation of the two axes is supposed to show changes in certain characteristics as a function of "age." Such visualizations presuppose that "aging" processes can be clearly and unequivocally related to chronological age, although what are presented are mostly unexplained data and merely possible connections.

The chronological identification of "aged" research populations presupposes an organization of the life course in which chronological time has become an important instrumental perspective (Kohli, 1986; Mayer & Müller, 1986). Concepts such as "age-groups," "age norms," and "age grading" presuppose chronological age, which has become the typical instrument to regulate many transitions or entitlements. Concepts used in the discussions of "aging" societies, such as "age structure," "birth cohorts," "dependency ratio," "age–cost profile," and "age-associated diseases" and all kinds of tables in which ages are associated with particular characteristics, pretending to give a quick informative overview, have become so general that their *gerontological* meaning is too seldomly questioned.

However, aging cannot be simply conceptualized as "attaining a higher chronological age." This does not imply that chronological time is not an important analytical tool for many purposes or that chronological age should be banned. For gerontological purposes, however, the significance of chronological age is limited, and its use often serves to *evade* the question of what aging actually is. That aging is poorly indicated by higher chronological ages may often be admitted, but this does not appear to lead to much change in research practices, resulting in an accumulation of data but not in *explanatory* knowledge (Bengtson, Putney, & Johnson, 2005).

This confronts us not only with theoretical questions but also with many practical issues, as studies about "aging" and "the aged" are used to inform or guide manifold practical arrangements for "the aged." Just like societies organize ways to educate children to prepare them for active adult lives, they tend to organize aging processes, especially when a relatively large part of the population counts as "aged." Gerontology cannot be held responsible for this organization of the life course, but it does have some responsibility where this organization is informed by scientific overviews that are just based on chronological age.

Mistaken Associations: Time Working as a Regular Cause

Generalizations about people with a certain calendar age actually presuppose a *causal* concept of time: because time has worked for a certain duration in aging people, certain inevitable effects should be reckoned with. Moreover, the effects are assumed to develop steadily and universally according to the rhythm of the clock. However, such a causal concept of time can never generate knowledge that might explain something of the *differences* that exist between human beings of the same age or allow us to understand that aging is a generalizing concept that is actually composed of many specific processes. While it is true that all causal relations are *also* temporal relations, or relations working "in time," it would be wrong to identify causality with time or to reduce the process of aging to the causal effects of time.

However, the grand ambition of gerontology still seems to be to establish how this chronological or calendar age of persons determines the characteristics of aging persons or even of all humans. This would eventually reduce gerontology to a straightforward set of simple formulas in which scientific precision and practical use would be united. In the early days of gerontology, this option was stated with much self-assurance: "Chronological age is one of the most useful single items of information about an individual if not the *most* useful. From this knowledge alone an amazingly large number of general statements or predictions can be made about his anatomy, physiology, psychology and social behavior" (Birren, 1959, p. 8). Its author has later dealt with time extensively and has expressed serious reservations about them: "By itself, the collection of large amounts of data showing relationships with chronological age does not help, because chronological age is not the cause of anything. Chronological age is only an index, and unrelated sets of data show correlations with chronological age that have no intrinsic or causal relationship with each other" (Birren, 1999, p. 460). Nevertheless, explicit analysis of concepts of time that are inevitably used in the study of aging has been scarce, although there have been some notable exceptions (cf. Baars & Visser, 2007). Interestingly, the sixth edition of the *Handbook of Aging and the Social Sciences* (Binstock & George, 2006) opens with a section titled "Aging and Time." However, in the title of the second chapter of that volume, "Modeling the Effects of Time" (Alwin, Hofer, & McCammon, 2006), we can see how causality and time are still unjustifiably connected and distort the analysis of aging and time.

Aging, Time, and Constitutive Contexts

We can begin to address the problems of interdisciplinary theorizing aging and time at different levels: constructing interdisciplinary paradigms, organizing interdisciplinary cooperation, and designing models for research or analysis. Another approach would be an anthropological reflection of the human or, rather, the *interhuman condition*. According to such a reflection, we could broadly distinguish three domains or aspects of human life that, however, present themselves in changing configurations of the gerontological spectrum.

To begin, our existence as *bodily* beings connects us with a natural environment that is not only very different in different parts of the world but also changing because of human interventions. This implies that our existence cannot be seen as purely natural; it must also be socially and historically situated. This introduces the second aspect, *social* existence, which means that we not only are born from our parents but also have been nourished, have learned to speak and understand a language, and numerous "things" that we may take for granted and others that we do not. This social context is also changing constantly and has led in late modern societies to extremely differentiated patterns. Finally, we are individual *persons* who can be distinguished from other humans—living singular lives while being dependent on and contributing to the environmental contexts.

In this fundamental sense, there is no human being who is not, at the same time, bodily, social, and a singular person; consequently, these aspects of human life, with all their complexity and changing contexts, will be intertwined from the beginning until the end. If these simple assumptions are correct, we can begin to understand why studying aging processes might be a very complicated endeavor. We cannot study processes of aging as we would study other processes because we cannot isolate "aging" in an experimental group and compare the results with a control group that does not age. Moreover, all aging takes place in specific contexts that co-constitute its outcomes, without being able to include them fully into our research (Baars, 1991). Human aging cannot be studied in a *pure* form: even a scientifically controlled life in a laboratory would be a life in a specific context that would co-constitute the processes that would take place. In this way, bodily functioning presents a context for the organization of care, nourishment and lifestyle present a context for research on aging cells, the organization of the labor market presents a context for research on cognitive aging, and so on. And all these interrelated processes and contexts do not remain the same but keep on changing. Of course, it remains possible to measure the *duration* of all processes in chronological time, but this does not give us much understanding.

Aging means living in a changing bodily–social–personal world. This fundamental human condition haunts even the most sophisticated research strategies (cf. Baars, 2007a; Schaie, 2007). The notorious age–period–cohort problem confronts us with the question of what we have actually established when we have found, for instance, that a high percentage of a group of 70-year-olds suffers from obesity. Is this because of their age? Is it part of their specific "cohort identity"? Is it because they lived for a certain period of years in a culture of fast junk food? Is it "a little bit of all that"?

Intrinsic Time and Intrinsic Malleability

There have been some attempts to emancipate the study of aging from this "external" chronological time and develop an "intrinsic" time perspective for aging processes. Departing from physics as the basic discipline for such an integrative perspective, the Second Law of Thermodynamics has been drawn on to develop a general theory of aging processes. Roughly, this law states in its classical form that systems in an equilibrium state can be characterized by a quantity called "entropy," which cannot decrease during the transitions of such systems. Its gerontological application has, however, been taken from later varieties of thermodynamics dealing with open, or "dissipative," systems that are far from equilibrium, although they still aim at clarifying aging (in a biological, social, and psychological sense) as an accumulation of entropy (Prigogine, 1955; Schroots & Birren, 1988; Yates, 2007a, 2007b). The ensuing problems (Uffink, 2007) demonstrate the antagonistic nature of two basic concepts: "openness" and "intrinsicalness." As soon as a certain system or organism is in any way open to its environment, its processes are no longer autonomous or intrinsic, as the environment will influence and co-constitute them. Another antagonism reigns between "intrinsicalness" and "generality": when we find an intrinsic quantity that can be calibrated as the "age" of some finite entity that changes over time, this intrinsic age can hardly form the basis for a general scale with which we could measure the "intrinsic age" of other systems. In other words, there may be as many "intrinsic" ages as there are (sub)systems (Uffink, 2007).

Although physical laws are certainly relevant to understanding the natural contexts in which we live, it remains unclear in what way they could be relevant for human aging. Therefore, at gerontological conferences, we encounter few physicists. Whereas fundamental physical theories appear to be time symmetric and, consequently, the reversibility, or "anisotropy," of time remains an important subject of theoretical debate, biology has more affinity with the irreversible processes we associate with aging: growth, decay, and death. The antagonism between "intrinsicalness," "openness," and "generality" remains, however, hard to reconcile when we go from physics to biology.

An intrinsic measure of aging, at least in a biological perspective, would require establishing clear indicators of "normal" functioning. Differently marked *ages* would ideally have to be synthesized in a continuum, as subsequent *phases* that would demonstrate a structured development away from a state of adult "health" or "normality." It is doubtful whether all biological processes can be adequately seen as *continuous* functional deterioration; some may just suddenly collapse. If we define aging in terms of biological reliability theory (Gravilov & Gravilova, 2006) as a phenomenon of increasing risk of failure with the passage of time, the question returns in what way the statistical notion of increasing risk can lead to an understanding of aging processes. Even if we would have reliable biomarkers of *age,* such as the aspartate racemization in the teeth that is used in forensics, this would not allow us to explain human *aging* in a broader sense.

From a biological perspective, human aging appears to imply many distinct but interrelated processes that are relatively independent but that also interact with other processes in the same body (Kirkwood et al., 2006). Arriving at a more general biological understanding of aging is complicated because the many possibly relevant processes of aging (genes, cells, mitochondria, organs, and so on) not only may have their own specific dynamical properties but also usually *include* an openness to the environments inside and outside the human body, possibly including ecological or social contexts and personal lifestyles. Tensions between intrinsicalness, specific contexts, and generality are also manifest in the experiments with fruit flies, nematodes, mice, rats, birds, and monkeys, as their aging processes are influenced in laboratory contexts to investigate whether their specific, intrinsic aging processes can be generalized to include human aging (cf. Masoro & Austed, 2006).

This illustrates the *intrinsic malleability* of aging processes (Kirkwood, 2005; Westendorp & Kirkwood, 2007), which is also demonstrated in the large differences in life expectancy that we can observe when we compare several historical and contemporary countries or regions with each other. We know from demographic research on mortality rates and life expectancy what impressive changes have taken place in the rich countries during the past 150 years, changes that cannot be explained by a major evolutionary shift or mutation in the bodily substrate of human life. Seen from an evolutionary perspective, our bodies have not changed since the ancient Greeks, let alone since the 19th century. Projections of life expectancy and mortality rates offer, however, no explanation of aging processes. Although they have their own right and relevance, they also play an underreflected role in the institutionalized overemphasis on chronological age.

Projections about life expectancy should also not be used implicitly as pseudoscientific estimates of the quality of human lives. The measurement of chronological ages cannot replace thinking about the classical question of what a *good* life might be, which includes the pressing contemporary question of how we can *age well.* For this, we need other concepts of time and temporal living, like the ones I will turn to at the end of this chapter. But first, I will complete my short overview of the many ways in which aging is one-sidedly approached from the perspective of chronological time.

The Chronologization of Aging and the Life Course

According to Kohli (1986), a historical process of "chronologization" would have resulted in a "chronologically standardized 'normative life course'" (p. 272). Although this proposition has encountered some historical criticism (cf. Grillis, 1987), it has been fruitful in many debates about the life course (Levy, Ghisletta, Le Goff, Spimi, & Widmer, 2005; Settersten, 1999, 2001; Vickerstaff, 1995). In this context, it may be helpful to make some distinctions.

First, we would have to distinguish a tendency toward a chronologization of *aging* in gerontological research. This centers around the complex question addressed previously: how can aging be approached from the perspective of chronological age, and what are the possibilities and, especially, the limitations and consequences of this approach?

Second, I would propose to distinguish the chronologization of the life course from its possible *standardization.* This last aspect of Kohli's proposal has aroused much debate, as standardization does not harmonize well with processes of individualization (cf. Uhlenberg & Mueller, 2004) or the many effects of international migration (Vincent, 1995, 2006). I propose that "chronologization of the life course" can also mean that, to the degree that persons participate in institutions and organizations, the *duration* of these participations will be not only registered bureaucratically but also organized, such as being limited to certain periods. We can also think of the duration of responsibilities for children or the duration of a mortgage. In other words, life courses may be very different and, thus, far from standardized, but they could still be structured chronologically. The chronological durations of education or employment not only may structure the way they remember, evaluate, or plan their lives but also can have many consequences in later life, such as in terms of pensions. This interpretation of the chronologization of the life course can easily be connected to research of *event* time (Schaie, 2007).

Third, although careers tend to become less standardized, the idea of a "late modern" or "postmodern" destandardization of the life course appears to be more adequate for *personal* relationships, where traditional family patterns have become much less dominant in a few decades, or for the changing lifestyles of well-to-do (early) retired elderly (Gilleard & Higgs, 2000, 2005) than for careers in *education* or *employment* (cf. Henretta, 2003). The effects of these careers can remain very important during later life, as they are connected with the distribution of (pension) income and related life chances (cf. Dannefer, 2003).

As institutions and organizations in late modern societies tend to use chronological time to control and coordinate their actions and processes, aging persons will also be confronted with the different "chronological regimes" (Baars, 2007a) that combine chronological age and duration of participations in areas such as employment, social services, and care (Leisering & Leibfried, 1999).

Chronological Regimes

All adults have a chronological age that may not be worth mentioning apart from festive occasions, yet it becomes suddenly a distinctive characteristic. This cultural relocation from "normal" adulthood into the category of the "aged" or "older" may take place at the age of 40 years, when the stigma of the "older worker" begins to hit especially those who have become unemployed (Hardy, 2006). In many Western countries, persons who have lived for 50 years are invited to join organizations such as the American Association of Retired Persons that will support their, apparently, suddenly weakened existence with age-specific benefits that may partly compensate for the negative effects of the age segregation these organizations paradoxically emphasize. The media confront us with scientifically based reports about the things these seniors are doing, what they prefer and desire, and what they still are or not capable of, although this category of people may represent in some countries a third or more of the adult population.

It does not take more than a few moments to realize the absurdity of this situation, which could be interpreted as typical of a culture that is so obsessed with youth that a distinction between "normal" and "older" adults is made as soon as possible, followed by indifference regarding the many possible differences between those who deviate from "normality." This awkward status of being "aged" may remain with them for several decades, much longer than their "normal" adulthood, although they are likely to change and to "fan out," becoming even more different from other members of their birth cohorts because they tend to follow their specific interests without being tied down by the institutional regularities of education, work, or raising children.

This paradoxical *acceleration of chronologically ascribed aging* in the labor markets of most Western countries stands in strong contrast with the risen and still rising life expectancy (Oeppen & Vaupel, 2002), which can be interpreted as a *slowing down* of the aging processes. Here, the inner contradictions surrounding chronological age illustrate that it serves as a pseudoexact labeling device that has been programmed by cultural trends that are easily obfuscated by it. This paradoxical development may offer attractive perspectives of many "golden years" to persons who can afford them but also enforces age segregation and even excludes many aging people from important possibilities to gain a decent income (Baars, 2007b; Walker & Maltby, 1997). Women who want to return to the labor market after having raised their children are particularly disadvantaged, as they are right from the start labeled "older workers" (Ginn, Street, & Arber, 2001). Finally, this acceleration of ascribed aging has increased the pressure on the lives of "normal adults" (25 to 45 years of age) to combine family life with a short and intense career during which the income of a long life must be gathered. When such long-term overburdening eventually leads to health problems, these are too often "explained" by referring to the *ages* of the persons concerned, offering another superficial argument to legitimate an early exit from the labor market.

In countries where retirement is still mandatory, such as the European Union, the labor market position of older workers fluctuates with the general economic situation, but investment in updating or retraining their capacities tends to slow down or stop as soon as they have reached the status of an "older worker" (Baars, 2006). But even in the United States, where mandatory retirement does not exist, older workers have the lowest rates of reemployment, which will typically be in part-time positions or jobs with low skill and training requirements, resulting in large wage losses (Chan & Stevens, 1999; Hirsch, MacPherson, & Hardy, 2000). Melissa Hardy (2006) concludes in her recent overview that research on the relationship between age and job performance fails to include contextual factors, thus resulting in little understanding of the relationship that should be clarified (Avolio, 1992; Czaja, 1995). The main reason is again a narrow focus on chronological age, although age accounts for only a fraction of the interindividual variability in performance (Avolio, Waldman, & McDaniel, 1990).

This situation leads to many unfortunate conflicts, as the abilities and needs of numerous people clash with implicit or explicit prejudice or regulations regarding their calendar age. As populations age, they are confronted with life course structures that are lagging behind differentiated processes of population aging—problems of "structural lag" that play a central role in the later work of Mathilda Riley (cf. Riley, Kahn, & Foner, 1994).

Given these circumstances, knowing the chronological age of persons in such contexts can be quite informative because ages can easily be related to certain characteristics. We can predict that the unemployment of older workers will tend to be longer than the unemployment of "normal" workers. The point is, however, that this does not demonstrate that older workers are "slower" or "less flexible" than younger ones. Given the tendency to exclude older workers from the labor market and the importance of work for income, housing, health, social contacts, participation, and the articulation of personal identities, these important aspects of life may become increasingly at risk as people reach higher ages. These increasing risks of loss and failure cannot be understood as being caused by aging processes per se; they are to a large degree constituted by age-related processes in the labor market. For aging studies, to focus on age without analyzing the processes that constitute many of the characteristics associated with these ages, merely because chronological age has been institutionalized in the societies in which people live, enforces the chronological regimes of these societies and does nothing to advance our understanding of human aging.

One of the principal issues at stake is whether gerontology does not, by establishing unclear links between chronological age and characteristics, introduce new generalizations or reinforce conventional generalizations about aging and the aged. Furthermore, even unfounded generalizations about categories of people with certain ages can be implemented in policies regarding, for instance, specific forms of care or housing for "the aged" and thus contribute to a reality that forces aging people to fit in because such generalizations may limit the options that are available. Consequently, later research can affirm the earlier generalizations not because they grasped the realities of aging but because gerontological expertise has again played its unreflected role in constituting the realities of aging. In such cases, the analytical apparatus of gerontology runs the danger of becoming an uncritical instrument catering to all kinds of organizational contexts in which aging people are relevant mainly as the subjects of planning procedures and statistical estimates even if the objective is to help and support them. Unfounded age-related generalizations may be practical for certain purposes but should not guide and certainly should not dominate the way aging is approached or understood; for gerontological purposes, this can hardly be satisfactory.

Personal Perspectives of Temporal Living

The chronologization of time, which is one of the typical aspects of contemporary culture, tends to occlude the richness of experiences and reflections of time that we can still find in many traditions. In the context of this chapter, we can distinguish three approaches to living in time that allow more elaboration of personal experiences of aging as living in time. One was initially developed by the fifth-century philosopher Augustine and had a major influence on such contemporary philosophers as Husserl, Heidegger, and Merleau-Ponty (Augustine, 1961; Baars, 2007b; Ricoeur, 1988). This approach offers opportunities to understand that we experience a *present* in which we read a text, speak with somebody, or listen to music. Such a "broad" experience of the present gets completely lost in the blur of rapidly rolling digital numbers. Moreover, although the duration of each event or experience could be measured, such measurements are completely irrelevant for the intensity of the experience. Even short moments in which "time seems to stand still" may be unforgettable and life changing.

This experience of the present is inherently connected with a remembrance of the *past* and an anticipation of the *future*. This opens a different perspective on time as becomes clear when we experience that something that happened "a long time ago" (from a chronological perspective) can be vividly remembered as if it happened yesterday, whereas something (e.g., a personal relationship) that was important a year ago can be experienced as way back in the past. Experiences of the past, present, and the future do not follow the orderly arrangements of chronological time. This does not exclude the possibility of locating the situations and experiences in chronological time, but this occurs in another perspective, and consequently we can wonder about the differences between them.

Memory as presence of the past does not comprise only what or how we *want* to remember. We evoke only a part of our memories consciously; a much greater part evokes us or keeps asking our attention, although we might prefer to forget it. In this context, Hannah Arendt (1958) referred not only to memory as a typically interhuman characteristic but also to forgiveness. Resentment or bitterness can be a destructive form of what Augustine called the presence of the past, in which painful events remain as vivid as if they took place only recently and no time seems to have passed since. Ultimately, nonforgiving obstructs one's openness to the present and to the future so that the past cannot be a source of inspiration for the future.

We may be able to understand our lives backwards, but we must, as Kierkegaard (1987) remarked, live forward and are inevitably confronted with uncertainty about the future, an uncertainty that opens, however, the opportunity to live one's life. That there are today no generally accepted structures of meaning in aging can be seen as a loss, but the obligation to follow fixed patterns or phases of life might weigh heavily and frustrate creativity. The awareness that our confrontations with the contingencies of life are not based on unquestioned structures of meaning makes life more insecure but also potentially richer. We may not know how to live with fundamental uncertainty, but we cannot live well without it either.

A second temporal concept is even older than Augustine's pathbreaking work and can be found in Hesiod (2006). This is the idea of "*kairos,*" which plays an important role in early Greek Pythagorean philosophy and in Stoic thought: the idea that the present offers or denies a particular opportunity. The idea has clearly pragmatic origins in experiences of sailing, fishing, and agriculture. For the Stoics, it was important to live according to what opportunities were given (ευκαιρια) or denied (ακαιρια) by the gods or the course of nature. This concept of time is still presupposed when we are thinking about when the "time is ripe" or not to do or say something. We know this from everyday expressions, such as "If you want to do it, do it now," "It's now or never," and "Now is not the right time." This sensitivity for the right moment cannot be derived from chronological time. The idea of *kairos* has in the past often been interpreted in relation to life's phases, or "seasons," which may be adequate if it does not unnecessarily limit the opportunities of persons. It is more generally relevant for important situations in life.

One of the remarkable aspects of a *narrative,* a third major form to articulate temporality, is its ability to integrate in a loose but potentially meaningful way the most diverse events and actions and their evaluations. According to Ricoeur, a central role in composing loosely integrative configurations is played by the *act* of *emplotment,* whereby unrelated incidents are integrated into a meaningful whole, making it part of a story that progresses with a beginning and an end.

Through the plot, *events and story* are connected reciprocally so that the story changes when other events or interpretations are introduced and vice versa. This implies that the "same" events can be integrated into different stories where the elements are arranged differently, with other emphases or from other points of view. Such differences are not due to a lack of precision, as it may appear from the point of view of methodically controlled intersubjectivity. Different stories may express other experiences, other evaluations, or different points of view very precisely. Another important achievement of emplotment is the integration of the *configurational* dimension of the narrative (where the emphasis falls on the meaningful pattern) with its *chronological* dimension (where the emphasis falls on the timing and succession of events). In the words of Ricoeur (1991), "Narrativity and temporality are as closely linked as a 'language-game' in Wittgenstein's terms is to a 'form of life.' . . . Narrativity is the mode of discourse through which the mode of being which we call temporality or temporal being, is brought to language" (p. 99).

As chronological time can easily be used in bureaucratic calculations, it will tend to dominate other perspectives on time and aging. The necessity to respect these not only is a moral imperative but also indispensable to understand what aging *means* to the persons concerned. Human aging is, inevitably, interpreted and connected with narratives about the value, glory, misery, happiness, and finitude of human life. When aging is approached only from a chronological perspective, the necessarily abstract character of chronological time discussed previously will empty human aging from the meaningful contents that are essential to understand it. Once time perspectives have been emptied of all content, commercial images tend to fill up the void. Many contemporary narratives about aging that are based on an idealization of youth—resulting in ideas of aging as "staying young" or submitting aging to standards of "success" or "productivity"—can hardly be seen as adequate for an inspiring and supportive culture of aging where people can continue to participate actively but where limitations and loss are *dignified* and not seen as failure (Baars, 2006, in press). In spite of their chronologization, calendars not only are used to count the years as we do when we speak of calendar age but also meaningfully structure the year with religious holidays or the remembrance of major historical events, such as wars, disasters, declarations, or constitutions. The yearly cycles and the rhythms of the natural environment are coordinated with specific seasonal activities such as fishing, sowing, harvesting, or socializing in warm homes during cold and dark winters, usually combined with seasonal festivities, markets, contests, and holidays (Zerubavel, 1981). Such cyclical representations of time are also implicit in social settings in which human beings are born, grow up, begin their own adult lives, get older, and eventually die. When cultural ideas, images, and metaphors about aging are not generally shared anymore, this does not necessarily imply that such interpretations are absent. The perspective of human aging is too rich to be reduced to chronological age, life expectancy, or mortality rates. It also requires a constantly renewed interpretation through stories that may offer inspiration, warning, or consolation as memories are evoked to face the future.

References

Alwin, D. F., Hofer, S. M., & McCammon, R. J. (2006). Modelling the effects of time: Integrating demographic and developmental perspectives. In R. H. Binstock & L. K. George (Eds.), *Handbook of aging and the social sciences* (6th ed., pp. 20–38). Boston: Academic Press.

Arendt, H. (1958). *The human condition.* Chicago: University of Chicago Press.

Augustine, A. (1961). *Confessions* (R. S. Pine-Coffin, Trans.). London: Penguin.

Avolio, B. J. (1992). A levels of analysis perspective of aging and work research. In K. W. Schaie & M. P. Lawton (Eds.), *Annual review of gerontology and geriatrics* (pp. 239–260). New York: Springer Publishing.

Avolio, B. J., Waldman, D. A., & McDaniel, M. A. (1990). Age and work performance in nonmanagerial jobs: The effects of experience and occupational type. *Academy of Management Journal, 33,* 407–422.

Baars, J. (1991). The challenge of critical gerontology: The problem of social constitution. *Journal of Aging Studies, 5,* 219–243.

Baars, J. (2006). *Het nieuwe ouder worden: Perspectieven en paradoxen van leven in de tijd.* Amsterdam: Humanistics University Press.

Baars, J. (2007a). Introduction. Chronological time and chronological age—Problems of temporal diversity. In J. Baars & H. Visser (Eds.), *Aging and time: Multidisciplinary perspectives* (pp. 1–14). Amityville, NY: Baywood Publishing.

Baars, J. (2007b). A triple temporality of aging: Chronological measurement, personal experience and narrative articulation. In J Baars & H. Visser (Eds.), *Aging and time: Multidisciplinary perspectives* (pp. 15–42). Amityville, NY: Baywood Publishing.

Baars, J. (in press). *Philosophy of aging, time and finitude.* In T. Cole, R. Ray, & R. Kastenbaum (Eds.), *A guide to humanistic studies in aging.* Baltimore: Johns Hopkins University Press.

Baars, J., & Visser, H. (Eds.). (2007). *Aging and time: Multidisciplinary perspectives.* Amityville, NY: Baywood Publishing.

Bengtson, V. L., Putney, N. M., & Johnson, M. L. (2005). The problem of theory in gerontology today. In M. L. Johnson (Ed.), *The Cambridge handbook of age and aging* (pp. 3–20). Cambridge: Cambridge University Press.

Binstock, R. H., & George, L. K. (2006). *Handbook of aging and the social sciences* (6th ed.). Boston: Academic Press.

Birren, J. (1959). Principles of research on aging. In J. Birren (Ed.), *Handbook of aging and the individual: Psychological and biological aspects* (pp. 2–42). Chicago: University of Chicago Press.

Birren, J. (1999). Theories of aging: A personal perspective. In V. L. Bengtson & K. W. Schaie (Eds.), *Handbook of theories of aging* (pp. 459–471). New York: Springer Publishing.

Chan, S., & Stevens, A. H. (1999). Employment and retirement following a late-career job loss. *American Economic Review, 70,* 355–371.

Czaja, S. J. (1995). Aging and work performance. *Review of Public Personnel Administration, 15,* 46–61.

Dannefer, D. (2003). Cumulative advantage/disadvantage and the life course: Cross-fertilizing age and social science theory. *Journal of Gerontology: Social Sciences, 58,* S327–S337.

Gilleard, C., & Higgs, P. (2000). *Cultures of aging: Self, citizen and the body.* Harlow: Prentice Hall.

Gilleard, C., & Higgs, P. (2005). *Contexts of aging: Class, cohort and community,* Malden, MA: Polity Press.

Ginn, J., Street, D., & Arber, S. (Eds.). (2001). *Women, work and pensions: International issues and prospects.* Buckingham: Open University Press.

Gravilov, L. A., & Gravilova, N. S. (2006). Reliability theory of aging and longevity. In E. J. Masoro & S. N. Austed (Eds.), *Handbook of the biology of aging* (6th ed., pp. 3–42). London: Academic Press.

Grillis, J. R. (1987). The case against chronologization: Changes in the Anglo-American life cycle 1600 to the present. *Etnologia Europaea, 17,* 97–106.

Hardy, M. (2006). Older workers. In R. H. Binstock & L. K. George (Eds.), *Handbook of aging and the social sciences* (6th ed., pp. 201–218). Boston: Academic Press.

Henretta, J. C. (2003). The life course perspective on work and retirement. In R. A. Settersten (Ed.), *Invitation to the life course: Toward new understandings of later life* (pp. 85–106). Amityville, NY: Baywood Publishing.

Hesiod. (2006). *Theogony, works and days: Vol. 1. Tesimonia* (G. W. Most, Ed.). Cambridge, MA: Loeb Classical Library.

Hirsch, B., MacPherson, D., & Hardy, M. (2000). Occupational age structure and access for older workers. *Industrial and Labor Relations Review, 42,* 401–418.

Kierkegaard, S. (1987). *Either-or.* Princeton, NJ: Princeton University Press.

Kirkwood, T. B. L. (2005). Understanding the odd science of ageing. *Cell, 120,* 437–447.

Kirkwood, T. B. L., Boys, R. J. , Gillespie, C. S., Procter, C. J., Shanley, D. P., & Wilkenson, D. J. (2006). Computer modelling in the study of aging. In E. J. Masoro & S. N. Austed (Eds.), *Handbook of the biology of aging* (6th ed., pp. 334–359). London: Academic Press.

Kohli, M. (1986). The world we forgot: A historical review of the life course. In V. Marshall (Ed.), *Later life: The social psychology of aging* (pp. 271–303). London: Sage.

Leisering L., & Leibfried, S. (1999). *Time and poverty in Western welfare states.* Cambridge: Cambridge University Press.

Levy, R., Ghisletta, P., Le Goff, J.-M., Spimi, D., & Widmer, E. (Eds.). (2005). *Towards an interdisciplinary perspective on the life course: Vol. 10. Advances in life course research.* Amsterdam: Elsevier.

Masoro, E. J. (2006). Are age-associated diseases an integral part of aging? In E. J. Masoro & S. N. Austed (Eds.), *Handbook of the biology of aging* (6th ed., pp. 43–62). London: Academic Press.

Masoro, E. J., & Austed, S. N. (Eds.). (2006). *Handbook of the biology of aging* (6th ed.). London: Academic Press.

Mayer, K. U., & Müller, W. (1986). The state and the structure of the life course. In A. B. Sorensen, F. E. Weinert, & L. R. Sherrod (Eds.), *Human development and the life course: Multidisciplinary perspectives* (pp. 217–245). London: Lawrence Erlbaum.

Oeppen, J., & Vaupel, J. (2002). Broken limits to life expectancy. *Science, 296,* 1029–1031.

Prigogine, I. (1955). *Introduction to thermodynamics of irreversible processes.* Springfield, IL: Charles C. Thomas.

Ricoeur, P. (1988). *Time and narrative* (3 vols.). Chicago: University of Chicago Press.

Ricoeur, P. (1991). *A Ricoeur reader* (M. J. Valdés, Ed.). New York: Harvester Wheatsheaf.

Riley, M. W., Kahn, R. L., & Foner, A. (1994). *Age and structural lag.* New York: Wiley.

Schaie, K. W. (2007). The concept of event time in the study of adult development. In J. Baars & H. Visser (Eds.), *Aging and time: Multidisciplinary perspectives* (pp. 121–136). Amityville, NY: Baywood Publishing.

Schroots, J. F., & Birren, J. E. (1988). The nature of time: Implications for research on aging. *Comprehensive Gerontology. Section C, Interdisciplinary Topics, 2,* 1–29.

Settersten, R. A. (1999). *Living in time and place: The problems and promises of developmental science.* Amityville, NY: Baywood Publishing.

Settersten, R. A. (Ed.). (2001). *Invitation to the life course: Toward new understandings of later life.* Amityville, NY: Baywood Publishing.

Uffink, J. (2007). Whence an emergence of biological time? In J. Baars & H. Visser (Eds.), *Time and aging: Multidisciplinary perspectives* (pp. 169–176). Amityville, NY: Baywood Publishing.

Uhlenberg, P., & Mueller, M. (2004). Family context and individual well-being: Patterns and mechanisms in life course perspective. In J. T. Mortimer & M. J. Shanhan (Eds.), *Handbook of the life course* (pp. 123–148). New York: Springer Publishing.

Vickerstaff, S. (1995). Life course, youth and old age. In P. Taylor-Gooby & J. O. Zinn (Eds.), *Risk in social science* (pp. 180–201). Oxford: Oxford University Press.

Vincent, J. A. (1995). *Inequality and old age.* London: UCL Press.

Vincent, J. A. (2006). Globalization and critical theory: Political economy of world population issues. In J. Baars, D. Dannefer, C. Phillipson, & A. Walker (Eds.), *Aging, globalization and inequality: The new critical gerontology* (pp. 245–272). Amityville, NY: Baywood Publishing.

Walker, A., & Maltby, T. (1997). *Ageing Europe.* Buckingham: Open University Press.

Westendorp, R. G. J., & Kirkwood, T. B. L. (2007). The biology of aging, In J. Bond, S. Peace, F. Dittmann-Kohli, & G. Westerhof (Eds.), *Ageing in society: European perspectives on gerontology* (pp. 15–37). London: Sage.

Yates, F. E. (2007a). Biological time as emergent property. In J. Baars & H. Visser (Eds.), *Time and aging: Multidisciplinary perspectives* (pp. 161–168). Amityville, NY: Baywood Publishing.

Yates, F. E. (2007b). Further conjectures on the nature of time in living systems: Causes of senescence. In J. Baars & H. Visser (Eds.), *Time and aging: Multidisciplinary perspectives* (pp. 177–186). Amityville, NY: Baywood Publishing.

Zerubavel, E. (1981). *Hidden rhythms: Schedules and calendars in social life.* Berkeley: University of California Press.

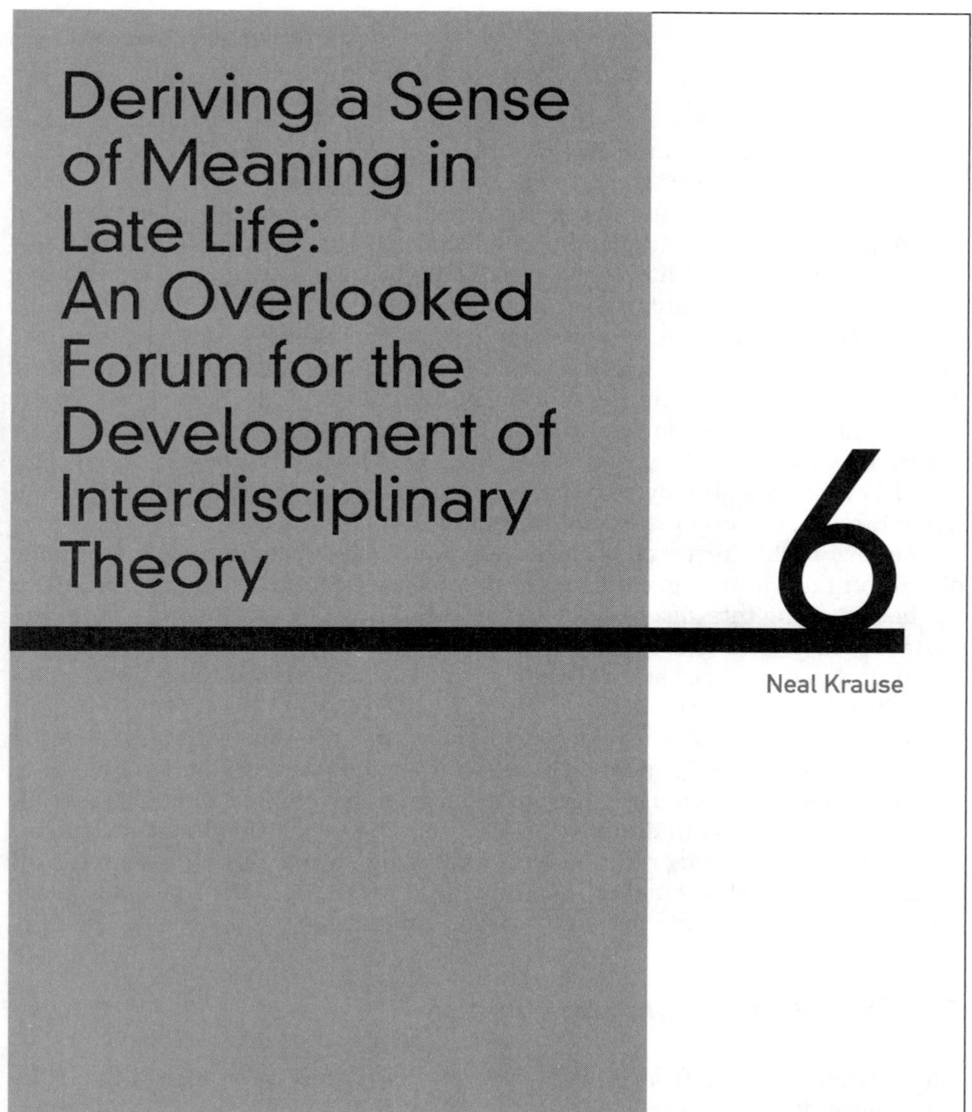

6 Deriving a Sense of Meaning in Late Life: An Overlooked Forum for the Development of Interdisciplinary Theory

Neal Krause

The purpose of this chapter is to show how research on meaning in life can be used to develop multidisciplinary theory in gerontology. Although it is difficult to find a good definition of meaning in life, a number of investigators rely on the one proposed by Reker. He defines meaning as "the cognizance of order, coherence, and purpose in one's existence, the pursuit and attainment of worthwhile goals, and an accompanying sense of fulfillment" (Reker, 2000, p. 41).

The discussion that follows is divided into four main sections. First, it is important to begin by showing why meaning should be used to form the cornerstone of a multidisciplinary theory. This is accomplished by turning to the work of theorists from sociology, psychology, and psychiatry who argue that deriving a sense of meaning is the ultimate goal of life and represents the highest state of human development. And as the work of other social and behavioral scientists will reveal, it is especially important to find a sense of meaning in late life. But a good theory must do more than provide an intuitively pleasing set of conceptual linkages. Instead, it must also be practical (it must address real-world problems). Consequently, the first section also contains a brief review of findings from empirical studies that speak directly to the practical implications of studying meaning in life. More specifically, this work suggests that meaning may be a key determinant of the physical and mental health of older people.

A necessary first step in developing a theory involves clearly defining the key constructs that are embedded in it. Unfortunately, the nature and content domain of meaning in life is notoriously difficult to grasp. Consequently, the goal of the second section is to address this problem by clarifying the basic nature of meaning in life. This is accomplished by moving beyond the verbal definition that has already been provided to an operational definition of meaning in life (i.e., the way meaning is measured).

Following this, research on meaning that has been conducted in a number of different disciplines is reviewed in the third section in order to demonstrate the bourgeoning interdisciplinary interest in this core construct. But more important, staking out the range of substantive disciplines that have contributed to our understanding of meaning helps get the basic building blocks of a multidisciplinary theory in place.

The fourth section forms the conceptual core of this chapter. The goal of this section is to look for logical linkages and connections among studies of meaning that have been conducted in different disciplines. Given the current state of the literature on meaning in life, it will not be possible to provide a well-articulated and fully developed theoretical framework. Even so, integrating research from a number of disciplines makes it possible to show that developing a multidisciplinary theory is not only possible but also advantageous.

The Pivotal Role of Meaning in Life

For decades, scholars from a wide range of disciplines have argued that finding a sense of meaning in life constitutes the pinnacle of human development. For example, Victor Frankl (1984), a widely cited psychiatrist, maintained that, "man's search for meaning is the primary motivation in his life" (p. 121). The same notion is evident in the work of sociologist Peter Berger (1967), who argued that there is "a human craving for meaning that appears to have the force of instinct" (p. 22). And Abraham Maslow (1968), a former president of the American Psychological Association, captured the essence of this perspective when he observed that "the human needs a framework of values, a philosophy of life . . . in about the same sense that he needs sunlight, calcium, and love" (p. 206). In fact, the emphasis that Maslow placed on meaning in life became even more pronounced toward the end of his career. As Koltko-Rivera (2006) points out, late in his life Maslow proposed a new level of development that he placed at the top of his hierarchy of needs ahead of self-actualization. He called this new stage "self-transcendence." Self-transcendence involves deriving a more comprehensive sense of meaning in life by moving beyond purely personal interests to more extrapersonal interests that include contributing to the community and being more concerned about the welfare of others.

If all these researchers are correct and the attainment of meaning is the ultimate goal of life, then evidence of efforts to attain this goal should be apparent in many human activities. The underlying importance of meaning for all human endeavors was captured succinctly by Carl Jung (1953), a noted psychiatrist, when he observed that "the least of things with a meaning is always worth more in life than the greatest of things without it" (p. 285).

Although deriving a sense of meaning may be important for people of all ages, there is some evidence that finding meaning in life may become increasingly important as people grow older. Turning to the work of Erikson (1959), Tornstam (2005), and Carstensen, Fung, and Charles (2003) helps show why this is so.

Erikson (1959) provided a widely cited argument for why it may be especially important for people to derive a sense of meaning when they reach late life. He divided the life span into eight stages. He proposed that a unique developmental challenge or crisis must be resolved as people move through each stage. The final stage, which is typically reached at the end of life, is characterized by the crisis of integrity versus despair. This is a time of deep introspection when people review their lives and try to reconcile the inevitable gap between what they set out to do and what they were actually able to accomplish. Viewed more broadly, this means that as people grow older, they try to weave the stories of their lives into a more coherent whole. Ultimately, the goal of this process is to imbue life with a deeper sense of meaning and significance.

Tornstam (2005) also provides evidence for the increasing importance of meaning with advancing age. His theory of gerotranscendence specifies that as people grow older, they experience a major shift in the way they view the world. This shift is characterized by a move away from a materialistic and pragmatic view of the world to more transcendent and cosmic concerns. This cosmic dimension involves an exploration of one's own inner space and, consistent with the work of Erikson (1959), a search for greater integrity. The process of gerotranscendence also involves a desire for maintaining fewer but more meaningful social relationships as well as a greater preference for and appreciation of solitude. Although Tornstam (2005) did not cast his theory explicitly in terms of meaning in life, issues involving the search for meaning clearly lie behind his discussion of introspection, integrity, and the desire for deeper personal relationships.

Like Tornstam (2005), Carstensen and her colleagues propose that as people grow older, they experience a shift away from obtaining more pragmatic knowledge and the development of new skills to seeking close emotional relationships with a smaller circle of family members and friends (Carstensen et al., 2003). This shift in priorities is driven by a growing awareness of the shortness of life and a greater desire to derive a sense of meaning in life. As these investigators note, "What characterizes old age is not hedonism, but a desire to derive a meaning and satisfaction through life" (Carstensen et al., 2003, p. 108).

Consistent with the theoretical perspectives that were devised by Erikson (1959), Tornstam (2005), and Carstensen et al. (2003), findings from several studies suggest that people who are currently older tend to have a greater sense of meaning in life than individuals who are currently younger. For example, Van Ranst and Marcoen (1997) report that younger adults tend to experience less meaning in life than older people. Similarly, Reker and Fry (2003) found a greater tendency for older adults to experience meaning in life than younger people.

But rather than being a purely academic curiosity, research on meaning in life is important because it speaks directly to key issues that face our aging population. More specifically, a growing number of studies suggest that people who have found a sense of meaning in life tend to enjoy better physical health (Krause, 2004; Parquart, 2002), and they tend to experience fewer symptoms of depression than individuals who have not been able to derive a sense that their lives have meaning. In addition, there is some evidence that people with a stronger sense of meaning also tend to be happier and report higher levels of satisfaction with their lives (Debats, 1990).

Identifying the Essence of Meaning in Life

In addition to clearly specifying the conceptual linkages among the various constructs in a theory, our understanding of the underlying theoretical processes is greatly enhanced by paying careful attention to operational definitions of key study constructs. Operational definitions refer to the procedures that are used to measure a construct. In the social and behavioral sciences, this typically involves the survey items that are used to assess a construct, such as meaning in life. Operational definitions form a vitally important bridge between data with theory. The essence of this key step in the research process was identified some time ago by Blalock (1982). He referred to operational definitions as auxiliary measurement theories. In so doing, he wanted to underscore the point that as in the development of substantive theories, the process of measurement also requires a set of theoretical assumptions. Viewed in this way, it is not hard to see why Blalock (1982) maintained that "the process of theory construction and measurement cannot be seen as distinctly different" (p. 25).

There are two reasons why operational definitions are important. The first was discussed by Blalock (1982). He argued that if subsequent empirical tests of a theory are inconclusive, "we will not know if the substantive theory, the auxiliary measurement theory, or both [are] at fault" (p. 25). The second reason why devising sound operational definitions is an indispensable part of the theory construction process is more subtle but equally important. By focusing on how a construct is measured, researchers are better able to grasp the content domain of a construct. And when the dimensions and elements of a construct are better understood, it is possible to more precisely specify the linkages between a construct and other theoretically relevant variables. Because meaning in life is notoriously difficult to define, assessing how it is measured makes it easier to grasp. Moreover, having clear operational definitions of meaning provides a rich conceptual arena for linking meaning with other outcomes, such as health and well-being.

A number of different operational definitions of meaning appear in the literature (Debats, 1998). No attempt is made to review them here. Instead, a recent effort to measure meaning in life that was devised by Krause (2004) is examined briefly because this measure of meaning was intended specifically for older adults. Based on the work of a number of investigators, Krause (2004) proposed that meaning in life is a complex multidimensional construct comprising four factors or dimensions: having a clear set of values, a sense of purpose, goals, and the ability to reconcile things that have happened in the past. These dimensions of meaning and examples of items that were devised to measure them are provided next.

A system of values helps guide behavior. In a world where the utility and worthiness of specific thoughts and behaviors are often unclear and uncertain, values provide the basis for selecting among different options by giving the assurance that personal choices are, in the words of Baumeister (1991), right, good, and justifiable. Among the indicators used by Krause (2004) to assess this dimension of meaning is the following: "I have a system of values and beliefs that guide my daily activities."

Although clearly linked to values, a sense of purpose is conceptually distinct. It has to do with believing that one's actions have a place in the order of things and that one's behavior fits appropriately into a larger and more important social whole. Values are codes or standards that define which thoughts and actions are desirable, whereas a sense of purpose carries evaluative and affective connotations that arise from the successful completion or execution of actions that comply with underlying values. Put another way, a sense of purpose cannot arise without action or effort because these actions affirm the underlying worth of held values. Krause (2004) used the following item to measure this facet of meaning: "I have discovered a satisfying life purpose."

A sense of meaning also involves expectations for the future or goals for which to strive. Goals help a person organize current activities and provide a conduit for focusing and implementing energies, efforts, and ambitions. But even though goals are oriented toward the future, they also provide more immediate rewards by giving rise to a sense of hope and by reinforcing and building on a sense of past achievements. This aspect of meaning was measured in the following way by Krause (2004): "In my life I have clear goals and aims."

The final dimension of meaning that is discussed by Krause (2004) has to do with the ability to reconcile things that have happened in the past. This facet of meaning builds on the work of Erikson (1959) that was discussed earlier. Recall that Erikson (1959) proposed that older adults tend to derive a sense of meaning by reflecting on the past and thinking about how their lives have unfolded. But this task is complicated because everyone falls short of the goals they set. Being able to work through and process these inconsistencies by finding a larger sense of order or purpose in the way one's life has been lived tends to infuse life with a greater sense of meaning. The following indicators illustrate how Krause (2004) assessed this dimension of meaning: "I am able to make sense of the unpleasant things that have happened in the past."

Interdisciplinary Research on Meaning in Life

A thorough review of the literature reveals that investigators from a wide range of disciplines have conducted research on meaning in life. Findings from studies by investigators in four different disciplines are reviewed next.

First, several studies have been conducted to see if various dimensions of personality are related to a person's sense of meaning in life. For example, Schnell and Becker (2006) recently found that about 16% of the variance in meaning in life is explained by personality dispositions. These findings were confirmed in another study by Halama (2005). Although researchers have devised a number of ways to measure personality traits (see Mroczek, Spiro, & Griffin, 2006), one trait has consistently emerged in research on meaning. More specifically, these studies suggest that extroverts are more likely to derive a greater sense of meaning in life than introverts.

But research on the sources of meaning in life is not confined to personality theorists. Instead, a number of studies suggest that a wide range of social factors may influence an older person's sense of meaning as well. More specifically, a growing body of research reveals that social relationships may exert an important influence on whether an older person is able to derive a sense of meaning in life. Finding a sense of purpose and order in life, as well as deriving a sense of fulfillment by reflecting on the past, is often an abstract and cognitively challenging process. In fact, Frankl (1984) maintains that a person must often experience a certain amount of suffering and conflict before they can find a sense of meaning in life. Consequently, it is not surprising to find that older people frequently turn to significant others for assistance when they are faced with the difficult task of finding a sense of meaning in life. Evidence of this may be found in a study by Krause (2004). His research suggests that older people who receive emotional support from family members and close friends are more likely to find a sense of meaning in life than older adults who do not have well-developed social support systems. The findings from this study are consistent with the work of Debats (1999), who reports that social relationships are an important source of meaning for people of all ages. Researchers in the field of communications and linguistics have also expressed interest in the study of meaning in life. Stated simply, one goal of the research in this important discipline is to study how the language that people use and the discourse in which they engage shape the perceptions of the world in which they live. Eisenberg (1998) put it this way: "The express purpose of communication is to discover what is true about the world and transmit this valuable information to others" (p. 98). Investigators in this branch of research strive to find how meaning is determined by the precise words that people use and the way in which these words and phrases change and are jointly constructed in the meaning-making process.

But research on meaning has not been restricted solely to social and behavioral sciences issues. Instead, inroads have been made recently in research on the physiological correlates of meaning in life. For example, a study by Bower, Kemeny, Taylor, and Fahey (2003) reveals that women who experienced a positive change in meaning over the course of their study showed an increase in natural killer cell cytotoxicity. These findings are noteworthy because an extensive body of research links increased natural killer cell activity with better health (e.g., Herberman, 2002).

Toward a Preliminary Theory of Meaning and Health in Late Life

It is encouraging to see that investigators from so many different disciplines are interested in studying meaning in life. However, the diverse findings from this research make it difficult to grasp and summarize the process of meaning making, and, as a result, it is hard to see how a sense of meaning in life may influence the health of older people. One way to resolve these problems is to look for logical connections among the elements in the conceptual frameworks that have driven studies in different disciplines. Doing so makes it possible to derive a rudimentary multidisciplinary theory of meaning in life. Although the findings from this work may be integrated in a number of ways, a potentially useful conceptual scheme is devised here by focusing on the following key linkages: (a) personality traits shape the nature of social relationships that are formed by older adults; (b) relationships with significant others, in turn, help determine an older person's sense of meaning in life; (c) the social process of meaning making is influenced, in part, by the language that actors use as they jointly create a sense of meaning in life; and (d) once a sense of meaning has been negotiated and is firmly in place, findings from research in biology and physiology help show how it may affect health in late life.

Personality Traits and Social Relationships

There are two reasons why it is important to begin constructing an interdisciplinary theory of meaning in life by focusing on the influence of personality traits. Both reasons are controversial. However, no attempt is made here to resolve the long-standing debates that swirl around them. Instead, the intent is simply to use the arguments that are developed by some investigators as a logical point of departure for weaving the diverse findings from research on meaning in life into a more coherent whole.

First, some researchers maintain that personality traits are highly stable across the life course (McCrae & Costa, 2003). More specifically, these investigators argue that "personality traits do not change much after about age 30" (McCrae & Costa, 2003, p. 206). This is not a new idea. Writing in 1892, William James came to precisely the same conclusion when he observed that "it is well for the world that in most of us, by age thirty, the character is set like plaster, and will never soften again" (James, 1961, p. 11).

Second, the presumed stability of personality traits is due, in part, to the fact that it is genetically determined. Research supporting this view is summarized by McCrae and Costa (2003). These investigators report that a large number of studies have been done on the genetic basis of personality traits, and the findings from this research "are remarkably consistent. They suggest that about half the variance in personality trait scores is attributable to genes, and that almost none is attributable to a shared family environment" (McCrae & Costa, 2003, p. 194).

Given the plausible reasons for beginning a multidisciplinary theory of meaning by focusing on personality traits, the next step involves showing how these traits may influence the social relationships that are maintained by older people. In order to address this issue, it is helpful to examine the ways in which personality traits are assessed. For years, the Five-Factor Theory devised by McCrae and Costa (2003) has dominated research in this field. However, as Mroczek et al. (2006) point out, controversy continues to engulf efforts to identify the full spectrum of personality traits. No attempt is made here to resolve this ongoing debate. Instead, it makes more sense to show how one specific personality trait may affect the nature of social ties that are formed in late life (extraversion). Focusing on this trait is justified because it often appears in the formulations of many personality theorists (e.g., Eysenck, 1998; McCrae & Costa, 2003).

McCrae and Costa (2003) argue that extraversion comprises three components: warmth, gregariousness, and assertiveness. Warmth refers to "a friendly, cordial, intimately involved style of personal interaction" (McCrae & Costa, 2003, p. 49). Gregariousness has to do with the desire for social stimulation and a drive to interact with others on a frequent basis. Assertiveness is concerned with the willingness to readily express one's own feelings and desires and a tendency to step up and take charge in social situations.

Extraversion is especially important for the purposes of this chapter because a number of studies suggest that extraverts are embedded in more active social networks than introverts. For example, a study by Swickert, Rosentreter, Hittner, and Mushrush (2002) suggests that extraverts have more frequent contact with social network members. Moreover, the results from this study indicate that compared to introverts, extraverts report receiving more emotional and tangible support from significant others. Although a good deal of the research on personality and social support has been conducted with younger adults, it is especially important to point out that some studies have focused specifically on older people. For example, Krause, Liang, and Keith (1990) found that compared to introverts, extraverts have more frequent contact with family members and friends. The findings from this study further suggest that extraverts are also more likely to receive emotional support from others, and they are more likely to believe that social network members will be willing to help out in the future should the need arise.

Social Support and Meaning in Life

Deriving a sense of meaning in life is hard work because the world is a complex and often confusing place. Moreover, this task is complicated by the fact that there are no absolute criteria for determining whether the sense of meaning in life that has been derived by an older person is adequate or sufficient. Consequently, it is not surprising to find that people often turn to family members and close friends to help them work through the questions and uncertainties that arise during their search for meaning. In the process, a close social network member is likely to serve as a role model by sharing his or her own experiences with finding a sense of meaning in life. This argument may be found in the work of a number of social theorists. For example, the essence of this perspective was succinctly captured some time ago by Berger and Pullberg (1965). These investigators forcefully and convincingly maintain that "the human enterprise of producing a world is not comprehensible as an individual project. Rather, it is a social process: *men together* engage in constructing a world, which then becomes their common dwelling. Indeed, since sociality is a necessary element in the human being, the process of world production is necessarily a social one (Berger & Pullberg, 1965, p. 201, emphasis in original).

Although the insights provided by Berger and Pullberg (1965) are noteworthy, there is a problem with the way in which their theoretical perspective is developed. Social relationships are a complex, multidimensional conceptual domain in their own right. Therefore, in order to see how social relationships influence meaning, it is important to first identify the types of social ties that are likely to be involved in this process. Although it is not possible to examine the linkages between a full range of social relationships and meaning in life in this chapter, three types of social ties that appear to play a key role in the meaning-making process are examined briefly next: receiving emotional support from others, anticipated support, and negative interaction.

A special emphasis is placed on emotional support in the current discussion because, as noted earlier, there is some evidence that as people grow older, they prefer to develop and maintain relationships that are emotionally close (Carstensen et al., 2003). Emotional support is defined as the provision of empathy, caring, love, and trust (Barrera, 1986). Research reveals that the subtle emotions that are conveyed in the process of providing emotional support are likely to make an older person feel that he or she is esteemed and valued (e.g., Krause & Borawski-Clark, 1994). This may, in turn, help older people feel as though they have a set place in the wider social order. Simply put, receiving emotional support from close others make older people feel as though they belong. Carrier (1965) captured the essence of this construct when he argued that the person who feel that he belongs "sees himself as taking part in his group; he identifies with it, he participates in it, he receives his motivation from it; in a word, he is in a state or disposition of interaction with the group, which understands, inspires, and welcomes him" (p. 58). Being part of a welcoming social network imbues life with a sense of order and purpose and in the process helps an older person derive a deeper sense of meaning in life. This perspective provides a way to show how focusing on operational definitions helps sharpen a theoretical framework. More specifically, this theoretical rationale suggests that social ties help forge a sense of meaning in life (i.e., a more general proposition) because the emotional support provided by significant others helps older people find a sense of purpose (i.e., a more focused hypothesis).

Researchers have demonstrated for some time that social relationships are not always positive and that at times older people may experience negative interaction with their social network members (Rook, 1984). If social interaction has negative as well as positive qualities, then a more balanced approach to the study of social relationships and meaning in life requires that both positive and negative interaction be taken into account. Negative interaction is characterized by disagreements, criticism, rejection, and the invasion of privacy (Rook, 1984). Sometimes excessive helping is subsumed under the broad rubric of this construct as well.

In order to see why negative interaction may compromise an older person's sense of meaning in life, it is important to reflect on how the unsettling effects of unpleasant interaction arise. Some insight into this issue may be found by turning to the basic tenets of expectancy theory (Olson, Roese, & Zanna, 1996). Cast within the context of social interaction, expectancies are beliefs about how people will think, feel, and act in the future. As Rook and Pietromonaco (1987) point out, most people encounter more positive than negative interaction over the course of their lives. This creates the impression (i.e., the expectancy) that social relationships will continue on a positive course. However, when unpleasant interaction arises, these expectancies are shattered, often stunning the recipient. And as Olson et al. (1996) observe, the disconfirmation of cherished expectancies may be a source of significant psychological distress. But negative interaction may do more than this. The expectancies that surround social relationships provide a sense that life is orderly and predictable. When negative interaction arises, these expectancies are crushed, and the resulting loss of predictability and order may threaten an older person's sense of meaning in life.

Anticipated support is defined as the belief that significant others will provide assistance in the future should the need arise (Wethington & Kessler, 1986). Anticipated support may be an important determinant of meaning for the following reason. As discussed previously, one dimension of meaning in life involves having plans and goals to strive for in the future. However, the loss of physical and cognitive abilities in late life may make these goals more difficult to attain (see Schulz & Heckhausen, 1996). Consequently, older people will be more likely to have greater faith in their ability to reach their goals if they believe that family members and close friends stand ready to help if they need assistance in attaining them. Once again, this theoretical specification shows how focusing on operational definitions of meaning in life foster the development of more focused research hypotheses.

Findings from a recent longitudinal survey by Krause (2007b) provide support for the linkages between meaning and each of the social relationship measures that are discussed in this section. More specifically, the data suggest that older people who receive more emotional support from family members and friends tend to have a greater sense of meaning in life. In addition, the findings reveal that more anticipated support at the baseline survey is associated with an increase in meaning over time. But in contrast, the results further indicate that older people who encounter negative interaction with their social network members are more likely to experience a diminished sense of meaning in life than older adults who are not exposed to interpersonal conflict. Taken together, these findings are important because they show how social support networks may promote as well as inhibit the meaning-making process.

Integrating Insights From Communications Research

Research reveals that the social support process is fragile and that even well-intentioned efforts to help others may go awry (Coyne, Wortman, & Lehman, 1988). Although there are a number of reasons why this may be so, one factor involves the way in which support is offered and the way in which it is perceived by potential help recipients. More specifically, social support is likely to be effective only if it is offered in a way that is sensitive to the needs of the recipient. For example, members of the current cohort of older adults value independence highly, and they want to avoid becoming overly dependent on others (Meredith & Schewe, 2002). Consequently, when help is provided, it must be given in a way that does not make it seem as though an older recipient has been given something for nothing. Research on linguistics and communications can help investigators better understand these finer nuances of the social support process by showing the specific words and phrases that help maximize the effectiveness of assistance that one person provides to another. Moreover, by exploring these issues, it is possible to find additional ways in which assistance that is provided by significant others may enhance an older person's sense of meaning in life.

At several points in this chapter, it has been noted that older people must often grapple with complex and abstract issues in order to derive a sense of meaning in life. Evidence of this may be found, for example, in the following item that is contained in the scale to measure meaning in life that was devised by Krause (2004): "In terms of my life, I see a reason for being here." Older adults may be uncertain about the conclusions they have reached regarding this issue, and they may question the rationale they have relied on to reach them. Having a trusted other help them reflect on these deliberations can be quite important. However, helping an older person work through complex issues involving meaning in life requires a good deal of understanding, patience, and interpersonal warmth. Focusing on the discourse that takes place during these interpersonal exchanges may provide valuable insight into how this helping process actually transpires.

Earlier, when the measurement of meaning was discussed, a component of meaning that has to do with reflecting on the past was introduced. When older people reflect on things that have happened earlier in their lives, they are likely to recall some of the unpleasant experiences they have encountered. Reexamining stressful events may raise a host of sensitive and painful issues. Evidence of this may be found in a study by Krause (2005) that involved assessing the relationship between exposure to traumatic life events and meaning in life. Wheaton (1994) defines trauma as events that are "spectacular, horrifying, and just deeply disturbing experiences" (p. 90). Included among traumatic events are sexual and physical abuse, witnessing a violent crime, the premature loss of a parent, and participation in combat. Because they are so severe, research reveals that the deleterious effects of trauma may last a lifetime (e.g., Krause, Shaw, & Cairney, 2004). Krause (2005) argues that efforts to reconcile the way a person has lived his or her life may be greatly complicated if the person has been exposed to a traumatic event. Under these circumstances, it may be difficult for older people to understand why an event happened, and it may be especially hard for them to see how the event fits into and plays a role in the larger course of their lives. If significant others aim to help an older person process past events that are especially painful, then the assistance they provide must be offered in a highly sensitive way.

Insights provided by communications research help show how the discourse that is initiated by social network members may play a key role in helping older people reconcile things that have happened in the past. Based on the comforting model that was developed by Burleson and Goldsmith (1998), Jones and Wirtz (2006) show how two facets of the communications process facilitate adjustment to troubling circumstances. The first is person centeredness. This refers to the degree to which a helper validates a target person's feelings and encourages him or her to talk about a challenging event. This may be accomplished by asking simple questions, such as "What happened?" and "How do you feel about the event now?" Moreover, an effective helper might further demonstrate person centeredness by asking, "So, what about this event made you feel angry?" The second facet of an effective communication process involves nonverbal intimacy. This refers to things like establishing close proximity during interaction, leaning forward at key points in a discussion, facial expressiveness, and an overall reflection of interpersonal warmth.

Knowing the precise verbal and nonverbal communication that makes up the help-giving process provides greater insight into the inner workings of a potentially important social determinant of meaning in life. Moreover, the knowledge that is gleaned from studying these precise communication skills provides a clear set of criteria for developing interventions to help older people find a sense of meaning in life.

Meaning in Life, Physiological Change, and Health

Up to this point, the discussion has been concerned solely with describing how a sense of meaning in life may arise. Although this is an important part of deriving an interdisciplinary theory, it does not go far enough because it is important to show how meaning may, in turn, affect health. The purpose of the discussion that is provided in this section is to address this issue. However, it is not possible to review all the ways in which meaning may influence health. Instead, in an effort to build wider interdisciplinary linkages, the discussion that follows will focus solely on physiological mechanisms. This makes sense because if meaning affects health, then it must ultimately do so by bringing about some sort of physiological changes in the body.

Recall the study by Bower et al. (2003) suggesting that women who experienced an increased sense of meaning in life showed subsequent increases in natural killer cell cytotoxicity. Although the findings in this study are provocative, it is not entirely clear how the potentially beneficial effects of meaning arise. Fortunately, some insight into this issue may be found by turning to research that reveals that positive emotions may have a beneficial effect on a wide range of physiological processes. More specifically, research reviewed by Salovey, Rothman, Detweiler, and Steward (2000) reveals that a number of positive emotions have been shown to exert a beneficial effect on a range of markers of immune functioning, including secretory immunoglobulin A, lymphocyte proliferation, and natural killer cell activity. The emphasis in this literature review on positive emotions is important because there is some evidence that positive emotions are an integral facet of the meaning-making process. Evidence of this may be found by returning to the definition of meaning and the discussion of the nature of meaning that was provided earlier. Recall that in defining a sense of meaning in life, Reker (2000) argues that it includes "an accompanying sense of fulfillment" (p. 41). Clearly, finding a sense of fulfillment is a positive emotion. In addition, having a sense of purpose in life was identified earlier as an important component of a sense of meaning. One of the items used by Krause (2004) to assess a sense of purpose in life states, "I have discovered a satisfying life purpose." Once again, the ability to find a satisfying purpose in life is a positive emotion. Taken together, these observations suggest that the positive emotions that arise in the meaning-making process are likely to generate the beneficial immune responses that are discussed by Salovey et al. (2000). And to the extent that this is true, older adults who find a sense of meaning in life should experience better health than older people who are unable to find that their lives have meaning.

Conclusions

Viewed broadly, the perspective that was devised in this chapter weaves together research in psychology, sociology, communications, and physiology to show how one of the most important goals in life can be attained and how it may affect health in late life. However, this conceptual framework is far from complete. Work in a number of other disciplines and fields should be integrated into this conceptual framework. Two examples of the research that should be taken into consideration are provided next.

First, a number of studies suggest that religion may play an especially important role in shaping an older person's sense of meaning in life (Krause, 2003, 2008). Focusing on religion is important because it highlights a distinction made by Reker (2000) between general and context-specific measures of meaning in life. General measures of meaning in life have been discussed throughout this chapter. This type of measure aims to assess a sense of meaning in life as a whole. In contrast, context-specific measures refer to a sense of meaning that arises within a specific social setting or social context. So, for example, people may derive a sense of meaning in life that arises specifically from their involvement in religion. Looking at one of the items that was devised by Krause (2008) makes it easier to grasp the content domain that is encompassed by measures of religious meaning in life: "My faith gives me a sense of direction in my life."

There are two reasons why context-specific measures of meaning in life are useful. To begin with, focusing on the interface between general and context-specific measures of meaning provides new ways of thinking about how a sense of meaning in life arises. If a person derives a sense of meaning in a number of life domains, such as religion, then researchers need to know if these various context-specific sources of meaning form the genesis of and give rise to a more general sense of meaning in life. Alternatively, the linkage between the two types of measures can be reversed to, instead, specify that a general sense of meaning in life appears first in time and subsequently shapes the way context-specific assessments of meaning in life are made. These two scenarios represent an extension of the "top-down" and "bottom-up" theoretical perspective that Diener (1984) devised to explain the interface between a general sense of life satisfaction and feelings of life satisfaction that arise in specific domains of life (e.g., financial satisfaction).

The second reason why context-specific measures of meaning in life are important has to do with the opportunity they provide to bring wider social structural issues to the foreground. Some social gerontologists may feel uneasy with the emphasis that was placed on personality traits in the conceptual perspective that was developed for this chapter. They may feel as though this view constitutes an overly reductionist approach to the study of the meaning-making process. Taking a sense of religious meaning into account should help allay these concerns because it shows how a sense of meaning may also be fostered by key social institutions (e.g., the church) as well.

But focusing on religion represents only one way to integrate research from other disciplines into the study of meaning in life. Another way involves returning to studies of the stress process. Earlier, the way in which lifetime trauma may complicate the process of meaning making was discussed. However, there is some evidence that meaning is involved in the stress process in another way. More specifically, a small cluster of studies suggest that a sense of meaning in life may also be an important resource for buffering or offsetting the deleterious effects of stress on health in late life. The intellectual roots of this approach may be traced back to the work of Frankl (1984), who maintained that "suffering ceases to be suffering at the moment it finds meaning" (p. 135). But instead of arguing that meaning is merely one of several useful coping resources, Frankl (1984) went on to argue that it may be the most important resource of all: "There is nothing in the world, I would venture to say, that would so effectively help one survive even the worst of conditions as the knowledge that there is meaning in one's life" (p. 126). Consistent with these insights, an empirical study by Krause (2007a) reveals that a strong sense of meaning in life tends to offset the noxious effects of lifetime trauma on depressive symptoms among older people.

Even though the conceptual framework that was developed in this chapter is incomplete, it nevertheless provides a useful point of departure for approaching a literature that is underdeveloped and fractured into a number of different disciplinary perspectives. Including the work of investigators from diverse substantive backgrounds helped infuse the framework that was developed with a richness and depth that would have otherwise been impossible.

If Frankl (1984), Berger (1967), and Maslow (1968) are correct in arguing that the ability to derive a sense of meaning in life represents the high-water mark of human development, then many, if not most, of the biological, psychological, and sociological processes that researchers study should somehow contribute to the attainment of this ultimate goal. To the extent that this is true, it is then possible to chart a new and exciting research agenda. More specifically, researchers should look across diverse disciplines to show how the work in these fields feeds into and contributes to the development of a sense of meaning in life and the health-related outcomes that arise from it. Viewing meaning in this way helps revive the ambitions of the early social theorists, such as Auguste Comte (see Wernick, 2001) and Lester Ward (1883), who steadfastly maintained that the work of all sciences fits together and converges on a common end point. Unfortunately, the vision of these early social scientists was never fully realized because they failed to specify precisely how research in fields like the bench sciences and the social sciences can be merged to form a coherent whole. Although a number of different constructs may provide a strategic context for accomplishing this task, the goal of this chapter has been to show how a sense of meaning in life may function in this capacity. By highlighting the pivotal role that is played by meaning in this respect, it is hoped that investigators will be encouraged to delve more deeply into this core construct and explore the ways in which the findings from their own studies speak to the work of researchers in other fields.

References

Barrera, M. (1986). Distinctions between social support concepts, measures, and models. *American Journal of Community Psychology, 14,* 413–425.

Baumeister, R. F. (1991). *Meanings in life.* New York: Guilford.

Berger, P. L. (1967). *The sacred canopy: Elements of a sociological theory.* New York: Doubleday.

Berger, P. L., & Pullberg, S. (1965). Reification and sociological critique of consciousness. *History and Theory, 4,* 196–211.

Blalock, H. M. (1982). *Conceptualization and measurement in the social sciences.* Beverly Hills, CA: Sage.

Bower, J. E., Kemeny, M. E., Taylor, S. E., & Fahey, J. L. (2003). Finding positive meaning and its association with natural killer cell cytotoxicity among participants in a bereavement-related disclosure intervention. *Annals of Behavioral Medicine, 25,* 146–155.

Burleson, B. R., & Goldsmith, D. J. (1998). How the comforting process works: Alleviating emotional distress through conversationally induced reappraisals. In P. A. Andersen & L. K. Guerrero (Eds.), *Communication and emotion* (pp. 246–275). Orlando, FL: Academic Press.

Carrier, H. (1965). *The sociology of religious belonging.* New York: Herder and Herder.

Carstensen, L. L., Fung, H. H., & Charles, S. T. (2003). Socioemotional selectivity theory and the regulation of emotion in the second half of life. *Motivation and Emotion, 27,* 103–203.

Coyne, J. C., Wortman, C. B., & Lehman, D. R. (1988). The other side of support: Emotional overinvolvement and miscarried helping. In B. H. Gottlieb (Ed.), *Marshaling social support: Formats, processes, and effects* (pp. 305–350). Newbury Park, CA: Sage.

Debats, D. L. (1990). The Life Regard Index: Reliability and validity. *Psychological Reports, 67,* 27–34.

Debats, D. L. (1998). Measurement of personal meaning: The psychometric properties of the Life Regard Index. In P. T. P. Wong & P. S. Fry (Eds.), *The human quest for meaning* (pp. 237–259). Mahwah, NJ: Lawrence Erlbaum Associates.

Debats, D. L. (1999). Sources of meaning: An investigation of significant commitments in life. *Journal of Humanistic Psychology, 29,* 30–57.

Diener, E. (1984). Subjective well-being. *Psychological Bulletin, 95,* 542–575.

Eisenberg, E. M. (1998). Flirting with meaning. *Journal of Language and Social Psychology, 17,* 97–108.

Erikson, E. (1959). *Identity and the life cycle.* New York: International University Press.

Eysenck, H. (1998). *Dimensions of personality.* New Brunswick, NJ: Transaction.

Frankl, V. E. (1984). *Man's search for meaning.* New York: Washington Square Press. (Original work published 1946)

Halama, P. (2005). Relationship between meaning in life and the Big Five personality traits in young adults and the elderly. *Studia Psychologica, 47,* 167–178.

Herberman, R. B. (2002). Stress, natural killer cell activity, and cancer. In H. G. Koenig & H. J. Cohen (Eds.), *The link between religion and health: Psychoneuroimmunology and the faith factor* (pp. 69–83). New York: Oxford University Press.

James, W. (1961). *Psychology: The briefer course.* New York: Harper & Row. (Original work published 1892)

Jones, S. M., & Wirtz, J. G. (2006). How does the comforting process work? An empirical test of an appraisal-based model of comforting. *Human Communication Research, 32,* 217–243.

Jung, C. G. (1953). *C. G. Jung psychological reflections* (J. Jacobi & R. F. C. Hull, Eds.). Princeton, NJ: Princeton University Press.

Koltko-Rivera, M. E. (2006). Rediscovering the later version of Maslow's hierarchy of needs: Self-transcendence and opportunities for theory, research, and unification. *Review of General Psychology, 10,* 302–317.

Krause, N. (2003). Religious meaning and subjective well-being in late life. *Journal of Gerontology: Social Sciences, 58,* S160–S170.

Krause, N. (2004). Stressors in highly valued roles, meaning in life, and the physical health status of older adults. *Journal of Gerontology: Social Sciences, 59,* S287–S297.

Krause, N. (2005). Traumatic events and meaning in life: Exploring variations in three age cohorts. *Ageing & Society, 25,* 501–524.

Krause, N. (2007a). Evaluating the stress-buffering function of meaning in life among older people. *Journal of Aging and Health, 19,* 792–812.

Krause, N. (2007b). Longitudinal study of social support and meaning in life. *Psychology and Aging, 22,* 456–469.

Krause, N. (2008). The social foundations of religious meaning in life. *Research on Aging, 30*(4), 395–427.

Krause, N., & Borawski-Clark, E. (1994). Clarifying the functions of social support in late life. *Research on Aging, 16,* 251–279.

Krause, N., Liang, J., & Keith, V. M. (1990). Personality, social support, and psychological distress in later life. *Psychology and Aging, 5,* 315–326.

Krause, N., Shaw, B. A., & Cairney, J. (2004). A descriptive epidemiology of lifetime trauma and the physical health status of older adults. *Psychology and Aging, 19,* 637–648.

Maslow, A. H. (1968). *Toward a psychology of being.* New York: Van Nostrand.

McCrae, R. R., & Costa, P. T. (2003). *Personality in adulthood: A Five-Factor Theory perspective.* New York: Guilford.

Meredith, G. E., & Schewe, C. D. (2002). *Defining markets, defining moments.* New York: Hungry Minds, Inc.

Mroczek, D. K., Spiro, A., & Griffin, P. W. (2006). Personality and aging. In J. E. Birrin & K. W. Schaie (Eds.), *Handbook of the psychology of aging* (pp. 363–377). San Diego, CA: Academic Press.

Olson, J. M., Roese, N. J., & Zanna, M. P. (1996). Expectancies. In E. T. Higgins & A. W. Kruglanski (Eds.), *Social psychology: Handbook of basic principles* (pp. 211–238). New York: Guilford.

Parquart, M. (2002). Creating and maintaining purpose in life in old age: A meta-analysis. *Aging International, 27,* 90–114.

Reker, G. T. (2000). Theoretical perspectives, dimensions, and measurement of existential meaning. In G. T. Reker & K. Chamberlain (Eds.), *Exploring existential meaning: Optimizing human development across the life span* (pp. 39–55). Thousand Oaks, CA: Sage.

Reker, G. T., & Fry, P. S. (2003). Factor structure and invariance of personal meaning measures in cohorts of younger and older adults. *Personality and Individual Differences, 35,* 977–993.

Rook, K. S. (1984). The negative side of social interaction: Impact on psychological well-being. *Journal of Personality and Social Psychology, 46,* 1097–1108.

Rook, K. S., & Pietromonaco, P. (1987). Close relationships: Ties that heal or ties that bind? In W. H. Jones & D. Perlman (Eds.), *Advances in personal relationships* (pp. 1–35). Greenwich, CT: JAI Press.

Salovey, P., Rothman, A. J., Detweiler, J. B., & Steward, W. T. (2000). Emotion states and physical health. *American Psychologist, 55,* 110–121.

Schnell, T., & Becker, P. (2006). Personality and meaning in life. *Personality and Individual Differences, 41,* 117–129.

Schulz, R., & Heckhausen, J. (1996). A life span model of successful aging. *American Psychologist, 51,* 702–714.

Swickert, R. J., Rosentreter, C. J., Hittner, J. B., & Mushrush, J. E. (2002). Extraversion, social support processes, and stress. *Personality and Individual Differences, 32,* 877–891.

Tornstam, L. (2005). *Gerotranscendence: A developmental theory of positive aging.* New York: Springer Publishing.

Van Ranst, N., & Marcoen, A. (1997). Meaning in life of young and older adults: An examination of the factorial validity and invariance of the Life Regard Index. *Personality and Individual Differences, 22,* 877–884.

Ward, L. F. (1883). *Dynamic sociology or applied social science as based upon statistical sociology and the less complex sciences* (Vol. 1). New York: D. Appleton and Company.

Wernick, A. (2001). *Auguste Comte and the religion of humanity: The post-theistic program of French social theory.* New York: Cambridge University Press.

Wethington, E., & Kessler, R. C. (1986). Perceived support, received support, and adjustment to stressful life events. *Journal of Health and Social Behavior, 27,* 78–89.

Wheaton, B. (1994). Sampling the stress universe. In W. R. Avison & I. H. Gottlib (Eds.), *Stress and mental health: Contemporary issues and prospects for the future* (pp. 77–114). New York: Plenum Press.

7 Understanding Healthy Aging: Key Components and Their Integration

Carol D. Ryff
Burton Singer

The central premise of this chapter is that that there is no single fundamental cause of healthy aging but rather a multiplicity of factors working together to facilitate optimal functioning well into later life. Trying to understand the interplay among these multiple influences is a key scientific challenge in terms of both formulating guiding theory and executing and interpreting empirical studies. In what follows, we first offer a definition of healthy aging, framed at two different levels of analysis. We then delineate three broad categories of influence on healthy aging: social structural factors, individual-level factors, and biological factors. Each of these covers wide territories, and all have been shown to contribute to variation in how people age. We then set forth five guiding propositions that are intended to advance hypothesis-testing research on healthy aging as a *biopsychosocial process*. We conclude with recommended future directions for theory building and empirical research.

Healthy Aging: What Is It?

We define healthy aging at two different but parallel levels of analysis. At the level of basic biological processes, healthy aging can be defined as *fending off of cellular and molecular damage for the longest possible period of the life course.* This definition draws on impressive advances in the biology of aging, including the growing recognition that there is *no single cause* of biological aging per se but rather that it occurs via multiple mechanisms (e.g., free radical damage or DNA damage) (Finch, 2007) that themselves have become the focus of integrative science (Kirkwood, 2008; Kirkwood et al., 2003). Healthy aging research in humans could benefit from incorporating knowledge at this level, which is frequently conducted with animal models. However, our definition seeks to shift or at least augment the focus in this research toward the factors that *prevent or delay deleterious processes.* Doing so requires conceptualizations of and empirical measures for protective factors (internal or external to the organism) that work against processes of biological decline and deterioration.

At a more molar level of analysis involving biomedical processes and behavioral capacities, we define healthy aging as *the maximal delay of illness, disease, disability, and hence mortality.* In this realm, the overwhelming focus of scientific interest has been on factors that predict morbidity, disability, and mortality rather than the factors that keep the organism *functioning optimally for the longest period of time.* Here we note that optimal functioning is not equivalent to longevity per se because it requires maintenance of capacities needed for quality, not just length, of life. Multiple systems (neuroendocrine, inflammatory, metabolic, cardiovascular, and musculoskeletal) are likely implicated in this broad definition. The central question across these systems and their interplay is what factors contribute to maintenance of normal, healthy functioning? We maintain that many influences, including social structural and individual-level factors, are involved.

Both of the preceding definitions build on the fact that aging occurs at different rates for different organisms. It is this variation in timing, richly verifiable in both human and animal models, that affords great opportunities to advance knowledge of healthy aging. Doing so requires identification of the factors and mechanistic processes that enable some organisms to remain functional and without signs of biological wear and tear for lengthy periods of the life span. As people enter the later decades of life and chronic conditions begin to emerge, there is also the capacity to remain functional in the face of these changes. Importantly, many of the influences on how healthy aging unfolds do not occur in old age per se but rather begin in earlier decades, sometimes even in childhood. Thus, the task of understanding healthy aging demands a long-term perspective.

From a scientific perspective, we suggest that the focus on protective influences is brought into high empirical relief via *challenge paradigms*—that is, naturalistic or experimental studies that examine the organism under conditions of challenge, threat, or adversity while simultaneously seeking to identify factors that prevent the occurrence of damaging biological processes or promote rapid recovery from any losses incurred along the way. Considerable scientific strides in understanding healthy aging could follow from these kinds of inquiries.

We acknowledge that many in the field of aging have asked similar questions to those posed here. Indeed, efforts to formulate successful, healthy, optimal, productive, exceptional aging abound (e.g., Baltes & Baltes, 1990; Bond, Cutler, & Grams, 1995; Rowe & Kahn, 1987; Schulz & Heckhausen, 1996). Our guiding definitions of healthy aging strongly converge with the growing literature on centenarians and old-aged survival (e.g., Danner, Snowden, & Friesen, 2001; Poon, Bramlett, Holtzberg, Johnson, & Martin, 1996; Vaupel et al., 1998), which also concerns itself with the factors (biological, psychological, and sociological) that enable some to survive for remarkably longer periods of time than is the norm. At more basic levels of biological aging, we further note the remarkable advances occurring in the search for genes, signaling pathways, and stress-resistant processes that extend the life span in more simple organisms, such as *Caenorhabditis elegans* (Kenyon, 2006). That is, we make no claim to novelty in invoking the central questions of healthy aging around which much of the field of gerontology revolves. Rather, our objective is to promote an *integrative approach* to the task of understanding the causes, processes, and pathways of healthy aging given the growing evidence that factors at multiple levels of influence are involved. Such multiplicity requires guiding frameworks that conceptualize how these influences work together and from which testable propositions can be derived. In our view, integrative inquiry sits in contrast to much prevailing work, including well-orchestrated studies of single influences that seek to "control for" (experimentally or statistically) numerous extraneous factors. While contributing important advances, such approaches are inherently inadequate to the task of understanding healthy aging as an integrative process. Our sense is that many shy away from that task given its daunting complexity, but we consider it an unavoidable challenge in making progress toward understanding the conditions under which and for whom healthy aging occurs. In the following section, we begin this integrative journey by delineating broad levels of influence that make up the overarching formulation.

How Does Healthy Aging Come About? Contributing Influences

As stated previously, healthy aging is fundamentally a *biopsychosocial process* involving multiple contributing factors. How such multiplicity is organized could be accomplished in numerous ways (i.e., there is no single right way to depict the elements involved). We have chosen to partition the contributing factors into three broad categories on the grounds that they (a) provide links to prior disciplinary-specific theories of aging and (b) can be usefully illustrated with ongoing lines of empirical research. Here we seek to articulate what these influences are—to get our arms around the relevant scientific territory. We then examine what, if any, prior efforts have been made to conceptualize linkages across these levels of influence. For the most part, relevant empirical findings are not detailed here but rather are covered in a later section on guiding propositions and emerging evidence.

It is important to reiterate that the three levels of influence on healthy aging detailed here are operative *across the life span*. This necessitates examining temporally distal factors that may create early vulnerability or, alternatively, convey early resistance to later-life health problems. Adopting a life course approach also calls attention to the importance of *cumulative processes* whereby influences of adversity or advantage persist and accumulate over time (Hatch, 2005; O'Rand & Hamil-Luker, 2005).

Social Structural Influences

Social structural influences, existing outside the organism, refer to the surrounding social context, which can be characterized in terms of how resources and opportunities are allocated as well as what normative guidelines and behavioral expectations shape daily practices, including related socialization processes. This domain is the purview largely of sociology and related population-based disciplines (demography, epidemiology, and some aspects of economics). In empirical studies, social structural influences are frequently indexed by one's location in the social structure, defined by factors such as age, gender, socioeconomic status (educational attainment, income, and occupational status), race/ethnicity, and cultural context (e.g., Asian versus Western societies). Socialization mechanisms, although frequently included in theories about social structural influences, are less prominently employed as empirical indicators.

There is considerable evidence in humans that rates of morbidity, disability, and mortality vary across different social strata, indexed by the previously mentioned sociodemographic variables (e.g., Adler et al., 1994; Hayward, Crimmins, Miles, & Yu, 2000; House et al., 1994; Ross & Wu, 1996; Sapolsky, 2005; Smith, 1998; Williams & Wilson, 2001). Age of onset of disabilities and chronic conditions also shows important and systematic variation across social strata (Jagger et al., 2007; Matthews, Smith, Hancock, Jagger, & Spiers, 2005). Gender is also prominently implicated in healthy aging given that women have longer life expectancy despite having greater morbidity than men (Rieker & Bird, 2005). These observations are self-evident among those who work in the previously mentioned disciplines. What we are calling for, however, is greater recognition of the need to link such social structural factors to the two other levels of analysis—individual-level factors and biological factors—detailed next. Such bridge building is needed for the simple reason that social structure, while undeniably important in understanding healthy aging or, alternatively, who succumbs to early morbidity, disability, and mortality, cannot in itself fully account for outcomes of interest. Socioeconomic disparities, for example, constitute one influence among many in accounting for health outcomes. In this sense, the integrative agenda we are advancing is at odds with "fundamental cause" formulations of illness and disease (e.g., Phelan & Link, 2005). Although analyses can be generated to show that certain causes prevail after other causes have been "adjusted for," such inquiries fail to capture the complex interplay of antecedent influences and, most important, ignore the wide variation around the average story in the data (a point elaborated on in a later section on methodological and analytic issues). Stated otherwise, we strongly agree with those calling for more complex models that integrate biological and social explanations to account for differences in health (Rieker & Bird, 2005), and, further, we assert that many efforts to understand complex processes have been obscured by conventions focused on the mean rather than the variability in the data.

Not explicitly mentioned thus far is a further level of social context that is part of delineating environmental influences on healthy aging—namely, the neighborhoods and communities in which individuals live. These constitute important components in the ecology of human development (Bronfenbrenner, 1979; Sampson & Sharkey, 2008; Sampson, Sharkey, & Raudenbush, 2008), and they have increasingly been viewed as relevant to understanding social inequalities in health. That is, socioeconomic characteristics of neighborhoods (crime, pollution, and crowding on the negative side or social cohesion and availability of parks and grocery stores on the positive side) have consequences for health (e.g., Chen & Paterson, 2006; Feldman & Steptoe, 2004) and, as such, must be incorporated into an integrative approach.

Individual Influences (Psychosocial and Behavioral Factors)

Although "individual influences" could refer to any number of factors about the person, including biology, we employ the phrase here in a more circumscribed fashion to refer to psychosocial and behavioral factors. Much of this extremely wide territory is the purview of personality psychology (e.g., McAdams, 2006), which elaborates many characteristics of individuals, such as their enduring traits (e.g., neuroticism, extraversion, and conscientiousness); their goals, needs, strivings, and motivations; and their self-concepts, coping strategies, and profiles of well-being, distress, and emotion regulation. Writ large, this is the realm of "individual differences" in psychology. Also included at this level of analysis are social characteristics, such as the nature and extent of social ties with others (in contexts of family, work, and community), along with behavioral practices related to health (e.g., patterns of exercise, nutrition, smoking, and drinking).

Given the enormous scope of influences at the individual level, a central challenge in rendering this realm useful for healthy aging research is to formulate integrative conceptions that put these many characteristics of the person together. That is not to deny the merits of research focused on particular characteristics, such as individual differences in neuroticism or social support, and how such profiles change with aging and/or how they influence health (e.g., Gorman & Sivaganesan, 2007; Mroczek & Spiro, 2007). However, accompanying these valuable endeavors is the need for more holistic, integrative conceptions of persons, particularly in building bridges to biology. We note that although the field of personality research has traditionally disaggregated the person into a large array of traits, emotions, and motives, there is increasing emphasis on the need to put the pieces of the person together (see McAdams & Pals, 2006; Ryff, 2008). Similarly, in aging research, there is growing recognition of the need to create whole-person perspectives (Gerstorf, Smith, & Baltes, 2006; Singer & Ryff, 2001).

Such integrative endeavors are especially useful in health research for reasons paralleling the observation provided in the preceding section—namely, although single characteristics predict important outcomes, including morbidity and mortality, they never fully account for who lives or dies or for who is healthy or ill. This is because people are complex combinations of many psychosocial strengths and vulnerabilities. Although we are confronted with this reality in daily life, as observed in interactions with friends, family, and coworkers, its complexity has posed thorny challenges for empirical research. Some solutions have been forged by typological approaches (e.g., Robins, John, & Caspi, 1998; Shmotkin, 2005; Singer, Ryff, Carr, & Magee, 1998), while others have pursued integrative analyses via the use of recursive partitioning to generate *person-centered pathways* (i.e., combinations of co-occurring conditions) to particular outcomes (see Gruenewald, Seeman, Ryff, Karlamangla, & Singer, 2006; Gruenewald, Mroczek, Ryff, & Singer, 2008).

Biological Influences

Biological influences on healthy aging occur at molecular and cellular levels as well as at more molar levels of biological systems and their interplay. Our objective here is to distill essential features of biological aging, as currently understood, in order that this level of analysis can be better linked to the previously mentioned influences. We note at the outset that much of what is covered here is about unhealthy aging—that is, damaging and degenerative processes that account for why organisms do not survive indefinitely. Nonetheless, these constitute extremely valuable routes into research on factors that prevent and protect or promote repair and rejuvenation in relation to such deleterious processes.

A large evidential base shows that what drives the acceleration toward mortality occurring with increasing age is inflammatory and oxidative damage accumulated by long-lived molecules and cells that in turn promotes dysfunction in physiological systems (Finch, 2007). Such degenerative change results from agents acting both outside and within the organism. Extant views of external agents focus on infections and physical trauma, although drawing on the two preceding sections, we would advocate for a notably wider array of external influences (e.g., location in the social hierarchy and psychosocial experience). Internal agents include free radicals produced by macrophages in the host's immune system and, subcellularly, by mitochondria involved in normal metabolism. Importantly, later-life dysfunction of the vasculature, brain, and cell growth may be traced to subclinical inflammatory changes from early life, thus underscoring the need for attention to temporally distal antecedents.

Bystander events and bystander damage are important concepts in understanding how the degenerative processes work. Bystander events are passively incurred, meaning that long-lived molecules accumulate damage over time from chemical agents in their immediate fluid environment, particularly glucose and free radicals, such as reactive oxygen species. Bystander damage, a fundamental feature of aging, occurs when the rate of incident damage exceeds the rate of molecular repair by enzymes or by rejuvenation from new molecular synthesis with turnover of an old molecule. At a different level, this might be likened to a time–dose relationship in epidemiology, such as pack years of exposure to tobacco smoke, which becomes a source of bystander damage to lung tissue that eventually culminates in lung cancer and possibly death.

Four primary types of bystander damage have been identified in the contemporary aging literature (Cho, Zhang, & Kleeberger, 2001; Dai et al., 2004;

Finch, 2007; Lakatta, 2003): (a) free radical damage, which is intensified by inflammation and attenuated by dietary restriction; (b) glyco-oxidation of proteins and DNA, which occurs by spontaneous reaction with sugars that are omnipresent in extracellular fluids; (c) chronic cell proliferation, which can be stimulated by inflammation and oxidative stress; and (d) mechanical trauma, which accumulates through accidents, wear and tear, and violence consequential to predation and social conflict.

In contrast to bystander damage, two other types of molecular aging changes must be considered: spontaneous conversion of L-amino acids from one form to another (racemization) and template errors in DNA synthesis. These molecular aging changes are less dependent on the immediate environment than bystander changes and occur at irreducible rates that may be considered "intrinsic aging." In particular, racemization of amino acids is an intrinsic feature of molecular instability and would occur in pure water. Mutations and others errors in DNA replication, transcription, and translation are inevitable because enzymes have intrinsic and irreducible errors in templating.

Without elaborating on the details, it can be said that in most chronic diseases of aging, oxidative stress and inflammation play prominent roles. It is also the case that many tissues not showing specific pathology nonetheless show modest inflammatory changes with aging. The substantial upward trends with increasing age in blood inflammatory markers, such as C-reactive protein and interleukin-6 (IL-6) (Finch, 2007), may be driven by vascular disease, although there is considerable evidence for the role of inflammation in degenerative neurological disorders (Schmidt et al., 2002). In the main, however, the general mechanisms of biological aging can be resolved as involving three interacting processes: (a) oxidative damage and inflammation, (b) damage to irreplaceable molecules and cells, and (c) physiological set points for food intake, locomotor activity, and blood metabolic hormones.

Linkages between immune and other biological systems must also be considered, such as the considerable literature on neuroendocrine systems as pacemakers of aging (Finch & Rose, 1995; Finch & Ruvkun, 2001). Also relevant are heavily documented pathways of communication between the neuroendocrine and immune systems, including signaling between the brain and the periphery (Besedovsky & Del Ray, 1996; Dhabhar & McEwen, 2001; Maier & Watkins, 1998; Sapolsky, Romero, & Munck, 2000), that clarify how, starting from the brain as the initial responder to external stimuli, linkages might be established between psychosocial factors and biological aspects of aging.

Returning to the theme of healthy aging per se, a central challenge is to understand the relative magnitude of the "forces of damage," by which cells age, compared to the "forces of prevention and repair," by which the process is slowed. The search for genes that extend the life span (Hsin & Kenyon, 1999) has made clear that functionally significant genes turned on in long-lived mutants, in fact, prevent or repair damage (Kenyon, 2006). Also relevant are DNA repair mechanisms (Hoeijmakers, 2001; Loizidou et al., 2008; Sancar, Lindsey-Boltz, Unsal-Kacmaz, & Linn, 2004), which are dependent on many factors, including cell type, age of cell, and extracellular environment. For example, the behavior of many genes involved in DNA repair is altered favorably under caloric restriction (Lopez-Torres, Grecilla, Sanz, & Barja, 2002). Other instances of repair and rejuvenation processes pertain to endothelial apoptosis (programmed cell death) (Conti et al., 2004), where it has been determined that insulin-like growth factor (IGF-1) strongly promotes survival of vascular smooth muscle cells. That is, high plasma IGF-1 is cardioprotective through increasingly understood mechanistic pathways. As described in later sections, many of these processes (e.g., inflammation, oxidative stress, and IGF-1) are increasingly studied in humans and, more important, are being connected to both psychosocial factors and social structural influences (socioeconomic standing). Thus, it is not far-fetched to anticipate ever more detailed quantitative specifications of causal pathways that contribute to the maintenance of good health via promotion of effective physiological functioning that is rooted in basic biological processes, some of which are shaped by inputs at these other levels of analysis.

Conceptualizing Linkages Across Levels of Influence

The field of aging has a history of attempts to connect the first two of the three previously mentioned levels of influence—namely, how societal factors and individual influences come together. Disengagement theory (Cumming & Henry, 1961), arguably the first theory in social gerontology, postulated that with aging there is a mutual severing of ties between the individual and society. The individual's withdrawal, manifest by the giving up of social roles and responsibilities, was purportedly good for society because it opened up roles for younger individuals but was also good for the older person by helping in the preparation for mortality. Empirical translations and tests of the theory were not extensive, although it prompted vigorous debate, including advocacy for alternative conceptions, such as activity theory, which, as the name suggested, defined positive aging in terms of remaining actively engaged in significant roles.

Later formulations continued to articulate how social structures impinge on the lives of aging individuals. The social breakdown syndrome (Kuypers & Bengtson, 1973) focused on shrinkage of social roles and reference groups that accompany old age as well as the presence of negative behavioral expectations. These were hypothesized to lead to negative self-attitudes and, ultimately, a reduced sense of competence among the elderly. How such processes bear on physical health was also considered (Heidrich & Ryff, 1993a). Another conception, the structural lag hypothesis (Riley, Kahn, & Foner, 1994), emphasized that social institutional structures lag behind the added years of life that many people now experience, thereby prompting diminished opportunities for continued productivity and meaningful life engagement among the elderly. Documented age differences in psychological well-being, particularly downward trajectories of purpose in life and personal growth among the elderly, are consistent with the structural lag formulation (Ryff & Singer, 2008).

Outside the aging field were other notable efforts to join individual and societal levels of analysis, such as the tradition of research on personality and social structure (House, 1981; Inkeles, 1959; Smelser & Smelser, 1970). Broad objectives of this work were to link characteristics of the individual (e.g., values, attitudes, beliefs, and needs) to aspects of the social structure (e.g., roles, norms, organizational features, and socialization processes). In the main, these efforts were limited for not being strongly empirical and for failing to explicate how and why relationships between individuals and society come about (House, 1981; Ryff, 1987; Ryff, Marshall, & Clarke, 1999).

Little if any prior work on individual–societal linkages has involved biology or even health. That is, by far the most neglected territory in biopsychosocial aging is in conceptualizing and testing linkages between the social structural–level and/or individual-level influences and biological factors (molecular or biomedical) (for efforts to link demographic behavior to biological levels of analysis, see Hobcraft, 2006). We underscore this omission in research of the biology of aging as well. That is, while overarching conceptual frameworks frequently include formulations of the "external environment" (Finch, 2007; Kirkwood, 2008), this is rarely explicated. By far, it is the most undeveloped part of integrative biological models. Thus, studies of core mechanisms that contribute to aging decline and deterioration could be greatly enriched by consideration of social organizational features of surrounding environment (e.g., dominance hierarchies; see Sapolsky, 2005) and even "individual differences" among animals (e.g., variability in reactivity to stress, a characteristic that can be richly manipulated in animal studies; see Liu et al., 1997). Doing so would greatly facilitate parallels with the human studies while simultaneously advancing comprehensive, multi-influence approaches to healthy aging.

Studying the Organism Under Challenge

We offer a further observation about the conditions under which the three previously mentioned influences are fruitfully investigated—namely, studying the organism (animal and human via experimental or naturalistic designs) *under conditions of challenge*. By this, we mean probing the impact of external threats, stressors, or cumulative adversity on the interplay of these three levels of influence. Challenge comes in many varieties: some following from social inequality and related discrepancies in opportunities to get ahead in life and others reflecting proximal role demands, such as responsibilities of caregiving for a loved one or conflict between work and family commitments. Loss events (death and unemployment) constitute other categories, as do natural disasters and major societal challenges (wars and economic depressions). Stress can also be construed in interpersonal terms, such as perceiving oneself as the target of discriminatory, unfair treatment by others. This multiplicity of stressors is increasingly studied in terms of implications for biology, such as regulation of the hypothalamic–pituitary–adrenal (HPA) axis (Miller, Chen, & Zhou, 2007).

External stressors are also extensively invoked in studies of biological aging with animal models. Stressors in those investigations also come in multiple varieties, such as dietary restriction paradigms, forced swimming, water immersion, intermittent electric shocks, and restraint stress. Experimental manipulation of stress is not, however, an exclusive purview of animal studies. It is also prominently used in human research, such as studies involving cognitive stress (e.g., math or memory tasks) or social stress (e.g., public speaking) and their effects on HPA activity (see Miller et al., 2007).

The reason we advocate for challenge paradigms in research on healthy aging is that such designs afford sharper tests of a key element in the integrative formulation, particularly the proposition that positive psychosocial factors are protective of good health. That is, good-quality social relationships and high life purpose are hypothesized to contribute to healthy aging via their contributions to maintaining and regulating biological systems. The condition under which these influences are most usefully investigated is when the individual or animal is confronted with challenge. Stated otherwise, protective psychosocial influences are thought to exert their beneficial effects particularly in the confrontation with challenge.

Healthy Aging as an Integrative Process: Testable Propositions and Emerging Evidence

Because this chapter is written for a collection on aging theories, we organize this section around *guiding propositions* that will usefully advance scientific knowledge of healthy aging. These do not constitute an integrative theory per se, but they do move the research toward hypothesis-testing inquiries about how multiple levels of influence come together to promote or undermine healthy aging. We present five such propositions and in each examine relevant extant empirical findings. The first pertains to *health promotion processes* and asserts that positive psychosocial factors contribute to better biological regulation. This is a testable hypothesis for which we summarize growing empirical evidence. The second proposition pertains to *resilience processes* and asserts that positive psychosocial factors protect against damaging health effects (including at the cellular and molecular levels) ensuing from external challenge (adverse events). Although increasingly studied in early and later life, such resilience investigations rarely include biology, despite growing interest in the neurobiological mechanisms that underlie it. One example ripe for greater empirical study involves those at the low end of the socioeconomic hierarchy who show strong profiles of psychosocial strengths. Whether these factors afford protection against damaging neurobiological processes is an important empirical question.

The third proposition pertains to *recovery and repair processes* and asserts that when health damage has occurred (e.g., heart attack at the biomedical level or oxidative stress at the cellular level), those with better psychosocial or behavioral strengths will recover more quickly and/or more completely. Thus, this proposition is about mechanistic processes that facilitate the regaining of lost or compromised capacities. The fourth proposition addresses *compensation processes* and asserts that liabilities in one realm (e.g., neuroticism at the psychosocial level or elevated cortisol levels at the neuroendocrine level) can be offset by strengths at the same level (e.g., extraversion modulates the negative impact of neuroticism, and high dehydroepiandrosterone [DHEA] helps down-regulate cortisol) or at a different level (e.g., the negative influence of poor sleep on inflammatory processes is offset by having good quality social relationships). Compensation processes are thus about the interplay (interactions) among different factors and levels of influence on health. We provide multiple empirical examples and call for greater ways in which strengths/assets offset vulnerabilities/weaknesses.

Our last proposition pertains to *gene expression processes,* which are fundamentally about transactions with environmental inputs. Here we distinguish between two types of influence, one having to do with environments that *prevent* the expression of genetic markers for disease or dysfunction and the other involving environments that *promote* the expression of genetic markers for healthy biological regulation and longevity. Both have received limited attention and are particularly promising realms for future integrative inquiries.

Proposition 1. Health Promotion Processes: Positive Psychosocial Factors Predict Better Biological Regulation

Some years ago, we called for a reformulation of human health as the presence of well-being or flourishing (Ryff & Singer, 1998) and asked what physiological substrates underlie positive psychosocial functioning. That is, we proposed that studying well-being at psychological and social levels could provide an alternative to medical models of health, which are fundamentally about illness, disease, and disability. True understanding of "positive health," we claimed, required a different starting point—namely, assessment of multiple aspects of well-being (e.g., positive relations with others, purpose in life, and environmental mastery) in people's lives and then probing the neural circuitry and physiological systems that underlie these psychosocial strengths.

A growing empirical literature now documents that those with higher levels of well-being show better health and better biological regulation. Positive affect (feeling happy and contented), for example, has been linked with lower morbidity, decreased health symptoms and pain, and increased longevity (Pressman & Cohen, 2005), resistance to illness (Cohen, Alpen, Doyle, Treanor, & Turner, 2006), decreased stroke incidence (Ostir, Markides, Peek, & Goodwin, 2001; Ostir, Raji, & Ottenbacher, 2003), and better glycemic control (Feldman & Steptoe, 2003; Tsenkova, Love, Singer, & Ryff, 2008). Measures of happiness obtained several times over the course of the workday have also been linked with lower ambulatory systolic blood pressure, lower ambulatory heart rate, and reduced fibrinogen stress responses (Steptoe & Wardle, 2005) as well as lower salivary cortisol and lower blood pressure response to laboratory stressors (Steptoe, Gibson, Hamer, & Wardle, 2006).

The previously mentioned "hedonic" aspects of well-being have been contrasted with "eudaimonic" components, which assess people's engagement in life and their sense of self-realization (Keyes, Shmotkin, & Ryff, 2002; Ryan & Deci, 2001; Ryff, 1989). Data from older women have shown that those with higher levels of eudaimonic well-being, such as purpose in life, personal growth, and positive relations with others, show lower cardiovascular risk (lower glycosylated hemoglobin, lower weight, lower waist-to-hip ratios, and higher high-density-lipoprotein cholesterol) as well as better neuroendocrine regulation (lower salivary cortisol throughout the day) (Ryff, Singer, & Love, 2004; Ryff et al., 2006). The latter finding was also obtained by Lindfors and Lundberg (2002). Higher profiles on positive relations with others and purpose in life have also been linked with lower inflammatory factors—IL-6 and its soluble receptor (sIL-6r) (Friedman, Hayney, Love, Singer, & Ryff, 2005; Friedman,

Hayney, Love, Singer, & Ryff, 2007). Quality interpersonal ties to others and their related emotions have been prominent psychosocial factors in building bridges to health (Ryff & Singer, 2000, 2001).

Research on affective neuroscience has also linked positive psychological characteristics with the brain. For example, well-being has been linked with asymmetric activation of the prefrontal cortex—specifically, greater left than right prefrontal activation was associated with higher levels of both hedonic and eudaimonic well-being (Urry et al., 2004), although it was only with eudaimonic well-being that the link to electroencephalographic asymmetry persisted after adjusting for hedonic well-being (i.e., the reverse was not true). Using functional magnetic resonance imaging, van Reekum et al. (2007) also showed that those with higher eudaimonic well-being effectively recruited the ventral anterior cingulate cortex when confronted with aversive laboratory stimuli and also showed reduced amygdala activity.

Health behaviors, such as exercise, are also relevant in positive health promotion via multiple biological pathways. For example, intensive-training exercise raises serum IGF-1, which has been increasingly documented as vascular protective (Conti et al., 2004; Finch, 2007). In prospective studies, higher IGF-1 levels have been shown to protect against heart disease, even after adjusting for body mass index, smoking, cholesterolemia, menopause, alcohol intake, physical activity, sex, age, social class, previous diabetes, family history of ischemic heart disease, self-rated health, use of antihypertensive agents, and circulating IGFBP-3 levels (which lower IGF-1 bioavailability) (Juul et al., 2002; Kloner & Jennings, 2001; Laughlin, Barrett-Connor, & Criqui, 2004). As such, in addition to assessing conventional cardiovascular risk factors, future studies would wisely include circulating IGF-1 levels (Rosen & Pollak, 1999). This is because elevated levels of the usual risk factors accompanying high levels of IGF-1 may be protective against heart disease (Conti et al., 2004). Further evidence about the importance of this biological pathway derives from the fact that healthy centenarians have high serum IGF-1 concentrations.

Regarding links with psychosocial factors, we note a recent study of a randomly selected nondisease population in Sweden that showed consistent age-related IGF-1 concentrations in both men and women that accompanied different association patterns relative to disease risk (Unden, Elofsson, Knox, Lewitt, & Brismar, 2002). In the younger age-group (20 to 44), there were positive correlations between IGF-1 and quality of life and well-being indicators. In the middle age-group (45 to 59), higher IGF-1 levels were related to better physical health, higher education, and higher concentrations of lipoprotein Lp(a). In the older age-group (59 and older), higher levels of low-density-lipoprotein cholesterol and lower levels of sex hormone–binding globulin were associated with higher levels of IGF-1. Viewed in life course perspective, high quality of life and well-being at younger ages may help to maintain higher IGF-1 levels in subsequent years and thereby prevent or delay potential vascular disease problems at older ages (Carter, Ramsey, & Sonntag, 2002).

Taken together, the previously mentioned studies document the biological underpinnings of positive psychosocial and behavioral influences. The general direction of findings is that strengths at the individual level help keep biological systems in normally functioning zones, although much is still unknown both about the pervasiveness of these effects and about how they come about (underlying mechanisms). The extent to which the nexus of positive psychosocial factors and healthy biological regulation prevents the emergence of disease processes is largely uncharted territory.

Proposition 2. Resilience Processes: Positive Psychosocial Factors Protect Against the Damaging Effects of External Adversity

Studies of the organism under challenge, which come in many varieties, bring into high relief the hypothesized *protective features* of psychosocial strengths—that is, do they help maintain good health (from molecular to molar levels) in the confrontation with adversity? Here we briefly describe research on resilience in both early and later life. This work clearly documents that many individuals do not succumb to maladjustment or illness and disease in the face of major challenges. However, little is known about underlying neurobiological mechanisms and processes.

We have previously reviewed studies of resilience in childhood and later life (Ryff & Singer, 2002; Ryff, Singer, Love, & Essex, 1998). The former include studies of children growing up under severe poverty or in negative family environments (parental psychopathology or discord) who nonetheless are competent, confident, and caring as judged by their teachers, peers, and school records. Protective factors in this literature have included personality attributes, intellectual abilities, and external social supports (Luthar, Cicchetti, & Becker, 2000; Masten, 1999). Biology is largely nonexistent in such investigations.

At the other end of the life span, there has been considerable emphasis on older persons' reserve capacity, defined as the potential for change and especially continued growth (Staudinger, Marsiske, & Baltes, 1995) with related assessment of positive psychological functioning in multiple domains (cognition, self, and social transactions) but limited assessment of actual life challenges. In both childhood and adulthood, resilience has also been viewed as a personality type (e.g., Klohnen, 1996; Robins, John, Caspi, Moffitt, & Stouthamer-Loeber, 1996). Our studies have formulated resilience as the capacity to maintain or regain high levels of well-being in the face of life challenges or transitions, such as caregiving and community relocation (Kling, Seltzer, & Ryff, 1997; Kwan, Love, Ryff, & Essex, 2003), recovering from major depression (Singer et al., 1998), or dealing with increased chronic conditions that accompany aging (Heidrich & Ryff, 1993b).

How psychological resilience in relation to challenge is linked to biology is a much-needed direction to add to the previously mentioned research. Here we note the work of Charney (2004), who has elaborated mechanisms of resilience at psychobiological levels—specifically delineating 11 neurochemical response patterns to acute stress (i.e., cortisol, DHEA, corticotropin-releasing hormone, locus coeruleus–norepinephrine system, neuropeptide Y, galanin, dopamine, serotonin [5-HT], benzodiazepine receptors, testosterone, and estrogen). While many of these have been associated with psychopathology, Charney connects them to neural mechanisms of reward and motivation processes (hedonia, optimism, and learned helplessness), fear responsiveness (effective behaviors despite fear), and adaptive social behavior (altruism, bonding, and teamwork), all relevant characteristics of resilience.

The work of Dienstbier (1989) on "physiological toughness" is also relevant for understanding, at a mechanistic level, a pattern of arousal that works in combination with effective psychological coping to comprise positive physiological reactivity. This involves low sympathetic nervous system (SNS) arousal base rates combined with strong, challenge-induced SNS–adrenal–medullary arousal, with resistance to brain catecholamine depletion and suppression of pituitary adrenal–cortical responses. Probing the connections between these patterns and psychosocial strengths in the face of adversity is an excellent future direction for resilience research.

In humans, one promising direction pertains to the large and growing literature on social inequalities in health, which has extensively documented that lower socioeconomic standing contributes to greater risk of illness, disease, and disability and earlier mortality (Adler, Marmot, McEwen, & Stewart, 1999; Alwin & Wray, 2005; House et al., 1994; Kawachi, Kennedy, & Wilkinson, 1999; Lantz et al., 2001; Marmot & Wilkinson, 1999; Preston & Taubman, 1994; Ross & Mirowsky, 1999). Important progress is also afoot in identifying the biological pathways through which these effects occur, such as heightened cardiovascular risk, elevated neuroendocrine activity, increased inflammatory processes, and poorer bone health (Bacon & Hadden, 2000; Brunner et al., 1997; Dyer et al., 1999; Karlamangla et al., 2005; Lupien, King, Meaney, & McEwen, 2001; Lynch, Kaplan, Cohen, Tuomilehto, & Salonen, 1996; Steptoe, Owen, Kunz-Ebrecht, & Mohamed-Ali, 2002). Many of these same biological risk factors, we note, have also been linked with poorer psychosocial functioning.

Notwithstanding such important strides in social inequalities research, we draw attention to the great variability *within* socioeconomic strata. In fact, in our analyses, psychological well-being factors show predicted downward trajectories when comparing higher versus lower educational groups (Ryff & Singer, 2008). However, in many instances, the within-grade variability is actually greater than the between-grade variability. This observation is relevant for resilience research and would advance understanding of social inequalities and *health (not illness)*. It requires attending to the psychosocial strengths among subgroups of the socioeconomically disadvantaged (see Markus, Ryff, Curhan, & Palmersheim, 2004), along with recognition that psychological advantage does not always accrue to privileged segments of society (Ryff, Keyes, & Hughes, 2003). More important, it requires linking these psychosocial strengths to biological processes to assess whether they afford protective benefits.

Our work has begun to address these questions. Emphasizing the importance of cumulative, long-term processes, we have shown, for example, that those with persistently low socioeconomic standing from childhood to adulthood had greater likelihood of biological wear and tear (high allostatic load) compared to those with persistent economic advantage. However, the more important finding was that this negative effect was *not* evident among those with persistently positive social relationships across time (Singer & Ryff, 1999). More recently, we have shown that persistently high psychological well-being over time shows as prominent a gradient in health as do differences in educational attainment (Ryff, Radler, & Singer, 2008). That is, persistent psychological strengths are linked with better health (better subjective health, fewer chronic conditions, and fewer health symptoms), even among those with low educational status. Probing the biological and neurological concomitants of these profiles is part of our ongoing inquiry.

Proposition 3. Recovery and Repair Processes: Positive Psychosocial Factors Facilitate the Regaining of Functional and/or Biological Capacities

At the human level, psychosocial resources have been studied for their influence on recovery processes. For example, mounting evidence points to the importance of optimism and hope in the face of health challenges (Scheier & Carver, 1992; Taylor, Kemeny, Reed, Bower, & Gruenewald, 2000). Positive expectations have been shown to predict better health after heart transplantation (Leedham, Meyerowitz, Muirhead, & Frist, 1995), and optimists have also been shown to have quicker recovery from coronary bypass surgery and have less severe anginal pain than pessimists (Fitzgerald, Tennen, Affleck, & Pransky, 1993). In men who are positive for human immunodeficiency virus (HIV), those who were asymptomatic and did not have negative expectations showed less likelihood of symptom development during follow-up (Reed, Kemeny, Taylor, Wang, & Visscher, 1994). Importantly, HIV-positive men with unrealistically optimistic beliefs about their own survival actually lived longer (Reed et al., 1994). Social support and emotional expression have also been linked with longer survival times among women with breast cancer (Spiegel, Sephton, Terr, & Stites, 1998) as well as with survival after myocardial infarction, even after controlling for severity of disease, comorbidity, and functional status (Berkman, Leo-Summers, & Horwitz, 1992).

At the biological level, further examples of repair processes are related to DNA damage. In human cells, both normal metabolic activities and environmental factors such as ultraviolet light can cause DNA damage resulting in as many as 1 million individual molecular lesions per cell per day. Many of these lesions cause structural damage to the DNA molecule and thereby alter or eliminate the cell's ability to transcribe the gene that the affected DNA encodes. Other lesions induce potentially harmful mutations in the cell's genome that affect the survival of its daughter cells after it undergoes mitosis. DNA repair, in turn, refers to a collection of processes by which a cell identifies and corrects damage to the DNA molecules that encode its genome. The rate of DNA repair is dependent on many factors, including the cell type, the age of the cell, and the extracellular environment. A cell that has accumulated a large amount of DNA damage or one that no longer repairs damage incurred to its DNA can enter one of three possible states: (a) an irreversible state of dormancy (senescence), (b) cell suicide (apoptosis or programmed cell death), and (c) unregulated cell division, which can lead to the formation of a cancerous tumor.

Although limited evidence to date links psychosocial and behavioral factors to DNA damage and repair, studies of this nature have begun to emerge (Gidron, Russ, Tissarchondou, & Warner, 2006). For example, Irie, Asami, Nagata, Miyata, and Kasai (2002) found an association between poor relationships with parents and DNA damage. It is possible that the sympatho–adrenal–medullary axis may mediate the effects of stress on DNA damage if activated for a long period. That is, psychological factors may lead to DNA damage via sympathetic induction of oxidative stress. For example, factors such as hostility can increase levels of norepinephrine (Malarkey, Kiecolt-Glaser, Pearl, & Glaser, 1994), and norepinephrine can induce DNA damage, causing oxidative stress (Okamoto et al., 1996). Notably lacking in consideration of these processes is the positive side of psychosocial experience and its possible roles in promoting DNA repair. This is a research frontier particularly in need of development.

It is also worth noting the link between caloric restriction, a phenomenon implicated in increased life span, and the rate of base excision repair in the nuclear DNA of rodents (Finch, 2007). If the behavior of many genes involved in DNA repair is altered (favorably) under caloric restriction, it raises important questions about caloric restriction at the human level. We would submit that many of the critical questions in this realm are psychosocial in nature. That is, if caloric restriction or even weight loss among those who are overweight (a growing segment of the population) is health promoting, we must examine why so few practice such behaviors. Presumably, this requires attending to the hedonic consequences of food, to say nothing of the extent to which meals, for many, are social relational experiences. Reducing food intake to a level at which persistent hunger is present and for which food-related social interaction is greatly diminished may substantially compromise whatever benefits of DNA repair and extended longevity that caloric restriction might afford for humans.

Proposition 4. Compensation Processes: Psychological or Biological Strengths Can Offset the Negative Consequences of Psychological or Biological Weaknesses

Ideas of compensation are particularly relevant in studying the interplay of psychosocial factors on healthy aging. Because people are complex combinations of many traits, coping strategies, affective styles, and the like, there can be instances wherein an otherwise negative vulnerability factor can be minimized or offset by the presence of a protective factor. Such compensation processes are fundamentally about the *interplay* among positive and negative psychosocial factors (although they may be relevant for interplay between positive and negative biological factors as well). Such effects in human studies are typically illustrated via moderating influences (i.e., interaction terms in statistical analyses). We note that researchers of aging have also been interested in compensation, primarily as it relates to managing age-related psychological losses and deficits (e.g., Dixon & Bäckman, 1995; Freund & Baltes, 2002).

We provide several examples from our prior research on healthy aging, some involving biological assessments as well. For example, in predicting inflammatory processes (IL-6) among older women, we have documented the importance of behavioral influences (i.e., sleep efficiency) and psychosocial influences (i.e., positive relationships with others)—those with the highest IL-6 levels were women with both poor sleep efficiency and poor social relationships (Friedman et al., 2005). However, the findings also revealed compensation processes. That is, lower levels of IL-6 were also observed among older women with poor sleep but good relationships as well as among those with poor relationships but good sleep profiles.

In predicting glycosylated hemoglobin (HbAlc, a marker for diabetes) in older women, we also found that positive affect moderated the effects of problem-focused coping strategies on *cross-time changes* in HbAlc (after controlling for sociodemographic and health factors). The interplay in this instance did not show compensatory influences, however, but rather amplification of the negative: namely, the degree to which poor coping strategies predicted greater increments in HbAlc was heightened among older women who also had low levels of positive affect (Tsenkova et al., 2008).

Shifting to the prediction of psychological outcomes, we have also shown that personality traits interact to predict well-being and distress following later-life relocation (Bardi & Ryff, 2007). For example, although high openness to experience amplified the negative effects of neuroticism on postmove well-being, high agreeableness and conscientiousness were found to reduce postmove distress but only among women who were low on extraversion, thus suggesting possible compensatory processes. Using data from the MIDUS (Midlife in the United States), we have further shown the interplay of traits (e.g., neuroticism and extraversion) and sociodemographic factors in predicting different levels of positive and negative affect among three age-groups of adults (Gruenewald et al., 2008). Numerous patterns of amplification and compensation were evident among these interacting influences (e.g., for some, neuroticism's negative effects were amplified by also having low extraversion profiles, while for others, good marital or partner relationships offset neuroticism's negative influence). Also demonstrated with data from MIDUS is the finding that sense of control moderates the effects of socioeconomic standing on health and well-being (Lachman & Weaver, 1998)—that is, low-income respondents with a high sense of control reported levels of health and well-being comparable to high-income respondents. These results represent but a limited subset of like findings in aging research. They constitute important future directions for advancing knowledge of healthy aging.

We would also note that compensation processes are relevant at the level of DNA repair where there is evidence of detection mechanisms (damage screens) operating around the genome that identify damage very quickly and then proceed to carry out repair. Protection from sources of damage should facilitate longer spans of healthy life, as trouble occurs only when the damage rate (and extent) is sufficiently high that it overwhelms the repair processes. Sancar et al. (2004) present an informative review of DNA repair mechanisms, although a precise linkage to psychosocial and social structural environments via the neuroendocrine and immune systems remains to be elucidated.

Proposition 5. Gene Expression Processes: Psychosocial Factors as Mitigating Against the Negative and Promoting the Positive

Most of what we have covered in this chapter is not about genetic influences, although they are obviously central to understanding healthy aging. We offer observations in this realm having to do with environmentally induced gene expression and the growing focus on gene–environment interactions (behavioral and molecular) for diverse mental and physical health outcomes (e.g., Moffitt,

Caspi, & Rutter, 2006). Because nearly all of current genomic science is focused on genetic influences on disease, we also underscore the need for genetic studies of health, even in the face of known genetic and/or environmental risk factors.

One route to healthy aging might involve psychosocial environments that *prevent the expression of genetic markers of disease.* We previously conducted a review of several disease outcomes for which there are known markers to make the point that many people with genetic susceptibility never actually develop the disease (Ryff & Singer, 2005). For example, and pertinent to aging, the risk for Alzheimer's disease among carriers of the apolipoprotein E gene diminishes sharply after age 85 (Finch & Kirkwood, 2000)—thus, centenarians appear to have genetic and/or environmental protective factors that are yet to be identified. We called for focused attention on enriched environments, especially social environments, to illuminate whether positive psychosocial influences could prevent the development of disease phenotypes.

Work with animal models (rats) shows how maternal behavior programs the expression of genes that regulate neuroendocrine responses to stress in their offspring (Caldji et al., 1998; Francis, Champagne, Liu & Meaney, 1999; Francis, Diorio, Liu, & Meaney, 1999; Liu et al., 1997; Meaney & Szyf, 2005; Szyf, McGowan, & Meaney, 2008). Specifically, mothers showing limited licking and grooming as well as arched-back nursing produce offspring who are more fearful as adults and who show numerous signs of elevated reactivity to stress (e.g., increased corticotrophin-releasing factor receptor levels in the locus ceruleus, decreased benzodiazepine receptors in the amygdala, and increased levels of norepinephrine in the paraventricular nucleus of the hypothalamus). More important, cross-fostering paradigms demonstrate the plasticity of these effects—namely, that genetically determined trajectories can be modified by new environmental signals. Offspring from the previously mentioned mothers show behavioral and biological stress responses that are indistinguishable from offspring of high licking/grooming and arched-back nursing mothers when they have been cross-fostered by mothers showing the same high licking/grooming and arched-back nursing behaviors (Francis, Champagne et al., 1999; Francis, Diorio et al., 1999).

Recently, Szyf et al. (2008) have proposed a theory in which the genome is programmed by the epigenome, which consists of chromatin and its modification by methylation of cytosine rings found at the dinucleotide sequence CG (Razin, 1998). In this formulation, the social environment gets "under the skin" when perceptions of it fire signaling pathways in the brain that in turn activate sequence specific factors that target the class of proteins known as histone acetyltransferases—a class of proteins that includes many known transcription factors—to specific sites facilitating DNA demethylation. Thus, the relationship between chromatin state and DNA methylation forms a molecular link through which environmental signals alter DNA methylation in specific genes in post-mitotic neurons.

The basic idea is that the epigenome, triggered by signaling pathways in the brain that are activated by environmental inputs, determines the accessibility of the transcription machinery, which, in turn, transcribes the genes into messenger RNA. The important point is that the fate of a gene is determined not by the DNA sequence per se but also by the manner in which the gene is marked and programmed by chromatin modification, DNA methylation, and noncoding RNA. This means that a change in gene programming by chromatin could have the same impact as a genetic polymorphism (which gets the lion's share of current scientific attention), leading to either enhancing or silencing of gene expression. Empirical support for the Szyf et al. (2008) framework is almost entirely grounded in animal studies. The analogues of the licker/groomer rat studies mentioned previously play heavily in the social environment–epigenome formulation and have, thus far, no counterparts in human studies.

In considering these genetic influences on healthy aging, our central objective is to bring the psychosocial environment into play. Such inquiry is in progress, as illustrated by studies of social environments and stress working in interaction with genetic polymorphisms to predict antisocial behavior (Caspi et al., 2002) or depression (Caspi et al., 2003). These studies strengthen the scientific evidence that it is not simply genetic vulnerability that is critical but also the interplay of such vulnerability with the surrounding social contexts. Returning to our theme of health rather than disease, distress, and dysfunction, we also note that even with *both* genetic and environmental risk factors present, many individuals do not show adverse outcomes. For example, carrying the short allele for the 5-HTT serotonin transporter gene may convey increased risk for depression, but negative environmental inputs (e.g., childhood maltreatment and adult stressful events) also matter (Caspi et al., 2003). However, among those with both risk factors, the majority did not become depressed. Thus, extensive opportunities are available to probe the factors (environmental or genetic) that afford protection against negative outcomes in the face of known risk. This is a place where the social environment–epigenome agenda can be substantially expanded and deepened.

Regrettably, there is little to be said on the topic of psychosocial environments that *promote healthy gene expression* for the simple reason that research is overwhelmingly focused on understanding disease and the mechanistic pathways through which genes have their effects (e.g., Meyer-Lindenberg & Weinberger, 2006). Even in work focused on the prevention of cancer, the emphasis is on the *breakdown* of DNA maintenance mechanisms (Hoeijmakers, 2001). A notable exception is a recent paper by Loizidou et al. (2008) where an association between the XRCC2 Arg188His polymorphism and epithelial ovarian cancer was considered. Here women carrying one His allele had a 20% reduction in risk, and those carrying two His alleles had a 50% reduction in risk of epithelial ovarian cancer in comparison with those homozygous for the Arg allele. Further, in a Polish population, homozygotes for the 188His variant showed a decreased risk for breast cancer. Additional research is needed to understand the mechanisms by which such protection might be afforded. Such inquiries are tremendously valuable and in no way diminish the remarkable strides in understanding the complex processes through which genetic factors contribute to disease. Nonetheless, genetic integrity—that is, the processes by which genes contribute to the normal, healthy development of the organism and healthy aging—is also worthy of inquiry.

Summary

We have called for the study of healthy aging as an integrative biopsychosocial process. The rationale underlying such an approach stems from the ever-accumulating evidence that there are numerous influences on how aging unfolds—some ensuing from one's location in the social structure and others following from psychosocial and behavioral factors at the individual level. These levels of analysis need to be connected to each other, but, more important, they must be linked with neural mechanisms and related biological and genetic processes. This is a tall order and, even among believers on a difficult day, may seem overwhelming in scope. However, to ignore the integrative challenge is, in our view, to accept a perpetually piecemeal understanding of human health and well-being over the life course.

Although we offer no overarching theory that assembles the full story, we have set forth five guiding propositions with supporting evidence that are intended to advance knowledge of healthy aging as a multilevel and multifaceted process. Throughout, we have tried to promote greater cross talk between human and animal studies (Singer, Friedman, Seeman, Fava, & Ryff, 2005) and, importantly, to augment the prevailing foci on pathways to disease, disability, and death with elaboration of influences that extend length and quality of life for the maximal number of years (our core definition of healthy aging).

Focusing on health promotion, we drew on largely associational evidence to support the claim that positive psychosocial factors predict better biological regulation (proposition 1). Here there is need for far more empirical study, including deeper understanding of pathways from the psychosocial environment, through perceptions in the brain, and their contribution to regulatory mechanisms at molecular levels. The start of such pathway specification has begun in the context of epigenomics (Szyf et al., 2008), although, as cautionary remarks by the authors indicate, a substantial research agenda involving interplay between human and animal studies is needed to rigorously support and, en route, refine the pathways of linkages between the social environment and the epigenome.

Understanding how positive psychological factors serve to protect against the damaging effects of external adversity requires a deeper understanding of biopsychosocial mechanisms of resilience (proposition 2). Here we see great opportunities for scientific advancement built on studies of the organism under challenge (including social structural challenge, such a low standing in the socioeconomic hierarchy), with attendant tracking of the relevant brain mechanisms and biological processes by which some continue to flourish. Similarly, our focus on recovery and repair processes (proposition 3) identified multiple examples of psychosocial influences that contribute to the regaining of lost capacities. Of particular interest in this realm are DNA repair processes, which have only in the most preliminary of ways been linked to psychosocial factors. Designing human studies where assessment of recovery and repair can be ascertained at both the molecular and the psychological level will require some ingenuity. The payoff would be a vastly enriched and more tightly integrated understanding of how the organism avoids damage under challenge (resilience) or, if damage occurs, is able to regain prior capacities (recovery and repair).

We also elaborated ideas of compensation processes (proposition 4) wherein strengths (psychosocial or biological) can offset weaknesses (psychosocial or biological). Most evidence in this realm has involved the interplay of psychological factors. The challenge of linking psychological compensation processes to biological processes, such as DNA repair mechanisms, represents essentially uncharted terrain.

We emphasize that genetic influences need to be incorporated into the previously mentioned inquiries as well. In building this interface, we again called for more research on health in juxtaposition to the preeminence of the genetics of disease. Here there are notable opportunities to investigate psychosocial environments as relevant influences on preventing the progression toward disease symptoms among those with known genetic risk as well as the more rarified idea of salubrious environments promoting genetic integrity (how genes contribute to normal, healthy functioning).

Undoubtedly, any effort to cast a wide net in understanding the forces that conspire to promote healthy aging will give insufficient attention to some important influences. That is, integrative approaches are inherently vulnerable to what they have left out. As such, we characterize what has been put forth in this chapter as the opening discussion, which will undoubtedly benefit from the critical commentary of others.

ACKNOWLEDGMENT. This research was supported by a grant from the National Institute on Aging (PO1-AG020166).

References

Adler, N. E., Boyce, T., Chesney, M. A., Cohen, S., Folkman, S., Kahn, R. L., et al. (1994). Socioeconomic status and health: The challenge of the gradient. *American Psychologist, 49,* 14–24.

Adler, N. E., Marmot, M. G., McEwen, B. S., & Stewart, J. (1999). *Socioeconomic status and health in industrialized nations: Social, psychological, and biological pathways* (Vol. 896). New York: New York Academy of Sciences.

Alwin, D. F., & Wray, L. A. (2005). A life-span developmental perspective on social status and health. *Journal of Gerontology: Social Sciences, 60*(Special Issue 2), 7–14.

Bacon, W. E., & Hadden, W. C. (2000). Occurrence of hip fractures and socioeconomic position. *Journal of Aging & Health, 12,* 193–203.

Baltes, P. B., & Baltes, M. M. (Eds.). (1990). *Successful aging: Perspectives from the behavioral sciences.* New York: Cambridge University Press.

Bardi, A., & Ryff, C.D. (2007). Interactive effects of traits on adjustment to a life transition. *Journal of Personality, 75,* 955–984.

Berkman, L. F., Leo-Summers, L., & Horwitz, R. I. (1992). Emotional support and survival after myocardial infarction: A prospective, population-based study of the elderly. *Annals of Internal Medicine, 117,* 1003–1009.

Besedovsky, H. O., & Del Rey, A. (1996). Immune-neuro-endocrine interactions: Facts and hypotheses. *Endocrine Review, 17,* 64–102.

Bond, L. A., Cutler, S. J., & Grams, A. (Eds.). (1995). *Promoting successful and productive aging.* Thousand Oaks, CA: Sage.

Bronfenbrenner, U. (1979). *The ecology of human development.* Cambridge, MA: Harvard University Press.

Brunner, E. J., Marmot, M. G., Nanchahal, K., Shipley, M. J., Stansfeld, S. A., Juneja, M., et al. (1997). Social inequality in coronary risk: Central obesity and the metabolic syndrome. Evidence from the Whitehall II study. *Diabetologia, 40,* 1341–1349.

Caldji, C., Tannenbaum, B., Sharma, S., Francis, D., Plotsky, P. M., & Meaney, M. J. (1998). Maternal care during infancy regulates the development of neural systems mediating the expression of fearfulness in the rat. *Proceedings of the National Academy of Sciences of the United States of America, 95,* 5335–5340.

Carter, C. S., Ramsey, M. M., & Sonntag, W. E. (2002). A critical analysis of the role of growth hormone and IGF-1 in aging and lifespan. *Trends in Genetics, 18,* 295–301.

Caspi, A., Mclay, J., Moffitt, T. E., Mill, J., Martin, J., Craig, I. W., et al. (2002). Role of genotype in the cycle of violence in maltreated children. *Science, 297,* 851–854.

Caspi, A., Sugden, K., Moffitt, T., Taylor, A., Craig, I. W., Harrington, H., et al. (2003). Influence of life stress on depression: Moderation by polymorphism in the 5-HTT gene. *Science, 301,* 386–389.

Charney, D. S. (2004). Psychobiological mechanisms of resilience and vulnerability: Implications for successful adaptation to extreme stress. *American Journal of Psychiatry, 161,* 195–215.

Chen, E., & Paterson, L. Q. (2006). Neighborhood, family, and subjective socioeconomic status: How do they relate to adolescent health? *Health Psychology, 25,* 704–714.

Cho, H. Y., Zhang, L. Y., & Kleeberger, S. R. (2001). Ozone-induced lung inflammation and hyperreactivity are mediated via tumor necrosis factor-alpha receptors. *American Journal of Physiology Lung Cell Physiology, 280,* L537–L546.

Cohen, S., Alpen, C. M., Doyle, W. J., Treanor, J. J., & Turner, R. B. (2006). Positive emotional style predicts resistance to illness after experimental exposure to rhinovirus or influenza A virus. *Psychosomatic Medicine, 68,* 809–815.

Conti, E., Carrozza, C., Capoluongo, E., Volpe, M., Crea, F., Zuppi, C., et al. (2004). Insulin-like growth factor-1 as a vascular protective factor. *Circulation, 110,* 2260–2265.

Cumming, E., & Henry, W. E. (1961). *Growing old: The process of disengagement.* New York: Basic Books.

Dai, G., Kaazempur-Mofrad, M. R., Natarajan, S., Zhang, Y., Vaughn, S., Blackman, B. R., et al. (2004). Distinct endothelial phenotypes evoked by arterial wareforms derived from atherosclerosis-susceptible and resistant regions of human vasculature. *Proceedings of National Academy of Sciences of the United States of America, 101,* 14871–14876.

Danner, D. D., Snowden, D. A., & Friesen, W. V. (2001). Positive emotions in early life and longevity: Findings from the Nun Study. *Journal of Personality and Social Psychology, 80,* 804–813.

Dhabhar, F. S., & McEwen, B. S. (2001). Bidirectional effects of stress and glucocorticoid hormones on immune function: Possible explanations for paradoxical observations. In R. Ader, D. L. Felten, & N. Cohen (Eds.), *Psychoneuroimmunology* (3rd ed., pp. 301–338). San Diego, CA: Academic Press.

Dienstbier, R. A. (1989). Arousal and physiological toughness: Implications for mental and physical health. *Psychological Review, 96,* 84–100.

Dixon, R. A., & Bäckman, L. (Eds.). (1995). *Compensating for psychological deficits and declines: Managing losses and promoting gains.* Mahwah, NJ: Lawrence Erlbaum Associates.

Dyer, A. R., Liu, K., Walsh, M., Kiefe, C. I., Jacobs, D. R., Jr., & Bild, D. E. (1999). Ten-year incidence of elevated blood pressure and its predictors: The CARDIA Study. Coronary Artery Risk Development in (Young) Adults. *Journal of Human Hypertension, 13,* 13–21.

Feldman, P. J., & Steptoe, A. (2003). Psychosocial and socioeconomic factors associated with glycated hemoglobin in nondiabetic middle-aged men and women. *Health Psychology, 22,* 398–405.

Feldman, P. J., & Steptoe, A. (2004). How neighborhoods and physical functioning are related: The roles of neighborhood socioeconomic status, perceived neighborhood strain, and individual health risk factors. *Annals of Behavioral Medicine, 27,* 91–99.

Finch, C. E. (2007). *The biology of human longevity: Inflammation, nutrition, and aging in the evolution of lifespans.* San Diego, CA: Academic Press.

Finch, C. E., & Kirkwood, T. B. L. (2000). *Chance, development, and aging.* New York: Oxford University Press.

Finch, C. E., & Rose, M. R. (1995). Hormones and the physiological architecture of life history evolution. *Quarterly Review of Biology, 70,* 1–52.

Finch, C. E., & Ruvkun, G. (2001). The genetics of aging. *Annual Review of Genomics & Human Genetics, 2,* 435–462.

Fitzgerald, T. E., Tennen, H., Affleck, G., & Pransky, G. S. (1993). The relative importance of dispositional optimism and control appraisals in quality of life after coronary artery bypass surgery. *Journal of Behavioral Medicine, 16,* 25–43.

Francis, D. D., Champagne, F. A., Liu, D., & Meaney, M. J. (1999). Maternal care, gene expression, and the development of individual differences in stress reactivity. In N. E. Adler,

M. Marmot, B. S. McEwen, & J. Stewart (Eds.), *Socioeconomic status and health in industrial nations: Social, psychological, and biological pathways* (pp. 66–84). New York: New York Academy of Sciences.

Francis, D., Diorio, J., Liu, D., & Meaney, M. J. (1999). Nongenomic transmission across generations of maternal behavior and stress responses in the rat. *Science, 286,* 1155–1158.

Freund, A. M., & Baltes, P. B. (2002). Life-management strategies of selection, optimization, and compensation: Measurement by self-report and construct validity. *Journal of Personality and Social Psychology, 82,* 642–662.

Friedman, E. M., Hayney, M., Love, G. D., Singer, B. H., & Ryff, C. D. (2005, March). *Serum interleukin-6 and soluble IL-6 receptors are modulated by psychological well-being in aging women.* Paper presented at the annual meeting of the American Psychosomatic Society, Vancouver, BC.

Friedman, E. M., Hayney, M., Love, G. D., Singer, B. H., & Ryff, C. D. (2007). Plasma interleukin-6 and soluble IL-6 receptors are associated with psychological well-being in aging women. *Health Psychology, 26,* 305–313.

Gerstorf, D., Smith, J., & Baltes, P. B. (2006). A systemic-wholistic approach to differential aging: Longitudinal findings from the Berlin Aging Study. *Psychology & Aging, 21,* 645–663.

Gidron, Y., Russ, K., Tissarchondou, H., & Warner, J. (2006). The relation between psychological factors and DNA-damage: A critical review. *Biological Psychology, 72,* 291–304.

Gorman, B. K., & Sivaganesan, A. (2007). The role of social support and integration for understanding socioeconomic disparities in self-rated health and hypertension. *Social Science & Medicine, 65,* 958–975.

Gruenewald, T. L., Mroczek, D. K., Ryff, C. D., & Singer, B. H. (2008). Diverse pathways to positive and negative affect in adulthood and later life: An integrative approach using recursive partitioning. *Developmental Psychology, 44,* 330–343.

Gruenewald, T. L., Seeman, T. E., Ryff, C. D., Karlamangla, A. S., & Singer, B. (2006). Combinations of biomarkers predictive of later life mortality. *Proceedings of the National Academy of Sciences of the United States of America, 103,* 14158–14163.

Hatch, S. L. (2005). Conceptualizing and identifying cumulative adversity and protective resources: Implications for understanding health inequalities. *Journal of Gerontology: Social Sciences, 60*(Special Issue 2), 130–134.

Hayward, M. D., Crimmins, E. M., Miles, T. P., & Yu, Y. (2000). The significance of socioeconomic status in explaining the racial gap in chronic health conditions. *American Sociological Review, 65,* 910–930.

Heidrich, S. M., & Ryff, C. D. (1993a). Physical and mental health in later life: The self-system as mediator. *Psychology & Aging, 8,* 327–338.

Heidrich, S. M., & Ryff, C. D. (1993b). The role of social comparison processes in the psychological adaptation of elderly adults. *Journal of Gerontology, 48,* P127–P136.

Hobcraft, J. (2006). The ABC of demographic behavior: How the interplays of alleles, brains, and contexts over the life course should shape research aimed at understanding population processes. *Population Studies, 60,* 153–187.

Hoeijmakers, J. H. (2001). Genome maintenance mechanisms for preventing cancer. *Nature, 421,* 366–374.

House, J. S. (1981). Social structure and personality. In M. Rosenberg & R. H. Turner (Eds.), *Social psychology: Sociological perspectives* (pp. 525–561). New York: Basic Books.

House, J. S., Lepkowski, J. M., Kinney, A. M., Mero, R. P., Kessler, R. C., & Herzog, A. R. (1994). The social stratification of aging and health. *Journal of Health & Social Behavior, 35,* 213–234.

Hsin, H., & Kenyon, C. (1999). Signals from the reproductive system regulate the lifespan of *C. elegans. Nature, 399,* 362–366.

Inkeles, A. (1959). Personality and social structure. In R. K. Merton, L. Broom, & J. L. S. Contrell (Eds.), *Sociology today: Problems and prospects* (pp. 249–276). New York: Basic Books.

Irie, M., Asami, S., Nagata, S., Miyata, M., & Kasai, H. (2002). Psychological mediation of a type of oxidative DNA damage, 8-hydroxydeoxyguanosine, in peripheral blood leukocytes of non-smoking and non-drinking workers. *Psychotherapy Psychosomatics, 71,* 90–96.

Jagger, C., Matthews, R., Meetzer, D., Matthews, F., Brayne, C., & MRC Cognitive Function and Ageing Study. (2007). Educational differences in the dynamics of disability incidence, recovery and mortality: Findings from the MRC Cognitive Function and Ageing Study (MRC CFAS). *International Journal of Epidemiology, 36,* 358–365.

Juul, A., Scheike, T., Davidsen, M., Brown, J., Adams, H., Zablosky, H., et al. (2002). Low serum insulin-like growth factor-1 is associated with increased risk of ischemic heart disease: A population-based case-control study. *Circulation, 106,* 939–944.

Karlamangla, A. S., Singer, B. H., Williams, D. R., Schwartz, J. E., Matthews, K., Kiefe, C. I., et al. (2005). Impact of socioeconomic status on longitudinal accumulation of cardiovascular risk in young adults: The CARDIA study (USA). *Social Science & Medicine, 60,* 999–1015.

Kawachi, I., Kennedy, B. P., & Wilkinson, R. C. (1999). *The society and population health reader: Vol. 1. Income inequality and health.* New York: New Press.

Kenyon, C. (2006). My adventures with genes from the fountain of youth. *Harvey Lecture Series, 100,* 29–70.

Keyes, C. L. M., Shmotkin, D., & Ryff, C. D. (2002). Optimizing well-being: The empirical encounter of two traditions. *Journal of Personality & Social Psychology, 82,* 1007–1022.

Kirkwood, T. B. (2008). A systematic look at an old problem. *Nature, 451,* 644–647.

Kirkwood, T. B. L., Boys, R. J., Gillespie, C. S., Proctor, C. J., Shanley, D. P., & Wilkinson, D. J. (2003). Towards an e-biology of ageing: Integrating theory and data. *Nature Reviews: Molecular Cell Biology, 4,* 243–248.

Kling, K. C., Seltzer, M. M., & Ryff, C. D. (1997). Distinctive late-life challenges: Implications for coping and well-being. *Psychology & Aging, 12,* 288–295.

Klohnen, E. C. (1996). Conceptual analysis and measurement of the construct of ego-resiliency. *Journal of Personality & Social Psychology, 70,* 1067–1079.

Kloner, R. A., & Jennings, R. B. (2001). Consequences of brief ischemia: Stunning, preconditioning, and their clinical implications: Part 1. *Circulation, 104,* 2981–2989.

Kuypers, J. A., & Bengtson, V. L. (1973). Social breakdown and competence: A model of normal aging. *Human Development, 16,* 181–201.

Kwan, C. M. L., Love, G. D., Ryff, C. D., & Essex, M. J. (2003). The role of self-enhancing evaluations in a successful life transition. *Psychology & Aging, 18,* 3–12.

Lachman, M. E., & Weaver, S. L. (1998). The sense of control as a moderator of social class differences in health and well-being. *Journal of Personality and Social Psychology, 74,* 763–773.

Lakatta, E. G. (2003). Arterial and cardiac aging: Major shareholders in cardiovascular disease enterprises: Part III: Cellular and molecular clues to heart and arterial aging. *Circulation, 107,* 490–497.

Lantz, P. M., Lynch, J. W., House, J. S., Lepkowski, J. M., Mero, R. P., Musick, M. A., et al. (2001). Socioeconomic disparities in health change in a longitudinal study of U.S. adults: The role of health-risk behaviors. *Social Science & Medicine, 53,* 29–40.

Laughlin, G. A., Barrett-Connor, E., & Criqui, M. H. (2004). The prospective association of serum insulin-like growth factor-1 (IGF01) and IGF-binding protein-1 levels with all cause and cardiovascular disease mortality in older adults: The Racho Bernardo Study. *Journal of Clinical Endocrinology and Metabolism, 89,* 114–120.

Leedham, B., Meyerowitz, B. E., Muirhead, J., & Frist, W. H. (1995). Positive expectations predict health after heart transplantation. *Health Psychology, 14,* 74–79.

Lindfors, P., & Lundberg, U. (2002). Is low cortisol release an indicator of positive health? *Stress & Health: Journal of the International Society for the Investigation of Stress, 18,* 153–160.

Liu, D., Diorio, J., Tannenbaum, B., Caldji, C., Francis, D., Freedman, A., et al. (1997). Maternal care, hippocampal glucocorticoid receptors, and hypothalamic-pituitary-adrenal responses to stress. *Science, 277,* 1659–1662.

Loizidou, M. A., Michael, T., Neuhausen, S. L., Newbold, R. F., Marcou, Y., Kakouri, E., et al. (2008). Genetic polymorphisms in the DNA repair genes XRCC1, XRCC2 and XRCC3 and risk of breast cancer in Cyprus. *Breast Cancer Research & Treatment,* DOI 10.1007/s10549–007–9881–4.

Lopez-Torres, M., Grecilla, R., Sanz, A., & Barja, G. (2002). Influence of aging and long term caloric restriction on oxygen and radical generation and oxidative DNA damage in rat liver mitochondria. *Free Radical Biology & Medicine, 32,* 882–889.

Lupien, S. J., King, S., Meaney, M. J., & McEwen, B. S. (2001). Can poverty get under your skin? Basal cortisol levels and cognitive function in children from low and high socioeconomic status. *Development & Psychopathology, 13,* 653–676.

Luthar, S. S., Cicchetti, D., & Becker, B. (2000). The construct of resilience: A critical evaluation and guidelines for future work. *Child Development, 71,* 543–562.

Lynch, J. W., Kaplan, G. A., Cohen, R. D., Tuomilehto, J., & Salonen, J. T. (1996). Do cardiovascular risk factors explain the relation between socioeconomic status, risk of all-cause mortality, cardiovascular mortality, and acute myocardial infarction? *American Journal of Epidemiology, 144,* 934–942.

Maier, S. F., & Watkins, L. R. (1998). Cytokines for psychologists: Implications of bidirectional immune-to-brain communication for understanding behavior, mood, and cognition. *Psychological Review, 105,* 83–107.

Malarkey, W. B., Kiecolt-Glaser, J. K., Pearl, D., & Glaser, R. (1994). Hostile behavior during marital conflict alters pituitary and adrenal hormones. *Psychosomatic Medicine, 56,* 41–51.

Markus, H. R., Ryff, C. D., Curhan, K. B., & Palmersheim, K. A. (2004). In their own words: Well-being at midlife among high school-educated and college-educated adults. In O. G. Brim, C. D. Ryff, & R. C. Kessler (Eds.), *How healthy are we?: A national study of well-being at midlife* (pp. 273–319). Chicago: University of Chicago Press.

Marmot, M. G., & Wilkinson, R. G. (1999). *Social determinants of health.* Oxford: Oxford University Press.

Masten, A. S. (1999). Resilience comes of age: Reflections on the past and outlook for the next generation of research. In M. D. Glantz & J. L. Johnson (Eds.), *Resilience and development: Positive life adaptations* (pp. 281–296). New York: Kluwer Academic/Plenum Press.

Matthews, R. J., Smith, L. K., Hancock, R. M., Jagger, C., & Spiers, N. A. (2005). Socioeconomic factors associated with the onset of disability in older age: A longitudinal study of people aged 75 and over. *Social Science & Medicine, 61,* 1567–1575.

McAdams, D. P. (2006). *The person: A new introduction to personality psychology* (4th ed.). New York: Wiley.

McAdams, D. P., & Pals, J. L. (2006). A new big five: Fundamental principles for an integrative science of personality. *American Psychologist, 61,* 204–217.

Meaney, M. J., & Szyf, M. (2005). Maternal care as a model for experience-dependent chromatin plasticity? *Trends in Neuroscience, 28,* 456–462.

Meyer-Lindenberg, A., & Weinberger, D. R. (2006). Intermediate phenotypes and genetic mechanisms of psychiatric disorders. *Nature Reviews: Neuroscience, 7,* 818–827.

Miller, G. E., Chen, E., & Zhou, E. S. (2007). If it goes up, must it come down? Chronic stress and the hypothalamic-pituitary-adrenocortical axis in humans. *Psychological Bulletin, 133,* 25–45.

Moffitt, T. E., Caspi, A., & Rutter, M. (2006). Measured gene-environment interactions in psychopathology: Concepts, research strategies, and implications for research, intervention, and public understanding of genetics. *Perspectives on Psychological Science, 1,* 5–27.

Mroczek, D. K., & Spiro, A. I. (2007). Personality change influences mortality in older men. *Psychological Science, 18,* 371–376.

Okamoto, T., Adachi, K., Muraishi, A., Seki, Y., Hidaka, T., & Toshima, H. (1996). Induction of DNA breaks in cardiac myoblast cells by norepinephrine. *Biochemistry & Molecular Biology International, 38,* 821–827.

O'Rand, A. M., & Hamil-Luker, J. (2005). Processes of cumulative adversity: Childhood disadvantage and increased risk of heart attack across the life course. *Journals of Gerontology: Social Sciences, 60*(Special Issue 2), 117–124.

Ostir, G. V., Markides, K. S., Peek, M. K., & Goodwin, J. S. (2001). The association between emotional well-being and the incidence of stroke in older adults. *Psychosomatic Medicine, 63,* 210–215.

Ostir, G. V., Raji, M. A., & Ottenbacher, K. J. (2003). Cognitive function and incidence of stroke in older Mexican Americans. *Journal of Gerontology: Biological Sciences, 58,* 531–535.

Phelan, J. C., & Link, B. G. (2005). Controlling disease and creating disparities: A fundamental cause perspective. *Journal of Gerontology: Social Sciences, 60*(Special Issue 2), 27–33.

Poon, L. W., Bramlett, M. H., Holtzberg, P. A., Johnson, M. A., & Martin, P. (1996). Who will survive to 105? In *1997 medical & health annual* (pp. 62–77). Chicago: Encyclopaedia Britannica.

Pressman, S. D., & Cohen, S. (2005). Does positive affect influence health? *Psychological Bulletin, 131,* 925–971.

Preston, S. H., & Taubman, P. (1994). Socioeconomic differences in adult mortality and health status. In L. G. Martin & S. H. Preston (Eds.), *Demography of aging* (pp. 279–318). Washington, DC: National Academies Press.

Razin, A. (1998). CpG methylation, chromatin structure and gene silencing a three-way connection. *EMBO Journal, 17,* 4905–4908.

Reed, G. M., Kemeny, M. E., Taylor, S. E., Wang, H.-Y., & Visscher, B. R. (1994). Realistic acceptance as a predictor of decreased survival time in gay men with AIDS. *Health Psychology, 13,* 299–307.

Rieker, P. P., & Bird, C. E. (2005). Rethinking gender differences in health: Why we need to integrate social and biological perspectives. *Journal of Gerontology: Social Sciences, 60*(Special Issue 2), 40–47.

Riley, M. W., Kahn, R. L., & Foner, A. (1994). *Age and structural lag.* New York: Wiley.

Robins, R. W., John, O. P., & Caspi, A. (1998). The typological approach to studying personality. In R. B. Cairns, L. R. Bergman, & J. Kagan (Eds.), *Methods and models for studying the individual* (pp. 135–160). Thousand Oaks, CA: Sage.

Robins, R. W., John, O. P., Caspi, A., Moffitt, T. E., & Stouthamer-Loeber, M. (1996). Resilient, overcontrolled, and undercontrolled boys: Three replicable personality types. *Journal of Personality & Social Psychology, 70,* 157–171.

Rosen, C. J., & Pollak, M. (1999). Circulating IGF-I: New perspectives for a new century. *Trends in Endocrinology and Metabolism, 10,* 136–141.

Ross, C. E., & Mirowsky, J. (1999). Refining the association between education and health: The effects of quantity, credential, and selectivity. *Demography, 36,* 445–460.

Ross, C. E., & Wu, C.-L. I. (1996). Education, age, and the cumulative advantage in health. *Journal of Health & Social Behavior, 37,* 104–120.

Rowe, J. W., & Kahn, R. L. (1987). Human aging: Usual and successful. *Science, 237,* 143–149.

Ryan, R. M., & Deci, E. L. (2001). On happiness and human potentials: A review of research on hedonic and eudaimonic well-being. *Annual Review of Psychology, 52,* 141–166.

Ryff, C. D. (1987). The place of personality and social structure research in social psychology. *Journal of Personality & Social Psychology, 53,* 1192–1202.

Ryff, C. D. (1989). Happiness is everything, or is it? Explorations on the meaning of psychological well-being. *Journal of Personality & Social Psychology, 57,* 1069–1081.

Ryff, C. D. (2008). Challenges and opportunities at the interface of aging, personality, and well-being. In O. P. John, R. W. Robins, & L. A. Pervin (Eds.), *Handbook of personality: Theory and research* (3rd ed.) (pp. 339–418). New York: Guilford.

Ryff, C. D., Keyes, C. L. M., & Hughes, D. L. (2003). Status inequalities, perceived discrimination, and eudaimonic well-being: Do the challenges of minority life hone purpose and growth? *Journal of Health & Social Behavior, 44,* 275–291.

Ryff, C. D., Love, G. D., Urry, H. L., Muller, D., Rosenkranz, M. A., Friedman, E. M., et al. (2006). Psychological well-being and ill-being: Do they have distinct or mirrored biological correlates? *Psychotherapy & Psychosomatics, 75,* 85–95.

Ryff, C. D., Marshall, V. W., & Clarke, P. J. (1999). Linking the self and society in social gerontology: Crossing new territory via old questions. In C. D. Ryff, V. W. Marshall, & P. J. Clarke (Eds.), *The self and society in aging processes* (pp. 3–41). New York: Springer Publishing.

Ryff, C. D., Radler, B., & Singer, B. (2008, February 9). *Known and unknown health gradients in MIDUS.* Paper presented at the annual meeting of the Society for Personality and Social Psychology, Albuquerque, NM.

Ryff, C. D., & Singer, B. H. (1998). The contours of positive human health. *Psychological Inquiry, 9,* 1–28.

Ryff, C. D., & Singer, B. H. (2000). Interpersonal flourishing: A positive health agenda for the new millennium. *Personality and Social Psychology Review, 4,* 30–44.

Ryff, C. D., & Singer, B. H. (2001). (Eds.). *Emotion, social relationships, and health.* Chicago: University of Chicago Press.

Ryff, C. D., & Singer, B. H. (2002). Flourishing under fire: Resilience as a prototype of challenged thriving. In C. L. M. Keyes & J. Haidt (Eds.), *Flourishing: Positive psychology and the life well-lived* (pp. 15–36). Washington, DC: American Psychological Association.

Ryff, C. D., & Singer, B. H. (2005). Social environments and the genetics of aging: Advancing knowledge of protective health mechanisms. *Journal of Gerontology: Social Sciences, 60*(Special Issue 1), 12–23.

Ryff, C. D., & Singer, B. H. (2008). Know thyself and become what you are: A eudaimonic approach to psychological well-being. *Journal of Happiness Studies, 9,* 13–39.

Ryff, C. D., Singer, B. H., & Love, G. D. (2004). Positive health: Connecting well-being with biology. *Philosophical Transactions of the Royal Society of London. Series B, Biological Sciences, 359,* 1383–1394.

Ryff, C. D., Singer, B. H., Love, G. D., & Essex, M. J. (1998). Resilience in adulthood and later life: Defining features and dynamic processes. In J. Lomranz (Ed.), *Handbook of aging and mental health: An integrative approach* (pp. 69–96). New York: Plenum Press.

Sampson, R. J., & Sharkey, P. (2008). Neighborhood selection and the social reproduction of concentrated racial inequality. *Demography, 45,* 1–29.

Sampson, R. J., Sharkey, P., & Raudenbush, S. W. (2008). Durable effects of concentrated disadvantage on verbal ability among African-American children. *Proceedings of the National Academy of Sciences of the United States of America, 105,* 845–852.

Sancar, A., Lindsey-Boltz, L. A., Unsal-Kacmaz, K., & Linn, S. (2004). Molecular mechanisms of mammalian DNA repair and the DNA damage checkpoints. *Annual Review of Biochemistry, 73,* 39–85.

Sapolsky, R. M. (2005). The influence of social hierarchy on primate health. *Science, 308,* 648–652.

Sapolsky, R. M., Romero, L. M., & Munck, A. U. (2000). How do glucocorticoids influence stress responses? Integrating permissive, suppressive, stimulatory, and preparative actions. *Endocrine Reviews, 21,* 55–89.

Scheier, M. F., & Carver, C. S. (1992). Effects of optimism on psychological and physical well-being: Theoretical overview and empirical update. *Cognitive Therapy & Research, 16,* 201–228.

Schmidt, R., Schmidt, H., Curb, J. D., Masaki, K., White, L. R., & Launer, L. J. (2002). Early inflammation and dementia: A 25-year follow-up of the Honolulu-Asia Aging Study. *Annals of Neurology, 52,* 168–174.

Schulz, R., & Heckhausen, J. (1996). A life span model of successful aging. *American Psychologist, 51,* 702–714.

Shmotkin, D. (2005). Happiness in the face of adversity: Reformulating the dynamic and modular bases of subjective well-being. *Review of General Psychology, 9,* 291–325.

Singer, B., Friedman, E., Seeman, T., Fava, G. A., & Ryff, C. D. (2005). Protective environments and health status: Cross-talk between human and animal studies. *Neurobiology of Aging, 26S,* S113–S118.

Singer, B. H., & Ryff, C. D. (1999). Hierarchies of life histories and associated health risks. In N. E. Adler & M. Marmot (Eds.), *Socioeconomic status and health in industrial nations: Social, psychological, and biological pathways* (Vol. 896, pp. 96–115). New York: New York Academy of Sciences.

Singer, B. H., & Ryff, C. D. (2001). Person-centered methods for understanding aging: The integration of numbers and narratives. In R. H. Binstock & L. K. George (Eds.), *Handbook of aging and the social sciences* (5th ed., pp. 44–65). San Diego, CA: Academic Press.

Singer, B. H., Ryff, C. D., Carr, D., & Magee, W. J. (1998). Life histories and mental health: A person-centered strategy. In A. Raftery (Ed.), *Sociological methodology* (pp. 1–51). Washington, DC: American Sociological Association.

Smelser, N. J., & Smelser, W. T. (1970). *Personality and social systems* (2nd ed.). Oxford: Wiley.

Smith, J. P. (1998). Socioeconomic status and health. *American Economic Review, 88,* 192–196.

Spiegel, D., Sephton, S. E., Terr, A. L., & Stites, D. P. (1998). Effects of psychosocial treatment in prolonging cancer survival may be mediated by neuroimmune pathways. *Annals of the New York Academy of Sciences, 840,* 674–683.

Staudinger, U. M., Marsiske, M., & Baltes, P. B. (1995). Resilience and reserve capacity in later adulthood: Potentials and limits of development across the life span. In D. Cicchetti & D. Cohen (Eds.), *Developmental psychopathology: Vol. 2. Risk, disorder and adaptation* (pp. 801–847). New York: Wiley.

Steptoe, A., Gibson, E. L., Hamer, M., & Wardle, J. (2006). Neuroendocrine and cardiovascular correlates of positive affect measured by ecological momentary assessment and by questionnaire. *Psychoneuroendocrinology, 32,* 56–74.

Steptoe, A., Owen, N., Kunz-Ebrecht, S., & Mohamed-Ali, V. (2002). Inflammatory cytokines, socioeconomic status, and acute stress responsivity. *Brain, Behavior & Immunity, 16,* 774–784.

Steptoe, A., & Wardle, J. (2005). Positive affect and biological function in everyday life. *Neurobiology of Aging, 26*(Suppl. 1), S108–S112.

Szyf, M., McGowan, P., & Meaney, M. J. (2008). The social environment and the epigenome. *Environmental and Molecular Mutagenesis, 49,* 46–60.

Taylor, S. E., Kemeny, M. E., Reed, G. M., Bower, J. E., & Gruenewald, T. L. (2000). Psychological resources, positive illusions, and health. *American Psychologist, 55,* 99–109.

Tsenkova, V., Love, G. D., Singer, B. H., & Ryff, C. D. (2008). Coping and positive affect predict longitudinal change in glycosylated hemoglobin. *Health Psychology, 27,* 2(Suppl.), S163–S171.

Unden, A.-L., Elofsson, S., Knox, S., Lewitt, M. S., & Brismar, K. (2002). IGF-1 in a normal population: Relation to psychosocial factors. *Clinical Endocrinology, 57,* 593–803.

Urry, H. L., Nitschke, J. B., Dolski, I., Jackson, D. C., Dalton, K. M., Mueller, C. J., et al. (2004). Making a life worth living: Neural correlates of well-being. *Psychological Science, 15,* 367–372.

van Reekum, C. M., Urry, H. L., Johnstone, T., Thurow, M. E., Frye, C. J., Jackson, C. A., et al. (2007). Individual differences in amygdala and ventromedial prefrontal cortex activity are associated with evaluation speed and psychological well-being. *Journal of Cognitive Neuroscience, 19,* 237–248.

Vaupel, J. W., Carey, J. R., Christensen, K., Johnson, T. E., Yashin, A. I., Holm, N. V., et al. (1998). Biodemographic trajectories of longevity. *Science, 280,* 855–860.

Williams, D. R., & Wilson, C. M. (2001). Race, ethnicity and aging. In R. H. Binstock & L. K. George (Eds.), *Handbook of aging and the social sciences* (5th ed., pp. 160–178). New York: Academic Press.

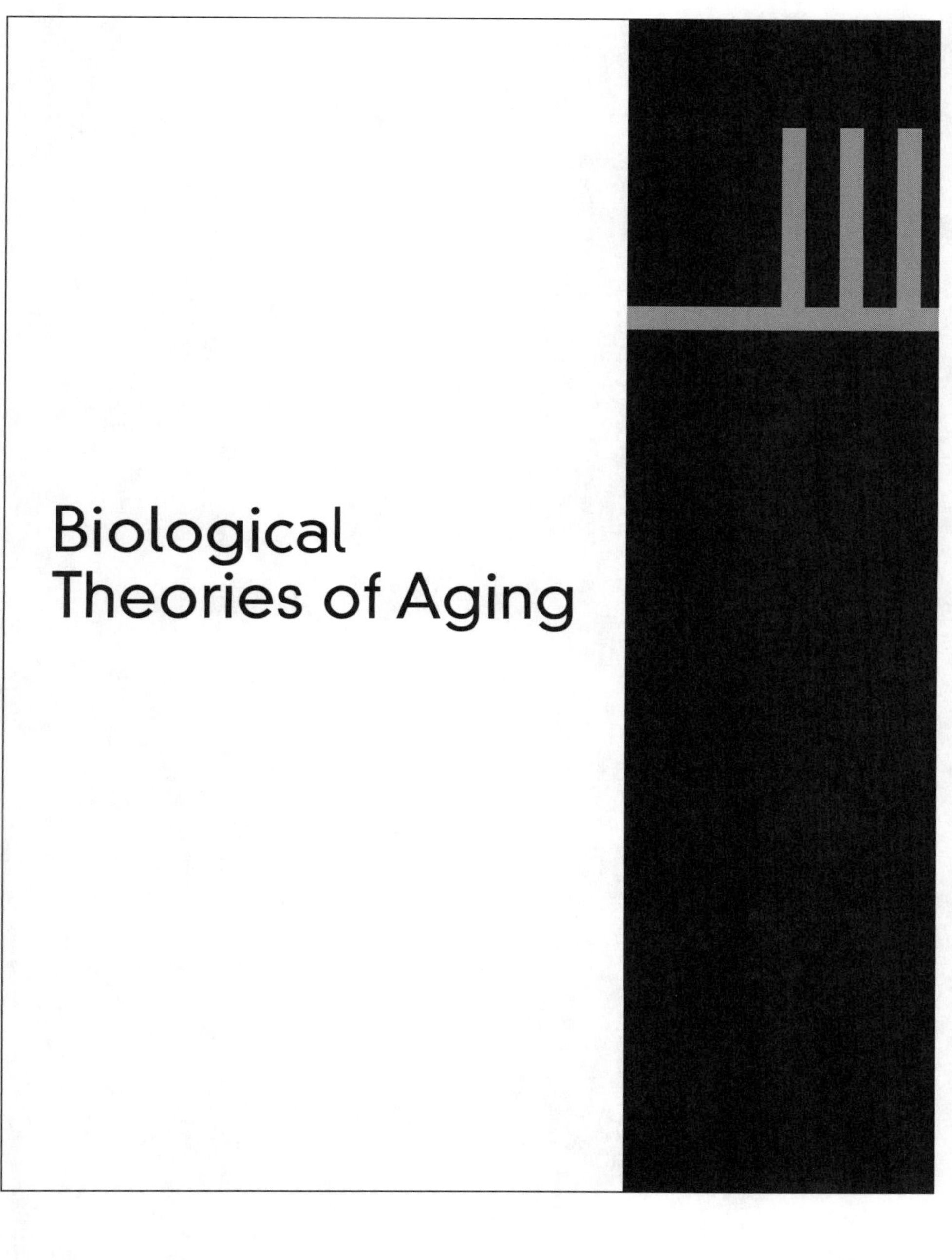

Biological Theories of Aging

Making Sense of Biological Theories of Aging

8

Steven N. Austad

Biological aging is the gradual and progressive decay in physical function that begins in adulthood and ends in death in virtually all animal species. The demographic consequences of aging are an increasing probability of death and decreasing reproductive rate with advancing age. Various statistical measures of age at death are frequently used as surrogates for the rate of aging. This clearly makes a certain degree of sense. Animals that physically deteriorate rapidly would not be expected to have a long life, whereas those that decay more slowly are likely to live longer. A caveat worth noting with respect to this simple relation between aging and longevity can conflate two distinct issues. Death can be the result of extrinsic environmental events that have little to do with the intrinsic degenerative process that most people consider to be aging. Thus, during the 20th century, life expectancy in the United States increased by about

30 years, yet it is scarcely conceivable that the intrinsic biology of humans changed much over those four to five generations. The change in longevity was brought about by a combination of better public health measures, improved nutrition, and enhanced medical knowledge and technology (Austad, 2005).

There is something of a biological paradox inherent in the phenomenon of aging. Although one could almost define a biological organism as any entity that is capable of self-repair, what is aging except the ultimate failure of self-repair? One goal of a general theory of aging would be to resolve this paradox, explaining why aging exists in the first place. To the extent that some organisms may not age (a controversial issue to be addressed later), a general theory of aging would also explain why these species fail to do so.

As everyone who has had a pet appreciates, different animal species can age at dramatically different rates. A fly becomes frail, feeble, and dies in several months, a mouse in several years, a horse in several decades, and a bowhead whale in more than a century (George et al., 1999). An informative general theory of aging should also be capable of explaining why some species age more slowly than others and make sense of broad patterns of aging across large groups of species.

In recent years, researchers have discovered that a species' rate of aging can be altered, sometimes quite dramatically, by manipulating animals' environmental conditions or nutrition or by altering a single gene (Kaeberlein et al., 2006; Magwere, Chapman, & Partridge, 2004; Weindruch, Walford, Fligiel, & Guthrie, 1986). Some species appear more malleable than others in this respect. For instance, the longevity of the nematode *Caenorhabditis elegans* has been extended nearly 10-fold by the alteration of a single gene (Ayyadevara, Alla, Thaden, & Shmookler Reis, 2008). Mammals appear to be considerably less flexible in this respect. The largest change in life span I am aware of in mammals is the Ames dwarf mouse, a single gene mutant that, when placed on a calorically restricted diet, has lived about 75% longer than fully fed nondwarf controls (Bartke et al., 2001). Might a general theory of aging help us predict the extent to which the life span of a particular species could be altered by these simple manipulations?

There has never been a shortage of theories to explain aging. In the absence of understanding, theories are prone to proliferate. Almost two decades ago, Russian geneticist Zhores Medvedev (1990) made a heroic attempt to assemble and categorize existing theories of aging and found more than 300 of them sprawled throughout the literature from Weismann's first evolutionary theory in 1882 to more molecular theories such as Orgel's error catastrophe theory, in which a positive feedback of errors in protein synthesis led to organismal deterioration. Of course, many of these hundreds of theories are overlapping or closely related to one another. But even assuming that the real number of distinct theories is far less than 300, this still represents a bewildering welter of concepts and ideas. Additionally, I would argue that we have learned more about the basic biology of aging since the publication of Medvedev's paper than we had learned over the centuries prior to it, so we might easily imagine that an updated list of aging theories would be considerably larger.

If there are truly hundreds or even several scores of tenable biological theories of aging, then the field is in a bad state. Given the numerous possibilities, what ideas will guide our research and organize our findings? Thus, it becomes necessary to ask ourselves, Are there really this many theories, or have we perhaps been misled?

What Is a Theory?

The *Oxford English Dictionary* defines a scientific theory as "a statement of what are held to be the general laws, principles, or causes of known or observed phenomena" (Anonymous, 2002). Contrast this definition with the idea of a hypothesis, defined by the same dictionary as "a supposition or conjecture put forth to account for known facts." A critical additional criterion to define a scientific hypothesis is that this supposition or conjecture needs to be stated in such a way that it is potentially falsifiable (Popper, 1959).

Consider then the difference between a hypothesis and a theory. A hypothesis is a falsifiable statement consistent with what is already known from which a prediction or predictions can be made, and these predictions can be empirically supported or falsified. By contrast, a theory is something considerably larger—a "general principle" as opposed to a "conjecture or supposition." Thought of in another way, a theory contains within it numerous related hypotheses, all of which need to be consistent with the known facts for the theory to be valid. It is important to note that there is no unique, clean, and sharp dividing line between theories and hypotheses. It depends on the level of generality one seeks. However, a reasonable distinction might be that no two valid theories can explain the same set of observations. Theories necessarily compete. If two theories exist for the same set of observations, then one must be wrong. On the other hand, multiple hypotheses about a set of observations may be simultaneously correct because each represents a contributing causal factor.

To take a specific example, Galileo in his famous, possibly apocryphal, experiment of simultaneously dropping a large and a small cannonball from the Leaning Tower of Pisa was testing Aristotle's reasonably general theory that the speed at which an object falls is directly proportional to its weight and inversely proportional to the density of the medium through which it is falling. A hypothesis contained within that theory was that in the same medium (air, in this case), an object weighing 10 times as much as a second object should fall 10 times as fast. By falsifying the hypothesis, Galileo invalidated Aristotle's theory. If his experiment had supported the theory, it still would have required testing of other hypotheses (the effect of the density of the medium) to establish strong support for the theory.

Aristotle's theory, however, seems like little more than a glorified hypothesis compared with Newton's universal theory of gravitation. That theory can be encapsulated in a simple equation in which gravitational force between two objects is predicted to be proportional to the product of the masses of those objects and inversely proportional to the square of the distance between them. Notice that although this theory applies to falling cannonballs, it also applies to much more. It applies to the orbits of planets around stars and stars and galaxies around one another. It addresses how the angle of repose of a pile of sand would differ on a large planet like Jupiter versus a small planet like Mercury. It truly is a grand theory (even if Einstein later discovered it was incomplete).

In this sense, are there really 300 theories of aging? I think the clear answer is no. For one thing, most of the so-called theories of aging are not mutually exclusive. Picking a few of Medvedev's theories at random, we see that aging has been attributed to the accumulation of cross-links in collagen, to the accumulation of DNA damage in somatic cells, and to the accumulation of random errors in protein synthesis. Clearly, all these processes might contribute to aging, might contribute more in some organs compared to others, and might contribute more in some organisms compared to others. Evidentiary support in favor of one of these ideas does not necessarily lessen support for the others. By any reasonable standard, each of these is really a hypothesis about the mechanisms underlying the observed phenomenon of aging. Dozens of them (at least) could be simultaneously valid. We in the aging research community have been playing fast and loose with our terminology.

Real Theories of Aging

Before we can separate real theories of aging from hypotheses or glorified hypotheses, we need to define the range of observations that a general theory of aging ought to address. I believe there are at least three such observations. First, a general theory of aging should address why biological organisms age at all. If there are organisms that do not age, their existence and general biological characteristics should be predicted by a general theory. If there are expected to be no such organisms, the reason behind such an expectation should be clear. Second, flies age more quickly than mice. Dogs age more slowly than mice but more quickly than horses or humans. Among mammals generally, large species age more slowly than small species. Similar patterns hold among birds (Calder, 1996). A satisfactory theory of aging ought to be able to explain these general patterns. Finally, there are major exceptions to the general pattern that larger mammals live longer. Bats and primates, for instance, live substantially longer than other mammals of the same body size (Austad & Fischer, 1991). An acceptable theory of aging ought to inform us as to the reasons these major exceptions to the general patterns exist.

As noted previously, virtually all mechanistic explanations of aging turn out to be noncompeting hypotheses rather than theories. The fact that one investigator feels strongly and has empirical support for the idea that the efficacy of genome maintenance is a key determinant of aging rate does not exclude or necessarily even affect the possibility that maintenance of membrane integrity and stability also contributes to aging. To the extent that mechanistic hypotheses have been expanded to become general theories, they have already been falsified, as I will show later.

From the preceding perspective, I believe that only three ideas qualify at our current state of knowledge as general theories of aging—two evolutionary in nature, one mechanistic—and two of the three have already been convincingly falsified. However, since this is not generally appreciated, I consider each of these three in some detail.

The Rate-of-Living Theory

Raymond Pearl (1928) gave the mechanistic rate-of-living theory its catchy name after several decades of research seemingly offered abundant evidence of its validity. The fundamental idea is that life itself, as embodied in the use of energy to support life's cellular and molecular processes, is inherently destructive and that consequently the more quickly energy is expended, the more rapidly tissue and organ damage will accumulate and thus the more rapidly aging occurs. This idea is intuitively quite satisfying, and it in fact pre-dated any significant supporting evidence (Weismann, 1882). By early in the 20th century, however, Max Rubner (1906) had measured resting energy expenditure in five species of mammal that differed by a 1,000-fold in body size and five-fold in life span and discovered that they used roughly the same amount of energy per kilogram of body mass in a lifetime. At about the same time, researchers studying ectothermic animals, such as insects, in the laboratory noticed that the warmer the temperature at which they were maintained, the shorter were their lives and conversely. It was these observations, combined with what he knew from Rubner's work, which convinced Pearl (1928) that "the duration of life varies inversely as the rate of energy expenditure during life" (p. 145). Several decades later, Denham Harman (1956) developed his free radical "theory," which, because oxygen radicals are an inevitable by-product of metabolism, seemed to provide a general mechanism for the rate-of-living effect. Soon after this, it was noticed that for a large selection of mammal species the rate at which longevity increased with body size matched almost exactly the rate at which metabolic rate per gram of body mass decreased with body size (Sacher, 1959), suggesting that all mammals had about the same energetic expenditure per cell per lifetime. Some species, such as mice, used up their energetic allotment quickly and died young, and others, such as elephants, used it slowly and survived for decades. Even the life-prolonging effect of food restriction in laboratory rodents was at one time attributed to a consequent decrease in metabolic rate (Sacher, 1977).

Rarely has a theory that we now know to be as thoroughly wrong as it is intuitively satisfying been so productive at inspiring research. We could say that the entire study of oxygen radical production and antioxidant defenses grew out of the rate-of-living theory. Scarcely a disease is now without its "oxidative stress" theory. At the same time, the major role of oxidative stress in aging is increasingly beleaguered (Austad, 2008).

Why do I say that the rate-of-living theory is now acknowledged by virtually everyone to be wrong? First, now that we know much more than earlier researchers about the longevity and metabolic rate of increasing numbers of species, the apparent constancy of cellular metabolic expenditure over a lifetime turns out to be illusory.

Lifetime energetic expenditure per gram body size varies by almost 30-fold among different mammal species (Austad & Fischer, 1991). Furthermore, some general species patterns of longevity directly conflict with predictions from the rate-of-living theory. For instance, marsupials have only 70% to 80% the metabolic rate of similar-sized eutherian mammals. The rate-of-living theory therefore predicts that marsupials should be longer lived than eutherians. In fact, the opposite is true. In addition, birds typically have higher metabolic rates than mammals of the same size yet on average live about three times longer (Holmes, Fluckiger, & Austad, 2001).

Perhaps even more damaging to the rate-of-living theory is recent work of John Speakman (2005), who not only considers how longevity relates to resting or basal metabolic rate, as most previous research has done, but instead considers actual daily energy expenditure under field conditions using doubly labeled water. His analyses reveal that lifetime energy expenditure is not independent of body mass but that small mammals typically expend more energy per gram of tissue per lifetime than do large mammals. Moreover, when he examines energy expenditure within a species—dogs—with abundant variation in body size and longevity, he finds that his smallest breed (Papillon) had nearly a 60% higher daily energy expenditure than his largest breed (Great Dane) yet lived more than 60% longer (Speakman, van Acker, & Harper, 2003).

Several other general observations also conflict with the rate-of-living theory. For one thing, because all animals have metabolic processes, then all animals should age. Whether all animals do in fact age is still controversial. Certainly there have been reports of some species, such as hydra, some worms, and even some fish and mammals, which do not appear to age (Bell, 1984; Buffenstein, 2008; Guerin, 2004; Martinez, 1998). However, whether these reports represent real nonaging animals or simply the lack of detailed information about them is not clear at this point. For decades it was assumed that bacteria, particularly those that reproduced by binary fission, did not age, but recently that was shown not to be true (Stewart, Madden, Paul, & Taddei, 2005). Additionally, it turns out that the robust life-extending and health-preserving effect of food restriction in laboratory rodents is not associated with reduced metabolic rate. Food restriction results in either no change or a slight increase in mass-specific metabolic rate (McCarter & Palmer, 1992; Selman et al., 2005). Thus, the rate-of-living theory fails to predict differences in aging rate between species or within species.

The rate-of-living theory has been reformulated for the molecular biology era and reborn as the oxidative stress theory of aging. Put succinctly by Sohal (1986), this idea states that aging "is directly related to the rate of unrepaired molecular damage inflected by the by-products of oxygen metabolism" (p. 26). However, even in this contemporary form, the rate-of-living theory fails. For instance, we now know that some long-lived mammals and birds survive quite nicely with higher levels of unrepaired oxidative molecular damage than their shorter-lived relatives (Andziak et al., 2006; Hamilton et al., 2001).

Aging as an Adaptive Program

The first evolutionary theory of aging considered it to be an adaptive process in the same sense that development and morphogenesis are considered to be adaptively programmed. In fact, whether aging is programmed or simply a nonadaptive by-product of adaptation for something else is a controversy that continues to bedevil the field (Austad, 2004; Bredesen, 2004). Weismann (1882) originated the idea of adaptive senescence, asserting that aging is beneficial in that it rids a species of old and decrepit individuals who would otherwise compete for resources with the young. Notice that there is an inherent circularity —a question begging—in this argument, as old individuals are assumed to be decrepit even though without aging they would not be. Weismann is to be credited, however, with the first serious thought on the evolution of aging.

The other problem with Weismann's theory is that it requires something called group selection, an evolutionary process in which traits spread during evolution because of their benefit to the group (population or species) rather than their benefit to the individual. When a trait is beneficial to both the individual and the group, it will certainly be favored evolutionarily. No one disputes that. The problem comes when something is detrimental to the individual (like aging) but beneficial to the group or beneficial to the individual but detrimental to the group. This particular issue was an area of virulent disagreement among evolutionary biologists in the 1960s and 1970s, but that disagreement has largely died away (albeit with an occasional spark from a dying ember) as mathematical modeling defined the conditions favoring and disfavoring group selection (Maynard Smith, 1976).

As we all learned in introductory biology, evolution by natural selection operates by differential survival and reproduction of individuals carrying different genetic traits. Group selection requires the fate of genetic traits to be due to differential survival and reproduction among groups or populations of individuals. But differential survival and reproduction of groups is typically a much slower process than differential survival and reproduction of individuals; thus, the effects of selection on individuals tend to swamp out selection on groups (Futuyma, 1986). Furthermore, group selection requires that groups have considerable genetic integrity; otherwise, traits favored within a group can be vitiated by the genes of immigrants. This is not to say that one cannot envision highly plausible scenarios in which group selection may operate, particularly when populations are structured in kin groups (Wilson, 1997). But to explain a virtually ubiquitous phenomenon such as aging, conditions favoring group selection would need to be virtually ubiquitous, something that virtually all evolutionary biologists reject (Rose, 1991).

Perhaps the easiest way to contrast aging as an adaptive program with aging as a nonadaptive accumulation of damage is to consider a species in which aging might possibly be adaptively programmed. Such a species could be any of the semelparous Pacific salmon (*Onchorhychus* spp.). As everyone knows, these fishes leave their natal streams and migrate to the ocean as young fry and return to their natal streams as adults, reproduce once, and then die. Their deterioration and death is highly stereotyped. They experience an extreme increase in circulating concentrations of the stress hormone cortisol, leading to the degeneration of multiple organs, and death is due to multiple organ failure. This series of events can be experimentally induced in young fish by the exogeneous administration of cortisol and can be avoided in mature fish by removing the gonads or the cortisol-producing glands.

A possible scenario by which this unique manifestation of aging could have evolved by group selection depends on the fact that juvenile fish return with very high fidelity to their natal stream (making each stream a genetically homogeneous population distinct from other genetically homogeneous stream populations) and that the advantage to postreproductive death is that the decomposing bodies of the parents increase food availability for the offspring of themselves and their close genetic relatives (Finch, 1990). Whether this scenario actually explains semelparity in salmon is not known. Note, however, that this is a highly specialized scenario and a stylized form of deterioration and death not seen frequently in other animals. Aging, on the other hand, is pervasive if not ubiquitous.

The other problem with the theory of aging as an adaptive program is that while it does address why aging exists, at its current state of development it does not address whether all species are expected to age, why certain species should age faster or slower than others, or why we might expect large species to generally live longer than small species.

Evolutionary Senescence Theory

The theory of aging that I will call evolutionary senescence theory and that has gained general acceptance over the past several decades grew out of a casual conversation between evolutionary biologist J. B. S. Haldane and immunologist Peter Medawar in the late 1940s. That discussion concerned why a fatal, dominant genetic allele that causes Huntington's disease (HD) was so common, roughly 1 case per 20,000 persons in northern European populations (Rose, 1991). Although this prevalence may not intuitively seem high, a reasonable expectation would be that an inevitably fatal allele would be subject to extreme selection pressure to remove it and would therefore be observed at little more than the recurring mutation frequency. However, only about 3% of cases occur in individuals without a family history of HD (Kremer et al., 1995), so clearly selection against it is weaker than one might imagine. Haldane's contribution was to point out that because the average age of onset of HD symptoms is late 40s to early 50s, those bearing the disease alleles would have had most if not all of the children they were likely to have before the disease was manifest. To the extent that the disease does not affect number of descendants left by its sufferers, then the disease alleles will be neither disfavored nor favored by natural selection. Despite its devastating effects on health, this allele would be evolutionarily neutral because it does not affect the number of descendants one leaves.

Medawar (1952) pondered this insight for a long time and finally published a long theoretical paper outlining a general theory of aging. His basic idea was that the power of natural selection to favor or disfavor genetic traits depends on the age at which those traits begin to affect Darwinian fitness, or the number of offspring produced. The later in life this happens, the weaker natural selection's impact. Assume, for instance, that you carried a gene that killed you immediately and inescapably on your 100th birthday. For several reasons, that gene will have no impact on the number of children you leave behind. First, you are very unlikely to still be alive for that gene to kill you. Only about 1 in 10,000 people in modern societies live to the age of 100. Second, even if you survived that long, you would certainly have long since ceased reproducing or even contributing to survival or reproduction of your children or grandchildren. The same logic would apply if the gene in question were beneficial to your personal health. Perhaps it might, on your 100th birthday, suddenly begin protecting you from ever dying from a heart attack. Natural selection would not affect the fate of that gene either for the same reason—it does not affect the number of offspring you leave.

By contrast, if our hypothetical gene killed you on your 15th birthday, you would be unlikely to leave any descendants at all. Natural selection would immediately make that gene disappear from the population, and it would reappear only when someone else in the population had a new mutation of the same sort in one of her germ cells. If on your 15th birthday a hypothetical gene protected you forever after from dying of a heart attack, then it might very well affect the number of descendants you left behind. If so, natural selection would see that over generations it became more and more common in the population. So traits affecting survival and reproduction early in life are strongly affected by natural selection, and to the extent that these effects appear later, natural selection will affect them more weakly. If reproduction and survival are affected by a gene sufficiently late in life, natural selection will be blind to the fate of that gene.

Medawar also addressed the subtle point of what "early in life" versus "late in life" means in this scenario. He noted trenchantly that "early" and "late" in life can be defined even for an animal that does not age because even nonaging organisms are not immortal. They still can be killed by external catastrophes, such as foul weather, famine, or disease. Early and late in life are defined by the likelihood that individuals will survive to that age regardless of whether they age.

Medawar's largely verbal theory implied that if there existed genes that had no effect on survival or reproduction until late in life but then had a horribly deleterious effect, those genes could become common because of very weak selection against them. If there were lots of such genes, then over time they would accumulate in the genome. This is Medawar's mutation accumulation hypothesis.

Medawar's basic idea had another implication that he noted in passing but was picked up and elaborated on by evolutionary biologist George C. Williams (1957) some years later. Williams noted that a hypothetical allele that had a beneficial effect on fitness early in life but a deleterious one later could actually be favored by natural selection because selection was powerful early in life and weak later on. This could be true even if the early life benefit was relatively small and the later effect large. This genetic effect came to be known as antagonistic pleiotropy. As an example of the type of effect he envisioned, Williams imagined an allele that would have a favorable effect on the calcification of bone during development but that later on might lead to calcification within arterial walls. Kirkwood (1977) later developed a closely related idea that he called the "disposable soma" theory of aging. According to this idea, aging is due to energetic trade-offs between growth, reproduction, and cellular maintenance activities. Evolution will work to optimize reproductive function even to the detriment of the soma.

Hamilton (1966) formulated the verbal models of Medawar and Williams in quantitative terms, showing how different age-specific effects on reproduction and survival can affect overall Darwinian fitness, thus theoretically confirming many of the predictions from the earlier models. He also showed that either form of gene action—mutation accumulation and antagonistic pleiotropy—could lead to the evolution of aging. The relative contribution of one form compared with the other was an empirical issue that required finding specific genes affecting aging. Others elaborated and refined Hamilton's model (Charlesworth, 1980; Rose, 1991).

Over the past 15 years, as alleles of more and more genes affecting aging rate have come to light, virtually all of them have been found to have detrimental early life fitness effects exactly as predicted by antagonistic pleiotropy theory. For instance, all the dwarfing genes in mice that extend life cause developmental delay, sterility, or subfertility. Sometimes these effects are subtle. For instance, the life extending worm gene *age-1* has no apparent antagonistically pleiotropic effect when worms are fed ad libitum as is typical in the lab, but when subjected to periodic food shortage as in nature, *age-1* mutants are quickly outcompeted by wild-type worms (Walker, McColl, Jenkins, Harris, & Lithgow, 2000). Support for mutation accumulation has remained weak, although it is inherently somewhat more difficult to empirically evaluate (Kirkwood & Austad, 2000).

But what about the strength of evidence for the general evolutionary theory of aging regardless of the form of gene action, driven by the declining power of natural selection with age? That theory makes a variety of predictions. First, it predicts that aging will evolve only in populations that have an age structure and not in populations that lack such structure. What sort of populations might lack age structure? Potentially, species in which there is no distinction between reproductive and somatic cells might lack age structure. Similarly, single-cell organisms that reproduce by binary fission might lack age structure.

In support of this idea, Bell (1984) followed laboratory populations of six species of asexually reproducing aquatic invertebrates, four of which reproduced by laying eggs and two of which reproduced by fission. He found that survival of individuals in all four egg-producing species declined with age but found no change or a small increase of survival with age in the species that reproduced by fission. Also supporting this idea was a report that hydra, which have no distinction between germ and somatic cells, did not senesce in the sense of showing a decline in reproduction or increase in mortality rate with age (Martinez, 1998). Among single-cell organisms, it was reported that those that reproduced asymmetrically, such as by budding, where a clear distinction between parent and offspring was possible, did indeed undergo aging, whereas those that reproduced by symmetric division did not.

Overlooked in these reports was that determining whether in symmetrically dividing species aging occurred was difficult because of problems with tracking individuals. Recently a remarkable study of *Escherichia coli,* the laboratory bacterium that reproduces by binary fission and had always been assumed to be the classic case of an organism that did not senesce, actually does so (Stewart et al., 2005). *Escherichia coli* are shaped like sausages. To reproduce, a cell lengthens until it is about twice its original length and then pinches off in the middle. These researchers realized that the recently pinched-off ends represent "new" cellular poles, whereas the original ends of the cell represent poles that were already in existence. Thus, after numerous divisions, some cells would consist of a new pole and a pole that had been in existence through many divisions, whereas others would consist of a new pole and a slightly less new pole, that is, a pole that had been in existence through only one or a few divisions. From this perspective, *E. coli* did have an age structure. Did the age of part of a cell matter? The answer turned out to be yes. By following more than 90 individual cell colonies as they repeatedly divided going from one to about 500 cells, researchers found that cells consisting of one very old pole grew and divided more slowly than cells without very old poles; that is, they did age. Moreover, they found that when cells divided, damaged proteins within the original cell were preferentially segregated into the new cell with the older pole (Lindner, Madden, Demarez, Stewart, & Taddei, 2008). In fact, new theoretical work suggests that in single-cell organisms, unless molecular damage can be completely avoided, such "rejuvenating reproduction" should be the norm (Ackermann, Chao, Bergstrom, & Doebeli, 2007). The new empirical and theoretical work does not specifically address whether some multicellular animals do indeed fail to age. However, these new data should give us pause about concluding without extensive evidence that any species does not age.

So whether there are populations lacking age structure or populations lacking senescence is no longer clear. However, the evolutionary prediction is still that if there are populations lacking age structure, they should indeed lack senescence as well.

What about the other phenomenon that a general theory should address—patterns of aging and longevity among species? Recall that larger mammal species generally live longer than small species (Figure 8.1). A second prediction from evolutionary senescence theory is that species that have evolved with a low level of environmental hazards should age more slowly than those that have evolved in high-hazard environments because the power of selection declines more slowly when the risk of nonsenescent death is low (Edney & Gill, 1968). This prediction has been supported both by experimental laboratory evolution (Stearns, Ackermann, Doebeli, & Kaiser, 2000) and by a natural experiment in the field (Austad, 1993).

One possible interpretation of the relationship between body size and longevity in mammals (and birds) is that body size inherently creates a safer environment for an animal. This would be due to larger animals having fewer potential predators, to their enhanced thermal inertia and hence greater resistance to temperature fluctuations, and to their lower metabolic rate, which would enhance their resistance to short-term food and water shortages. In addition, because larger animals typically live at lower population densities, their exposure to infectious agents might be reduced.

If this interpretation of the body size–longevity relation is valid, then it might be expected that animals that lived in safer environments for other reasons would be longer lived than expected. Generally, animals that are protected from predators by spines, armor, or venom are longer lived than similar-sized animals lacking protection (Austad & Fischer, 1991; Blanco & Sherman, 2005). Another trait that can affect animal safety from environmental hazards is aerial flight. Flight allows animals to avoid terrestrial predators and move long

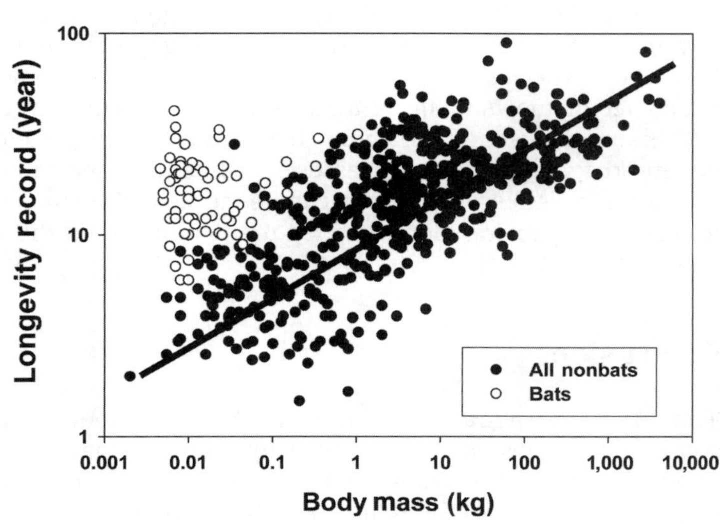

8.1

Record longevities for 623 mammal species. Note that all bats are exceptionally long lived for their body size.

distances quickly if local environmental conditions deteriorate. Among birds, species that are strong fliers are longer lived than species that are weak fliers (Holmes & Austad, 1995). Birds generally are substantially longer lived than mammals of similar body size (Calder, 1996). Therefore, one might predict that flying mammals would also be longer lived than expected for their body size, something that is clearly true (Figure 8.1). Bats are the longest-lived mammalian order, even though most longevity records for bats come from wild populations, whereas most such records in other mammals come from zoo records (Wilkinson & South, 2002).

Evolutionary senescence theory appears to be largely successful at addressing three of the large questions I previously mentioned—explaining why animals age at all, explaining large patterns in aging rate across species, and predicting exceptions to these patterns. However, several studies have appeared recently that seem to conflict with these predictions. For instance, guppies from natural streams lacking predators do not age more slowly when brought into the laboratory than guppies from streams with high-predation (Reznick, Bryant, Roff, Ghalambor, & Ghalambor, 2004), and fecundity continually increases with age in both slow-growing, long-lived populations and fast-growing, short-lived populations of garter snakes (Sparkman, Arnold, & Bronikowski, 2007).

The Medawar–Williams–Hamilton paradigm from which the classic evolutionary predictions evaluated in this section derive depends on a variety of assumptions about the effect of a change in extrinsic mortality on the population in question (Abrams, 1993). It has been known for some time that under different assumptions, differ predictions obtain (Rose, 1991). For instance, altered predation rate can affect not only extrinsic mortality but also fecundity as, say, population density is affected, which may in turn affect food availability (hence fecundity) for the survivors. These complex scenarios were not addressed by the original models but can easily be incorporated into them (Abrams, 1993). The full richness of evolutionary senescence theory has not yet been thoroughly worked out, although progress is being made (Abrams, 1993; Baudisch, 2005). It is rather remarkable that a simple population genetic model worked out more than 40 years ago has retained such powerful predictive power.

I also noted that it would be useful if a general theory of aging predicted how malleable to environmental or genetic manipulation the rate of aging might be within a species. Alas, current evolutionary theory, which remains divorced from specific mechanisms of aging, has not yet been developed to the point of addressing this issue. One hopes that with the emergence of deeper molecular genetic knowledge about processes of cellular damage and resistance to it, basic evolutionary senescence theory can be merged with molecular systems biology to ultimately provide more detailed predictions about the modulation of aging (Promislow & Pletcher, 2002).

Conclusions

Thankfully, there are not really more than 300 theories of aging, as has been sometimes suggested (Medvedev, 1990). Most of what are glibly called theories of aging is in fact mechanistic hypotheses that do not directly compete with one another. Many of them may be valid simultaneously. There are, however, at least three general theories of aging that make predictions about the ubiquity of senescence, broad patterns among species in the rate of aging, and when we might expect major exceptions to these patterns. Of these, evolutionary senescence theory is the only one with broad and deep evidentiary support. Empirical evidence to date strongly supports antagonistic pleiotropy as the form of gene action underlying the determination of aging rate. Evolutionary senescence theory still requires further elaboration, however, and would benefit enormously from a quantitative merging with modern molecular genetic systems biology—a development that could possibly emerge over the next few years.

References

Abrams, P. A. (1993). Does increased mortality favor the evolution of more rapid senescence? *Evolution, 47,* 877–887.

Ackermann, M., Chao, L., Bergstrom, C. T., & Doebeli, M. (2007). On the evolutionary origin of aging. *Aging Cell, 6,* 235–244.

Andziak, B., O'Connor, T. P., Qi, W., DeWaal, E. M., Pierce, A., Chaudhuri, A. R., et al. (2006). High oxidative damage levels in the longest-living rodent, the naked mole-rat. *Aging Cell, 5,* 463–471.

Anonymous. (2002). *Oxford English Dictionary* (2nd ed.). Oxford: Oxford University Press.

Austad, S. N. (1993). Retarded senescence in an insular population of Virginia opossums. *Journal of Zoology, 229,* 695–708.

Austad, S. N. (2004). Is aging programmed? *Aging Cell, 3,* 249–251.

Austad, S. N. (2005). A biologist's perspective: Whence come we, where are we, whither go we? In D. J. Sheets, D. B. Bradley, & J. Hendricks (Eds.), *Enduring questions and changing perspectives in gerontology* (pp. 29–62). New York: Springer Publishing.

Austad, S. N. (2008). Hot topics in vertebrate aging research 2007. *Aging Cell, 7,* 119–124.

Austad, S. N., & Fischer, K. E. (1991). Mammalian aging, metabolism, and ecology: Evidence from the bats and marsupials. *Journal of Gerontology: Social Sciences, 46,* 47–53.

Ayyadevara, S., Alla, R., Thaden, J. J., & Shmookler Reis, R. J. (2008). Remarkable longevity and stress resistance of nematode PI3K-null mutants. *Aging Cell, 7,* 13–22.

Bartke, A., Wright, J. C., Mattison, J. A., Ingram, D. K., Miller, R. A., & Roth, G. S. (2001). Extending the lifespan of long-lived mice. *Nature, 414,* 412.

Baudisch, A. (2005). Hamilton's indicators of the force of selection. *Proceedings of the National Academy of Sciences of the United States of America, 102,* 8263–8268.

Bell, G. (1984). Evolutionary and nonevolutionary theories of senescence. *American Naturalist, 124,* 600–603.

Blanco, M. A., & Sherman, P. W. (2005). Maximum longevities of chemically protected and non-protected fishes, reptiles, and amphibians support evolutionary hypotheses of aging. *Mechanisms of Ageing and Development, 126,* 794–803.

Bredesen, D. E. (2004). The non-existent aging program: How does it work? *Aging Cell, 3,* 255–259.

Buffenstein, R. (2008). Negligible senescence in the longest living rodent, the naked mole-rat: Insights from a successfully aging species. *Journal of Comparative Physiology. B, Biochemical, Systemic, and Environmental Physiology, 178,* 439–445.

Calder, W. A. I. (1996). *Size, function, and life history* (New ed.). Mineola, NY: Dover.

Charlesworth, B. (1980). *Evolution in age-structured populations.* Cambridge: Cambridge University Press.

Edney, E. B., & Gill, R. W. (1968). Evolution of senescence and specific longevity. *Nature, 220,* 281–282.

Finch, C. E. (1990). *Longevity, senescence, and the genome.* Chicago: University of Chicago Press.

Futuyma, D. J. (1986). *Evolutionary biology* (2nd ed.). Sunderland, MA: Sinauer Associates.

George, J. C., Bada, J., Zeh, J., Scott, L., Brown, S. E., O'Hara, T., et al. (1999). Age and growth estimates of bowhead whales (*Balaena mysticetus*) via aspartic acid racemization. *Canadian Journal of Zoology, 77,* 571–580.

Guerin, J. C. (2004). Emerging area of aging research: Long-lived animals with "negligible senescence." *Annals of the New York Academy of Sciences, 1019,* 518–520.

Hamilton, M. L., Guo, Z., Fuller, C. D., Van, R. H., Ward, W. F., Austad, S. N., et al. (2001). A reliable assessment of 8-oxo-2-deoxyguanosine levels in nuclear and mitochondrial DNA using the sodium iodide method to isolate DNA. *Nucleic Acids Research, 29,* 2117–2126.

Hamilton, W. D. (1966). The moulding of senescence by natural selection. *Journal of Theoretical Biology, 12,* 12–45.

Harman, D. (1956). Aging: A theory based on free radical and radiation chemistry. *Journal of Gerontology, 11,* 298–300.

Holmes, D. J., & Austad, S. N. (1995). Birds as animal models for the comparative biology of aging: A prospectus. *Journal of Gerontology: Biological Sciences, 50,* 59–66.

Holmes, D. J., Fluckiger, R., & Austad, S. N. (2001). Comparative biology of aging in birds: An update. *Experimental Gerontology, 36,* 869–883.

Kaeberlein, T. L., Smith, E. D., Tsuchiya, M., Welton, K. L., Thomas, J. H., Fields, S., et al. (2006). Lifespan extension in *Caenorhabditis elegans* by complete removal of food. *Aging Cell, 5,* 487–494.

Kirkwood, T. B. (1977). Evolution of ageing. *Nature, 270,* 301–304.

Kirkwood, T. B., & Austad, S. N. (2000). Why do we age? *Nature, 408,* 233–238.

Kremer, B., Almqvist, E., Theilmann, J., Spence, N., Telenius, H., Goldberg, Y. P., et al. (1995). Sex-dependent mechanisms for expansions and contractions of the CAG repeat on affected Huntington disease chromosomes. *American Journal of Human Genetics, 57,* 343–350.

Lindner, A. B., Madden, R., Demarez, A., Stewart, E. J., & Taddei, F. (2008). Asymmetric segregation of protein aggregates is associated with cellular aging and rejuvenation. *Proceedings of the National Academy of Sciences of the United States of America, 105,* 3076–3081.

Magwere, T., Chapman, T., & Partridge, L. (2004). Sex differences in the effect of dietary restriction on life span and mortality rates in female and male *Drosophila melanogaster. Journals of Gerontology: Biological Sciences, 59,* 3–9.

Martinez, D. E. (1998). Mortality patterns suggest lack of senescence in hydra. *Experimental Gerontology, 33,* 217–225.

Maynard Smith, J. (1976). Group selection. *Quarterly Review of Biology, 51,* 277–283.

McCarter, R. J., & Palmer, J. (1992). Energy metabolism and aging: A lifelong study of Fischer 344 rats. *American Journal of Physiology, 263,* E448–E452.

Medawar, P. B. (1952). *An unsolved problem in biology.* London: H. K. Lewis.

Medvedev, Z. A. (1990). An attempt at a rational classification of theories of ageing. *Biological Reviews of the Cambridge Philosophical Society, 65,* 375–398.

Pearl, R. (1928). *The rate of living.* New York: A. A. Knopf.

Popper, K. (1959). *The logic of scientific discovery.* New York: Basic Books.

Promislow, D. E., & Pletcher, S. D. (2002). Advice to an aging scientist. *Mechanics of Ageing and Development, 123,* 841–850.

Reznick, D. N., Bryant, M. J., Roff, D., Ghalambor, C. K., & Ghalambor, D. E. (2004). Effect of extrinsic mortality on the evolution of senescence in guppies. *Nature, 431,* 1095–1099.

Rose, M. R. (1991). *Evolutionary biology of aging.* Oxford: Oxford University Press.

Rubner, M. (1906). *Das Problem der Lebensdauer und seine Beziehungen zum Wachstum und Ernahrung.* Munich: Oldenbourg.

Sacher, G. A. (1959). Relation of life span to brain weight and body weight in mammals. In G. E. W. Wolstenholme & M. O'Connor (Eds.), *CIBA Foundation Colloquia on Ageing* (pp. 115–141). London: Churchill.

Sacher, G. A. (1977). Life table modification and life prolongation. In L. Hayflick & C. E. Finch (Eds.), *Handbook of the biology of aging* (pp. 69–82). New York: Van Nostrand Reinhold.

Selman, C., Phillips, T., Staib, J. L., Duncan, J. S., Leeuwenburgh, C., & Speakman, J. R. (2005). Energy expenditure of calorically restricted rats is higher than predicted from their altered body composition. *Mechanics of Ageing and Development, 126,* 783–793.

Sohal, R. S. (1986). The rate of living theory: A contemporary interpretation. In K.-G. Collatz & R. S. Sohal (Eds.), *Insect aging* (pp. 23–44). Berlin: Springer-Verlag.

Sparkman, A. M., Arnold, S. J., & Bronikowski, A. M. (2007). An empirical test of evolutionary theories for reproductive senescence and reproductive effort in the garter snake *Thamnophis elegans. Proceedings Biological Science, the Royal Society, 274,* 943–950.

Speakman, J. R. (2005). Body size, energy metabolism and lifespan. *Journal of Experimental Biology, 208,* 1717–1730.

Speakman, J. R., van Acker, A. A., & Harper, E. J. (2003). Age-related changes in the metabolism and body composition of three dog breeds and their relationship to life expectancy. *Aging Cell, 2,* 265–275.

Stearns, S. C., Ackermann, M., Doebeli, M., & Kaiser, M. (2000). Experimental evolution of aging, growth, and reproduction in fruitflies. *Proceedings of the National Academy of Sciences of the United States of America, 97,* 3309–3313.

Stewart, E. J., Madden, R., Paul, G., & Taddei, F. (2005). Aging and death in an organism that reproduces by morphologically symmetric division. *Public Library of Science Biology, 3*(e45), 295–300.

Walker, D. W., McColl, G., Jenkins, N. L., Harris, J., & Lithgow, G. J. (2000). Evolution of lifespan in *C. elegans*. *Nature, 405,* 296–297.

Weindruch, R., Walford, R. L., Fligiel, S., & Guthrie, D. (1986). The retardation of aging in mice by dietary restriction: Longevity, cancer, immunity and lifetime energy intake. *Journal of Nutrition, 116,* 641–654.

Weismann, A. (1882). *Über die Dauer des Lebens.* Jena: G. Fischer.

Wilkinson, G. S., & South, J. M. (2002). Life history, ecology and longevity in bats. *Aging Cell, 1,* 124–131.

Williams, G. C. (1957). Pleiotropy, natural selection, and the evolution of senescence. *Evolution, 11,* 398–411.

Wilson, D. S. (1997). Human groups as units of selection. *Science, 276,* 1816–1817.

The Immunological Theory of Aging Revisited

9

Rita B. Effros

Biological aging is intrinsically linked to multiple and bidirectional interactions between organisms and their environment. Indeed, it is probable that these interactions played a central role in the evolution of life span. One of the key components of the interplay between the internal and external environments is the immune system, which enables multicellular organisms to effectively deal with the extensive array of pathogens to be encountered throughout life.

As early as 1961, the late Roy Walford proposed the novel hypothesis that normal aging is pathogenically related to faulty immunological processes.

Acknowledgments: The research described in this chapter was supported by the following funding sources: NIH AG 023720 and AI 060362 and the Plott Endowed Chair in Gerontology.

To explore this paradigm shift in the field of gerontology, he submitted a National Institutes of Health grant titled "The Role of Immune Phenomena in the Aging Process" and in 1969 further expanded this notion in his now-classic book *The Immunologic Theory of Aging* (Walford, 1969).

Research over the nearly 50 years since those ideas were first suggested has confirmed this farsighted vision regarding the central role of the immune system in aging. Indeed, several longitudinal studies in elderly humans have documented significant correlations between specific immune functional traits and early mortality regardless of the cause of death (Wayne, Rhyne, Garry, & Goodwin, 1990; Wikby, Maxson, Olsson, Johansson, & Ferguson, 1998). Even in the simple organism *Caenorhabditis elegans,* longevity is associated with increased resistance to bacteria (Garsin et al., 2003), underscoring the evolutionarily conserved link between immunity and life span. Doubtless, the original immunological theory of aging was based on information that is far less sophisticated than what is currently known about the immune system, yet its basic tenets have withstood the test of time.

This chapter first reviews the major characteristics of the immune system and then provides some illustrative examples of important connections between immune function and biological aging. Revisiting the original immunological theory of aging from the vantage point of more recent research on the process of aging and the intricate workings of the immune system not only confirms the validity of the theory but also provides a scientific framework for developing novel immune-based approaches for increasing human health span.

Immunology 101

Innate Versus Adaptive Immunity

The immune system, which is central to our ability to deal with the external environment, has two main components, one that is considered to be innate and the other that is known as "adaptive." Innate immunity in mammals closely resembles the immune systems of lower organisms, from which it undoubtedly evolved. This type of immunity is fairly nonspecific but, nonetheless, constitutes a rapid and fairly efficient first line of defense. By contrast, adaptive immunity requires more time to develop an optimal response and is characterized by its exquisite specificity and the capacity to develop memory, features that form the basis for successful vaccination, and rapid immune reactivity to repeatedly encountered pathogens. The combined activities of the innate and adaptive immune systems provide excellent coverage against the myriad of different bacteria, viruses, and parasites that we encounter throughout life.

Specificity Within the Adaptive Immune System

The two major cellular components of the adaptive immune system are T and B lymphocytes, cells that derive from hematopoietic stem cells within the marrow of our long bones. Each T and B cell has on its surface a unique receptor by which it can recognize a specific foreign substance, or "antigen." The intricate genetic mechanism by which these antigen receptors are formed leads to the generation of an immune system with an enormous range of specificities.

Briefly, during the development of each lymphocyte, one member of a set of gene segments is joined to other gene segments by an irreversible process of DNA recombination. The selection of the particular gene segment for each juxtaposition event is totally random, so that the final antigen-receptor molecule is unique to that particular B or T cell. The consequence of this intricate mechanism is that just a few hundred different gene segments can combine in a variety of ways to create thousands of receptor chains. Moreover, since functional antigen receptors are composed of two different receptor chains, each encoded by distinct sets of gene segments, an additional level of diversity is added during the random pairing of two different chains. By these mechanisms, a small amount of genetic material is utilized to generate at least 10^8 different specificities. The unique antigen specificity of the individual lymphocytes combines to create an immune system that is capable of responding to the nearly infinite number of foreign antigens that could be encountered over a lifetime.

Clonal Expansion

Each lymphocyte expresses many copies of its antigen receptor on the cell surface, and once generated, the receptor specificity of a particular lymphocyte (and its progeny) does not change (Janeway, Travers, McClemments, & Wellcome, 1997). When an antigen interacts with receptors expressed on a mature lymphocyte, that lymphocyte becomes activated and starts dividing, giving rise to a clone of identical progeny bearing identical receptors for antigen. Antigen specificity is thereby maintained as the dividing cells continue to proliferate and differentiate into effector cells that function to eliminate the foreign pathogen. Once the antigen is cleared, a small number of memory cells persist, all expressing the same antigen receptor. If the same antigen is encountered again, the process of activation and clonal expansion is repeated.

The two main components of the adaptive immune system perfectly complement each other in their activities. B cells secrete a soluble protein known as antibody, which can essentially "neutralize" or inactivate pathogens that are still in the bloodstream. However, once a bacterium or virus infects a cell, it is essentially invisible to antibodies. At this point, the T cell arm of the immune system takes over. In particular, cytotoxic T cells are the effector cells within the immune system that are able to recognize and kill infected cells. However, because of the enormous antigenic receptor repertoire, the number of cells that can recognize and respond to any single antigen is extremely small. Thus, to generate a sufficient quantity of specific effector cells to fight an infection, the few cytotoxic T cells that recognize a particular virus, for example, must undergo massive clonal expansion. For this reason, the process of proliferation (i.e., cell division) is a critical component of successful immunity, and the natural barrier to unlimited cell division, known as the Hayflick limit, is highly relevant to cells of the immune system. Indeed, the intrinsic cellular program that limits the number of cell divisions before the cells reach a state of irreversible growth arrest, known as replicative senescence, could potentially have devastating consequences on immune function, as is discussed later.

Replicative Senescence and the Immune System

In Vitro Models

The process of replicative, or cellular, senescence has been studied extensively in a variety of cell types since the original observations of Hayflick (Hayflick & Moorhead, 1961). Although some of the early research in this area had been based on the naive notion that aging at the organismic levels was due to aging at the level of individual cells, it is now clear that the relationship is far more subtle and complex. In the case of fibroblasts, for example, it has been shown that senescent fibroblasts may create a suitable microenvironment for cancer development and thereby indirectly affect life span (Campisi & d'Adda, 2007). Similarly, other types of senescent cells within specific organ systems may exert negative influences and exacerbate or initiate pathological changes (Chang & Harley, 1995).

Given the importance of adequate clonal expansion in generating T cell responses, the potential barrier of replicative senescence would be predicted to play a pivotal role in immune function, especially by old age. To test this possibility, cell culture models of T cell replicative senescence were established by several different groups with the goal of identifying the specific characteristics associated with lymphocyte senescence (Pawelec, Rehbein, Haehnel, Meri, & Adibzadeh, 1997; Perillo, Walford, Newman, & Effros, 1989). It is now clear that T cell senescence shares some characteristics with other cell types that reach senescence and also displays some unique features. Similar to other cell types that reach replicative senescence in vitro, cultures of senescent T cells show irreversible growth arrest, increased expression of several cell cycle inhibitors, inability to undergo apoptosis (a type of death that is initiated by the cell itself), and telomere shortening (Dagarag, Evazyan, Rao, & Effros, 2004; Spaulding, Guo, & Effros, 1999; Vaziri et al., 1993). Telomeres are the ends of chromosomes that shorten with each cell division and are believed to be the "clock" that keeps track of the number of divisions a cell has undergone. When a critically short telomere length is reached, the cell enters a state of irreversible growth arrest (Harley, Futcher, & Greider, 1990).

As T cells progress to senescence in culture, they also show altered secretion patterns of several key soluble mediators, known as cytokines. Specifically, with increasing numbers of population doublings, T cells secrete progressively higher titers of two proinflammatory cytokines, namely, tumor necrosis factor-alpha (TNFα) and interleukin-6 (IL-6), and reduced levels of a critical antiviral cytokine, interferon-gamma (IFNγ; Dagarag et al., 2004; Effros, Dagarag, Spaulding, & Man, 2005). Importantly, senescent T cells no longer express a key signaling surface receptor, CD28. After undergoing multiple rounds of antigen-driven cell division, cultures initiated from T cells that all expressed CD28 become nearly 100 percent CD28-negative (CD28–) at senescence (Effros et al., 1994).

Replicative Senescence Is a Physiological Process

The results of the in vitro studies paved the way for the in vivo analysis of this facet of immune function during normal aging. Based on the cell culture observation that absence of CD28 expression is a marker of senescence, analysis of this marker in blood samples provided a practical approach to determining whether senescent T cells accumulate with age. Several groups have shown that older persons have significant increases in the proportion of T cells lacking CD28 expression, with some aged individuals having >60% CD28– cells within the CD8+ T cell subset, compared to the mean young adult value of <10% (Effros et al., 1994). These putatively senescent T cells are often part of oligoclonal expansions, suggesting that they arose as a consequence of the immune response to specific antigens. Telomere studies have confirmed that the CD28– cells had undergone extensive cell division compared to other T cells from the same individual.

Importantly, cells lacking CD28 expression do not suddenly appear in old age; there is a progressive increase over the life span in the proportion of T cells that lack CD28 expression (Boucher et al., 1998). Moreover, chronological age is not unique in its association with T cell replicative senescence. T cells with the characteristics associated with senescence are seen in a variety of clinical situations that involve chronic stimulation of the immune system. Persons with rheumatoid arthritis, an autoimmune disease involving abnormal reactivity of T cells to self-antigens within the affected joints, have increased proportions of T cells lacking CD28. These cells secrete high titers of TNFα, one of the cytokines associated with replicative senescence in cell culture studies. Chronic infection with human immunodeficiency virus-1 (HIV-1) is also associated with the progressive accumulation over time of CD8+ T cells that are CD28– (Borthwick, Bofill, & Gombert, 1994). Telomere analysis on purified cell populations showed that the mean telomere length of the CD8+CD28– T cells from 43-year-old persons infected with HIV was the same range as that of lymphocytes isolated from (uninfected) centenarians (Effros et al., 1996).

Chronic Stimulation Drives Replicative Senescence In Vivo

It has been suggested that infection with herpes viruses may constitute the underlying cause for the accumulation of senescent CD8+ T cells during aging (Pawelec et al., 2004). Most humans become infected with herpesviruses, such as cytomegalovirus (CMV) or Epstein-Barr virus (EBV) early in life, and the viruses establish a persistent latent state, meaning that they are never eliminated from the body. Reemergence from the latent state does not generally occur, except in immunocompromised individuals, such as recipients of organ transplants who take immunosuppressive drugs to prevent rejection. Nevertheless, maintaining the latent state of these herpesviruses is not without cost. Indeed, it seems that the immune system is working overtime to keep herpesviruses latent over many decades.

Elderly persons have large numbers of dysfunctional CD8+ T cells bearing antigen receptors for a specific antigenic component of CMV (Ouyang et al., 2003). Even younger persons who are infected with HIV and whose immune systems are thought to age prematurely harbor substantial numbers of CD8+CD28– T cells that are specific for CMV and EBV. These sorts of data suggest that the long-term outcome of maintaining control over latent infections is the progressive generation of senescent CD8+ T cells (Pawelec et al., 2004). Since senescent cells are unable to undergo apoptosis, they persist and begin to occupy progressively more and more of the memory T cell pool in the elderly, restricting the repertoire of the remaining T cells. Since naive T cell production is reduced with age because of the reduced output by the thymus (Jamieson et al., 1999), the T cell population of elderly persons contains reduced proportions of cells that can respond to neoantigens and increased proportions of memory cells, many of which are senescent or are approaching senescence.

Latent herpesviruses are not the only driving force for the generation of senescent T cells. Cells with surface markers suggesting of senescence are observed in additional clinical situations that involve chronic antigenic stimulation. As noted previously, in rheumatoid arthritis, there are high proportions of senescent CD4 (helper) T cells in the affected joints. Tumor-associated antigens may also cause chronic stimulation of T cells. Indeed, in advanced cases of renal carcinoma, the proportion of CD8+ T cells with a senescent phenotype has been shown to have predictive value with respect to patient survival (Characiejus et al., 2002). Similarly, in patients with head and neck tumors, the proportion of CD8+CD28− T cells increases during the period of tumor growth and diminishes once the tumor has been removed (Tsukishiro, Donnenberg, & Whiteside, 2003). These studies provide further evidence in support of a role for chronic stimulation as the key factor in the accumulation of senescent T cells in vivo.

Immune System Involvement in Age-Related Pathologies

The beneficial effects of the immune system, which is devoted to the neutralization of harmful environmental agents early in life, may become detrimental during old age, a period not foreseen by evolution. Indeed, a variety of age-related pathologies are now understood to involve immune cell components. In some cases, there is evidence that the immune system is actually responsible for the disease, but in others, a causal role has not yet been established. Nonetheless, even if the immune system is only involved in disease progression, the link itself raises the possibility of immune-based therapeutic approaches that might limit disease severity or retard its progression.

Inflammation and Aging

It is through inflammation and its mediators that the immune system influences critical defense reactions against foreign pathogens. Nevertheless, *chronic* elevation of these mediators is known to have negative influences on a variety of organ systems and, indeed, on life span itself. Several studies have shown that increased levels of circulating proinflammatory cytokines, such as IL-6 and TNFα, and their receptors are strong independent risk factors of morbidity and mortality in the elderly (Bruunsgaard & Pedersen, 2003). Hyperproduction of proinflammatory cytokines in the elderly is also associated with increased production of several chemokines and C-reactive protein, which are correlated with multiple age-related pathologies (Appay & Rowland-Jones, 2002; Bo et al., 2005; Mariani et al., 2002).

In mice subject to the life span–extending regimen of caloric restriction, there is a reduction in T cell production of both TNFα and IL-6, suggesting that this cytokine profile change may play a role in the increased survival (Spaulding, Walford, & Effros, 1997). These and other studies have led to the term "inflamm-aging" to reflect the central role of inflammation in the age-associated immunological changes (De Martinis, Franceschi, Monti, & Ginaldi, 2006; Salvioli et al., 2006). This notion is further underscored by data from Swedish longitudinal studies on elderly humans that highlight the importance of low-grade inflammation in predicting mortality very late in life (Wikby et al., 2006).

Inflammation effects need not begin during the period of old age. Indeed, inflammatory exposure early in life can persist throughout adulthood and has been proposed as a major determinant of life span. The notion that reduction in lifetime exposure to infectious diseases and other sources of inflammation contributes to the historical decline in old-age mortality is supported by analysis of cohort mortality data spanning two centuries (Finch & Crimmins, 2004). These data are consistent with the hypothesis that the chronic inflammatory effects of infections during early life drive subsequent old-age morbidity and mortality.

Osteoimmunology

Bone homeostasis is the result of both local and systemic factors, and recent observations have documented that some of these mediators are produced by cells within the immune system. It is becoming increasingly clear that age-associated loss in bone mass is due not only to hormonal changes but also to immunological effects. Activated T cells secrete large amounts of RANKL (receptor-activator for NFkB ligand), which functions to drive the maturation and activation of osteoclasts, the cells responsible for bone resorption. Other factors produced by immune cells, such as TNFα, IL-6, and IFNγ, also play a role in bone homeostasis by tipping the balance between osteoclast and osteoblast activity. The emerging picture in the new and highly active field known as "osteoimmunology" (Arron & Choi, 2000) is that skeletal bone integrity results from complex regulatory interactions between bone-remodeling cells and immune cells. Clinical studies further reinforce this link, for example, by documenting the association between T lymphocytes with a senescent phenotype and osteoporotic fractures in elderly women (Pietschmann et al., 2001).

Decrease in bone density during aging is not restricted to skeletal bone. Reduced bone mass within the oral cavity is a major cause of tooth loss in the elderly and may also be linked to other age-related pathologies, such as atherosclerosis. Details of immune cell involvement in the loss of alveolar bone (bone within the jaw) are just beginning to emerge. For example, both helper (CD4+) and cytotoxic (CD8+) T lymphocytes are present in periodontal lesions (Lorenzo, 2000; Seguier, Godeau, Leborgne, Pivert, & Brousse, 1999), and these cells express markers indicative of memory and activation (Taubman & Kawai, 2001). Moreover, interference with RANKL, by systemic administration of osteoprotegerin, a decoy molecule that inhibits RANK binding to its RANKL, results in abrogation of periodontal disease, indicating that T cell mediated involvement in bone resorption is RANKL dependent (Taubman, Valverde, Han, & Kawai, 2005). Interestingly, the presence of CD8+ T cells lacking CD28 expression in gingival tissue was reported (Wassenaar, Reinhardus, Abraham-Inpijn, & Kievits, 1996). As noted previously, the CD8+CD28– phenotype is associated with replicative senescence, suggesting that chronic antigenic stimulation may play a role in alveolar bone loss. If the CD8+CD28– within the gingival tissue produce the same proinflammatory cytokines (TNFα and IL6) as T cells that reach replicative senescence in vitro, they may be contributing to alveolar bone loss.

Immune Cells and the Brain

Similar to age-related pathologies involving bone, Alzheimer's disease (AD) also involves a number of cells and proteins associated with the immune system (McGeer & McGeer, 1996). The interaction between the proinflammatory cytokine IL-6 with beta amyloid is thought to play an active role in the development of AD neuropathology; IL-6 is produced not only by astrocytes and microgila cells but also by several types of immune cells. The levels of IL-6 are known to increase within the central nervous system of AD patients (Blum-Degen et al., 1995). Importantly, IL-6 has numerous activities that may impact AD, such as modulating neuron differentiation (Satoh et al., 1988) and decreasing the integrity of the blood–brain barrier (de Vries et al., 1996). Moreover, IL-6 is directly involved in regulation of the Alzheimer's beta amyloid precursor protein (APP) production (Brugg et al., 1995; Del, Angeretti, Lucca, De Simoni, & Forloni, 1995).

An integral role of IL-6 in AD is also consistent with data showing association of a particular variant allele of IL-6 with delayed onset and reduced risk of AD (Papassotiropoulos et al., 1999). Moreover, since serum IL-6 levels are correlated with the severity of dementia, IL-6 may be useful as a biomarker of disease progression (Kaalmaan et al., 1997). Other immune system proteins, such as IL-1 and those of the classical complement pathway (Zanjani et al., 2005), are closely connected with beta-amyloid deposits, and high plasma concentration of TNFα is associated with dementia in centenarians (Bruunsgaard et al., 1999).

There is also evidence suggesting possible involvement of a specific adaptive immune response in AD. Activated microglia express high levels of MHC class II glycoproteins and could therefore theoretically function as antigen-presenting cells. T cells do, in fact, infiltrate the diseased tissue in AD, suggesting possible antigen recognition. Interestingly, activated T and B cells express high levels of surface APP expression, suggesting that the immune system may be regularly exposed to this AD precursor protein (Bullido, Muanoz-Fernandez, Recuero, Fresno, & Valdivieso, 1996). In that regard, it has been reported that T cells from healthy but not AD patients undergo increased proliferation and IL-2 production in response to APP peptides.

The previous observations raise the intriguing possibility that cellular immunity may normally function to protect against AD by helping to eliminate potentially amyloidogenic substances and that AD occurs when the system fails (Trieb, Ransmayr, Sgonc, Lassmann, & Grubeck-Loebenstein, 1996). The notion of normal immune system responses going awry in AD has also been suggested in studies on complement components in the brain where some of the normal regulators of complement were absent in the diseased brain (Zanjani et al., 2005).

Telomere studies on persons with AD are also consistent with immune system involvement. In a small study on community-dwelling persons with AD, it was shown that telomere length of T cells correlated with disease status, as determined by the Mini-Mental Status Exam. The association was true only for T cells and not for B cells or monocytes, eliminating the possibility that the telomere attrition was due to generalized oxidative stress (Panossian et al., 2002). Lymphocyte telomere dysfunction has also been reported in other studies on AD (Zhang et al., 2003). Interestingly, persons with Down syndrome, who universally develop AD by age 40, show accelerated lymphocyte telomere loss compared to age-matched controls (Vaziri et al., 1993). Further research is required to determine the underlying mechanism for the lymphocyte telomere length findings with respect to AD. At this point, it is unclear whether immune cells play a role in the initiation and/or progression of the disease.

Cardiovascular Disease

Epidemiological studies as well as laboratory experiments strongly support direct involvement of the immune system in cardiovascular disease (CVD). The role of monocytes, which develop into inflamed foam cells on exposure to oxidized lipids, has been well established (Libby, 2007). In addition, it has been shown that T cells are present in atherosclerotic lesions (Libby, Sukhova, Lee, & Galis, 1995; Schmitz, Herr, & Rothe, 1998; Seko et al., 1997; Zhdanov, Chumachenko, Cherpachenko, Beskrovnova, & Lavrova, 1995) and that there is direct interaction of CD40 on T cells with vascular endothelial cells, smooth muscle cells, and macrophages (Mach et al., 1997). Thus, several immune cell types have been implicated in CVD. Moreover, growing evidence suggests that cytokines participate as autocrine or paracrine factors in atherogenesis since immune cells in lesions can both produce and respond to these mediators (Libby et al., 1995).

The initiating events in CVD are unclear, but systemic inflammation or autoreactivity caused by chronic infections have been hypothesized to increase the risk of CVD. Cross-reactivity between the normal cellular heat shock protein 60 (hsp60) with bacterial antigens has been proposed by several investigators (George, Harats, Gilburd, & Shoenfeld, 1996; Mayr et al., 1999; Metzler, Xu, & Wick, 1998). This notion is consistent with studies on clinically healthy volunteers in whom sonographically documented carotid artery atherosclerosis is correlated with increased antibody titers to hsp65 compared to controls with no lesion. Follow-up studies showed that those with highest antibody titers showed highest mortality (Xu et al., 1999). In an animal model of atherosclerosis, the addition of hsp65 actually increases the severity of atherosclerotic lesions induced by high cholesterol diet alone (Xu & Wick, 1996). The blocking of the hsp65 effect by T cell immunosuppressive agents further implicates specific immunity in the pathogenesis of atherosclerosis (Metzler et al., 1998).

An increasing body of epidemiological evidence links immune reactivity, *Chlamidia pneumoniae* with CVD, consistent with studies showing antibiotics might reduce risks of CVD events (Gupta et al., 1997; Gurfinkel, Bozovich, Daroca, Beck, & Mautner, 1997; Halme & Surcel, 1997). In animal studies, immunization with myosin peptides that resemble those present in *Chlamidia* induces antigen-specific T cells that were able to transfer heart disease to fresh mice, consistent with an autoimmune response based on antigenic mimicry (Bachmaier et al., 1999).

Cancer

Cancer is a disease of old age. Indeed, being old confers an even greater risk for cancer development than smoking. There is increasing evidence that failure of adequate immunosurveillance may play a role in tumor initiation and progression, particularly for those cancers that have a viral etiology (Kreft et al., 2000). Indeed, tumors associated with latent viral infections frequently arise in persons with immunodeficiency. For example, in immunosuppressed individuals, virtually all lymphomas are EBV in origin, presumably resulting from the failure of T cells to effectively control EBV infection (Israel & Kenney, 2003; Pardoll, 2001). Kaposi's sarcoma is consequent to latent infection with another herpesvirus infection (HSV 8), and cervical cancer, which also increases during immune suppression, is associated with certain strains of human papillomavirus.

Even nonviral tumor-associated antigens have the potential to drive relevant antigen-reactive T cells to replicative senescence. For example, prostate-specific antigen (PSA), whose elevated blood levels are observed during prostate cancer, is also present in normal prostate tissue and is thus an antigen to which T cells have had prolonged exposure (Kennedy-Smith et al., 2002); CD8+ T cells from patients with prostate cancer do, in fact, show reactivity to PSA peptides (Chakraborty et al., 2003), consistent with the notion that they have been previously primed to this antigen. Thus, like antigens of viruses that establish latency, tumor-associated antigens have the potential to cause chronic T cell activation, possibly driving some antigen-specific cells to senescence.

Mortality

Recent longitudinal studies provide further support to the immunological theory of aging. In one study, lymphocyte telomere length at age 60 was shown to be predictive of subsequent life span. The immune involvement in these associations is underscored by that fact that the individuals with telomere lengths in the shortest quartile at age 60 had a seven- to eight-fold greater risk of dying from infection as compared with those in the longest telomere quartile group (Cawthon, Smith, O'Brien, Sivatchenko, & Kerber, 2003).

The Swedish OCTO and NONA longitudinal studies on elderly cohorts examined a variety of physiological parameters associated with life span and identified a cluster of immune parameters strongly predictive of early mortality, independent of the cause of death (Wikby et al., 2002; Wikby et al., 1998). This so-called immune risk phenotype consisted of a reversal of the normal ratio between helper and cytotoxic T cells, reduced T cell proliferative potential, increased proportion of CD8+ T cells lacking CD28 (i.e., senescent T cells), and evidence of CMV infection. The inclusion of high proportions of senescent T cells in immune risk phenotype has been viewed as a clinical confirmation of the importance of the Hayflick limit in human organismic aging (Effros & Pawelec, 1997).

The underlying mechanism for the associations between immune profiles and mortality is not known. Clearly, if the senescent T cells present in vivo have proinflammatory cytokine profiles that are similar to cells that are driven to senescence in cell culture, increased inflammation may play a role in the mortality data. Indeed, frailty and other deleterious outcomes in elderly humans are associated with serum markers of inflammation. Alternatively, there is accumulating evidence that CD8+CD28– T cells may function as suppressor cells, influencing a variety of immune functions (Cortesini, LeMaoult, Ciubotariu, & Cortesini, 2001). For example, several studies have shown a significant correlation between high proportions of senescent CD8 T cells and poor antibody responses to influenza vaccination (Goronzy et al., 2001; Saurwein-Teissl et al., 2002). Expanded populations of CD8+CD28– T cells also correlate with a more severe disease course in anklylosing spondylitis patients (Schirmer et al., 2002).

Concluding Remarks

The immune system devotes itself to combating harmful agents early in life. The success of this process results in increased life span, but old age is associated with a variety of detrimental immunological changes that are the outcome of properly coordinated immune function throughout life. Thus, appropriate immune responses that control infections and injury can become maladaptive over time. As has been previously suggested, the immune system is a double-edged sword that provides an ideal example of the evolutionary biology term "antagonistic pleiotropy," which describes processes that are beneficial during one life stage but that may exert negative effects at another point in the life span (Crimmins & Finch, 2006).

In conclusion, the immunological theory of aging has been validated by a large body of basic science and clinical studies performed since it was originally proposed nearly 50 years ago. Importantly, this theory of aging does not preclude other theoretical constructs but, rather, actually incorporates some of the other biological theories of aging. For example, oxidative stress, which accelerates telomere shortening, may enhance T cell replicative senescence and may also affect T cell membrane integrity required for appropriate signal transduction. Similarly, DNA damage and inadequate repair mechanisms may be particularly deleterious to the function of highly proliferative tissues, such as the cells involved in immune responses. Future studies will undoubtedly further elucidate the underlying mechanisms that link so many facets of biological aging with the immune system.

References

Appay, V., & Rowland-Jones, S. (2002). Premature ageing of the immune system: The cause of AIDS? *Trends in Immunology, 23,* 580–585.

Arron, J. R., & Choi, Y. (2000). Bone versus immune system. *International Immunology, 408,* 535–536.

Bachmaier, K., Neu, N., de la Maza, L. M., Pal, S., Hessel, A., & Penninger, J. M. (1999). Chlamydia infections and heart disease linked through antigenic mimicry [see comments]. *Science, 283,* 1335–1339.

Blum-Degen, D., Meuller, T., Kuhn, W., Gerlach, M., Przuntek, H., & Riederer, P. (1995). Interleukin-1 beta and interleukin-6 are elevated in the cerebrospinal fluid of Alzheimer's and de novo Parkinson's disease patients. *Neuroscience Letters, 202,* 17–20.

Bo, S., Gambino, R., Uberti, B., Mangiameli, M. P., Colosso, G., Repetti, E., et al. (2005). Does C-reactive protein identify a subclinical metabolic disease in healthy subjects? *European Journal of Clinical Investigation, 35,* 265–270.

Borthwick, N. J., Bofill, M., & Gombert, W. M. (1994). Lymphocyte activation in HIV-1 infection II. Functional defects of CD28– T cells. *AIDS, 8,* 431–441.

Boucher, N., Defeu-Duchesne, T., Vicaut, E., Farge, D., Effros, R. B., & Schachter, F. (1998). CD28 expression in T cell aging and human longevity. *Experimental Gerontology, 33,* 267–282.

Brugg, B., Dubreuil, Y. L., Huber, G., Wollman, E. E., Delhaye-Bouchaud, N., & Mariani, J. (1995). Inflammatory processes induce beta-amyloid precursor protein changes in mouse brain.

Proceedings of the National Academy of Sciences of the United States of America, 92, 3032–3035.

Bruunsgaard, H., Andersen-Ranberg, K., Jeune, B., Pedersen, A. N., Skinhj, P., & Pedersen, B. K. (1999). A high plasma concentration of TNF-alpha is associated with dementia in centenarians. *Journal of Gerontology: Biological Sciences, 54,* M357–M364.

Bruunsgaard, H., & Pedersen, B. K. (2003). Age-related inflammatory cytokines and disease. *Immunology and Allergy Clinics of North America, 23,* 15–39.

Bullido, M. J., Muanoz-Fernandez, M. A., Recuero, M., Fresno, M., & Valdivieso, F. (1996). Alzheimer's amyloid precursor protein is expressed on the surface of hematopoietic cells upon activation. *Biochimica et Biophysica Acta, 1313,* 54–62.

Campisi, J., & d'Adda, D. F. (2007). Cellular senescence: When bad things happen to good cells. *Nature Reviews: Molecular Cell Biology, 8,* 729–740.

Cawthon, R. M., Smith, K. R., O'Brien, E., Sivatchenko, A., & Kerber, R. A. (2003). Association between telomere length in blood and mortality in people aged 60 years or older. *Lancet, 361,* 393–395.

Chakraborty, N. G., Stevens, R. L., Mehrotra, S., Laska, E., Taxel, P., Sporn, J. R., et al. (2003). Recognition of PSA-derived peptide antigens by T cells from prostate cancer patients without any prior stimulation. *Cancer Immunology, Immunotherapy, 52,* 497–505.

Chang, E., & Harley, C. B. (1995). Telomere length as a measure of replicative histories in human vascular tissues. *Proceedings of the National Academy of Sciences of the United States of America, 92,* 11190–11194.

Characiejus, D., Pasukoniene, V., Kazlauskaite, N., Valuckas, K. P., Petraitis, T., Mauricas, M., et al. (2002). Predictive value of CD8highCD57+ lymphocyte subset in interferon therapy of patients with renal cell carcinoma. *Anticancer Research, 22,* 3679–3683.

Cortesini, R., LeMaoult, J., Ciubotariu, R., & Cortesini, N. S. (2001). CD8+CD28– T suppressor cells and the induction of antigen-specific, antigen-presenting cells-mediated suppression of Th reactivity. *Immunological Reviews, 182,* 201–206.

Crimmins, E. M., & Finch, C. E. (2006). Infection, inflammation, height, and longevity. *Proceedings of the National Academy of Sciences of the United States of America, 103,* 498–503.

Dagarag, M. D., Evazyan, T., Rao, N., & Effros R. B. (2004). Genetic manipulation of telomerase in HIV-specific CD8+ T cells: Enhanced anti-viral functions accompany the increased proliferative potential and telomere length stabilization. *Journal of Immunology, 173,* 6303–6311.

Del, B. R., Angeretti, N., Lucca, E., De Simoni, M. G., & Forloni, G. (1995). Reciprocal control of inflammatory cytokines, IL-1 and IL-6, and beta-amyloid production in cultures. *Neuroscience Letters, 188,* 70–74.

De Martinis, M., Franceschi, C., Monti, D., & Ginaldi, L. (2006). Inflammation markers predicting frailty and mortality in the elderly. *Experimental and Molecular Pathology, 80,* 219–227.

de Vries, H. E., Blom-Roosemalen, M. C., van Oosten, M., de Boer, A. G., van Berkel, T. J., Breimer, D. D., et al. (1996). The influence of cytokines on the integrity of the blood-brain barrier in vitro. *Journal of Neuroimmunology, 64,* 37–43.

Effros, R. B., Allsopp, R., Chiu, C. P., Wang, L., Hirji, K., Harley, C. B., et al. (1996). Shortened telomeres in the expanded CD28–CD8+ subset in HIV disease implicate replicative senescence in HIV pathogenesis. *AIDS/Fast Track, 10,* F17–F22.

Effros, R. B., Boucher, N., Porter, V., Zhu, X., Spaulding, C., Walford, R. L., et al. (1994). Decline in CD28+ T cells in centenarians and in long-term T cell cultures: A possible cause for both in vivo and in vitro immunosenescence. *Experimental Gerontology, 29,* 601–609.

Effros, R. B., Dagarag, M. D., Spaulding, C. C., & Man, J. (2005). The role of CD8 T cell replicative senescence in human aging. *Immunological Reviews, 205,* 147–157.

Effros, R. B., & Pawelec, G. (1997). Replicative senescence of T lymphocytes: Does the Hayflick limit lead to immune exhaustion? *Immunology Today, 18,* 450–454.

Finch, C. E., & Crimmins, E. M. (2004). Inflammatory exposure and historical changes in human life-spans. *Science, 305,* 1736–1739.

Garsin, D. A., Villanueva, J. M., Begun, J., Kim, D. H., Sifri, C. D., Calderwood, S. B., et al. (2003). Long-lived *C. elegans* daf-2 mutants are resistant to bacterial pathogens. *Science, 300,* 1921.

George, J., Harats, D., Gilburd, B., & Shoenfeld, Y. (1996). Emerging cross-regulatory roles of immunity and autoimmunity in atherosclerosis. *Immunologic Research, 15,* 315–322.

Goronzy, J. J., Fulbright, J. W., Crowson, C. S., Poland, G. A., O'Fallon, W. M., & Weyand, C. M. (2001). Value of immunological markers in predicting responsiveness to influenza vaccination in elderly individuals. *Journal of Virology, 75,* 12182–12187.

Gupta, S., Leatham, E. W., Carrington, D., Mendall, M. A., Kaski, J. C., & Camm, A. J. (1997). Elevated *Chlamydia pneumoniae* antibodies, cardiovascular events, and azithromycin in male survivors of myocardial infarction. *Circulation, 96,* 404–407.

Gurfinkel, E., Bozovich, G., Daroca, A., Beck, E., & Mautner, B. (1997). Randomised trial of roxithromycin in non-Q-wave coronary syndromes: ROXIS Pilot Study. ROXIS Study Group [see comments]. *Lancet, 350,* 404–407.

Halme, S., & Surcel, H. M. (1997). Cell mediated immunity to *Chlamydia pneumoniae. Scandinavian Journal of Infectious Diseases. Supplementum, 104,* 18–21.

Harley, C., Futcher, A. B., & Greider, C. (1990). Telomeres shorten during ageing of human fibroblasts. *International Immunology, 345,* 458–460.

Hayflick, L., & Moorhead, P. S. (1961). The serial cultivation of human diploid cell strains. *Experimental Cell Research, 25,* 585–621.

Israel, B. F., & Kenney, S. C. (2003). Virally targeted therapies for EBV-associated malignancies. *Oncogene, 22,* 5122–5130.

Jamieson, B. D., Douek, D.C., Killian, S., Hultin, L. E., Scripture-Adams, D. D., Giorgi, J. V., et al. (1999). Generation of functional thymocytes in the human adult. *Immunity, 10,* 569–575.

Janeway, C. A., Travers, P., McClemments, M., & Wellcome, C. (1997). *Immunobiology: The immune system in health and disease*. New York: Taylor & Francis.

Kaalmaan, J., Juhaasz, A., Laird, G., Dickens, P., Jaardaanhaazy, T., Rimanaoczy, A., et al. (1997). Serum interleukin-6 levels correlate with the severity of dementia in Down syndrome and in Alzheimer's disease. *Acta Neurologica Scandinavica, 96,* 236–240.

Kennedy-Smith, A. G., McKenzie, J. L., Owen, M. C., Davidson, P. J., Vuckovic, S., & Hart, D. N. (2002). Prostate specific antigen inhibits immune responses in vitro: A potential role in prostate cancer. *Journal of Urology, 168,* 741–747.

Kreft, B., Fischer, A., Kruger, S., Sack, K., Kirchner, H., & Rink, L. (2000). The impaired immune response to diphtheria vaccination in elderly chronic hemodialysis patients is related to zinc deficiency. *Biogerontology, 1,* 61–66.

Libby, P. (2007). Fat fuels the flame: Triglyceride-rich lipoproteins and arterial inflammation. *Circulation Research, 100,* 299–301.

Libby, P., Sukhova, G., Lee, R. T., & Galis, Z. S. (1995). Cytokines regulate vascular functions related to stability of the atherosclerotic plaque. *Journal of Cardiovascular Pharmacology, 25*(Suppl. 2), S9–S12.

Lorenzo, J. (2000). Interactions between immune and bone cells: New insights with many remaining questions. *Journal of Clinical Investigation, 106,* 749–752.

Mach, F., Scheonbeck, U., Sukhova, G. K., Bourcier, T., Bonnefoy, J. Y., Pober, J. S., et al. (1997). Functional CD40 ligand is expressed on human vascular endothelial cells, smooth muscle cells, and macrophages: Implications for CD40-CD40 ligand signaling in atherosclerosis. *Proceedings of the National Academy of Sciences of the United States of America, 94,* 1931–1936.

Mariani, E., Meneghetti, A., Neri, S., Ravaglia, G., Forti, P., Cattini, L., et al. (2002). Chemokine production by natural killer cells from nonagenarians. *European Journal of Immunology, 32,* 1524–1529.

Mayr, M., Metzler, B., Kiechl, S., Willeit, J., Schett, G., Xu, Q., et al. (1999). Endothelial cytotoxicity mediated by serum antibodies to heat shock proteins of *Escherichia coli* and *Chlamydia pneumoniae:* Immune reactions to heat shock proteins as a possible link between infection and atherosclerosis. *Circulation, 99,* 1560–1566.

McGeer, P. L., & McGeer, E. G. (1996). Anti-inflammatory drugs in the fight against Alzheimer's disease. *Annals of the New York Academy of Sciences, 777,* 213–220.

Metzler, B., Xu, Q., & Wick, G. (1998). The role of (auto-) immunity in atherogenesis. *Wiener Klinische Wochenschrift, 110,* 350–355.

Ouyang, Q., Wagner, W. M., Wikby, A., Walter, S., Aubert, G., Dodi, A. I., et al. (2003). Large numbers of dysfunctional CD8+ T lymphocytes bearing receptors for a single dominant CMV epitope in the very old. *Journal of Clinical Immunology, 23,* 247–257.

Panossian, L., Porter, V. R., Valenzuela, H. F., Masterman, D., Reback, E., Cummings, J., et al. (2002). Telomere shortening in T cells correlates with Alzheimer's disease status. *Neurobiology of Aging, 24,* 77–84.

Papassotiropoulos, A., Bagli, M., Jessen, F., Bayer, T. A., Maier, W., Rao, M. L., et al. (1999). A genetic variation of the inflammatory cytokine interleukin-6 delays the initial onset and reduces the risk for sporadic Alzheimer's disease. *Annals of Neurology, 45,* 666–668.

Pardoll, D. (2001). T cells and tumours. *International Immunology, 411,* 1010–1012.

Pawelec, G., Akbar, A., Caruso, C., Effros R. B., Grubeck-Loebenstein, B., & Wikby, A. (2004). Is immunosenescence infectious? *Trends in Immunology, 25,* 406–410.

Pawelec, G., Rehbein, A., Haehnel, K., Meri, A., & Adibzadeh, M. (1997). Human T cell clones in long-term culture as a model of immunosenescence. *Immunological Reviews, 160,* 31–42.

Perillo, N. L., Walford, R. L., Newman, M. A., & Effros, R. B. (1989). Human T lymphocytes possess a limited in vitro lifespan. *Experimental Gerontology, 24,* 177–187.

Pietschmann, P., Grisar, J., Thien, R., Willheim, M., Kerschan-Schindl, K., Preisinger, E., et al. (2001). Immune phenotype and intracellular cytokine production of peripheral blood mononuclear cells from postmenopausal patients with osteoporotic fractures. *Experimental Gerontology, 36,* 1749–1759.

Salvioli, S., Capri, M., Valensin, S., Tieri, P., Monti, D., Ottaviani, E., et al. (2006). Inflamm-aging, cytokines and aging: State of the art, new hypotheses on the role of mitochondria and new perspectives from systems biology. *Current Pharmaceutical Design, 12,* 3161–3171.

Satoh, T., Nakamura, S., Taga, T., Matsuda, T., Hirano, T., Kishimoto, T., et al. (1988). Induction of neuronal differentiation in PC12 cells by B-cell stimulatory factor 2/interleukin 6. *Molecular and Cellular Biology, 8,* 3546–3549.

Saurwein-Teissl, M., Lung, T. L., Marx, F., Gschosser, C., Asch, E., Blasko, I., et al. (2002). Lack of antibody production following immunization in old age: association with CD8(+)CD28(–) T cell clonal expansions and an imbalance in the production of Th1 and Th2 cytokines. *Journal of Immunology, 168,* 5893–5899.

Schirmer, M., Goldberger, C., Wurzner, R., Duftner, C., Pfeiffer, K. P., Clausen, J., et al. (2002). Circulating cytotoxic CD8(+) CD28(–) T cells in ankylosing spondylitis. *Arthritis Research, 4,* 71–76.

Schmitz, G., Herr, A. S., & Rothe, G. (1998). T-lymphocytes and monocytes in atherogenesis. *Herz, 23,* 168–177.

Seguier, S., Godeau, G., Leborgne, M., Pivert, G., & Brousse, N. (1999). Immunohistologic and morphometric analysis of cytotoxic T lymphocytes in gingivitis. *Journal of Periodontology, 70,* 1383–1391.

Seko, Y., Sato, O., Takagi, A., Tada, Y., Matsuo, H., Yagita, H., et al. (1997). Perforin-secreting killer cell infiltration in the aortic tissue of patients with atherosclerotic aortic aneurysm. *Japanese Circulation Journal, 61,* 965–970.

Spaulding, C. C., Walford, R. L., & Effros, R. B. (1997). Elevated serum TNFa and IL-6 levels in old mice are normalized by caloric restriction. *Mechanisms of Ageing and Development, 93,* 87–94.

Spaulding, C. S., Guo, W., & Effros, R. B. (1999). Resistance to apoptosis in human CD8+ T cells that reach replicative senescence after multiple rounds of antigen-specific proliferation. *Experimental Gerontology, 34,* 633–644.

Taubman, M. A., & Kawai, T. (2001). Involvement of T-lymphocytes in periodontal disease and in direct and indirect induction of bone resorption. *Critical Reviews in Oral Biology and Medicine, 12,* 125–135.

Taubman, M. A., Valverde, P., Han, X., & Kawai, T. (2005). Immune response: The key to bone resorption in periodontal disease. *Journal of Periodontology, 76,* 2033–2041.

Trieb, K., Ransmayr, G., Sgonc, R., Lassmann, H., & Grubeck-Loebenstein, B. (1996). APP peptides stimulate lymphocyte proliferation in normals, but not in patients with Alzheimer's disease. *Neurobiology of Aging, 17,* 541–547.

Tsukishiro, T., Donnenberg, A. D., & Whiteside, T. L. (2003). Rapid turnover of the CD8(+)CD28(–) T-cell subset of effector cells in the circulation of patients with head and neck cancer. *Cancer Immunology, Immunotherapy, 52,* 599–607.

Vaziri, H., Schachter, F., Uchida, I., Wei, L., Zhu, X., Effros, R., et al. (1993). Loss of telomeric DNA during aging of normal and trisomy 21 human lymphocytes. *American Journal of Human Genetics, 52,* 661–667.

Walford, R. L. (1969). *The immunologic theory of aging.* Copenhagen: Munksgaard.

Wassenaar, A., Reinhardus, C., Abraham-Inpijn, L., & Kievits, F. (1996). Type-1 and type-2 CD8+ T-cell subsets isolated from chronic adult periodontitis tissue differ in surface phenotype and biological functions. *Immunology, 87,* 113–118.

Wayne, S. J., Rhyne, R. L., Garry, P. H., & Goodwin, J. S. (1990). Cell-mediated immunity as a predictor of morbidity and mortality in subjects over 60. *Journal of Gerontology: Biological Sciences, 45,* M45–M48.

Wikby, A., Johansson, B., Olsson, J., Lofgren, S., Nilsson, B. O., & Ferguson, F. (2002). Expansions of peripheral blood CD8 T-lymphocyte subpopulations and an association with cytomegalovirus seropositivity in the elderly: The Swedish NONA immune study. *Experimental Gerontology, 37,* 445–453.

Wikby, A., Maxson, P., Olsson, J., Johansson, B., & Ferguson, F. G. (1998). Changes in CD8 and CD4 lymphocyte subsets, T cell proliferation responses and non-survival in the very old: The Swedish longitudinal OCTO-immune study. *Mechanisms of Ageing and Development, 102,* 187–198.

Wikby, A., Nilsson, B. O., Forsey, R., Thompson, J., Strindhall, J., Lofgren, S., et al. (2006). The immune risk phenotype is associated with IL-6 in the terminal decline stage: Findings from the Swedish NONA immune longitudinal study of very late life functioning. *Mechanisms of Ageing and Development, 127,* 695–704.

Xu, Q., Kiechl, S., Mayr, M., Metzler, B., Egger, G., Oberhollenzer, F., et al. (1999). Association of serum antibodies to heat-shock protein 65 with carotid atherosclerosis: Clinical significance determined in a follow-up study [see comments]. *Circulation, 100,* 1169–1174.

Xu, Q., & Wick, G. (1996). The role of heat shock proteins in protection and pathophysiology of the arterial wall. *Molecular Medicine Today, 2,* 372–379.

Zanjani, H., Finch, C. E., Kemper, C., Atkinson, J., McKeel, D., Morris, J. C., et al. (2005). Complement activation in very early Alzheimer disease. *Alzheimer Disease and Associated Disorders, 19,* 55–66.

Zhang, J., Kong, Q., Zhang, Z., Ge, P., Ba, D., & He, W. (2003). Telomere dysfunction of lymphocytes in patients with Alzheimer disease. *Cognitive and Behavioral Neurology, 16,* 170–176.

Zhdanov, V. S., Chumachenko, P. V., Cherpachenko, N. M., Beskrovnova, N. N., & Lavrova, N. F. (1995). [Subpopulations of lymphocytes and monocytes/macrophages at the early stages of human aorta atherosclerosis]. *Arkhiv Patologii, 57,* 67–71.

Modalities of Gene Action Predicted by the Classical Evolutionary Theory of Aging

10

George M. Martin

"Nothing in biology makes sense except in the light of evolution." This oft-quoted phrase was first enunciated by Theodosius Dobzhansky, a distinguished geneticist (1900–1975) (Fig. 10.1), in a presentation of the summer meeting of the American Society of Zoologists at Boulder, Colorado, on August 27, 1964 (Dobzhansky, 1964). Although Dobzhansky warned against "reckless generalizations," including his own famous pronouncement, it has nevertheless guided my thinking, first as a pathologist, then as a geneticist, and finally as a biogerontologist. It is the motivation behind this chapter, which summarizes and elaborates on

Acknowledgments: The author thanks his University of Washington colleague Joseph Felsenstein for historical information on the writings of Theodosius Dobzhansky and for an unpublished photograph (Fig. 10.1). He is also grateful to Steven N. Austad for helping him "bone up" on the bones of our ancient ancestors!

10.1

Theodosius Dobzhansky (center) together with his longtime collaborator at Columbia University, Howard Levine. The third individual may be Martin L. Tracey, Jr., who was then a postdoctoral fellow. The photograph was taken at a meeting on evolutionary biology (probably at Davis, CA) within a year of Dobzhansky's death from cancer in 1975. The author is indebted to Professor Joseph Felsenstein (University of Washington Department of Genome Sciences) for this unpublished photograph.

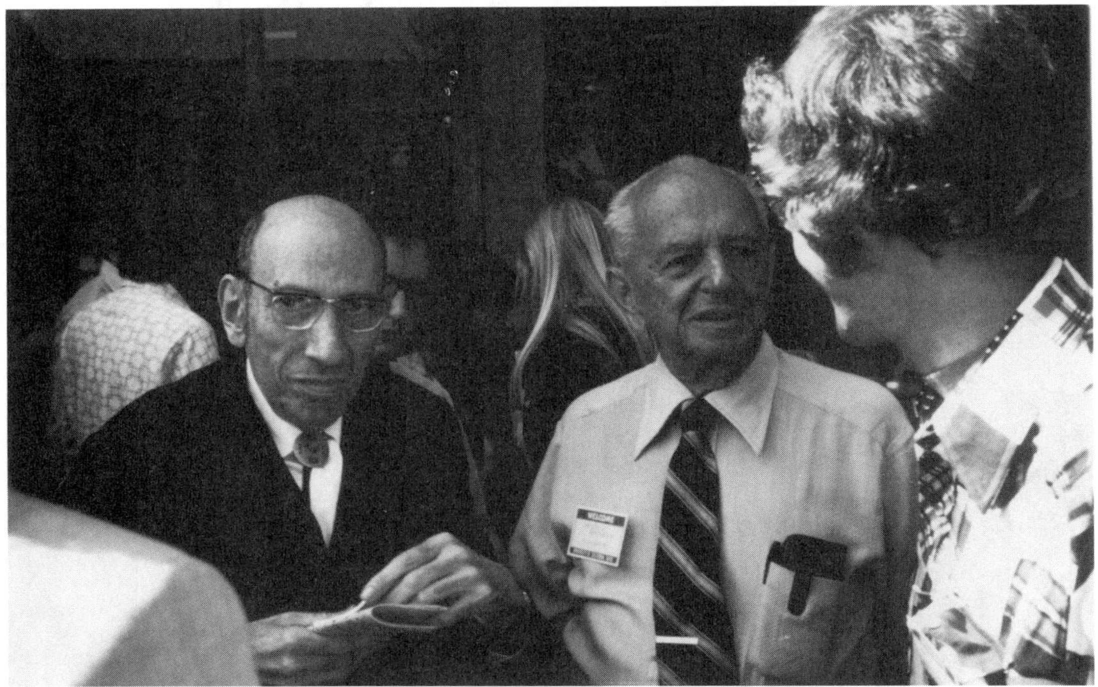

my earlier publications on this subject (Martin, 1979, 1996, 1997, 1998a, 1998b, 2000, 2002a, 2002b, 2002c, 2006, 2007a, 2007b; Martin, Austad, & Johnson, 1996; Martin, Bergman, & Barzilai, 2007; Ogburn et al., 2001). An additional reference is a charming "must-read" interchange with my colleagues, available to anyone with access to the Internet (http://www.americanaging.org/news/AGE%20News%20May%202005%20Martin%20Discussion.pdf).

But what does the title mean when it uses the adjective "classical" before "evolutionary theory of aging"? This will become clear when we discuss recent credible challenges to that theory, one of which is the subject of chapter 3 in this volume. To nonbiologists, the term "gene action" perhaps needs some clarification. In fact, given the recent spectacular progress in clarifying the functions of sequences of DNA that do not code for proteins, even professional biologists require such clarification. I use the term "gene action" to refer to the expression (that is, the translation into action, or function) of *all* the building blocks of the DNA of an organism—namely, the sequences of nucleotide base pairs and the alphabetic components of its informational content. This encompasses single-base-pair variations that are relatively common within a population, called polymorphisms; much rarer mutations, including single-base-pair substitutions (point mutations), deletions and insertions; and variations in the copy numbers of its components and in their arrangements (e.g., inversions in the order of the sequences or translocations of sets of sequences to different areas of the same or other chromosomes). Such spontaneously occurring variations are the "raw materials" for the processes of evolution—the results of environmental pressures that select either for or against a particular innovation or historical episodes that lead to small genetic isolates (genetic drift).

Genetics is all about variation—differences between the *phenotypes* of organisms (what can be seen in their behavior, anatomy, biochemistry, physiology, and pathology)—and how these can be related to their *genotypes* (the particular varieties of genes or, better, DNA sequences). It is important to keep in mind that DNA sequences do not act in a vacuum. Their contributions to a given phenotype can be dramatically modulated by other DNA sequences within the same organisms ("gene–gene interactions") and by interactions with the environment ("gene–environment interactions"). But there is also an important role of stochastic (chance) events in the determination of many phenotypes, including those associated with biological aging. Such contributions can be particularly important in explaining differences of life span *within* a species. This chapter devotes some special attention to this subject and presents a provocative theory as to the evolution of such "stochasticity" in gene actions. Let us begin, however, by briefly describing the phenotypes of interest to gerontologists.

The Complexity of Aging Phenotypes Seen in Our Species

We probably know more about the behavior, physiology, biochemistry, microbiology, pharmacology, pathology, ecology, and, surprisingly, the developmental biology of members of our species than that of any other species; until recently, genetics was strikingly absent from this partial list of disciplines, but, as suggested previously, this has changed dramatically in the past few years. One approach to testing the validity of this statement is to compare the number of relevant citations in the biomedical literature of two of the best-studied model organisms—the budding yeast (*Saccharomyces cerevisiae*) and the fruit fly (*Drosophila melanogaster*)—with *Homo sapiens;* the results strongly support the proposition (Martin et al., 2007). This statement does not in any way disparage the fantastic contributions of colleagues who have been laboring for many decades to elucidate the biology of yeast, flies, worms, mice, and other model organisms. They created a large segment of the foundations for the progress we have seen in human biology. Moreover, their contributions have typically been more incisive, in part because of the experimental tractability of their materials.

Beginning functional declines can be documented in virtually every organ system not long after sexual maturation, assuming that one employs sufficiently sensitive assays. Consider, for example, the world records of marathon runners, which select for the most robust, physically fit members of our population. This is an attractive assay, as it tests for fitness of multiple organ systems and one's ability to maintain metabolic homeostasis. Declines are observable during the fourth decade, later than what is the case for sprinters. This probably occurs, in part, because it takes considerably more training and experience in perfecting one's optimal pacing for a marathon. It also takes years for the gradual development of such compensatory processes as cardiac muscle hypertrophy. For a remarkably wide range of sports, peak activity occurs during the third decade (Schultz & Curnow, 1988).

These data were derived from a highly selected subset of individuals in whom one can assume a reasonably good deal of synchrony in the rates of decline of specific physiological systems. In other words, to achieve superathlete status, one should not have "an Achilles' heel," manifested as a particularly rapid rate of decline in one specific major organ system. To the best of my knowledge, however, that proposition has never been tested. It would ideally require quite sensitive assays. I would predict modest to moderate variations, not perfect synchrony, based on the classical evolutionary biological theory of aging (see the next section), the enormous genetic and environmental heterogeneity within our species, and the wide range of gene–gene and gene–environment interactions that have the potential to modulate rates of aging in various systems.

Declines in the various physiological processes (and underlying molecular and biochemical processes) that maintain optimum functions are likely to "set the stage" for the plethora of late-life disorders and diseases, some 87 of which have recently been tabulated, all of which are subject to both genetic and environmental modulations (Martin et al., 2007). Specific evidence for a highly polygenic basis for the emergence of a smaller subset of these senescent phenotypes has been published (Martin, 1978). The estimate of the number of genes involved in aging (about 7%) was almost certainly an underestimate. Technological advances are now leading to the identification of many new genetic loci, variations at which alter one's risk of such common late-life disorders as age-related macular degeneration, type 2 diabetes mellitus, and prostate cancer (Couzin & Kaiser, 2007).

The Classical Evolutionary Biological Theory of Aging

This theory was developed for the case of species with age-structured populations, a situation that occurs when there are serial episodes of reproduction as opposed to one massive "big-bang" production of progeny (Diamond, 1982). That means that, in any given population, there are admixtures of young, middle-aged, and old subjects. We have no reliable data on the precise age distributions within populations of our remote ancestors during the emergence of our species. What few skeletal remains can be found are consistent with death at a comparatively young age for the great majority of our remote progenitors; in one such study of a prehistoric site, the life expectancy at birth was calculated to be only 20 years (Lovejoy et al., 1977). One might expect that figure to be even lower among more ancient populations. Such short lives make sense if one considers the environments of these pioneers. Life was full of dangers—lethal predators; dangerous terrains conducive to accidents; uncontrolled viral, bacterial, and fungal infectious agents; and uncertain supplies of food and water, much of which might have been contaminated with infectious agents and toxic chemicals. Thus, it would be a difficult task indeed to achieve a ripe old age. Clearly, much younger cohorts would have dominated the population. Now let us imagine classes of gene action that would not reach some phenotypic level of expression until comparatively late in the life span. By not reaching a phenotypic level of expression, I mean that it is presumed not to make a significant impact on the body's structure and function during the early phases of the life course. The particular variety of genes ("alleles") or non–protein-coding DNA sequences that underlie such gene action might have neutral effects early in life or might in fact have been selected to enhance reproductive fitness in the environment in which they emerged. If one accepts the proposition that there were very few survivors during the establishment of our species, then what would be the chances that such gene actions would be passed on to subsequent generations? They would be very small indeed, as the genes that are passed on would be dominated by the much larger cohorts of young individuals. If the gene actions in question eventually had deleterious effects, given longer life spans such as we enjoy today, they will have contributed to senescent phenotypes. It is important to note that these arguments obtain for the theoretical situation in which a very favorable gene action emerges late in the life span. Such genes would also escape the force of natural selection. This is the essence of the classical evolutionary biologic theory of aging, as pioneered by J. B. S. Haldane (Haldane, 1942), Peter Medawar (Medawar, 1957), William D. Hamilton (Hamilton, 1966), Brian Charlesworth (Charlesworth, 1994), and George C. Williams (Williams, 1957) and brilliantly popularized, defended, questioned, or extended by Michael R. Rose (Rose, 1991), Thomas B. Kirkwood (Kirkwood, 1988; Kirkwood & Holliday, 1979), Steven N. Austad (Austad, 1997), Linda Partridge (Partridge, 2001), James W. Curtsinger (Curtsinger et al., 1995), Trudy F. C. Mackay (Nuzhdin, Pasyukova, Dilda, Zeng, & Mackay, 1997), Daniel E. Promislow (Promislow & Tatar, 1998), Marc Tatar (Packer, Tatar, & Collins, 1998), David N. Reznick (Reznick, Bryant, & Holmes, 2006; Reznick, Bryant, Roff, Ghalambor, & Ghalambor, 2004), and Leonid A. Gavrilov and Natalia S. Gavrilova (Gavrilova et al., 1998), among others.

This is not to say that, in modern times, gene actions that emerge comparatively late in the life span have little possibility of being passed on to subsequent generations. In chapter 3, Kaplan points out that the grandparental generation passes on wealth to the younger generations, thus contributing to their reproductive fitness. Moreover, he challenges the classical evolutionary biological theory by presenting evidence that some rare and remote extant "primitive" populations, possible surrogates for the structure of populations in ancient times, have significant numbers of elders, enough to measurably impact on the younger generations. This is thus a serious challenge to the classical theory. Unfortunately, it will be very difficult indeed to decide how closely these current primitive populations are valid surrogates for our remote progenitors, nor how well protected they really are from modern external forces. Moreover, some contemporary field studies with other mammalian species, including a primate species, fail to support the "grandmother" hypothesis (Packer et al., 1998). Other studies with live animals in the field have given conflicting results, one strongly supporting the theory (Austad, 1993) and the other giving unexpected results (Reznick et al., 2004).

A range of demographic observations seems inconsistent with the theory in that they provide evidence of a paradoxical decline in the force of mortality in very old age for a wide range of species (summarized by Vaupel et al., 1998).

My own view of these observations is that they may be largely related to behavioral differences that emerge in extreme old age, related mainly to dramatic declines in mobility. For the case of fruit flies and medflies, for example, perhaps the cessation of flight translates into less opportunity for injury and death. For the case of human subjects (where these declines in mortality rates are much more modest), perhaps it also reflects, in part, dramatic declines in mobility (which translates into fewer falls, fractures, and subsequent complications). It may also be the result, in part, of secular trends that have led to widespread immunization of older subjects (pneumococci and influenza) and the introductions of central heating and air conditioning, at least in most sectors of the developed societies. I call this my "cocoon" hypothesis.

More recently, a mathematically rigorous challenge to the theory, specifically to the assumptions made by Hamilton in his famous paper (Hamilton, 1966), has been published (Baudisch, 2005; Vaupel, Baudisch, Dolling, Roach, & Gampe, 2004). It describes a scenario whereby the force of natural selection can actually *increase* during aging. There are in fact some species of fish that continue to grow and, as such, become more like predators than prey. Under those circumstances, it is easy to imagine declines in the force of natural selection with age.

Some of my colleagues believe that the striking demonstration that single gene mutations can extend the life span of nematodes, fruit flies, and mice—sometimes dramatically—provides strong evidence against the classical theory. We have argued that rates of aging and, hence, life span is under polygenic controls. That a single gene can enhance longevity comes as a surprise to many. Moreover, we have known for many decades that a single environmental manipulation, caloric restriction (or, more conservatively, dietary restriction), can substantially enhance life span in a remarkably wide range of species (reviewed by Masoro, 2006). Some would argue that these observations support a "programmed" mechanism of aging—that is, something more in the line of sequential, determinative changes in gene expression that actively *produce* aging. This would clearly be an *adaptive* theory of aging, whereas the classical evolutionary theory quite clearly posits aging as being *nonadaptive*. It is interesting that one of the giants of 19th-century biology, August Weissmann, once embraced the idea that aging is good for the species in that it results in enhanced resources for the young. His work is reviewed in a scholarly publication that argues against this proposition and in fact suggests that Weissmann eventually changed his mind (Kirkwood & Cremer, 1982). Nevertheless, there remain some hardy champions of the idea that biological aging is "programmed," including the authors of chapter 12.

My interpretation of both the single gene mutation and caloric restriction experiments is that all or many of them are examples of *diapauses*—time-outs from the business of reproduction during "bad times"—be they nutritional, climatic, or other environmental challenges. While it is true that there are apparent examples of single gene mutations in which there seems to be no trade-off with reproduction, these experiments have been carried out under artificial laboratory conditions. For at least certain varieties of these mutations, when the experiments are conducted under sequential "feast-and-famine" conditions—a scenario much more likely to obtain in the wild—the mutant organism cannot compete with the wild type, thus losing the evolutionary race and disappearing from the natural world (Jenkins, McColl, & Lithgow, 2004). These experiments have been carried out with a mutant in the now famous IGF-1 signal transduction pathway (reviewed by Samuelson, Carr, & Ruvkun, 2007). But there are a plethora of different types of diapauses in nature, particularly within the insect world (Danks, 1987). These can provide major new avenues of investigation for the biochemical genetics of longevity. In the final analysis, however, all such temporary and partial reprieves from the ravages of aging are eventually "trumped" by the several classes of gene action that play out as a result of the evolutionary biological theory of aging, as I outline later in this chapter.

A final argument challenging the primacy of the evolutionary theory, apparently first put forth by an anthropologist, is that perhaps the theory is not at all necessary, as one might argue that *all* complex machines have characteristic half-lives to failure (Wood, Weeks, Bentley, & Weiss, 1994). This idea has come to be known as reliability theory (Gavrilov & Gavrilova, 1991). This begs the question, however, as to how some animal machines are built more reliably than others. Gavrilov and Gavrilova (2001) have tried to reconcile reliability theory with the evolutionary theory.

Types of Gene Action Predicted by the Classical Evolutionary Biological Theory of Aging

The great majority of publications on this subject specify only two classes of gene action that mediate the evolutionary biological theory of aging. The first, attributable mainly to Medawar, is generally referred to as "mutation accumulation." This is an unfortunate name, as the mutations in question are not somatic mutations developing during the life span but germ-line mutations (mutations that one is born with). These are rather special mutations in that they are thought to be benign early in the life span but with serious negative impacts on health and survival in middle age or later. Huntington's disease is the prototypical example. Haldane was puzzled by the surprisingly high frequency of this dominant mutation in the English population. Germ-line mutations typically have frequencies of about one in a million, whereas this genetic disorder exhibited frequencies of about one in a thousand. Haldane suggested that the reason the mutation survived in the population was because of its delayed manifestations, thus escaping the force of natural selection. It is interesting to note, parenthetically, that very recent experiments suggest that the mutation has much broader effects than on the basal ganglia of the central nervous system. The triplet repeats of nucleotides that code for polyglutamine have been shown to result in aberrations in mitochondrial metabolism in peripheral tissues (brown fat), with deleterious effects on energy metabolism (Weydt et al., 2006). Huntington's disease may thus be more relevant to basic mechanisms of aging than anyone could have imagined.

Medawar greatly elaborated these ideas of Haldane (Haldane, 1942; Medawar, 1957). For example, he pointed out that for at least a subset of such mutant alleles, they might well have had some significant but nonlethal deleterious effects in comparatively early stages of the life course. If that were the case, there would be selection for what geneticists call "suppressor alleles"—changes in other genes that bypass or repress or compensate for these deficiencies. Medawar concluded that many such suppressors might only delay these deleterious effects to the point at which there could no longer be further selection for suppressors, thus contributing to aging phenotypes. This scenario, especially when coupled with the other mechanisms discussed later, would result in an enormous degree of heterogeneity in patterns of aging among individuals in outbreeding populations. Thus, each of us may be essentially unique in precisely *how* we age. We may all have, for example, certain "private" intrinsic vulnerabilities that might accelerate specific aspects of aging in different ways.

The second major class of gene action that has attracted a great deal of attention derives from the work of George C. Williams (Williams, 1957) and is referred to as "antagonistic pleiotropy." By this view, some varieties of genes might have been selected because of good effects early in the life span but which may also have deleterious effects late in the life span, thus contributing to aging phenotypes. There have been many suggested examples in the literature, but they have been hard to definitively establish. The latest example that I am aware of provides some insight into the important phenotype of immunosenescence (Cicin-Sain et al., 2007). Other potential examples include atherosclerosis (Martin, 1998a), the role of the apolipoprotein E 4 allele in Alzheimer's disease (Martin, 1999), and common late-life cancers (Campisi, 2005).

A third class of gene action that is highly relevant to our understanding of the evolution of life spans is so obvious that it is not always mentioned. I refer to the fact that there are many genes that evolved to enhance macromolecular integrity, and, as such, they are both "good for us" when we are both young and old. Examples would include the hundreds of genes that detect and repair DNA damage and scavenge reactive oxygen species. These have been referred to as "longevity assurance genes" and are the basis for a program of research supported by the National Institute on Aging (Hodes, McCormick, & Pruzan, 1996).

I have recently reviewed additional varieties of gene action that could be invoked by the evolutionary biological theory of aging (Martin, 2007b); interested readers may wish to consult other references given in that review. These gene actions include variations on the theme of antagonistic pleiotropic gene action. One such example is the adaptive silencing of genes relatively early in the life span. Once such a mechanism is "engaged," however, it may have a "life of its own" since there would be no selective pressure to "put a brake" on the system. This could eventually lead to deleterious effects later in the life course. A possible example is the regulated decline in protein synthesis and turnover that is coupled with the cessation of the major epoch of somatic growth. Continued declines in synthesis and turnover could result in increases of posttranslational modifications of proteins, a generally accepted molecular mechanism of aging. Some genes are obviously up-regulated early in the life course in order to enhance reproduction yet may result in negative late-life phenotypes. A cogent example is the up-regulation of androgenic genes, which will ultimately contribute to the benign prostatic hypertrophy so common in older males, with consequent deleterious effects on renal function. There can also be a nonadaptive loss of gene silencing. These are "good" alleles that are inappropriately up-regulated late in life. There are well-documented examples involving genes on autosomes and sex chromosomes (Bennett-Baker, Wilkowski, & Burke, 2003). Studies of twins have also demonstrated that one can observe apparently nonadaptive losses of expression of many alleles (Fraga et al., 2005).

There appear to be rare forms of what one might refer to as paradoxical antagonistic pleiotropy (Mannucci et al., 1997). These would be alleles with deleterious effects early in the life span but that might exhibit good effects in older individuals who survive these bad effects.

A final type of gene action with an obvious impact on aging phenotypes is somatic mutation. This can involve both nuclear DNA (Martin, Ogburn, et al., 1996) and mitochondrial DNA (Kujoth, Bradshaw, Haroon, & Prolla, 2007).

The Role of Chance in Explaining Intraspecific Variations in Aging: Does This Too Have an Evolutionary Explanation?

All biogerontologists can agree that the major force responsible for the dramatic variations in life spans *between* animal species is the informational content of the genome. We can all agree that environmental factors also play an important role in the extent to which this informational content fulfills the messages of the genome, such as in the well-documented impact of caloric restriction. It seems unlikely, a priori, that chance events during the life course can explain much of this *interspecific* variation in life span. The situation seems to be quite different for the case of variations in life span *within* a species (i.e., *intraspecific* differences in how long individual animals may survive). Gerontologists have long been puzzled by the substantial differences in the length of life observed among individuals within populations of a variety of animal species despite apparently uniform genotypes and an experimentally controlled environment. Experiments with the humble roundworm *Caenorhabditis elegans* provide the best example. These worms are hermaphrodites; all their diploid loci are thus driven to homozygosity. As far as one can tell, therefore, they are, at birth, like identical twins. Moreover, one can control their environments to a much greater extent than is the case of inbred mice and rats. While for most routine experiments they are grown on Petri dishes with lawns of bacteria (*Escherichia coli*) as their food, they can also be grown in suspension cultures with reproducibly defined medium (although not yet fully chemically defined). Under such conditions (especially if "spinner" cultures are used to circulate the medium), we can be reasonably certain that each worm constantly experiences the identical temperature, the same source of calories, and the same degree of waste product contamination. Yet here again, one observes remarkable variations of life span (Vanfleteren, De Vreese, & Braeckman, 1998). Moreover, when one compares the range of life spans of wild-type worms with strains that have mutations that confer major increases in *average* life span, there is substantial overlap in the distributions (Kirkwood & Finch, 2002). An initial set of experiments from the laboratory of Thomas E. Johnson suggest that one mechanism for these variations might be epigenetic, nonheritable alterations in gene expression (Rea, Wu, Cypser, Vaupel, & Johnson, 2005). Epigenetic alterations are those that do not modify the sequence of DNA nucleotides, their arrangement, or their copy number but that are chemical changes "on top of" the basic genomic framework, changes that are essential if we are to make an organism with a range of different specialized cell types.

Why, then, should there be nonidentical shifts in gene expression within populations that are essentially like identical twins? One set of experiments, on real human identical twins, have suggested that these variations increase with aging and are likely to be attributable to different environmental experiences (Fraga et al., 2005). We have seen, however, that for the case of worms, the environment can be virtually identical. Moreover, the Johnson experiments noted previously gave results at day 1 of birth that could predict the life span. Why and how might such a situation evolve? Returning again to Dobzhansky, let's think first about *why* nature may have gotten into the business of playing dice with gene expression. To return to our wiggly worms, let us imagine them squirming in the dirt of a toxic dump in which there are random "hot spots" of highly toxic substances, such as cadmium or other heavy metals. We know of at least one protective class of gene products, metallothioneins (Henkel & Krebs, 2004). Now imagine that an entire population of worms with random variations in the expression of such gene products were to venture into such a hot spot. The lucky few with exceptionally strong expression of these genes would be likely to survive, while the vast majority of its brethren would likely succumb or, at the least, have dramatic decreases in their fertility. Very different patterns of selection might play out in different environments. I suggest that such a putative feature of evolution developed to enhance the reproductive fitness of populations of not only inbred organisms but also outbred organisms, including mammals like us. The precise molecular machinery for generating such putative random variations in gene expression at multiple loci is of course unknown but could conceivably involve multiple levels of gene action, including transcription, posttranscriptional modifications of RNA, variations in mRNA stabilization, translational controls, and posttranslational modifications. A surprising new mechanism, involving the differential transcription of the genetic material of an estimated 1,000 or more human autosomal loci (those on non–sex chromosomes), has just been published, lending partial support for the above hypothesis (Gimelbrant, Hutchinson, Thompson, & Chess, 2007). For reasons that are not understood, a subset of genetic loci may "fire" (transcribe) from only the paternally inherited chromosome, from only the maternally inherited chromosome, or from both of these chromosomes. These are random events that involve patches of tissues. Remarkably, one such locus is *APP*, which codes for the beta amyloid precursor protein. That protein is widely believed to be of central importance for the pathogenesis of dementias of the Alzheimer type (reviewed by Wolfe & Guenette, 2007). It is quite possible that the significant differences that have been observed in the ages of onset of Alzheimer's disease among pairs of identical twins can be at least partially explained by such stochastic events. A twin with haploinsufficiency (expression of only one allele) in a key area of the brain such as the entorhinal cortex or hippocampus would be expected to produce fewer molecules of beta amyloid, the toxic moiety made by certain modes of processing *APP*, its precursor protein. It had been known for some time that, for the case of the human X chromosome, there is random inactivation of a large segment of one of the two X chromosomes of females during a stage of early development, the famous Lyon hypothesis (Wutz & Gribnau, 2007). Since this is a random process, it is sometimes the case that a particular tissue or region within a tissue may reflect, predominantly, expression inherited from the father or vice versa. Genes that are inherited via the

X chromosome might also modulate one's influence to Alzheimer's disease, thus providing additional stochastic variables. On the positive side, the fact that the human female is a somatic mosaic could enhance survival. Imagine that one X chromosome had a gene mutation for a locus the product of which could be secreted. This deficiency would be potentially compensated by the secretion of the normal product from the unaffected X chromosome within a tissue that reflected a mixture of the two types of X chromosomes. Alas, males do not have this advantage, as they only have one X chromosome.

The challenge for the future will be to design experiments to falsify the hypothesis that stochastic variations are of major importance in explaining *intraspecific* variations in life spans and health spans. If the hypothesis can be sustained, much credit should go to Caleb Finch and Tom Kirkwood, who provided an early major review of this subject (Finch & Kirkwood, 2000).

References

Austad, S. N. (1993). Retarded senescence in an insular population of Virginia possums (*Didelphis virginiana*). *Journal of Zoology (London), 229,* 695–708.

Austad, S. N. (1997). *Why we age: What science is discovering about the body's journey through life.* New York: Wiley.

Baudisch, A. (2005). Hamilton's indicators of the force of selection. *Proceedings of the National Academy of Sciences of the United States of America, 102,* 8263–8268.

Bennett-Baker, P. E., Wilkowski, J., & Burke, D. T. (2003). Age-associated activation of epigenetically repressed genes in the mouse. *Genetics, 165,* 2055–2062.

Campisi, J. (2005). Aging, tumor suppression and cancer: High wire-act! *Mechanisms of Ageing and Development, 126,* 51–58.

Charlesworth, B. (1994). *Evolution in age-structured populations* (2nd ed.). Cambridge: Cambridge University Press.

Cicin-Sain, L., Messaoudi, I., Park, B., Currier, N., Planer, S., Fischer, M., et al. (2007). Dramatic increase in naive T cell turnover is linked to loss of naive T cells from old primates. *Proceedings of the National Academy of Sciences of the United States of America, 104,* 19960–19965.

Couzin, J., & Kaiser, J. (2007). Genome-wide association: Closing the net on common disease genes. *Science, 316,* 820–822.

Curtsinger, J. W., Fukui, H. H., Khazaeli, A. A., Kirscher, A., Pletcher, S. D., Promislow, D. E., et al. (1995). Genetic variation and aging. *Annual Review of Genetics, 29,* 553–575.

Danks, H. V. (1987). *Insect dormancy: An ecological perspective.* Ottawa: Biological Survey of Canada (Terrestrial Arthropods).

Diamond, J. M. (1982). Big-bang reproduction and ageing in male marsupial mice. *Nature, 298,* 115–116.

Dobzhansky, T. (1964). Biology, molecular and organismic. *American Zoologist, 4,* 443–452.

Finch, C. E., & Kirkwood, T. B. L. (2000). *Chance, development, and aging.* New York: Oxford University Press.

Fraga, M. F., Ballestar, E., Paz, M. F., Ropero, S., Setien, F., Ballestar, M. L., et al. (2005). Epigenetic differences arise during the lifetime of monozygotic twins. *Proceedings of the National Academy of Sciences of the United States of America, 102,* 10604–10609.

Gavrilov, L. A., & Gavrilova, N. S. (1991). *The biology of life span: A quantitative approach* (Rev. and updated English ed.). Chur: Harwood Academic Publishers.

Gavrilov, L. A., & Gavrilova, N. S. (2001). The reliability theory of aging and longevity. *Journal of Theoretical Biology, 213,* 527–545.

Gavrilova, N. S., Gavrilov, L. A., Evdokushkina, G. N., Semyonova, V. G., Gavrilova, A. L., Evdokushkina, N. N., et al. (1998). Evolution, mutations, and human longevity: European royal and noble families. *Human Biology, 70,* 799–804.

Gimelbrant, A., Hutchinson, J. N., Thompson, B. R., & Chess, A. (2007). Widespread monoallelic expression on human autosomes. *Science, 318,* 1136–1140.

Haldane, J. B. S. (1942). *New paths in genetics.* New York: Harper & Brothers.

Hamilton, W. D. (1966). The moulding of senescence by natural selection. *Journal of Theoretical Biology, 12,* 12–45.

Henkel, G., & Krebs, B. (2004). Metallothioneins: Zinc, cadmium, mercury, and copper thiolates and selenolates mimicking protein active site features—Structural aspects and biological implications. *Chemical Reviews, 104,* 801–824.

Hodes, R. J., McCormick, A. M., & Pruzan, M. (1996). Longevity assurance genes: How do they influence aging and life span? *Journal of the American Geriatrics Society, 44,* 988–991.

Jenkins, N. L., McColl, G., & Lithgow, G. J. (2004). Fitness cost of extended lifespan in *Caenorhabditis elegans. Proceedings of the Royal Society B: Biological Sciences, 271,* 2523–2526.

Kirkwood, T. B. (1988). The nature and causes of ageing. *Ciba Foundation Symposium, 134,* 193–207.

Kirkwood, T. B., & Cremer, T. (1982). Cytogerontology since 1881: A reappraisal of August Weismann and a review of modern progress. *Human Genetics, 60,* 101–121.

Kirkwood, T. B., & Finch, C. E. (2002). Ageing: The old worm turns more slowly. *Nature, 419,* 794–795.

Kirkwood, T. B., & Holliday, R. (1979). The evolution of ageing and longevity. *Proceedings of the Royal Society of London. Series B, Biological Sciences, 205,* 531–546.

Kujoth, G. C., Bradshaw, P. C., Haroon, S., & Prolla, T. A. (2007). The role of mitochondrial DNA mutations in mammalian aging. *Public Library of Science Genetics, 3*(e24), 161–173.

Lovejoy, C. O., Meindl, R. S., Pryzbeck, T. R., Barton, T. S., Heiple, K. G., & Kotting, D. (1977). Paleodemography of the Libben Site, Ottawa County, Ohio. *Science, 198,* 291–293.

Mannucci, P. M., Mari, D., Merati, G., Peyvandi, F., Tagliabue, L., Sacchi, E., et al. (1997). Gene polymorphisms predicting high plasma levels of coagulation and fibrinolysis proteins: A study in centenarians. *Arteriosclerosis, Thrombosis, and Vascular Biology, 17,* 755–759.

Martin, G. M. (1978). Genetic syndromes in man with potential relevance to the pathobiology of aging. *Birth Defects Original Article Series, 14,* 5–39.

Martin, G. M. (1979). Genetic and evolutionary aspects of aging. *Federation Proceedings, 38,* 1962–1967.

Martin, G. M. (1996). Somatic mutagenesis and antimutagenesis in aging research. *Mutation Research, 350,* 35–41.

Martin, G. M. (1997). The genetics of aging. *Hospital Practice (Minneapolis), 32,* 47–6, 59.

Martin, G. M. (1998a). Atherosclerosis is the leading cause of death in the developed societies. *American Journal of Pathology, 153,* 1319–1320.

Martin, G. M. (1998b). The genetics of aging. *Aging (Milano), 10,* 148–149.

Martin, G. M. (1999). APOE alleles and lipophylic pathogens. *Neurobiology of Aging, 20,* 441–443.

Martin, G. M. (2000). Molecular mechanisms of late life dementias. *Experimental Gerontology, 35,* 439–443.

Martin, G. M. (2002a). The evolutionary substrate of aging. *Archives of Neurology, 59,* 1702–1705.

Martin, G. M. (2002b). Gene action in the aging brain: An evolutionary biological perspective. *Neurobiology of Aging, 23,* 647–654.

Martin, G. M. (2002c). Keynote: Mechanisms of senescence—Complificationists versus simplificationists. *Mechanisms of Ageing and Development, 123,* 65–73.

Martin, G. M. (2006). Keynote lecture: An update on the what, why and how questions of ageing. *Experimental Gerontology, 41,* 460–463.

Martin, G. M. (2007a). Clonal attenuation of somatic cells in aging mammals: A review of supportive evidence and its biomedical significance. *Annals of the New York Academy of Sciences, 1119,* 1–8.

Martin, G. M. (2007b). Modalities of gene action predicted by the classical evolutionary biological theory of aging. *Annals of the New York Academy of Sciences, 1100,* 14–20.

Martin, G. M., Austad, S. N., & Johnson, T. E. (1996). Genetic analysis of ageing: Role of oxidative damage and environmental stresses. *Nature Genetics, 13,* 25–34.

Martin, G. M., Bergman, A., & Barzilai, N. (2007). Genetic determinants of human health span and life span: Progress and new opportunities. *PLoS Genetics, 3,* e125.

Martin, G. M., Ogburn, C. E., Colgin, L. M., Gown, A. M., Edland, S. D., & Monnat, R. J., Jr. (1996). Somatic mutations are frequent and increase with age in human kidney epithelial cells. *Human Molecular Genetics, 5,* 215–221.

Masoro, E. J. (2006). Dietary restriction-induced life extension: A broadly based biological phenomenon. *Biogerontology, 7,* 153–155.

Medawar, P. B. (1957). An unsolved problem of biology. In P. B. Medawar (Ed.), *The uniqueness of the individual* (pp. 44–70). London: Methuen & Co.

Nuzhdin, S. V., Pasyukova, E. G., Dilda, C. L., Zeng, Z. B., & Mackay, T. F. (1997). Sex-specific quantitative trait loci affecting longevity in *Drosophila melanogaster. Proceedings of the National Academy of Sciences of the United States of America, 94,* 9734–9739.

Ogburn, C. E., Carlberg, K., Ottinger, M. A., Holmes, D. J., Martin, G. M., & Austad, S. N. (2001). Exceptional cellular resistance to oxidative damage in long-lived birds requires active gene expression. *Journal of Gerontology: Biological Sciences, 56,* B468–B474.

Packer, C., Tatar, M., & Collins, A. (1998). Reproductive cessation in female mammals. *Nature, 392,* 807–811.

Partridge, L. (2001). Evolutionary theories of ageing applied to long-lived organisms. *Experimental Gerontology, 36,* 641–650.

Promislow, D. E., & Tatar, M. (1998). Mutation and senescence: Where genetics and demography meet. *Genetica, 102–103,* 299–314.

Rea, S. L., Wu, D., Cypser, J. R., Vaupel, J. W., & Johnson, T. E. (2005). A stress-sensitive reporter predicts longevity in isogenic populations of *Caenorhabditis elegans. Nature Genetics, 37,* 894–898.

Reznick, D., Bryant, M., & Holmes, D. (2006). The evolution of senescence and post-reproductive lifespan in guppies (*Poecilia reticulata*). *Public Library of Science Biology, 4*(e7), 136–143.

Reznick, D. N., Bryant, M. J., Roff, D., Ghalambor, C. K., & Ghalambor, D. E. (2004). Effect of extrinsic mortality on the evolution of senescence in guppies. *Nature, 431,* 1095–1099.

Rose, M. R. (1991). *Evolutionary biology of aging.* New York: Oxford University Press.

Samuelson, A. V., Carr, C. E., & Ruvkun, G. (2007). Gene activities that mediate increased life span of *C. elegans* insulin-like signaling mutants. *Genes and Development, 21,* 2976–2994.

Schultz, R., & Curnow, C. (1988). Peak performance and age among superathletes: Track and field, swimming, baseball, tennis, and golf. *Journal of Gerontology, 43,* 113–120.

Vanfleteren, J. R., De Vreese, A., & Braeckman, B. P. (1998). Two-parameter logistic and Weibull equations provide better fits to survival data from isogenic populations of *Caenorhabditis elegans* in axenic culture than does the Gompertz model. *Journal of Gerontology: Biological Sciences, 53,* B393–B403.

Vaupel, J. W., Baudisch, A., Dolling, M., Roach, D. A., & Gampe, J. (2004). The case for negative senescence. *Theoretical Population Biology, 65,* 339–351.

Vaupel, J. W., Carey, J. R., Christensen, K., Johnson, T. E., Yashin, A. I., Holm, N. V., et al. (1998). Biodemographic trajectories of longevity. *Science, 280,* 855–860.

Weydt, P., Pineda, V. V., Torrence, A. E., Libby, R. T., Satterfield, T. F., Lazarowski, E. R., et al. (2006). Thermoregulatory and metabolic defects in Huntington's disease transgenic mice implicate PGC-1alpha in Huntington's disease neurodegeneration. *Cell Metabolism, 4,* 349–362.

Williams, G. C. (1957). Pleiotropy, natural selection, and the evolution of senescence. *Evolution, 11,* 398–411.

Wolfe, M. S., & Guenette, S. Y. (2007). APP at a glance. *Journal of Cell Science, 120,* 3157–3161.

Wood, J. W., Weeks, S. C., Bentley, G. R., & Weiss, K. M. (1994). The population biology of human aging. In D. E. Crews & R. N. Garruto (Eds.), *Biological anthropology and aging: Perspectives on human variation over the life span* (pp. 19–75). Oxford: Oxford University Press.

Wutz, A., & Gribnau, J. (2007). X inactivation Xplained. *Current Opinion in Genetics and Development, 17,* 387–393.

Contribution of a Mouse Model System to Neuroscientific Theories of Learning, Memory, and Aging

11

Diana S. Woodruff-Pak
Michael R. Foy
Richard F. Thompson

Neuroscience is data driven rather than theory driven. The basis of the discipline is an inductive or "bottom-up" approach. As such, we might consider that the domain of neuroscience has more models (defined in this volume as descriptions or prototypes of empirical relationships) than theories (herein defined as explanations to account for the empirical relationships).

Pioneers in neuroscience such as Harvard neuroscientist Karl S. Lashley and McGill neuroscientist Donald O. Hebb built their theoretical perspective from empirical observations rather than formulating theories first and then marshaling support for them. Indeed, in his search for mechanisms and neural substrates of learning early in the 20th century, Lashley was frustrated,

Supported by grants from the National Institute on Aging, R01 AG021925 and R01 AG023742, to DSW-P and P01 AG026572 to RFT.

stating that his data on the localization of the memory trace led to the necessary conclusion that learning was just not possible. In the mid-20th century, Hebb developed theories about brain function and plasticity that were conceptual, based on naturalistic observation. This tradition has been maintained, although contemporary theories also incorporate computer models, simulations of brain function, and the model system approach.

Advantages of the Mouse as a Model System

A principle laid down in the 19th century in biology by Thomas Henry Huxley is that we are unlikely to ever know everything about every organism. Therefore, we should agree on some convenient organism(s) to study in great depth so that we can use the experience of the past (in that organism) to build on in the future. This will lead to a body of knowledge in that "model system" that we can then expand and generalize to other species.

Among the criteria for a model biological system are whether the organism is easy to rear, whether its size is manageable and convenient for research, whether it is inexpensive to maintain, whether it has a short life span, whether its genetics are known and manipulable, and whether studies of it are likely to generalize to other species. The mouse model system is ideal as a mammalian model on all the previously listed criteria. In particular, for studies of aging, the mouse has a relatively short life span, approximately 30 months, and its entire genome has been mapped. Mouse models also have utility from a cognitive standpoint. Mice have the capacity to perform a number of cognitive and behavioral tasks.

The Model System of Eyeblink Classical Conditioning

Eyeblink classical conditioning has become arguably the best-delineated model system for the study of learning and memory available today. The neural circuitry is almost completely mapped, and the behavioral and neurobiological parallels in this form of associative learning extend to all mammals that have been studied, including humans. Processes of normal aging affect eyeblink classical conditioning similarly in all species in which older organisms have been tested—mice, rats, rabbits, cats, and humans. Mouse models, with their short life span, mapped genome, and capacity to perform a number of cognitive and behavioral tasks, provide an important means to understand causes of age-related impairment in learning and memory.

More than two decades ago, we pointed to the promise of eyeblink classical conditioning as a model system for the study of learning and memory in aging (Woodruff-Pak & Thompson, 1985). Among the significant advantages of this model system for gerontology are (a) that age differences in the classically conditioned eyeblink responses are large and (b) that striking parallels exist between the age differences in eyeblink conditioning in nonhuman mammals and humans. Subsequently, we have documented behavioral and neurobiological parallels that generalize in aging to all mammals studied, including humans (Thompson & Woodruff-Pak, 1987; Vogel, Ewers, Ross, Gould, & Woodruff-Pak, 2002;

Weiss & Thompson, 1991; Woodruff-Pak, 2006; Woodruff-Pak, Cronholm, & Sheffield, 1990; Woodruff-Pak & Thompson, 1988). In 1985, we pointed out advantages of a mouse model of aging and eyeblink classical conditioning (Woodruff-Pak & Thompson, 1985). However, at that time the extensive database of neurobiological and behavioral experiments available with eyeblink conditioning in rabbits was not developed for rodents. Now techniques for behavioral and electrophysiological testing in rats (Rogers, Britton, & Steinmetz, 2001; Skelton, 1988), including neonatal rats (Stanton, Freeman, & Skelton, 1992), have been developed along with techniques to test eyeblink conditioning in normal, mutant, and transgenic mice (Aiba et al., 1994; Kim & Thompson, 1997; Woodruff-Pak, Green, Levin, & Meisler, 2006) and rodent slice preparations (Foy, 2001), including slice preparations comparing young adult and older rats (Foy, Baudry, Foy, & Thompson, 2008).

Delay and Trace Eyeblink Classical Conditioning Procedures

In the delay procedure, a neutral stimulus, such as a tone-conditioned stimulus (CS), is presented before the onset of a corneal airpuff–unconditioned stimulus (US). The organism learns to blink to the tone CS before the onset of the airpuff US, and the learned response is called the conditioned response (CR). The interval between the onset of the CS and the onset of the US is called the interstimulus interval (ISI). The length of this interval affects the rate of conditioning, with ISIs greater than 500 ms increasing difficulty level for rabbits and mice. In the trace procedure, the CS is presented and then turned off, and a blank period ("trace") ensues before the onset of the US. The trace procedure is called "hippocampus dependent" because organisms with bilateral hippocampal lesions do not acquire CRs. In rabbits, the hippocampus is essential when the trace interval exceeds 300 ms (Moyer, Deyo, & Disterhoft, 1990). In humans, the trace interval must be 1,000 ms for eyeblink conditioning to be abolished by bilateral hippocampal lesions (Clark & Squire, 1998). In mice, bilateral ibotinic acid lesions of hippocampus abolish eyeblink conditioning in a 500-ms trace procedure with a trace interval of 250 ms (Tseng, Guan, Disterhoft, & Weiss, 2004). The cerebellar interpositus nucleus is essential in all eyeblink conditioning procedures (Christian & Thompson, 2003; Green & Woodruff-Pak, 2000).

Brain Circuitry of Eyeblink Classical Conditioning

A variety of techniques, including electrophysiological recording of multiple and single units, electrolytic and chemical lesions, physical and chemical reversible lesions, neural stimulation, genetic mutations, and pharmacological manipulation, have been used to demonstrate that the dorsolateral interpositus nucleus ipsilateral to the conditioned eye is the essential site for acquisition and retention of conditioned eyeblink responses (Anderson & Steinmetz, 1994; Kim & Thompson, 1997; Lavond, Kim, & Thompson, 1993; Steinmetz, 1996; Steinmetz, Gluck, & Solomon, 2001; Thompson, 1986, 2000). Selective lesions (electrolytic or chemical) of the cerebellum prevent the acquisition and retention of conditioned eyeblink responses in the delay (Lavond, McCormick, & Thompson, 1984; Lincoln, McCormick, & Thompson, 1982; McCormick & Thompson, 1984a;

McCormick et al., 1981) or trace (Woodruff-Pak, Lavond, & Thompson, 1985) procedures. Electrophysiological recording of single and multiple-unit activity in the cerebellum indicated that cells in specific cerebellar regions undergo learning-induced changes during eyeblink conditioning (Gould & Steinmetz, 1994, 1996; McCormick & Thompson, 1984b; Thompson, 1990). The involvement of the cerebellum in eyeblink conditioning is also supported by studies that show that electrical stimulation of the two major afferents to the cerebellum—the mossy fibers from the pontine nuclei and the climbing fibers from the inferior olive—can substitute for the peripheral tone CS (Steinmetz, 1990; Steinmetz, Lavond, & Thompson, 1985; Steinmetz, Rosen, Chapman, Lavond, & Thompson, 1986) and corneal airpuff US (Mauk, Steinmetz, & Thompson, 1986), respectively. Stimulation of both the mossy fiber pontine CS pathway and the climbing fiber inferior olive US pathway also results in the acquisition of CRs (Steinmetz, Lavond, & Thompson, 1989). Reversible inactivation of the anterior interpositus nucleus and overlying cerebellar cortex by cooling or application of muscimol (a GABA-receptor agonist) or lidocaine (an open Na^{+}-channel blocker) during training completely prevents acquisition of CRs (Clark, Zhang, & Lavond, 1992; Hardiman, Ramnani, & Yeo, 1996; Krupa, Thompson, & Thompson, 1993). However, inactivation of the efferents (superior cerebellar peduncle and red nucleus) does not prevent acquisition (Clark & Lavond, 1993; Krupa & Thompson, 1995; Krupa, Weng, & Thompson, 1996).

A hypothetical model of the neural circuitry essential for eyeblink conditioning was presented (Thompson, 1986) and elaborated (Kim & Thompson, 1997; Thompson 1990) (Figure 11.1). According to the model, both the cerebellar cortex and the interpositus nucleus receive information about the CS, conveyed by the mossy fiber system emanating from the pontine nucleus, and information about the US, relayed by the climbing fiber system originating from the inferior olive. Converging CS and US signals are relayed to Purkinje cells in cerebellar cortex and principle cells in interpositus nucleus. The efferent (eyelid closure) CR pathway projects from the interpositus nucleus in cerebellum to the red nucleus and via the descending rubral pathway to act ultimately on motor neurons.

A cellular model system proposed as a mechanism for information storage in the cerebellum is long-term depression (LTD). In this model, coactivation of climbing fiber and parallel fiber inputs to a Purkinje cell induces a persistent, input-specific depression of the parallel fiber–Purkinje cell synapse (for a review, see Linden & Connor, 1995). Mouse models have been used in a series of collaborative studies in the Thompson lab to explore LTD and eyeblink conditioning. Motor coordination (rotorod), cerebellar cortical LTD, and eyeblink conditioning were tested in various mutant and knockout mice. Mutants that maintain multiple climbing fiber innervation of Purkinje neurons to adulthood showed impaired motor coordination (Offermanns et al., 1997, Gαq knockout; C. Chen et al., 1995, PKCλ knockout), normal cerebellar cortical LTD, and supernormal eyeblink conditioning (C. Chen et al., 1995). On the other hand, the GFAP knockout mouse showed normal motor coordination, impaired cerebellar cortical LTD, and impaired cerebellar eyeblink conditioning (Shibuki et al., 1996). There was a consistent correlation between impaired cerebellar cortical LTD and impaired eyeblink conditioning and a lack of correlation between LTD and rotorod performance (Kim & Thompson, 1997).

11.1

A putative eyeblink conditioning circuit based on experimental findings and gross anatomy of the cerebellum and brain stem. The conditioned stimulus (CS) pathway consists of excitatory mossy fiber projections from the pontine nuclei to the interpositus nucleus and to the cerebellar cortex (indicated with stars). In the cortex, the mossy fibers form synapses with granule cells that in turn send excitatory parallel fibers to the Purkinje cells. The Purkinje cells are the exclusive output neurons from the cortex, and they send inhibitory fibers to deep nuclei, such as the interpositus. The unconditioned stimulus (US) pathway consists of excitatory climbing fiber projections from the inferior olive (dorsal accessory olive) to the interpositus nucleus and to the Purkinje cells in cerebellar cortex. The efferent conditioned response (CR) pathway projects from the interpositus nucleus to the red nucleus and via the descending rubral pathway to act ultimately on the eyeblink reflex path. Additional abbreviations: NV = spinal fifth cranial nucleus; UR = unconditioned response (adapted from Thompson, 1990).

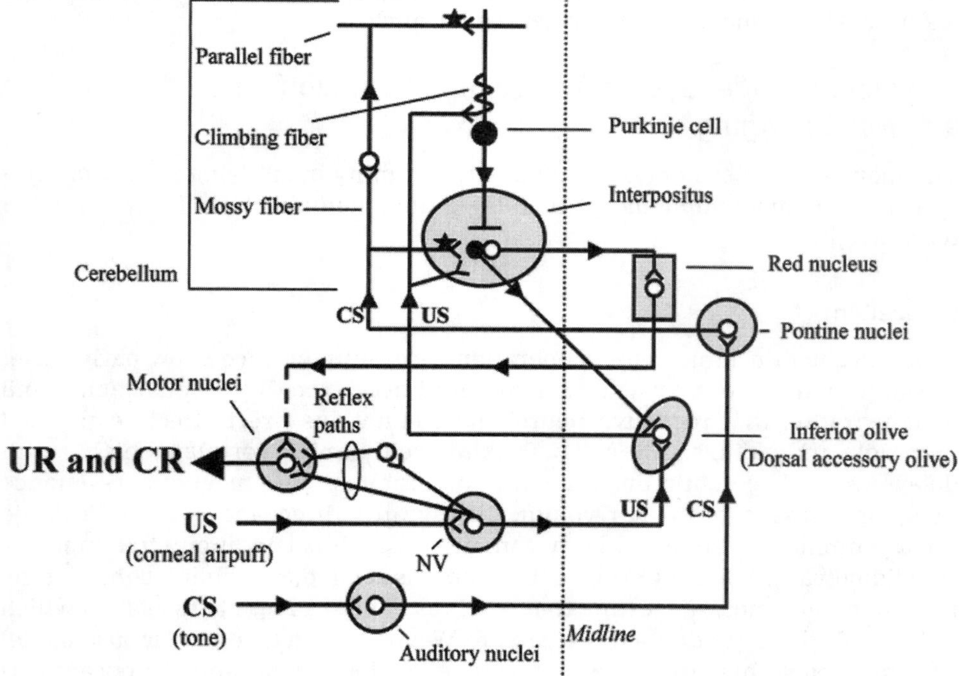

In a study examining how eyeblink conditioning affects synapse number in rat cerebellum, Kleim et al. (2002) found significantly more synapses per neuron within the interpositus nucleus in animals receiving paired presentations of CS and US than animals receiving explicitly unpaired or no stimulus presentations. The increase was caused by the addition of excitatory rather than inhibitory synapses. Failure to find increases in the number of inhibitory synapses per neuron in interpositus nucleus in conditioned rats suggests mechanisms for learning in the cerebellum in addition to LTD. The increase in interpositus nucleus synapses was caused by the addition of excitatory rather than inhibitory synapses. Thus, the increase is associated with strengthening of inputs from precerebellar nuclei that are excitatory in interpositus nucleus (most likely mossy fiber inputs) rather than with strengthening of intracerebellar inputs (from Purkinje cells) that are inhibitory. Whereas results from the analysis of synapse formation could be interpreted to suggest that input to the interpositus nucleus from Purkinje cells (the only cerebellar cortical input to deep nuclei) is not affected by conditioning, the cerebellar cortex is of demonstrated involvement during normal acquisition. Lesions of cerebellar cortex caused a transient but substantial impairment in the conditioned eyeblink response (Lavond & Steinmetz, 1989; Lavond, Steinmetz, Yokaitis, & Thompson, 1987; McCormick & Thompson, 1984a; Woodruff-Pak, Lavond, Logan, Steinmetz, & Thompson, 1993). The impairment was residual and never permanent, unless the interpositus nucleus was damaged. However, Yeo, Hardiman, and Glickstein (1985) claimed that such lesions abolished the CR. It was impossible to resolve this issue with the lesion method because complete removal of cerebellar cortex inevitably damaged the deep cerebellar nuclei.

The Mouse Model System of Eyeblink Conditioning and Normal Aging

The mouse model system is of demonstrated utility in studying neural mechanisms in learning and memory and has significant implications for research on normal aging.

Cerebellum

Heterozygous Purkinje cell degeneration (*pcd*) mutant mice show early-onset Purkinje neuron loss, providing a model of accelerated cerebellar aging and demonstrating that recessive neurological mutations exert effects expressed in middle and old age. Cerebellar Purkinje cell number correlates highly with delay eyeblink conditioning in mice and rabbits, and magnetic resonance imaging–assessed cerebellar volume (likely an indirect measure of Purkinje neuron number) correlates highly with delay eyeblink conditioning in humans. Individual variation in Purkinje cell number is related to eyeblink conditioning in young organisms, suggesting that reserves of neuron numbers against which individuals draw are defined early in life. We have been using the mouse model system to test hypotheses about cerebellar-dependent and hippocampus-dependent mechanisms responsible for age-related deficits in eyeblink conditioning and other forms of learning and memory.

The controversy about the role of the cerebellar cortex in acquisition of CRs is an instance in which the use of the mouse model system was helpful. The *pcd* mutant mouse model provided critical data for addressing this debate. In mice homozygous for the *pcd* mutation, the cerebellum develops normally until about 2 weeks after birth, at which point all Purkinje neurons die over a period of about 2 weeks. For the next 2 months, all other neuronal systems appear to be normal, but the cerebellar cortex is completely nonfunctional. At 4 months of age, during this period before other neural systems in the cerebellum deteriorated, *pcd* mice were tested on delay eyeblink conditioning (L. Chen,

Bao, Lockard, Kim, & Thompson, 1996). As shown in Figure 11.2, 4-month *pcd* mutant mice acquired CRs at a dramatically slower rate and to a lower maximal level than did their wild-type littermates (L. Chen et al., 1996). Extending deep cerebellar nucleus lesion effects shown in other mammals, cerebellar lesions that included the interpositus nucleus completely blocked eyeblink conditioning in wild-type mice (L. Chen et al., 1996) and in *pcd* mice (L. Chen, Bao, & Thompson, 1999). Tests of delay eyeblink classical conditioning in mice with a genetically induced "lesion" selective to sodium channels of Purkinje neurons demonstrated impaired acquisition (Woodruff-Pak et al., 2006). The results support the interpretation that loss or impairment of Purkinje neuron function disrupts acquisition of delay eyeblink conditioning.

Loss of Purkinje neurons in cerebellar cortex is associated with age-related deficits in eyeblink conditioning in mice (Woodruff-Pak, 2006) and in rabbits (Woodruff-Pak & Trojanowski, 1996; Woodruff-Pak et al., 1990), and the *pcd* mutation provides an accelerated aging model. It was demonstrated that mice heterozygous for the *pcd* mutation have significantly fewer Purkinje cells at 7 months earlier than wild-type mice (Doulazmi, Hadj-Sahraoui, Frederic, & Mariani, 2002). An apparently recessive neurological mutation may exert, in

11.2

Acquisition and extinction as measured by conditioned response (CR) percentage in Purkinje cell deficient (*pcd*) mutant mice and their wild-type littermates. Acquisition of CRs occurs in these *pcd* mutant mice in the total absence of Purkinje cells, but the rate and magnitude of conditioning is significantly impaired. These mutant mice show classic cerebellar symptoms, such as impaired motor coordination and mild ataxia, but reduction in eyeblink conditioning is not due to impairments in motor control. The *pcd* mutants did not differ from wild-type mice in terms of sensitivity to the shock unconditioned stimulus (US) or unconditioned response performance to the US. These results demonstrated that Purkinje cells are required for optimal learning, but some learning can occur in the interpositus nucleus in the complete absence of cerebellar cortical Purkinje cells. (L. Chen et al., 1996).

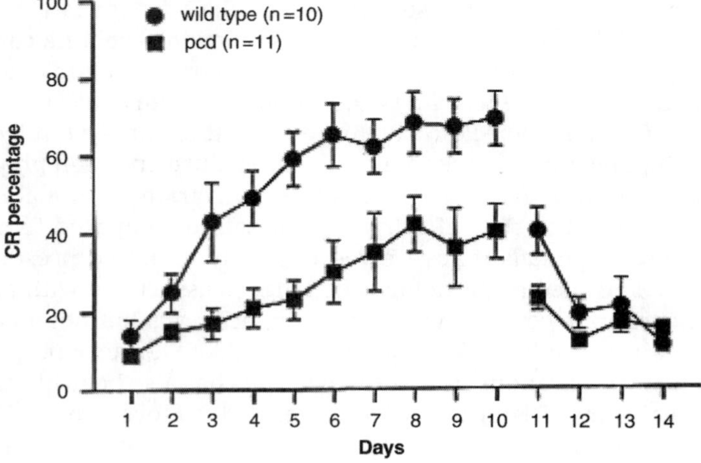

the heterozygous state, a deleterious effect on Purkinje neurons during the aging process. Other studies demonstrated that there is a progressive and age-related loss of Purkinje neurons in mice heterozygous for mutations classically viewed as recessive, such as staggerer and reeler, which begin much earlier in the life span than in C57BL/6 wild-type mice. For example, heterozygous staggerer (+/sg) mice exhibit a progressive and age-related loss of Purkinje cells by 12 months of age despite their apparent clinical normality (Zanjani, Mariani, Delhaye-Bouchaud, & Herrup, 1992). In heterozygous reeler mice (+/rl), there is a 16% deficit in the number of Purkinje cells in 3-month-old +/rl and a 24% deficit in 16-month-old animals, but the deficit is present only in +/rl males (Hadj-Sahraoui, Frederic, Delhaye-Bouchaud, & Mariani, 1996). These results illustrate a synergy between the aging process and the heterozygous genotype and provide a model for the genetic contribution to regressive age-related changes in the brain.

Hippocampus

The hippocampus and septohippocampal acetylcholine system is involved in basic associative learning of the sort represented by eyeblink conditioning (see Berger, Berry, & Thompson, 1986). In a series of studies using delay eyeblink classical conditioning in rabbits, it was observed that activity recorded in the CA1 pyramidal cell region of the hippocampus forms a predictive "model" of the amplitude–time course of the learned behavioral response but only under conditions where behavioral learning occurs (Berger, Alger, & Thompson, 1976; Berger & Thompson, 1978b). This response is generated largely by pyramidal neurons (Berger, Rinaldi, Weisz, & Thompson, 1983; Berger & Thompson, 1978a). The role of the hippocampus in classical conditioning of the eyeblink response is called "modulatory" because manipulations of the hippocampus can impair or enhance the rate of acquisition. The memory trace itself is not in the hippocampus, but the hippocampus can markedly influence the storage process.

Although the hippocampus is not necessary for normal acquisition in the delay procedure, it is necessary for discrimination reversal (Berger & Orr, 1983) and trace conditioning (Kaneko & Thompson, 1997; Kim, Clark, & Thompson, 1995; Moyer et al, 1990; Port, Romano, Steinmetz, Mikhail, & Patterson, 1986; Solomon, Vander Schaaf, Thompson, & Weisz, 1986). There is a long-lasting neuronal plasticity formed in the hippocampus following eyeblink conditioning. This change is essential for learning to occur in the trace eyeblink conditioning procedure, at least until the learning is consolidated (Kim et al., 1995).

Disterhoft, Coulter, and Alkon (1986) trained rabbits in eyeblink conditioning using the hippocampus-dependent trace procedure and then prepared hippocampal slices. Pyramidal neurons in slices from trained animals showed a marked reduction in the slow afterhyperpolarization compared to neurons in slices from control animals that received explicitly unpaired presentations of the CS and US. This electrophysiological change is associated with an increase in the area of synaptic contacts within the hippocampus but not an overall increase in synapse number (Geinesman et al., 2000). Afterhyperpolarization recorded in slice preparations from trained rabbits has also been observed in relation to normal aging (Disterhoft & McEchron, 2000; Moyer, Power, Thompson, & Disterhoft, 2000). Excitability of CA1 neurons was studied 24 hours after the last training session in aged rabbits that reached a 60% behavioral criterion ("learning intact"), rabbits trained for 30 days that never demonstrated more than 30% CRs per session ("failed to learn"), and naive aging rabbits. Aged CA1 neurons from learning-intact animals had significantly reduced postburst afterhyperpolarizations and reduced spike frequency adaptation compared with neurons from control groups of naive and aging rabbits that failed to learn. No differences were seen in resting potential characteristics after learning. The data suggest that postsynaptic excitability of CA1 neurons is correlated with learning hippocampus-dependent trace eyeblink conditioning in both young and older rabbits. In young and in learning-intact older rabbits, the data also suggest that a similar level of postsynaptic excitability is achieved at the time that learning has occurred regardless of rabbit age and regardless of the actual speed of acquisition of the CR. To identify the ion current(s) underlying the age-associated learning deficits and decreases in neuronal excitability reflected by an enhanced postburst afterhyperpolarization in CA1 hippocampal pyramidal neurons, whole-cell voltage-clamp recording experiments were carried out using hippocampal slices in young and older rabbits (Power, Wu, Sametsky, Oh, & Disterhoft, 2002). Aging neurons had an enhanced slow outward calcium-activated potassium current. The amplitude of this current was correlated at a significant level with the amplitude of the postburst afterhyperpolarization ($r = 0.63$, $p < 0.001$).

Normal Aging in the Hippocampus and Cerebellum

Individual variations in neuron cell numbers are likely related to outcomes of aging (Finch, 2003; Finch & Kirkwood, 2000). Neuron numbers vary widely among individuals, in part as a consequence of chance developmental variations. Individual variations are greatest in large populations of neurons arrayed in parallel, which in the neocortex exceed ±50% (Williams & Herrup, 1988). The neuron cell loss required for functional impact appears to differ widely among brain regions, and the magnitude of neuron loss in normal aging also varies among brain regions. Until recently, it was widely accepted that neuron death in most brain regions was an inevitable result of normal aging. The empirical bases for this perspective were a number of investigations based on techniques that introduced biases in assessment of tissue number (e.g., Brizzee & Ordy, 1979; Brody, 1955; Dayan, 1971). Parameters such as tissue fixation, neuronal shrinkage, and age-related changes in the volume of brain structures were confounding factors when the assumption was made that decreased neuron density equated with decreased neuron number (West, 1993a). The design of the early studies was to measure neuron density in a given structure rather than total neuron number. Problems with this common technique first became apparent in the 1980s when Haug, Kuhl, Mecke, Sass, and Wasner (1984) reported no age-related neuronal loss in human cerebral cortex. With the development of stereological methods for counting neurons and the application of these techniques to research on aging, it has now become apparent that in the neocortex and hippocampus of humans and many other species there is little age-related decline in neuron number (Gomez-Isla et al., 1996; Rapp & Gallagher, 1996; West, 1993b; West, Coleman, Flood, & Troncoso, 1994; West & Gundersen, 1990).

Research on Aging and Unbiased Stereology

The dissector principle as an unbiased method for estimating the total number of objects was introduced in the mid-1980s (Sterio, 1984). The dissector is a three-dimensional counting chamber with inclusion and exclusion planes that ensure that all objects have an equal probability of being sampled and are counted only once. Until the dissector was introduced, researchers often used counting profiles. This method is biased because taller objects can get counted in more than one profile, and smaller objects may never get counted at all. In the case of studies of age differences in cell number, differential shrinkage of brain tissue as it was being fixed for analysis added additional bias. Studies carried out during most of the 20th century reported significant loss of neurons with aging in many regions of the brain (for reviews, see Morrison & Hof, 1997, 2007).

Implementation of methods that have become known as stereology came slowly, but by the late 20th century these methods had reshaped perspectives of aging and the brain. Many brain regions assessed with unbiased stereology, including structures such as the hippocampus that are critically involved in learning and memory, showed little or no cell loss in rodents (Gallagher et al., 1996; West, Slimianka, & Gundersen, 1991) and modest and regionally circumscribed cell loss in humans (West, 1993b). Unbiased stereological techniques indicate that whereas neuron number is maintained in neocortex and hippocampus, there is significant Purkinje neuron loss associated with aging in the cerebellar cortex.

In a stereological study of the entire cerebellar cortex, Larsen, Skalicky, and Viidik (2000) reported 11% fewer Purkinje cells in 23-month-old Sprague-Dawley rats. Using unbiased stereological techniques, we counted Purkinje neurons in the entire cerebellar cortex of 25 C57BL/6 mice ranging in age between 4 and 24 months (Woodruff-Pak, 2006). Average estimates for mice in each age-group are presented in Figure 11.3. There is a statistically significant effect of age on Purkinje cell number in C57BL/6 mice. There were significantly fewer Purkinje cells in 18- and 24-month-old mice than in 4-, 8-, and 12-month-old mice. In Jean Mariani's laboratory, where unbiased stereology was not used, stability was observed in whole-cerebellum Purkinje cell numbers of C57BL/6 mice up to the age of 18 months with decline by 24 months (Table 11.1). Our results suggest that age-related loss of Purkinje cells in C57Bl/6 mice occurs earlier—between 12 and 18 months. Stereological Purkinje neuron counts in CBA mice indicate a later loss of Purkinje neurons, between the age of 18 and 24 months, and eyeblink conditioning over the life span of CBA mice is also impaired later—at the age of 24 months (Eagan, Zach, Roker, & Woodruff-Pak, 2007).

Although there is stability of neuron number in the older hippocampus, electrophysiological investigations of aging in the mammalian hippocampus have revealed that some aspects are compromised (Barnes, 1994). Place cells in the hippocampal CA1 region are less stable in older rats and are associated with poorer spatial learning (Barnes, Suster, Shen, & McNaughton, 1997). In learning-impaired older rabbits, single-unit records of clusters of pyramidal neurons in CA1 showed diminished responding (McEchron, Weible, & Disterhoft, 2001). Hippocampal glutamate receptors showed age-related decline (Clark et al., 1992). Calcium-dependent afterhyperpolarizations in hippocampal neurons of aged rats were abnormally prolonged (Landfield & Pitler, 1984).

11.3

The number of Purkinje cells in the whole cerebellum estimated with unbiased stereological techniques. There were a total of 25 C57BL/6 mice ranging in age from 4 to 24 months with five mice in each age-group. Error bars are standard error of the mean (Woodruff-Pak, 2006).

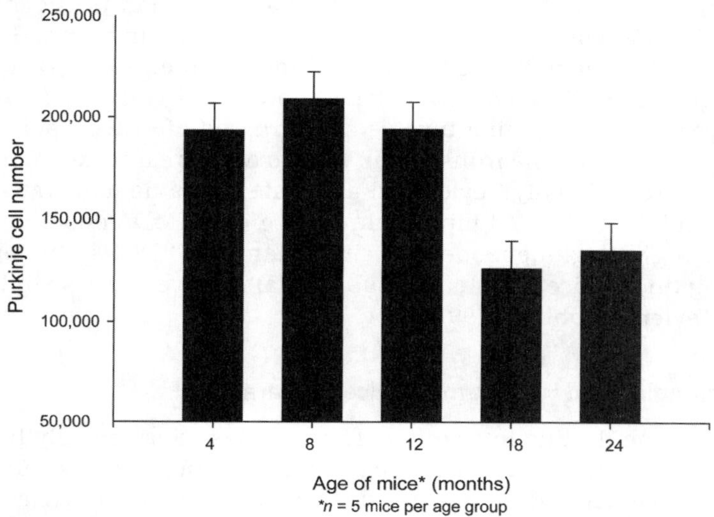

11.1 Estimates of Whole-Cerebellum Purkinje Cell Number in C57BL/6 Mice

Study	*n*/age-group	Gender	Mean (standard error of the mean) × 10^{-3} cerebellar Purkinje cell number				
			3–4 months	8–9 months	12–13 months	16–18 months	24–26 months
Hadj-Sahraoui et al. (1996)	3–4	M, F	149 (7)	—	—	173 (7)	151 (8)
Hadj-Sahraoui et al. (1997)	4	F	—	—	171 (2)	174 (1)	135 (5)
Doulazmi et al. (1999)	4	F	185 (5)	—	177 (1)	179 (1)	142 (5)
Doulazmi et al. (2002)	3–4	F	—	—	—	176 (1)	—
Woodruff-Pak (2006)	5	M, F	194 (13)	209 (13)	194 (13)	126 (13)	135 (13)

Considerable evidence supports a calcium dysregulation hypothesis of brain aging, and in the hippocampus this may be related to elevated postsynaptic calcium that is closely associated with altered neuronal plasticity. There is a dramatic increase in the amount of LTD induced in the CA1 hippocampal slice in the aged rat (see the following discussion and Norris, Korol, & Foster, 1996; Vouimba, Foy, Foy, & Thompson, 2000). The critical event in induction of both long-term potentiation (LTP) and LTD is increased intracellular calcium (Bear & Abraham, 1996). Landfield and associates have shown dramatic increases in calcium influx (L-type voltage-gated calcium channels) in pyramidal neurons in hippocampal slices from aged rats (Landfield & Pitler, 1984). Disterhoft and associates (Moyer & Disterhoft, 1994) have shown that age-related impairments in trace eyeblink conditioning involve an increased afterhyperpolarization in hippocampal pyramidal neurons due in turn to an increased calcium-activated potassium current. Finally, Teyler and associates have demonstrated two distinct forms of LTP in the CA1 hippocampal slice, one NMDA dependent and the other involving voltage-dependent calcium channels (VDCCs; Grover & Teyler, 1990). Aging (in rat slice) results in a substantial relative increase in VDCC LTP (Shankar, Teyler, & Robbins, 1998).

Research on Aging and Hippocampal Slice Preparations

During aging, the decline in cognitive function has most recently been attributed to alterations of cellular structure and function, presumably and ultimately affecting mechanisms of neural plasticity. In many cases, changes in neural plasticity during aging are quite subtle; however, in other cases, such as animal models that emulate age-associated disorders, they are more apparent. Here we discuss our work in aging animals involving the model systems approach to the neurobiology of learning and memory function using the strategy of studying well-characterized changes in electrophysiology and behavior in relatively simple and controlled preparations.

A primary model of neural plasticity used extensively in neurophysiology is hippocampal LTP, which consists of a long-lasting increase in neural efficacy at glutamatergic synapses, is viewed by many as a putative mechanism of memory storage, and has proven to be a valuable model for the study of synaptic plasticity at the cellular level (Bear & Malenka, 1994). Another model of neural plasticity and a counterpart to LTP is represented by hippocampal LTD. In hippocampal LTD, cumulative activation of specific inputs to hippocampal neurons leads to a long-lasting reduction in synaptic transmission of neuronal responses (Bear & Abraham, 1996). Hippocampal LTP and LTD have been extensively studied as potential mechanisms for learning and memory function and appear to be modified during aging.

For more than 30 years, age-related alterations in synaptic function within the hippocampus have been suggested to contribute to age-related memory impairment (Burke & Barnes, 2006; Geinisman, de Toledo-Morrell, Morrell, & Heller, 1995; Landfield, McGaugh, & Lynch, 1978). In aged rats, several alterations in the properties of hippocampal LTP and LTD have been reported. One of the most dramatic effects of aging on neural plasticity involves LTD. Compared to young adult male rats (3 to 5 months) that show little or no LTD, an increased magnitude of LTD and decreased threshold for LTD induction have been reported in hippocampal slices prepared from aged male rats (22 to 24 months) in which both adult and aged slices received the standard low-frequency stimulation protocol (1 Hz, 900 pulses) (Foster, 1999). We replicated this finding in our laboratory where both adult and aged groups exhibited an initial depression following low-frequency stimulation, but the aged animals maintained the depression, whereas the adult animals' excitatory postsynaptic potentials (EPSPs), slope, and amplitude recordings recovered within about 20 minutes (Foy et al., 2008; Vouimba et al., 2000) (compare artificial cerebrospinal fluid [aCSF] data between Figure 11.4 [adult rats] and Figure 11.5 [aged rats]). Further studies have found this aged effect presumably due to calcium dysregulation (Foster & Kumar, 2002; Kumar & Foster, 2004, 2005, 2007).

Using the rodent hippocampal slice preparation with both field potential and intracellular recording techniques, we have studied the effects of ovarian hormones, behavioral stress, and aging on neural plasticity. We have shown that acute administration of the ovarian hormone 17β-estradiol (E2) to hippocampal slices from adult rats enhances synaptic transmission, thus replicating Teyler's original observations (Foy, Chiaia, & Teyler, 1984; Foy & Teyler, 1983; Teyler, Vardaris, Lewis, & Rawitch, 1980) and also markedly enhances LTP involving both NMDA and AMPA receptor activation (Foy et al., 1999). The rapid estrogen action (<5 minutes) on NMDA receptors has also been found to be mediated

11.4

Plot of normalized fEPSP recordings in slices of hippocampal area CA1 from adult (3-month-old) male Sprague-Dawley rats. All hippocampal slices were perfused with aCSF for 10 minutes to obtain fEPSP amplitude percentage baseline data. After 10 minutes of baseline recording, experimental slices were perfused with 100 pM 17β-estradiol (E2). Control slices continued to be perfused with aCSF. After 30 minutes of either E2 or aCSF, slices received low-frequency stimulation to elicit hippocampal long-term depression. Error bars are standard error of the mean (Foy et al., 2008).

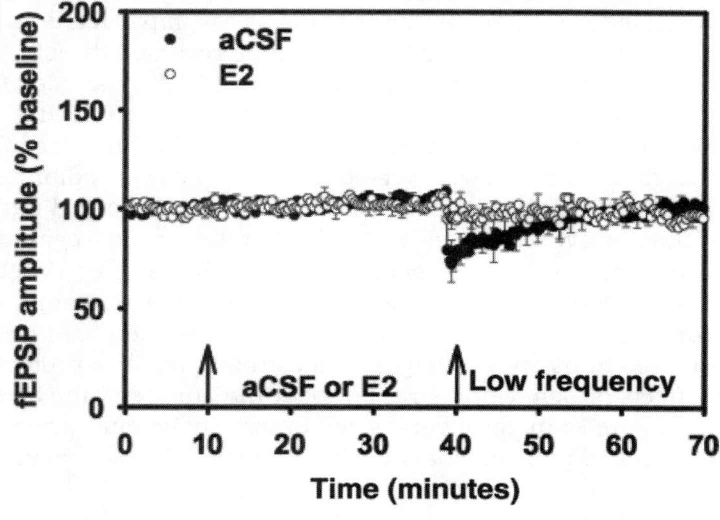

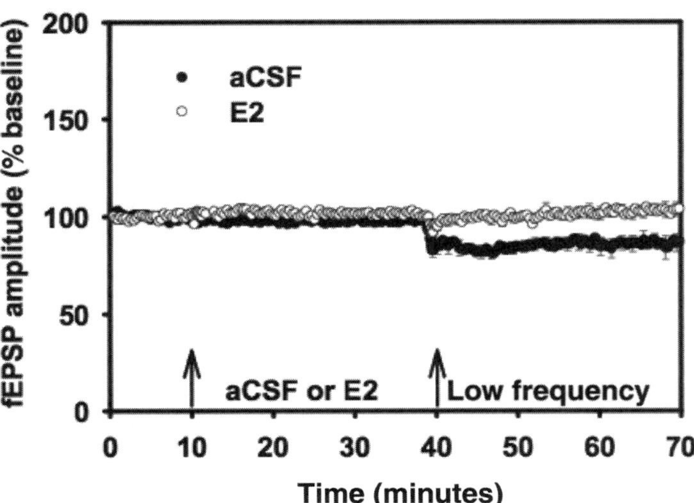

11.5

Plot of fEPSP recordings from hippocampal slices of aged (24-month-old) male Sprague-Dawley rats that were perfused with either 17β-estradiol E2 or aCSF (Foy et al., 2008).

by nongenomic activation of the ERK/MAP kinase pathway via tyrosine phosphorylation of NR2 subunits of NMDA receptors (Bi, Broutman, Foy, Thompson, & Baudry, 2000). In another series of studies on neural plasticity, an age-related increase in LTD was reversed by acute application of E2 in hippocampal slices (Foy et al., 2008; Vouimba et al., 2000) (Figure 11.5). Here, addition of E2 in the incubation medium of both adult and aged hippocampal slices somewhat attenuated the initial depression following low-frequency stimulation but completely suppressed the persisting depression in slices from the aged animals (Foy et al., 2008).

In an earlier series of studies, we have shown that behavioral stress (animal restraint plus tail shock) markedly impaired subsequent LTP in the rodent CA1 hippocampal slice preparation (Foy, Stanton, Levine, & Thompson, 1987; Kim, Foy, & Thompson, 1996; Shors, Foy, Levine, & Thompson, 1990). In a recent series of experiments, we have found that the stress impairment of LTP from adult animals exposed to behavioral stress can be reversed through acute application of E2 to the hippocampal slices from which LTP is recorded (Foy et al., 2008) (Figure 11.6). An investigation of the stress effect on LTD has also been done in which behavioral stress markedly enhances LTD in slices from both adult and aged rats, which is also reversed following the acute administration of E2 (Foy et al., 2008). Our results indicate that LTD was increased during aging and was blocked or even reversed in aged rats following estrogen treatment. Further, when comparing the estrogen effects in adult and aged behaviorally stressed groups with those in adult and aged control (vehicle) groups, LTD magnitude is strongest in the vehicle condition but becomes significantly decreased following estrogen infusion. We suggest that estrogen acts as a protective agent against the effects of behavioral stress in both the adult and the aged groups. The differential effects in adult versus aged rats may be due to age or stress-related differences in hippocampal neurons or some other mechanism involving estrogen.

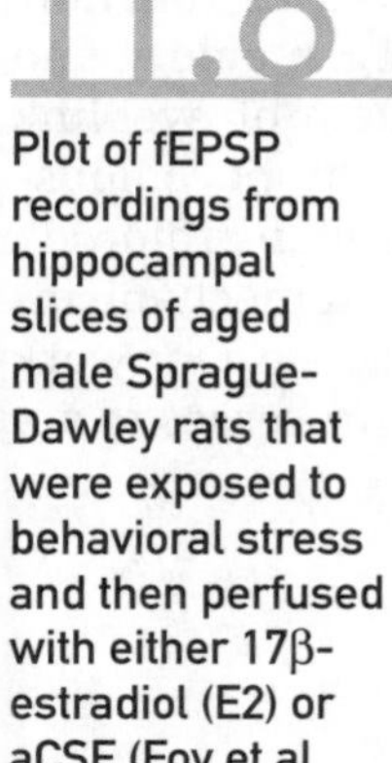

11.6

Plot of fEPSP recordings from hippocampal slices of aged male Sprague-Dawley rats that were exposed to behavioral stress and then perfused with either 17β-estradiol (E2) or aCSF (Foy et al., 2008).

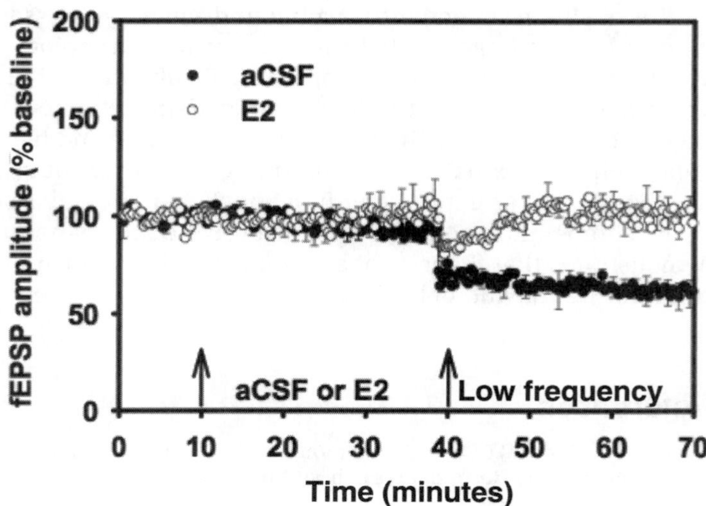

The recent development of a triple-transgenic mouse model of Alzheimer's disease has resulted in a report of an age-related and progressive neuropathological phenotype that includes both plaque and tangle pathology restricted mainly to the hippocampus, amygdala, and cerebral cortex (Oddo et al., 2003). An in vitro study examining synaptic dysfunction in these triple-transgenic mice (3x-Tg-AD) at 6 months of age reported lowered levels of hippocampal basal synaptic transmission and reduced levels of LTP compared to nontransgenic mice (Oddo et al., 2003). It was suggested that synaptic dysfunction found in the 3x-Tg-AD mouse model represents an early change in neural plasticity that precedes the accumulation of the hallmark pathological lesions that accompany Alzheimer's disease.

Collectively, electrophysiological results using the animal model systems approach indicate that both systemic and behavioral variables can have a significant impact on neural plasticity in rodent hippocampus. Prevention by estrogen of age-related enhancement of LTD, for example, might account for the protective effects of estrogen on memory function during aging recently reported in clinical studies (Henderson, 2006; Sherwin, 2006).

Conclusions

Brain memory systems and associated brain structures differ in the magnitude of age-related neuron loss. Aging in hippocampus-dependent learning and memory is associated with reduced functional capacity of pyramidal neurons in the CA fields, but neuron number is stable. Furthermore, estrogen acts as a protective agent in the hippocampus against the effects of behavioral stress in both the adult and the aged groups. The differential effects in adult versus aged rats may be due to age or stress-related differences in hippocampal neurons or some other mechanism involving estrogen.

Cerebellum-dependent learning and memory is associated with Purkinje neuron loss and age-related impairment in morphology as well as function. Traditionally, cerebellar and hippocampal substrates of learning, memory, and aging have been studied independently. Using the model system of eyeblink classical conditioning and other forms of learning and memory (hippocampus-dependent contextual fear conditioning and cerebellum-dependent rotorod), we investigated structural and functional changes and associated mechanisms in the cerebellum and hippocampus over the life span in the mouse. Our work demonstrates that theories of aging must embrace a variety of processes to account for neural and behavioral effects.

References

Aiba, A. M., Kano, M., Chen, C., Stanton, M. E., Fox, G. D., Herrup, K., et al. (1994). Deficient cerebellar long-term depression and impaired motor learning in mGluR1 mutant mice. *Cell, 79,* 377–388.

Anderson, B. J., & Steinmetz, J. E. (1994). Cerebellar and brainstem circuits involved in classical eyeblink conditioning. *Review of Neuroscience, 5,* 251–273.

Barnes, C. A. (1994). Normal aging: Regionally specific changes in hippocampal synaptic transmission. *Trends in Neuroscience, 17,* 13–18.

Barnes, C. A., Suster, M. S., Shen, J., & McNaughton, B. J. (1997). Multistability of cognitive maps in the hippocampus of old rats. *Nature, 388,* 272–275.

Bear, M. F., & Abraham, W. C. (1996). Long-term depression in hippocampus. *Annual Review of Neuroscience, 19,* 437–462.

Bear, M. F., & Malenka, R. C. (1994). Synaptic plasticity: LTP and LTD. *Current Opinion in Neurobiology, 4,* 389–399.

Berger, T. W., Alger, B. E., & Thompson, R. F. (1976). Neuronal substrate of classical conditioning in the hippocampus. *Science, 192,* 483–485.

Berger, T. W., Berry, S. D., & Thompson, R. F. (1986). Role of the hippocampus in classical conditioning of aversive and appetitive behaviors. In R. L. Isaacson & K. H. Pribram (Eds.), *The hippocampus* (pp. 203–239). New York: Plenum Press.

Berger, T. W., & Orr, W. B. (1983). Hippocampectomy selectively disrupts discrimination reversal conditioning of the rabbit nictitating membrane response. *Behavioural Brain Research, 8,* 49–68.

Berger, T. W., Rinaldi, P. C., Weisz, D. J., & Thompson, R. F. (1983). Single unit analysis of different hippocampal cell types during classical conditioning of the rabbit nictitating membrane response. *Journal of Neurophysiology, 50,* 1197–1219.

Berger, T. W., & Thompson, R. F. (1978a). Identification of pyramidal cells as the critical elements in hippocampal neuronal plasticity during learning. *Proceedings of the National Academy of Sciences of the United States of America, 75,* 1572–1576.

Berger, T. W., & Thompson, R. F. (1978b). Neuronal plasticity in the limbic system during classical conditioning of the rabbit nictitating membrane response. I. The hippocampus. *Brain Research, 145,* 323–346.

Bi, R., Broutman, G., Foy, M. R., Thompson, R. F., & Baudry, M. (2000). The tyrosine kinase and mitogen-activated protein kinase pathways mediate multiple effects of estrogen in hippocampus. *Proceedings of the National Academy of Science (U.S.A.), 97,* 3602–3607.

Brizzee, K. R., & Ordy, J. M. (1979). Age pigments, cell loss and hippocampal function. *Mechanisms of Ageing and Development, 9,* 143–162.

Brody, H. (1955). Organization of the cerebral cortex. III. A study of aging in the human cerebral cortex. *Journal of Comparative Neurology, 102,* 551–556.

Burke, S. N., & Barnes, C. A. (2006). Neural plasticity in the aging brain. *National Review of Neuroscience, 7,* 30–40.

Chen, C., Kano, M., Abeliovich, A., Chen, L., Bao, S., Kim, J. J., et al. (1995). Impaired motor coordination correlates with persistent multiple climbing fiber innervation in PKCγ mutant mice. *Cell, 83,* 1233–1242.

Chen, L., Bao, S., Lockard, J. M., Kim, J. J., & Thompson, R. F. (1996). Impaired classical eyeblink conditioning in cerebellar lesioned and Purkinje cell degeneration (*pcd*) mutant mice. *Journal of Neuroscience, 16,* 2829–2838.

Chen, L., Bao, S., & Thompson, R. F. (1999). Bilateral lesions of the interpositus nucleus completely prevent eyeblink conditioning in Purkinje cell-degeneration mutant mice. *Behavioral Neuroscience, 111,* 204–210.

Christian, K. M., & Thompson, R. F. (2003). Neural substrates of eyeblink conditioning: Acquisition and retention. *Learning & Memory, 11,* 427–455.

Clark, R. E., & Lavond, D. G. (1993). Reversible lesions of the red nucleus during acquisition and retention of a classically conditioned behavior in rabbit. *Behavioral Neuroscience, 107,* 264–270.

Clark, R. E., & Squire, L. R. (1998). Classical conditioning and brain systems: A key role for awareness. *Science, 280,* 77–81.

Clark, R. E., Zhang, A. A., & Lavond, D. G. (1992). Reversible lesions of the cerebellar interpositus nucleus during acquisition and retention of a classical conditioned behavior. *Behavioral Neuroscience, 106,* 879–888.

Dayan, A. D. (1971). Comparative neuropathology of ageing: Studies on the brains of 47 species of vertebrates. *Brain, 94,* 31–42.

Disterhoft, J. F., Coulter, D. A., & Alkon, D. L. (1986). Conditioning-specific membrane changes of rabbit hippocampal neurons *in vitro. Proceedings of the National Academy of Sciences of the United States of America, 83,* 2733–2737.

Disterhoft, J. F., & McEchron, M. D. (2000). Cellular alterations in hippocampus during acquisition and consolidation of hippocampus-dependent trace eyeblink conditioning. In D. S. Woodruff-Pak & J. E. Steinmetz (Eds.), *Eyeblink classical conditioning: Vol. 2. Animal models* (pp. 313–334). Boston: Kluwer Academic Publishers.

Doulazmi, M., Frederic, F., Lemaigre-Dubreuil, Y., Hadj-Sahraoui, N., Delhaye-Bouchaud, N., & Mariani, J. (1999). Cerebellar Purkinje cell loss during life span of the heterozygous staggerer mouse (Rora(+)/Rora(sg)) is gender-related. *Journal of Comparative Neurology, 411,* 267–273.

Doulazmi, M., Hadj-Sahraoui, N., Frederic, F., & Mariani, J. (2002). Diminishing Purkinje cell populations in the cerebella of aging heterozygous Purkinje cell degeneration but not heterozygous nervous mice. *Journal of Neurodegeneration, 16,* 111–123.

Eagan, D. E., Zach, J., Roker, L. A., & Woodruff-Pak, D. S. (2007). Age differences in eyeblink and fear classical conditioning in CBA mice using an orbicularis oculi unconditioned stimulus for both paradigms. Program No. 95.12. *2007 Abstract Viewer/Itinerary Planner.* Washington, DC: Society for Neuroscience.

Finch, C. E. (2003). Neurons, glia, and plasticity in normal brain aging. *Neurobiology of Aging, 24*(Suppl. 1), S123–S127.

Finch, C. E., & Kirkwood, T. B. L. (2000). *Chance, development, and aging.* New York: Oxford University Press.

Foster, T. C. (1999). Involvement of hippocampal synaptic plasticity in age-related memory decline. *Brain Research Review, 30,* 236–249.

Foster, T. C., & Kumar, A. (2002). Calcium dysregulation in the aging brain. *The Neuroscientist, 8,* 297–301.

Foy, M. R. (2001). 17beta-estradiol: Effect on CA1 hippocampal synaptic plasticity. *Neurobiology of Learning and Memory, 76,* 239–252.

Foy, M. R., Baudry, M., Foy, J. G., & Thompson, R. F. (2008). 17B-estradiol modifies stress-induced and age-related changes in hippocampal synaptic plasticity. *Behavioral Neuroscience, 122,* 301–309.

Foy, M. R., Chiaia, N. L., & Teyler, T. J. (1984). Reversal of hippocampal sexual dimorphism by gonadal steroid manipulation. *Brain Research, 321,* 311–314.

Foy, M. R., Stanton, M. E., Levine, S., & Thompson, R. F. (1987). Behavioral stress impairs long-term potentiation in rodent hippocampus. *Behavioral Neural Biology, 48,* 138–149.

Foy, M. R., & Teyler, T. J. (1983). 17-alpha-estradiol and 17-beta-estradiol in hippocampus. *Brain Research Bulletin, 10,* 735–739.

Foy, M. R., Xu, J., Xie, X., Brinton, R. D., Thompson, R. F., & Berger, T. W. (1999). 17beta-estradiol enhances NMDA receptor-mediated EPSPs and long-term potentiation. *Journal of Neurophysiology, 81,* 925–929.

Gallagher, M., Landfield, P. W., McEwen, B., Meaney, M. J., Rapp, P. R., Sapolsky, R., et al. (1996). Hippocampal neurodegeneration in aging. *Science, 274,* 484–485.

Geinesman, Y., de Toledo-Morrell, L., Morrell, F., & Heller, T. E. (1995). Hippocampal markers of age-related memory dysfunction: Behavioral, electrophysiological and morphological perspectives. *Progress in Neurobiology, 45,* 223–252.

Geinesman, Y., Disterhoft, J. F., Gundersen, H. J., McEchron, M. D., Persina, I. S., Power, J. M., et al. (2000). Remodeling of hippocampal synapses after hippocampus-dependent associative learning. *Journal of Comparative Neurology, 417,* 49–59.

Gomez-Isla, T., Price, J. L., McKeel, D. W. Jr., Morris, J. C., Growdon, J. H., & Hyman, B. T. (1996). Profund loss of layer II entorhinal cortex neurons occurs in vary mild Alzheimer's disease. *Journal of Neuroscience, 16,* 4491–4500.

Gould, T. J., & Steinmetz, J. E. (1994). Multiple unit activity from rabbit cerebellar cortex and interpositus nucleus during classical discrimination/reversal eyelid conditioning. *Brain Research, 652,* 98–106.

Gould, T. J., & Steinmetz, J. E. (1996). Changes in rabbit cerebellar cortical and interpositus nucleus activity during acquisition, extinction, and backward classical eyelid conditioning. *Neurobiology of Learning and Memory, 65,* 17–34.

Green, J. T., & Woodruff-Pak, D. S. (2000). Eyeblink classical conditioning: Hippocampus is for multiple associations as cerebellum is for association-response. *Psychological Bulletin, 126,* 138–158.

Grover, L. M., & Teyler, T. J. (1990). Two components of long-term potentiation induced by different patterns of afferent activation. *Nature, 347,* 477–479.

Hadj-Sahraoui, N., Frederic, F., Delhaye-Bouchaud, N., & Mariani, J. (1996). Gender effect on Purkinje cell loss in the cerebellum of the heterozygous reeler mouse. *Journal of Neurogenetics, 11,* 45–58.

Hadj-Sahraoui, N., Frederic, F., Zanjani, H., Herrup, K., Delhaye-Bouchaud, N., & Mariani, J. (1997). Purkinje cell loss in heterozygous staggerer mutant mice during aging. *Developmental Brain Research, 98,* 1–8.

Hardiman, M. J., Ramnani, N., & Yeo, C. H. (1996). Reversible inactivation of the cerebellum with muscimol prevents the acquisition and extinction of conditioned nictitating membrane responses in the rabbit. *Experimental Brain Research, 110,* 235–247.

Haug, H., Kuhl, S., Mecke, E., Sass, N. L., & Wasner, K. (1984). The significance of morphometric procedures in the investigation of age changes in cytoarchitectonic structures of human brain. *Journal of Hirnforsch, 25,* 353–374.

Henderson, V. W. (2006). Estrogen-containing hormone therapy and Alzheimer's disease risk: Understanding discrepant inferences from observational and experimental research. *Neuroscience, 138,* 1031–1039.

Kaneko, T., & Thompson, R. F. (1997). Disruption of trace conditioning of the nictitating membrane response in rabbits by central cholinergic blockade. *Psychophysiology, 131,* 161–166.

Kim, J. J., Clark, R. E., & Thompson, R. F. (1995). Hippocampectomy impairs the memory of recently, but not remotely, acquired trace eyeblink conditioned responses. *Behavioral Neuroscience, 109,* 195–203.

Kim, J. J., Foy, M. R., & Thompson, R. F. (1996). Behavioral stress modifies hippocampal plasticity through N-methyl-D-aspartate receptor activation. *Proceedings of the National Academy of Sciences of the United States of America, 93,* 4750–4753.

Kim, J. J., & Thompson, R. F. (1997). Cerebellar circuits and synaptic mechanisms involved in classical eyeblink conditioning. *Trends in Neuroscience, 20,* 177–181.

Kleim, J. A., Freeman, J. H., Bruneau, R., Nolan, B. C., Cooper, N. R., Zook, A., et al. (2002). Synapse formation is associated with memory storage in the cerebellum. *Proceedings of the National Academy of Sciences of the United States of America, 99,* 13228–13231.

Krupa, D. J., Thompson, J. K., & Thompson, R. F. (1993). Localization of a memory trace in the mammalian brain. *Science, 260,* 989–991.

Krupa, D. J., & Thompson, R. F. (1995). Inactivation of the superior cerebellar peduncle blocks expression but not acquisition of the rabbit's classically conditioned eyeblink response. *Proceedings of the National Academy of Sciences of the United States of America, 92,* 5097–5101.

Krupa, D. J., Weng, J., & Thompson, R. F. (1996). Inactivation of brainstem motor nuclei blocks expression but not acquisition of the rabbit's classically conditioned eyeblink response. *Behavioral Neuroscience, 110,* 219–227.

Kumar, A., & Foster, T. C. (2004). Enhanced long-term potentiation during aging is masked by processes involving intracellular calcium stores. *Journal of Neurophysiology, 91,* 2437–2444.

Kumar, A., & Foster, T. C. (2005). Intracellular calcium stores contribute to increased susceptibility to LTD induction during aging. *Brain Research, 1031,* 125–128.

Kumar, A., & Foster, T. C. (2007). Shift in induction mechanisms underlies an age-dependent increase in DHPG-induced synaptic depression at CA3 CA1 synapses. *Journal of Neurophysiology, 98,* 2729–2736.

Landfield, P. W., McGaugh, J. L., & Lynch, G. (1978). Impaired synaptic potentiation processes in the hippocampus of aged, memory-deficient rats. *Brain Research, 150,* 85–101.

Landfield, P. W., & Pitler, T. A. (1984). Prolonged Ca2+-dependent afterhyperpolarizations in hippocampal neurons of aged rats. *Science, 226,* 1089–1092.

Larsen, J. O., Skalicky, M., & Viidik, A. (2000). Does long-term physical exercise counteract age-related Purkinje cell loss? A stereological study of the rat cerebellum. *Journal of Comparative Neurology, 428,* 213–222.

Lavond, D. G., Kim, J. J., & Thompson, R. F. (1993). Mammalian brain substrates of aversive classical conditioning. *Annual Review of Psychology, 44,* 317–342.

Lavond, D. G., McCormick, D. A., & Thompson, R. F. (1984). A non-recoverable learning deficit. *Physiological Psychology, 12,* 103–110.

Lavond, D. G., & Steinmetz, J. E. (1989). Acquisition of classical conditioning without cerebellar cortex. *Behavioral Brain Research, 33,* 113–164.

Lavond, D. G., Steinmetz, J. E., Yokaitis, M. H., & Thompson, R. F. (1987). Reacquisition of classical conditioning after removal of cerebellar cortex. *Experimental Brain Research, 67,* 569–593.

Lincoln, J. S., McCormick, D. A., & Thompson, R. F. (1982). Ipsilateral cerebellar lesions prevent learning of the classically conditioned nictitating membrane/eyelid response. *Brain Research, 242,* 190–193.

Linden, D. J., & Connor, J. A. (1995). Long-term synaptic depression. *Annual Review of Neuroscience, 18,* 319–357.

Mauk, M. D., Steinmetz, J. E., & Thompson, R. F. (1986). Classical conditioning using stimulation of the inferior olive as the unconditioned stimulus. *Proceedings of the National Academy of Sciences of the United States of America, 83,* 5349–5353.

McCormick, D. A., Lavond, D. G., Clark, G. A., Kettner, R. E., Rising, C. E., & Thompson, R. F. (1981). The engram found? Role of the cerebellum in classical conditioning of the nictitating membrane and eyelid responses. *Bulletin of the Psychonomic Society, 18,* 103–105.

McCormick, D. A., & Thompson, R. F. (1984a). Cerebellum: Essential involvement in the classically conditioned eyelid response. *Science, 223,* 296–299.

McCormick, D. A., & Thompson, R. F. (1984b). Neuronal responses of the rabbit cerebellum during acquisition and performance of a classically conditioned nictitating membrane-eyelid response. *Journal of Neuroscience, 4,* 2811–2822.

McEchron, M. D., Weible, A. P., & Disterhoft, J. F. (2001). Aging and learning-specific changes in single-neuron activity in CA1 hippocampus during rabbit trace eyeblink conditioning. *Journal of Neurophysiology, 86,* 1839–1857.

Morrison, J. H., & Hof, P. R. (1997). Life and death of neurons in the aging brain. *Science, 278.* 412–418.

Morrison, J. H., & Hof, P. R. (2007). Life and death of neurons in the aging cerebral cortex. *International Review of Neurobiology, 81,* 41–57.

Moyer, J. R., Deyo, R. A., & Disterhoft, J. F. (1990). Hippocampectomy disrupts trace eye-blink conditioning in rabbits. *Behavioral Neuroscience, 104,* 243–252.

Moyer, J. R., Jr., & Disterhoft, J. F. (1994). Nimodipine decreases calcium action potentials in rabbit hippocampal CA1 neurons in age-dependent and concentration-dependent manner. *Journal of Neurophysiology, 68,* 2100–2109.

Moyer, J. R., Power, J. M., Thompson, L. T., & Disterhoft, J. F. (2000). Increased excitability of aged rabbit CA1 neurons after trace eyeblink conditioning. *Journal of Neuroscience, 20,* 5476–5482.

Norris, C. M., Korol, D. L., & Foster, T. C. (1996). Increased susceptibility to induction of long-term depression and long-term potentiation reversal during aging, *Journal of Neuroscience, 16,* 5382–5392.

Oddo, S., Caccamo, A., Shepherd, J. D., Murphy, M. P., Golde, T. E., Kayed, R., et al. (2003). Triple-transgenic model of Alzheimer's disease with plaques and tangles: Intracellular Abeta and synaptic dysfunction. *Neuron, 39,* 409–421.

Offermanns, S., Hashimoto, K., Watanabe, M., Sun, W., Kurihara, H., Thompson, R. F., et al. (1997). Impaired motor coordination and persistent multiple climbing fiber innervation of cerebellar Purkinje cells in mice lacking Gαq. *Proceedings of the National Academy of Sciences of the United States of America, 94,* 14089–14094.

Port, R. L., Romano, A. G., Steinmetz, J. E., Mikhail, A. A., & Patterson, M. M. (1986). Retention and acquisition of classical trace conditioned responses by rabbits with hippocampal lesions. *Behavioral Neuroscience, 100,* 745–752.

Power, J. M., Wu, W. W., Sametsky, E., Oh, M. M., & Disterhoft, J. F. (2002). Age-related enhancement of the slow outward calcium-activated potassium current in hippocampal CA1 pyramidal neurons in vitro. *Journal of Neuroscience, 22,* 7234–7243.

Rapp, P. R., & Gallagher, M. (1996). Preserved neuron number in the hippocampus of aged rats with spatial learning deficits. *Proceedings of the National Academy of Sciences of the United States of America, 93,* 9926–9930.

Rogers, R. F., Britton, G. B., & Steinmetz, J. E. (2001). Learning-related interpositus activity is conserved across species as studied during eyeblink conditioning in the rat. *Brain Research, 905,* 171–177.

Shankar, S., Teyler, T., & Robbins, N. (1998). Aging differentially alters forms of long-term potentiation in rat hippocampal area CA1. *Journal of Neurophysiology, 79,* 334–341.

Sherwin, B. B. (2006). Estrogen and cognitive aging in women. *Neuroscience, 138,* 1021–1026.

Shibuki, K., Gomi, H., Chen, L., Bao, S., Kim, J. J., Wakatuski, H., et al. (1996). Deficient cerebellar long-term depression, impaired eyeblink conditioning, and normal motor coordination in GFAP mutant mice. *Neuron, 16,* 587–599.

Shors, T. J., Foy, M. R., Levine, S., & Thompson, R. F. (1990). Unpredictable and uncontrollable stress impairs neuronal plasticity in the rat hippocampus. *Brain Research Bulletin, 24,* 663–667.

Skelton, R. W. (1988). Bilateral cerebellar lesions disrupt conditioned eyelid responses in unrestrained rats. *Behavioral Neuroscience, 102,* 586–590.

Solomon, P. R., Vander Schaaf, E. R., Thompson, R. F., & Weisz, D. J. (1986). Hippocampus and trace conditioning of the rabbit's classically conditioned nictitating membrane response. *Behavioral Neuroscience, 100,* 729–744.

Stanton, M. E., Freeman, J. H., Jr., & Skelton, R. W. (1992). Eyeblink conditioning in the developing rat. *Behavioral Neuroscience, 106,* 657–665.

Steinmetz, J. E. (1990). Classical nictitating membrane conditioning in rabbits with varying interstimulus intervals and direct activation of cerebellar mossy fibers as a CS. *Behavioural Brain Research, 38,* 97–108.

Steinmetz, J. E. (1996). The brain substrates of classical eyeblink conditioning in rabbits. In J. Bloedel, T. Ebner, & S. Wise (Eds.), *Acquisition of motor behavior in vertebrates* (pp. 89–114). Cambridge, MA: MIT Press.

Steinmetz, J. E., Gluck, M. A., & Solomon, P. R. (2001). *Model systems and the neurobiology of associative learning.* Mahwah, NJ: Lawrence Erlbaum Associates.

Steinmetz, J. E., Lavond, D. G., & Thompson, R. F. (1985). Classical conditioning of the rabbit eyelid response with mossy fiber stimulation as the conditioned stimulus. *Bulletin of the Psychonomic Society, 23,* 245–248.

Steinmetz, J. E., Lavond, D. G., & Thompson, R. F. (1989). Classical conditioning in rabbits using pontine nucleus stimulation as a conditioned stimulus and inferior olive stimulation as an unconditioned stimulus. *Synapse, 3,* 225–233.

Steinmetz, J. E., Rosen, D. J., Chapman, P. F., Lavond, D. G., & Thompson, R. F. (1986). Classical conditioning of the rabbit eyelid response with a mossy-fiber stimulation CS: I. Pontine nuclei and middle cerebellar peduncle stimulation. *Behavioral Neuroscience, 100,* 878–887.

Sterio, D. C. (1984). The unbiased estimation of number and sizes of arbitrary particles using the dissector. *Journal of Microscopy, 134,* 127–136.

Teyler, T. J., Vardaris, R. M., Lewis, D., & Rawitch, A. B. (1980). Gonadal steroids: Effects on excitability of hippocampal pyramidal cells. *Science, 209,* 1017–1018.

Thompson, R. F. (1986). The neurobiology of learning and memory. *Science, 233,* 941–947.

Thompson, R. F. (1990). Neural mechanisms of classical conditioning in mammals. *Philosophical Transactions of the Royal Society of London. Series B, Biological Sciences, 329,* 161–170.

Thompson, R. F. (2000). Discovering the brain substrates of eyeblink classical conditioning. In D. S. Woodruff-Pak & J. E. Steinmetz (Eds.), *Eyeblink classical conditioning: Vol. 2. Animal models* (pp. 17–49). Boston: Kluwer Academic Publishers.

Thompson, R. F., & Woodruff-Pak, D. S. (1987). A model system approach to age and the neuronal bases of learning and memory. In M. W. Riley, J. D. Matarazzo, & A. Baum (Eds.), *The aging dimension* (pp. 41–76). Hillsdale, NJ: Lawrence Erlbaum Associates.

Tseng, W., Guan, J. F., Disterhoft, J. F., & Weiss, C. (2004). Trace eyeblink conditioning is hippocampally dependent in mice. *Hippocampus, 14,* 58–65.

Vogel, R. W., Ewers, M., Ross, C., Gould, T. J., & Woodruff-Pak, D. S. (2002). Age-related impairment in the 250-millisecond delay eyeblink classical conditioning procedure in C57BL/6 mice. *Learning & Memory, 9,* 321–336.

Vouimba, R. M., Foy, M. R., Foy, J. G., & Thompson, R. F. (2000). 17beta-estradiol suppresses expression of long-term depression in aged rats. *Brain Research Bulletin, 53,* 783–787.

Weiss, C., & Thompson, R. F. (1991). The effects of age on eyeblink conditioning in the freely moving Fischer-344 rat. *Neurobiology of Aging, 12,* 249–254.

West, M. J. (1993a). New stereological methods for counting neurons. *Neurobiology of Aging, 14,* 275–285.

West, M. J. (1993b). Regionally specific loss of neurons in the aging human hippocampus. *Neurobiology of Aging, 14,* 287–293.

West, M. J., Coleman, P. D., Flood, D. G., & Troncoso, J. C. (1994). Differences in the pattern of hippocampal neuronal loss in normal aging and Alzheimer's disease. *Lancet, 344,* 769–772.

West, M. J., & Gundersen, H. J. (1990). Unbiased stereological estimation of the number of neurons in the human hippocampus. *Journal of Comparative Neurology, 296,* 1–22.

West, M. J., Slimianka, L., & Gundersen, H. J. G. (1991). Unbiased stereological estimation of the total number of neurons in the subdivisions of the rat hippocampus using the optical fractionator. *Anatomical Record, 231,* 482–497.

Williams, R. W., & Herrup, K. (1988). The control of neuron number. *Annual Review of Neuroscience, 11,* 423–453.

Woodruff-Pak, D. S. (2006). Stereological estimation of Purkinje neuron number in C57BL/6 mice and its relation to associative learning. *Neuroscience, 141,* 233–243.

Woodruff-Pak, D. S., Cronholm, J. F., & Sheffield, J. B. (1990). Purkinje cell number related to rate of eyeblink classical conditioning. *NeuroReport, 1,* 165–168.

Woodruff-Pak, D. S., Green, J. T., Levin, S. I., & Meisler, M. H. (2006). Inactivation of sodium channel Scn8A (NaV1.6) in Purkinje neurons impairs learning in Morris water maze and delay but not trace eyeblink classical conditioning. *Behavioral Neuroscience, 120,* 229–240.

Woodruff-Pak, D. S., Lavond, D. G., Logan, C. G., Steinmetz, J. E., & Thompson, R. F. (1993). Cerebellar cortical lesions and reacquisition in classical conditioning of the nictitating membrane response in rabbits. *Brain Research, 608,* 67–77.

Woodruff-Pak, D. S., Lavond, D. G., & Thompson, R. F. (1985). Trace conditioning: Abolished by cerebellar nuclear lesions but not lateral cerebellar cortex aspirations. *Brain Research, 348,* 249–260.

Woodruff-Pak, D. S., & Thompson, R. F. (1985). Classical conditioning of the eyelid response in rabbits as a model system for the study of brain mechanisms of learning and memory in aging. *Experimental Aging Research, 11,* 109–122.

Woodruff-Pak, D. S., & Thompson, R. F. (1988). Classical conditioning of the eyeblink response in the delay paradigm in adults aged 18–83 years. *Psychology and Aging, 3,* 219–229.

Woodruff-Pak, D. S., & Trojanowski, J. Q. (1996). The older rabbit as an animal model: Implications for Alzheimer's disease. *Neurobiology of Aging, 17,* 283–290.

Yeo, C. H., Hardiman, M. J., & Glickstein, M. (1985). Classical conditioning of the nictitating membrane response in the rabbit. II. Lesions of the cerebellar cortex. *Experimental Brain Research, 60,* 99–113.

Zanjani, H. S., Mariani, J., Delhaye-Bouchaud, N., & Herrup, K. (1992). Neuronal cell loss in heterozygous *staggerer* mutant mice: A model for genetic contributions to the aging process. *Developmental Brain Research, 67,* 153–160.

Programmed Longevity and Programmed Aging Theories

12

Stavros Gonidakis
Valter D. Longo

Major diseases such as cancer and Alzheimer's are likely to claim the lives of both us, the authors, and you, the reader. Understanding why aging is the major risk factor for these diseases is therefore of central importance not only for gerontologists but also for biomedical researchers. Hence, it is not unexpected that biologists have spent considerable intellectual energy in their effort to elucidate the molecular and evolutionary origin of the aging process.

Any theory aspiring to provide an evolutionary explanation for aging must accommodate the following three sets of observations: (a) nutrient-responsive signal transduction pathways modulate aging across phylogenetically distant organisms, and genetic inactivation of components of these pathways induces life span extension in a number of model systems (Longo & Finch, 2003); (b) reduction of caloric intake to 60% to 70% of ad libitum levels robustly retards the aging process in many species (Sohal & Weindruch, 1996); and (c) maximum life spans of living organisms range across several orders of magnitude.

Although the codiscoverers of natural selection, Charles Darwin and Alfred Wallace, recognized the possibility of aging having evolved as an adaptive trait that maximizes the fitness of a population, the orthodox evolutionary thinking that formed and prevailed during the latter part of the 19th century postulated that aging is a nonadaptive process escaping the force of natural selection.

We hereby review the theoretical considerations and experimental findings supporting the view that, under certain circumstances, age-dependent altruistic death has evolved as an adaptive trait increasing the fitness of a population at the expense of individual fitness, focusing our attention on recent data obtained with one of the workhorses of aging research, the budding yeast *Saccharomyces cerevisiae*. Toward this goal, we also attempt to clarify the fundamental distinction between programmed longevity and programmed aging; failure to do so has afflicted several past attempts to tackle the evolutionary origin of aging. It should be noted that the investigation of the distal, evolutionary causes of aging that this chapter examines is partly overlapping but quite distinct from the investigation of theories pertinent to the molecular causes of aging, such as the "free radical" or the "error catastrophe" theory.

The Force of Natural Selection

The realization by John Haldane in the 1940s that disorders like Huntington's disease persist in the human population because their effects are manifested toward the end of the reproductive life span provided the seed for evolutionary theories of aging based on the decline in the force of natural selection. This decline may be equated to the reduction of the reproductive probability of an individual with increasing adult age (Figure 12.1). Importantly, this decline does not assume an intrinsic senescence process since infections, predation, and any other aging-independent potential cause of death in a wild environment ("extrinsic senescence") result in a higher probability of survival and reproduction at age x than at age $x + a$.

Consequently, the later a deleterious mutation manifests itself during an individual's life, the smaller the chance that it will be removed by natural selection. According to the mutation accumulation theory proposed by Medawar

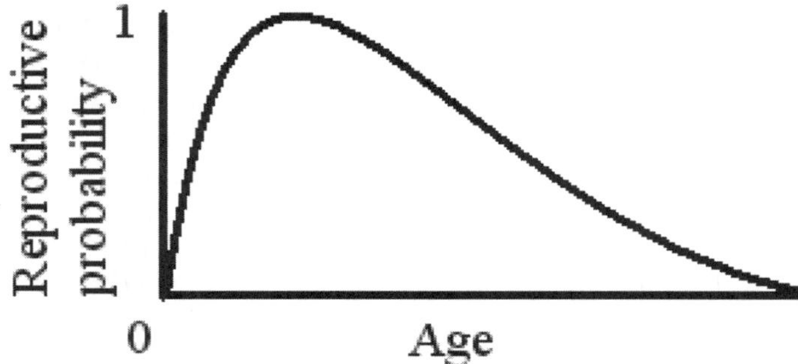

12.1

Generalized scheme of the age-dependent decline in reproductive probability and hence in the force of natural selection.

(1952), aging results from the collective effect of such late-acting deleterious alleles, created by de novo mutations in the germ line. Note that this theory should not be confused with the somatic mutation theory, according to which the accumulation of stochastic DNA damage in somatic cells is the underlying cause of the aging phenotype.

Trade-Off Theories

Almost every circumstance one can think of can be both "good" and "bad"; close examination of all the repercussions in the context of temporal change is bound to reveal the flip side of the coin. This fundamental duality of things in the form of inevitable genetic or metabolic trade-offs lies at the heart of the classical evolutionary theories of aging. George Williams (1957) recognized the possibility that alleles, having been fixed because of their fitness-enhancing effect early in life, actively contribute to the age-dependent demise of an organism later on. The antagonistic pleiotropy theory is built around this idea and postulates that aging is the combined result of (a) the indirect selection of late-acting deleterious alleles due to their salubrious effect early in life and (b) the reduced capacity of natural selection to remove the late-acting detrimental effect of these alleles. The theory places the cumulative effect of these late-acting genes in a centrally causal position to the aging rate characterizing each species. The theory predicts a positive correlation between the extrinsic mortality rate suffered by a population and its aging rate since increasing extrinsic mortality will expedite the rate of decline in reproductive probability (shown in Figure 12.1) and therefore compress the time window available for the expurgation of senescence-causing alleles. Despite the recent challenge in its generality (Reznick, Bryant, Roff, Ghalambor, & Ghalambor, 2004), this prediction provides a partial explanation for the vastly different life spans observed in nature by incorporating the effect of each species' ecological circumstances on aging rates through extrinsic mortality rates. Citing a specific natural instance, the exceptional longevity of bats for animals of their small size and high metabolic rate (Brunet-Rossinni & Austad, 2004) may be accounted for by the low extrinsic mortality enjoyed by these animals due to their ability to fly away from predators.

The antagonistic pleiotropy theory also predicts that any gene inactivation causing an extended life span must cause a physiological impairment early in life. Most long-lived model organisms grow more slowly or reproduce less vigorously than their wild-type counterparts. However, the existence of long-lived mutants, such as *Ras2* in yeast and *daf-2* in *Caenorhabditis elegans,* that grow and reproduce at a normal rate (Longo & Finch, 2003) suggests that a fitness cost is not a necessary requirement for extended life. Still, it is possible that the costs associated with life span extension are not apparent under standard laboratory conditions and require tests more closely resembling the organisms' natural environment, such as the resistance to feeding–starvation cycles that unveiled a nonobvious competitive disadvantage of long-lived *age-1* worms (Walker, McColl, Jenkins, Harris, & Lithgow, 2000) and the inability of long-lived yeast *Ras2* and *Sch9* mutants to compete against their wild-type counterpart (Fabrizio et al., 2004). Therefore, the balance of evidence tilts toward the existence of conditional trade-offs for extended life that are manifested under conditions specific to each species and life span–extending mutation.

According to another prediction of the antagonistic pleiotropy theory, rapid individual development should be correlated with rapid senescence. Since reproductive maturation marks the onset of senescence, the sooner it is reached, the sooner the effects of aging will become apparent. Most long-lived mutant animals develop at a slower rate than wild type; the theory could attribute their extended longevity to their delayed attainment of reproductive maturation. Contrary to this explanation, adult-specific inactivation of *daf-2* produced a life span extension similar to that produced by inactivation of the gene throughout development (Dillin, Crawford, & Kenyon, 2002). Observations of this sort injure the universality of another prediction of the antagonistic pleiotropy theory. Although the list of loci with seemingly antagonistically pleiotropic effects is growing (Leroi et al., 2005), the theory is not without problems, as shown previously.

The disposable soma theory overcomes some of those problems by invoking the existence of metabolic trade-offs as the distal reason for the evolution of aging. This theory proposes that aging is an inherently stochastic process caused by the accumulation of unrepaired molecular damage. The failure to repair this accumulated damage is a direct consequence of the fact that metabolic resources allocated to a certain physiological function are unavailable to another. Hence, the aging rate of each species is determined by the optimization over evolutionary time of the allocation of limited metabolic resources to growth and reproduction (germ-line maintenance and propagation) on the one hand and to somatic maintenance on the other (Kirkwood, 2005). The observation that limited food intake extends life span in all species thus far tested seems diametrically opposite to the major tenet of this theory. However, proponents of it have argued that over evolutionary time scales, the ability to adjust the previously mentioned metabolic allocations in the face of changing environmental conditions has evolved. Thus, the life span extension induced by dietary restriction may represent the adaptive readjustment of the organism's metabolic economy away from growth and reproduction and toward somatic maintenance (Shanley & Kirkwood, 2000). Although the theory predicts that aging is the result of stochastic molecular damage across different tissues inflicted and repaired through the action of several different gene products, it accommodates the findings summarized in point (a) at the beginning of this chapter by invoking a change in the allocation of metabolic resources toward maintenance functions through the perturbation of master regulators adapted to respond to changing nutrient availability.

Programmed Longevity

Although not explicitly stated or predicted by "antagonistic pleiotropy" and "disposable soma," both these classical theories of aging, as well as programmed aging, embrace the view that longevity is a trait under selective pressure. As mentioned previously, the disposable soma theory explains the apparently contradictory effect of reduced calories leading to/causing life span extension by suggesting that reduction in growth and reproduction may allow an increased investment of energy in protection even with reduced calories. The possibility that dietary restriction–induced life span extension is a mere physiological response and not an adaptive trait is distant, based on the frequency of starvation conditions for wild populations and also on mathematical models in favor of the adaptive hypothesis (Kirkwood & Shanley, 2005).

According to the programmed longevity theory (Longo, Mitteldorf, & Skulachev, 2005), the healthy portion of an organism's life span is programmed in order to optimize fitness. However, according to this theory, senescence occurs not because of trade-offs early or late in life but simply because the species reaches an evolutionarily stable strategy for life span that would be less or as stable if longevity were increased. In other words, a worm could gain a set of mutations that would make it live as long as a fly, but this does not happen because the worm is already adopting a strategy that is as stable as that of the fly. The extended life span of mutants in the insulin/IGF-signaling pathways is caused by a genetic simulation of the programmed longevity response that appears to have evolved as an adaptation to conditions of famine. In many cases, a longevity-extending mutation will cause a trade-off, but in some cases it will not. The programmed longevity theory provides a convenient link between the evolutionary and mechanistic theories of aging. For example, microarray analyses have revealed that daf-16, the transcription factor downstream of the *daf-2*–mediated life span extension in *C. elegans,* controls a number of genes involved in stress response, antioxidant and antimicrobial defense, and energy generation (Murphy et al., 2003). Of particular interest is the much more pronounced life span extension caused by inactivation of components of central nutrient-sensing pathways compared to the life span extension achieved in different model systems by the overexpression of specific genetic parts of the longevity program. For example, the yeast strain lacking *Sch9,* a conserved kinase that links nutrient status to cell size and growth rate (Toda, Cameron, Sass, & Wigler, 1988), lives three times longer than wild type (Fabrizio, Pozza, Pletcher, Gendron, & Longo, 2001), whereas overexpression of the mitochondrial superoxide dismutase causes only a 30% life span extension (Fabrizio et al., 2003). Similar results have been obtained with the worm, the fruit fly, and the mouse. Superoxide dismutases are proteins present in virtually all organisms with the conserved function of catalytically converting the damaging superoxide radical formed as a by-product of metabolism to hydrogen peroxide and water. Thus, it becomes apparent that the alleviation of reactive oxygen species (ROS)–induced stochastic damage is one among the several maintenance and repair functions contributing to the longevity extension program elicited by dietary restriction or genetic inactivation of components of the conserved insulin/IGF-signaling pathways.

Programmed Aging and Group/Kin Selection Theories

In contrast to programmed longevity, several theoretical and empirical objections can be raised against the notion of a set of specific, conserved, and stereotypical molecular mechanisms produced by natural selection that accelerate the senescence of an organism. The selection for alleles that enhance the fitness of a group at the expense of individual fitness is the most contentious prediction made by the programmed aging theory since several generations of evolutionary biologists have been propagating the near-universal application of selection at the level of the individual. The programmed aging theory posits that alleles have been fixed that cause the altruistic age-dependent death of an individual, enhancing the fitness of the group the individual belongs to (Longo et al., 2005). As mentioned at the beginning of this chapter, the possibility of selection operating at the level of the group and not of the individual was incorporated in the initial theories of evolution by natural selection proposed by Darwin and Wallace. However, group selection fell out of favor in the 1960s when the work of Williams, Maynard Smith, and Hamilton provided explanations for the instances of seemingly altruistic adaptations observed by Wynne-Edwards (1962) in wild populations. The major argument against the operation of group selection mechanisms in the evolution of aging is that its effect is too indirect and diffuse to compensate for the heavy cost of reduced individual fitness. However, mathematical models and experimental observations support the possibility of populations going extinct because of an unchecked consumption of the resources available to them for the purpose of maximizing reproductive output (Longo et al., 2005).

Another strong theoretical argument against group selection is the susceptibility of altruistic groups to intrusion by selfish cheaters who would rapidly dominate an altruistic environment. Group selectionists counter that a group of altruists overtaken by a selfish individual is doomed to extinction, rendering this scenario an evolutionarily unstable strategy. Moreover, coadaptations of altruistic traits with mechanisms minimizing the chances of invasion by selfish cheaters is not an implausible scenario.

Similar to the central dichotomous question permeating the entire discipline of biology (nature versus nurture), the conundrum presented by group versus individual selection is most satisfactorily resolved by conceding our uncertainties about the way in which nature works and by proposing a compromising model that is based on the two antithetical forces sharing dominance. The arbitrating model goes by the name of multilevel selection and owes much of its existence to David Sloan Wilson. As its name eloquently states, this model merges the orthodox view of selection operating at the gene and individual levels with the possibility of instances whereby selection forces at the group level overpower forces of the opposite selective direction at the gene and individual levels. Wilson (1997) has proposed that group selection has been an important driving force in human evolution, based on the observation that the majority of hunter-gatherer societies operate according to egalitarian social norms that minimize the chances of success of selfish individuals within a group composed of altruistic members.

In short, programmed aging can be well accommodated by an evolutionary worldview that uses the ability to adjust to different evolutionary environments as its cornerstone. Although several decades of work have focused on selection operating at the level of specific reproducing entities (be they genes, individuals, or groups), evolutionary thinking must incorporate the flexibility of living systems with respect to their "choice" of these entities as units of selection in the face of changing ecological circumstances.

The Arguments Against Programmed Aging and Group Selection

Aging is believed to be selectively irrelevant, based largely on the notion that almost all organisms in the wild die well before old age by non–aging-related causes, such as predation or infection. Although the obvious fallacy of this notion was exposed as early as 1957 (Williams, 1957), it still makes its way into lists of arguments against programmed aging published in the current millennium. As any honest and otherwise healthy 40-year-old man can attest, senescence produces a tangible effect on an organism's physical performance without provoking a specific age-related ailment. Paraphrasing the insightful comment of Williams, one should not confuse the process of senescence with the state of senility, as the former affects the survival and reproduction of an organism well before the latter is reached.

Opponents of the programmed aging theory claim that aging widely fails to meet the programmatic benchmarks set by the archetypal programmed biological process of development (Austad, 2004). According to this view, the obviously stochastic nature of the aging process in mice, where different tissues age at different rates by different mechanisms causing age-related disease at different times, even among genetically identical individuals (Turturro, Duffy, Hass, Kodell, & Hart, 2002), cannot be equated to the series of carefully orchestrated molecular events that contribute to the miraculous transformation of a single cell to an entity as complex as a fruit fly (Levine & Davidson, 2005). However, this is a potentially flawed argument since the generation of a highly complex organism that can grow, survive, and reproduce with extreme precision and reliability requires an equally complex and precise program, whereas the destruction of an organism can be much less orchestrated as it would be true for the construction and destruction of an automobile. The purpose of an aging program would be only to make the organism less competitive and more prone to death, not necessarily in a "carefully orchestrated" manner.

Particularly relevant to the current discussion are the following data adding credence to the potentially deterministic nature of the aging phenotype. Numerous microarray studies of old versus young organisms in different model systems have revealed certain commonalities in the aging transcriptome across different species. For example, a study comparing the gene expression profiles of the nematode *C. elegans* and the fruit fly *Drosophila melanogaster* identified a shared program of adult-onset gene expression that includes genes involved in mitochondrial metabolism, DNA repair, peptidolysis, and cellular transport (McCarroll et al., 2004). Furthermore, the identification of chronic inflammation as a common underlying mechanism contributing to the incidence of different kinds of age-related mammalian diseases, such as neoplasias, cardiovascular complications, and Alzheimer's disease, could reveal another mechanism consistent with an aging program (Finch & Crimmins, 2004).

Raising the Bar for Programmed Aging

We regard the fulfillment of the following criteria as necessary and sufficient for the demonstration of an instance of programmed and altruistic aging:

1. A programmed and reprogrammable mechanism of age-dependent death with clearly defined molecular components and phenotypic products
2. Multiple markers of programmed cell death, akin to mammalian apoptosis

3. A competitive advantage of a population undergoing programmed aging against a population undergoing stochastic aging
4. A reversible sub-optimal protection against cell damage and death in the absence of reproduction
5. Extrapolation of the validity of the previously mentioned findings with reasonable confidence to wild populations

The intensely scrutinized phenomenon of programmed cell death (PCD) has been a useful signpost for travelers of the programmed aging avenues. Apoptosis, the most well-studied among several forms of PCD, contributes to the morphogenesis of multicellular organisms by removing unwanted cells during tissue and organ formation and is also an important defense mechanism against the uncontrolled proliferation of damaged cells. Escaping the controlling hands of apoptosis is one of the crucial checkpoints in the path to carcinogenesis. One could, by indulging in a bout of anthropomorphism, envisage the removal of aging individuals from a population and of injured or potentially harmful cells from a multicellular organism as feats of biologically programmed altruism that benefit the "common good." Although PCD in multicellular organisms can easily be seen as an adaptive trait in light of its involvement in indispensable homeostatic functions such as those described previously, the existence of PCD in populations of unicellular organisms is much harder to account for in terms of classical evolutionary thinking that is bound to attribute some sort of individual fitness-enhancing function to every adaptation observed in living organisms. We are choosing to focus our attention on PCD in the budding yeast *S. cerevisiae* because of its more intimate bearing on the aging issue and direct the reader to a recent review of the extensive literature concerning instances of programmed death from the bacterial realm (Lewis, 2000).

Programmed Aging in Yeast: A Case Study

The combination of cheap and facile maintenance of aging populations in the lab, powerful genetic and genomic techniques, and remarkable similarity at the cellular level with higher eukaryotes have made *S. cerevisiae* one of molecular biogerontology's favorite model systems. In short, aging experiments are performed by allowing the establishment of nondividing populations following exponential proliferation using the carbon and energy available in a certain liquid nutrient medium (Fabrizio & Longo, 2003). These populations, the initial density of which is approximately 100 million organisms per milliliter of culture, are maintained in rotating flasks under constant temperature, humidity, and aeration. The declining survival of members of these populations over time is quantified by the ability of individual cells to form colonies when plated on rich nutrient plates. Yeast has proven its value as a powerful molecular platform for the discovery of mechanisms relevant to the control of senescence in higher eukaryotes through the realization that two salient features of the aging process, namely, the involvement of central nutrient sensing pathways in life span modulation and the role of superoxide signaling in the regulation of multiple maintenance and repair functions are remarkably well conserved from yeast to mice (Longo & Finch, 2003). Of paramount importance to the case for programmed aging in yeast is the discovery from multiple labs of telltale features of apoptosis induced by ROS during yeast aging. For example, Herker et al. (2004) showed an increase in the production of ROS associated with increased DNA cleavage and chromatin condensation during yeast aging; importantly, the same study reported better survival of aging cultures lacking the caspase YCA1, one of the proteins required for the execution of the apoptotic program. Overexpression in yeast of Bax, a conserved mammalian proapoptotic protein, has been shown to induce morphological changes typically observed in apoptotic metazoan cells, such as plasma membrane blebbing and DNA fragmentation (Ligr et al., 1998). Human Bcl-2, a conserved antiapoptotic regulator, was found to reverse the survival defects of yeast lacking the cytosolic superoxide dismutase and delay the age-dependent death of wild-type yeast (Longo, Ellerby, Bredesen, Valentine, & Gralla, 1997). The previously mentioned enumeration of a sample of the relevant experimental observations makes it hard to argue against the involvement of conserved apoptotic components and mechanisms in the physiological aging of the budding yeast, thus satisfying criterion (1) presented in the previous section.

Yeast populations tend to show a "regrowth" after the initial age-dependent mortality phase that has claimed the lives of 90% to 99% of individuals (Fabrizio et al., 2004). This resumption of proliferation toward the end of an aging experiment by a small number of cells (a subset of the 1 million to 10 million survivors from an initial population of 100 million organisms per milliliter of culture) feeding on the nutrients released by dead cells is reminiscent of the well-studied phenomenon of growth advantage in stationary phase (GASP) observed in stationary-phase populations of *Escherichia coli* (Zambrano, Siegele, Almiron, Tormo, & Kolter, 1993). This regrowth phenotype provides an excellent entry point in the search for a potentially adaptive role played by age-dependent death. The initial powerful observation made toward this end was that the wild-type strain exhibits the adaptive regrowth phenotype in 49% of the aging experiments performed, whereas the corresponding figure for long-lived strains is 6.8% (Fabrizio et al., 2004). Furthermore, short-lived strains lacking the cytosolic superoxide dismutase (SOD1) regrow in more than 80% of the experiments performed. When maintained in monoculture, regrowth mutants isolated from wild-type populations start regrowing earlier than wild types. Genetic analysis of these mutants confirms that the regrowth phenotype is indeed caused by a mutation obtained during the course of the aging experiment. The inverse correlation between longevity and adaptive regrowth incidence is immediately suggestive of specific genetic factors contributing both to the ROS-mediated age-dependent death of the majority of the population and to the subsequent proliferation of a certain fraction of the survivors. More specifically, it is possible that the aging and death occurring in the wild-type strain is part of an adaptive program that ensures the survival of the group in spite of changing environmental conditions. This scenario is consistent with a special case of group selection that goes by the name of kin selection since there is a high genetic similarity between the regrowing individuals and those that died during the course of the aging experiment. In fact, the entire aging population may be regarded as a "clone" since it was established by the asexual proliferation of a small number of "seed cells" inoculated in fresh nutrient medium. Conversely, inactivation of the putative aging program in the *Sch9Δ* strain produces a threefold extension in mean life span compared to wild type, but results in the extinction of the clone since no regrowth was observed in *sch9Δ* among 15 independent aging experiments (Fabrizio et al., 2004). The similar pattern observed in strains overexpressing superoxide dismutase and/or catalase (CTT1), two of the major antioxidant enzymes of organisms ranging from bacteria to mammals, implicates ROS in the regulation of age-dependent death and adaptive regrowth in yeast. Also consistent with a role of superoxide and hydrogen peroxide in the adaptive regrowth phenotype following aging are the data showing a competitive disadvantage of the strain overexpressing SOD1 and CTT1 when maintained in the same flask with the wild-type strain. Although the latter ages faster, it eventually drives its long-lived competitor to extinction since wild-type but not SOD1/CTT1-overexpressing cells are able to resume proliferation using the nutrients released from dead organisms. Reinforcing the same conclusion is the complementary observation of the strain lacking SOD1 outcompeting the wild-type strain when both are maintained in the same flask.

Age-dependent mutation frequency, a measure of the DNA damage accumulated during yeast aging partly because of oxidative metabolism, provides mechanistic links among ROS-induced molecular damage, aging, and adaptive regrowth. Extended life span achieved by means of antioxidant overexpression or gene inactivation is associated with decreased age-dependent mutation frequency (Fabrizio et al., 2004).

The extended life span of *sch9Δ* is also associated with a reduced age-dependent inactivation of the superoxide-sensitive enzyme aconitase (Fabrizio et al., 2001) and with a higher expression of the cytosolic superoxide dismutase (Fabrizio et al., 2003). By contrast, the early-regrowing mutants lacking SOD1 have a five-fold increase in mutation frequency (Fabrizio et al., 2004). These observations suggest that wild-type cells promote superoxide-dependent aging, DNA damage, and death to (a) generate better-adapted organisms by increasing mutation rate and (b) generate the nutrients required for the growth and survival of the better-adapted mutants by causing the premature death of the majority of the population. These pro-aging changes are achieved by signaling through conserved nutrient-responsive pathways such as that mediated by *sch9*, which actively down-regulates maintenance and repair functions, including but not limited to antioxidant enzymes. The same set of observations could be accounted for in the context of "disposable soma" by invoking a shift toward repair functions triggered by *sch9* deletion. However, since both wild-type and mutant populations are in a nonreproducing state under the experimental conditions, the physiological process favored over repair and maintenance in the wild-type strain is far from obvious.

Taken together, the data presented here are consistent with *S. cerevisiae* having evolved a superoxide-mediated adaptive program of altruistic aging and death that maximizes the fitness of a clonal population under changing environmental conditions. Inactivation of this program by genetic means brings about life span extension and a greatly reduced incidence of adaptive regrowth mutants, which can possibly be attributed to a generalized attenuation in age-dependent mutation frequency. Further reinforcing these data are in silico simulations of aging experiments under programmed or stochastic conditions. The pattern shown in Figure 12.2, whereby wild-type populations undergoing programmed aging favor the regrowth of better-adapted mutants, was observed

12.2

Fifty-two percent of computer simulations of programmed aging in wild-type populations result in the regrowth of better-adapted mutants (a). Instead, the regrowth frequency for *Sch9Δ* populations undergoing stochastic aging is 0.4% (b).

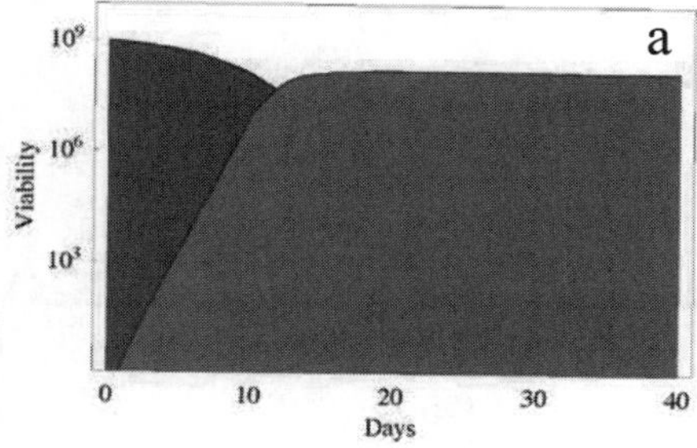

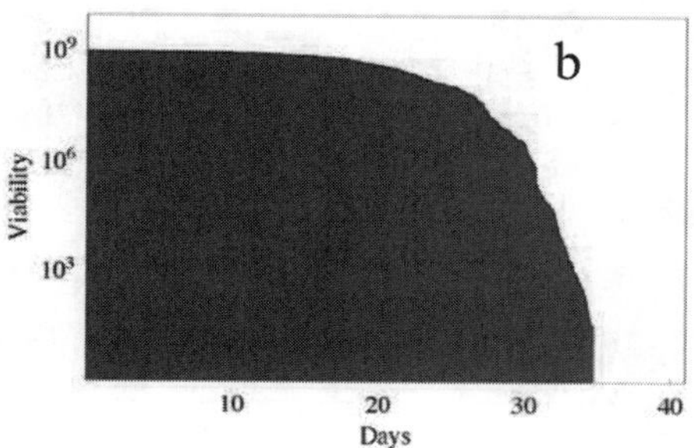

in 52% of the simulations done. On the other hand, stochastically aging populations of the long-lived *sch9Δ* strain showed the appearance of mutants with the potential to regrow in only four of the 1,000 simulations performed. Furthermore, the simulation suggests that these rare mutants would not be able to compete for nutrients with the billions of selfish long-lived yeast and therefore would die before taking over the population. Notably, the simulation experiments assumed experimentally determined values for age-dependent mutation frequencies in wild-type and *sch9Δ* populations.

The colonial population structure of yeast in the wild would be conducive to the operation of a group selection mechanism of the kind outlined here. Another aspect of the lifestyle of wild yeast populations simulated in the lab is the switching of an aging population from nutrient medium to sterile distilled water (Figure 12.3); this experiment resembles the "feast-and-famine" cycles the majority of microorganisms are thought to experience in nature. The incubation of yeast in water causes a major life span extension compared to continued maintenance in nutrient medium. This experimental regime, which is believed to be mechanistically and evolutionarily related to the dietary restriction response observed in multiple species, illustrates the flexibility of the "altruistic program" outlined earlier. In our experimental paradigm, dietary restriction can be thought of as an environmental cue for the inactivation of the aging program and the concomitant activation of an extended longevity program described previously, since no adaptive regrowth can be supported in the absence of nutrients. Yeast seems to have evolved the ability to couple its aging and longevity regulation to the environmental nutrient status by deploying the aging program in times of plenty and the extended longevity program in times of scarcity. Along the same vein runs the observation by Mair, Goymer, Pletcher, and Partridge (2003) that dietary restriction instigated at any age during the *Drosophila melanogaster* life span produces within 2 days the same mortality slope observed for flies subjected to long-term dietary restriction.

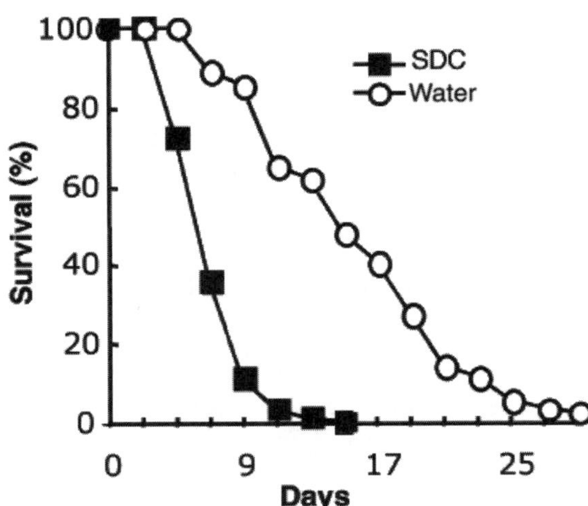

12.3

Survival of a wild-type yeast strain maintained in nutrient medium or in sterile water.

The Pacific Salmon—Not an Anecdote

The life histories of certain semelparous animals (reproducing only once in their lifetime) provide the most easily recognizable potential example of programmed aging in higher organisms. Pacific salmon species of the genus *Oncorhynchus* are the mostly cited such example since they die shortly after the first and last spawning bout of their lives (Finch, 1990). It has been argued that this phenomenon is a direct result of the excessive physical effort required to swim against the flow of the river before spawning. However, sudden postreproductive death is not observed when the gonad or adrenal glands are removed (Robertson & Wexler, 1962). Since invertebrates feed on the debris of dead salmon and young salmon feed on invertebrates, the rapid aging and death pattern observed in the Pacific salmon could be an adaptation ensuring the survival of its progeny by indirectly increasing the amount of nutrients available to it. In other words, physiological aging of this species is also consistent with the operation of a selection mechanism akin to the one described previously in *S. cerevisiae*.

Although the evidence for programmed aging in multicellular eukaryotes is scarce at best, evolutionary biologists and molecular biogerontologists need to accept the potentiality of programmed and altruistic aging operating at least in some organisms under certain specific circumstances.

References

Austad, S. N. (2004). Rebuttal to Bredesen: The non-existent aging program: How does it work? *Aging Cell, 3,* 253–254.

Brunet-Rossinni, A. K., & Austad, S. N. (2004). Ageing studies on bats: A review. *Biogerontology, 5,* 211–222.

Dillin, A., Crawford, D. K., & Kenyon, C. (2002). Timing requirements for insulin/IGF-1 signaling in *C. elegans*. *Science, 298,* 830–834.

Fabrizio, P., Battistella, L., Vardavas, R., Gattazzo, C., Liou, L. L., Diaspro, A., et al. (2004). Superoxide is a mediator of an altruistic aging program in *Saccharomyces cerevisiae*. *Journal of Cell Biology, 166,* 1055–1067.

Fabrizio, P., Liou, L. L., Moy, V. N., Diaspro, A., Valentine, J. S., Gralla, E. B., et al. (2003). SOD2 functions downstream of Sch9 to extend longevity in yeast. *Genetics, 163,* 35–46.

Fabrizio, P., & Longo, V. D. (2003). The chronological life span of *Saccharomyces cerevisiae. Aging Cell, 2,* 73–81.

Fabrizio, P., Pozza, F., Pletcher, S. D., Gendron, C. M., & Longo, V. D. (2001). Regulation of longevity and stress resistance by Sch9 in yeast. *Science, 292,* 288–290.

Finch, C. E. (1990). *Longevity, senescence, and the genome.* Chicago: University of Chicago Press.

Finch, C. E., & Crimmins, E. M. (2004). Inflammatory exposure and historical changes in human life-spans. *Science, 305,* 1736–1739.

Herker, E., Jungwirth, H., Lehmann, K. A., Maldener, C., Frohlich, K. U., Wissing, S., et al. (2004). Chronological aging leads to apoptosis in yeast. *Journal of Cell Biology, 164,* 501–507.

Kirkwood, T. B. (2005). Understanding the odd science of aging. *Cell, 120,* 437–447.

Kirkwood, T. B., & Shanley, D. P. (2005). Food restriction, evolution and ageing. *Mechanics of Ageing and Development, 126,* 1011–1016.

Leroi, A. M., Bartke, A., De Benedictis, G., Franceschi, C., Gartner, A., Gonos, E. S., et al. (2005). What evidence is there for the existence of individual genes with antagonistic pleiotropic effects? *Mechanics of Ageing and Development, 126,* 421–429.

Levine, M., & Davidson, E. H. (2005). Gene regulatory networks for development. *Proceedings of the National Academy of Sciences of the United States of America, 102,* 4936–4942.

Lewis, K. (2000). Programmed death in bacteria. *Microbiology and Molecular Biology Reviews, 64,* 503–514.

Ligr, M., Madeo, F., Frohlich, E., Hilt, W., Frohlich, K. U., & Wolf, D. H. (1998). Mammalian Bax triggers apoptotic changes in yeast. *FEBS Letters, 438,* 61–65.

Longo, V. D., Ellerby, L. M., Bredesen, D. E., Valentine, J. S., & Gralla, E. B. (1997). Human Bcl-2 reverses survival defects in yeast lacking superoxide dismutase and delays death of wild-type yeast. *Journal of Cell Biology, 137,* 1581–1588.

Longo, V. D., & Finch, C. E. (2003). Evolutionary medicine: From dwarf model systems to healthy centenarians? *Science, 299,* 1342–1346.

Longo, V. D., Mitteldorf, J., & Skulachev, V. P. (2005). Programmed and altruistic ageing. *Nature Reviews: Genetics, 6,* 866–872.

Mair, W., Goymer, P., Pletcher, S. D., & Partridge, L. (2003). Demography of dietary restriction and death in *Drosophila. Science, 301,* 1731–1733.

McCarroll, S. A., Murphy, C. T., Zou, S., Pletcher, S. D., Chin, C. S., Jan, Y. N., et al. (2004). Comparing genomic expression patterns across species identifies shared transcriptional profile in aging. *Nature Genetics, 36,* 197–204.

Medawar, P. (1952). *An unsolved problem of biology.* London: H. K. Lewis.

Murphy, C. T., McCarroll, S. A., Bargmann, C. I., Fraser, A., Kamath, R. S., Ahringer, J., et al. (2003). Genes that act downstream of DAF-16 to influence the lifespan of *Caenorhabditis elegans. Nature, 424,* 277–283.

Reznick, D. N., Bryant, M. J., Roff, D., Ghalambor, C. K., & Ghalambor, D. E. (2004). Effect of extrinsic mortality on the evolution of senescence in guppies. *Nature, 431,* 1095–1099.

Robertson, O. H., & Wexler, B. C. (1962). Histological changes in the organs and tissues of senile castrated kokanee salmon (*Oncorhynchus nerka kennerlyi*). *General and Comparative Endocrinology, 2,* 458–472.

Shanley, D. P., & Kirkwood, T. B. (2000). Calorie restriction and aging: A life-history analysis. *Evolution: International Journal of Organic Evolution, 54,* 740–750.

Sohal, R. S., & Weindruch, R. (1996). Oxidative stress, caloric restriction, and aging. *Science, 273,* 59–63.

Toda, T., Cameron, S., Sass, P., & Wigler, M. (1988). SCH9, a gene of *Saccharomyces cerevisiae* that encodes a protein distinct from, but functionally and structurally related to, cAMP-dependent protein kinase catalytic subunits. *Genes and Development, 2,* 517–527.

Turturro, A., Duffy, P., Hass, B., Kodell, R., & Hart, R. (2002). Survival characteristics and age-adjusted disease incidences in C57BL/6 mice fed a commonly used cereal-based diet modulated by dietary restriction. *Journal of Gerontology: Biological Sciences, 57,* B379–B389.

Walker, D. W., McColl, G., Jenkins, N. L., Harris, J., & Lithgow, G. J. (2000). Evolution of lifespan in *C. elegans. Nature, 405,* 296–297.

Williams, G. (1957). Pleiotropy, natural selection and the evolution of senescence. *Evolution, 11,* 398–411.

Wilson, D. S. (1997). Human groups as units of selection. *Science, 276,* 1816–1817.
Wynne-Edwards, V. (1962). *Animal dispersion in relation to social behaviour.* Edinburgh: Oliver & Boyd.
Zambrano, M. M., Siegele, D. A., Almiron, M., Tormo, A., & Kolter, R. (1993). Microbial competition: *Escherichia coli* mutants that take over stationary phase cultures. *Science, 2591,* 757–760.

Free Radicals and Oxidative Stress in Aging

13

Reshma Shringarpure
Kelvin J. A. Davies

Aging has been defined as the process that converts fit adults into frailer adults with a progressively increased risk of injury, illness, and death (Miller, 1999). Multiple theories of aging have been proposed: the free radical theory of aging (Harman, 1956, 1992) and the somatic mutation theory of aging (Morley, 1995) suggest that aging is the result of an accumulation of many deleterious changes over time, whereas the developmental theory of aging and the theory of antagonistic pleiotropy (Kirkwood & Rose, 1991) indicate that aging is intrinsically programmed and that life expectancy is at least partially specified by the genome (Wood, 1998). As portrayed by the evolutionary theory of aging, however, it appears that aging may be a balance (or lack thereof) between wear and tear and genetically controlled mechanisms of prevention and repair (Ricklefs, 1998). Although a direct causal relationship between increased oxidative stress and an effect on life span remains to be unequivocally established (Kregel & Zhang, 2007; Muller, Lustgarten, Jang, Richardson, & Van Remmen, 2007; Sohal, Mockett, & Orr, 2002), the importance of oxidative stress in aging and many age-related disease states is well recognized (Balaban, Nemoto, & Finkel, 2005; Cutler, 2005; Harman, 2006; Sohal, 2002; Sohal & Weindruch, 1996). This chapter briefly reviews the free radical theory of aging, describes the mechanisms of oxidative damage to macromolecules during aging, and discusses some of the evidence supporting or challenging the hypothesis that oxidative stress accelerates the process of aging.

The Free Radical Theory of Aging

Following on initial observations and suggestions by Rebecca Gershman and Dan Gilbert, Denham Harman formally proposed the free radical theory of aging, which suggested that free radicals produced during aerobic respiration cause cumulative oxidative damage, resulting in aging and death (Harman, 1956). Although the existence of highly reactive, damaging free radicals in vivo was questioned at the time, the detection of free radicals in biological systems (Commoner, Townsend, & Pake, 1954; Kenny & Commoner, 1969) and subsequent identification of the enzyme superoxide dismutase (SOD; McCord & Fridovich, 1969) provided confirmation that free radicals were generated in vivo during mitochondrial electron transport (Balaban et al., 2005). It is now well established that free radicals are generated in vivo by auto-oxidation and by a number of physiological processes, including mitochondrial electron transport (Chance, Sies, & Boveris, 1979; Dionisi, Galeotti, Terranova, & Azzi, 1975), the "respiratory burst" of phagocytic cells of the immune system (Nowak, 1990), cytochrome P-450 reactions (Zangar, Davydov, & Verma, 2004), and other reactions involving peroxisomal oxidases (Schrader & Fahimi, 2004), NAD(P)H oxidases (Li et al., 2001), and xanthine-xanthine oxidase (Rieger, Shah, & Gidday, 2002), to name but a few (Davies, 1995; Kregel & Zhang, 2007). Recognizing that mitochondria are major sources for the generation of reactive oxygen species, the free radical theory of aging was later extended by Harman (1972, 2006) to suggest that life span is determined primarily by the rate of oxidative damage to mitochondrial DNA.

Although the free radical theory of aging originally referred to the damaging power of free radicals, the phenomenon has now been extended to other reactive oxygen species that are generally nonradical products of radical chain reactions, such as hydrogen peroxide, lipid peroxides, various aldehydes, and so on. Such species are not free radicals because they do not contain an unpaired electron, but they are still highly products of free radical reactions. In addition to reactive oxygen species, reactive nitrogen species have also been implicated in oxidative injury. Nitric oxide, produced within cells by the actions of nitric oxide synthases, is a relatively unreactive radical but can form other reactive intermediates, such as nitrate, nitrite, peroxynitrite, and 3-nitrotyrosine (Drew & Leeuwenburgh, 2002), all of which are capable of causing oxidative damage. Considering the different reactive species involved, the free radical theory of aging might be more broadly referred to as the oxidative stress theory of aging or as the oxygen paradox (Davies, 1995). The oxygen paradox (Davies, 1995) refers to the conundrum that oxygen is essential for aerobic life but is also a direct danger to all organisms. The identification of antioxidants and the evolution of antioxidant enzymes support the notion that reactive oxygen species, generated as by products of metabolism, are a threat to survival. Nevertheless, direct evidence demonstrating that increased oxidative stress can accelerate aging and decrease life span is limited.

Cellular Antioxidant Defense Mechanisms

Most organisms are equipped with several lines of defense against oxidative stress that either minimize the generation of free radicals or enzymatically eliminate reactive oxygen species. A number of small molecules function as antioxidants or scavengers of free radicals: these include the antioxidants α-tocopherol (vitamin E), ascorbic acid (vitamin C), and glutathione (GSH), to name a few. Small-molecular-weight thiols like glutathione, as well as enzyme systems containing redox-active cysteines, such as thioredoxin/thioredoxin reductases and protein disulfide isomerases, enzymes responsible for facilitating proper protein folding by forming or rearranging disulfide bonds, also serve to maintain an overall reducing environment in the cell and reduce erroneously formed disulfide bridges between proteins (Berlett & Stadtman, 1997; Dean, Fu, Stocker, & Davies, 1997; Grune, Reinheckel, & Davies, 1997; Laboissiere, Sturley, & Raines, 1995).

In addition to the small-molecule antioxidants that minimize the formation of reactive oxygen species, most organisms are equipped with many antioxidant enzymes that actively deactivate or dismutate reactive oxygen species to stable, less reactive or unreactive moieties. These antioxidant enzymes include SOD, catalase, glutathione peroxidase, methionine sulfoxide reductase, and thioredoxin reductase, among others. The importance of each enzyme varies from organism to organism and from cell to cell and cell compartment to cell compartment in multicellular organisms. Specifically, SOD converts the superoxide anion into hydrogen peroxide, which is further inactivated by glutathione peroxidase or by catalase (Balaban et al., 2005; McCord & Fridovich, 1969; Radi et al., 1991) to water and oxygen.

A number of experiments in model organisms have attempted to elucidate the role of antioxidant enzymes in life span by genetic manipulation of these enzymes. Experiments in model organisms evaluating the effects of overexpressing antioxidant enzymes on life span provide the best evidence to date in support of the free radical theory of aging (Orr & Sohal, 1994; Sun, Folk, Bradley, & Tower, 2002; Sun & Tower, 1999). However, results of such experiments have been equivocal and have not been consistent across different species (Huang, Carlson, Gillespie, Shi, & Epstein, 2000; Seto, Hayashi, & Tener, 1990; Sun & Tower, 1999). Results of some of the studies evaluating effects of some of the most prominent antioxidant enzymes are discussed briefly here.

Role of Antioxidant Enzymes in Aging

Superoxide dismutase is generally thought to work with glutathione peroxidases or with catalase to convert superoxide to water and bypass the production of hydroxyl radical. There are two types of SOD enzymes within cells: SOD1, or Cu/ZnSOD, is present primarily in the cytosol, whereas SOD2, or MnSOD, is found predominantly in the mitochondrial matrix. Some mutations in Cu/Zn SOD are known to increase the extent of oxidative stress and have been associated with the neurodegenerative disease familial amyotrophic lateral sclerosis in humans (Deng et al., 1993; Sun & Tower, 1999). Similarly, a null mutation of Cu/Zn SOD in *Drosophila* has been shown to render such flies hypersensitive to oxidative stress with a reduction in longevity (Phillips, Campbell, Michaud, Charbonneau, & Hilliker, 1989). It was therefore hypothesized that overexpression of Cu/Zn SOD might result in increased resistance to oxidative stress, which, according to the free radical theory of aging, would lead to an increase in life span. However, overexpression of Cu/Zn SOD in *Drosophila* has yielded inconsistent results, possibly because of the use of different *Drosophila* strains and different methods of genetic manipulation (Orr & Sohal, 1993; Reveillaud, Niedzwiecki, Bensch, & Fleming, 1991; Seto et al., 1990; Stavely, Phillips, & Hilliker, 1990; Sun & Tower, 1999). While one *Drosophila* study showed a moderate increase in resistance to oxidative stress without a noticeable effect on life span (Reveillaud et al., 1991), another study demonstrated an increase in life span of 10% to 48% (Sun & Tower, 1999). Some *Drosophila* studies concluded that there was no effect of Cu/Zn SOD overexpression on life span (Orr & Sohal, 1993; Seto et al., 1990). Similar studies in mice found no effect of Cu/Zn SOD overexpression on life span (Huang et al., 2000).

Overexpression of catalase has also been studied; overexpression of catalase by itself in *Drosophila* was shown to increase resistance to oxidative stress but did not increase the life span (Sun & Tower, 1999). Simultaneous overexpression of both catalase and SOD has also yielded inconsistent results. While Sun and Tower (1999) found that catalase did not add to the life span–extending effects of SOD, Orr and Sohal (1994) reported that overexpressing the combination of SOD and catalase led to a 34% increase in mean life span, although neither of the individual genes had showed any effect on life span in their studies. These data, although compelling in some instances, have not been conclusive in demonstrating a causative effect for oxidative stress in the process of aging.

Oxidative Damage and Repair of Biological Macromolecules

Although elaborate, the previously discussed antioxidant defense mechanisms are not completely effective, and oxidative damage to cellular macromolecules is inevitable. Nucleic acids, lipids, and proteins are all susceptible to modification by reactive oxygen species; while most oxidation products of macromolecules are repaired or turned over in young, healthy cells, oxidatively damaged macromolecules accumulate with age, either because of enhanced production of reactive oxygen species, reduced efficiency of damage removal and repair systems, or both.

Oxidative Damage and Repair of Mitochondrial and Nuclear DNA

As stated by the extended free radical theory of aging (Harman, 1972), mitochondria are the main sites for the generation of reactive oxygen species, resulting in oxidative damage to mitochondrial DNA, and the rate of mitochondrial DNA damage may determine life span. This view has given rise to the mitochondrial theory of aging, and it is now recognized that mitochondrial DNA damage increases with age (Hagen et al., 2004; Miquel, Economos, Fleming, & Johnson, 1980; Muller et al., 2007) and is significantly greater than damage to nuclear DNA (Balaban et al., 2005; de Grey, 1997, 2002; Muller et al., 2007; Richter, Park, & Ames, 1988). A major product of oxidatively damaged DNA is 8-hydroxy-2-dexoxyguanosine, which is commonly used as a marker to assess the extent of oxidative DNA damage. However, many different oxidatively damaged products of DNA bases have been characterized (Cooke, Evans, Dizdaroglu, & Lunec, 2003). For example, the hydroxyl radical can react with the double bonds of DNA bases or abstract a hydrogen atom from the methyl groups of thymine, giving rise to C5-OH or C6-OH adduct radicals or the formation of the allyl radical (Cooke et al., 2003; Steenken, 1987). Some of these radicals have oxidizing properties and can form further oxidative damage, while others have reducing properties (Steenken, 1987).

Oxidized pyrimidine radicals can eventually yield many different products, such as cytosine glycol and thymine glycol (Breen & Murphy, 1995; Cooke et al., 2003; Dizdaroglu, 1992; Teoule, 1987). Products of thymine peroxyl radicals can yield thymine glycol, 5-hydroxymethyluracil, 5-formyluracil, and 5-hydroxy-5-methylhydantoin (Wagner, Van Lier, Berger, & Cadet, 1994), and products of cytosine glycol may further deaminate or dehydrate to yield uracil glycol, 5-hydroxycytosine, and 5-hydroxyuracil (Breen & Murphy, 1995; Dizdaroglu, 1992; Dizdaroglu, Holwitt, Hagan, & Blakely, 1986; Wagner, 1994). The most studied product of oxidative damage to DNA, 8-hydroxy-guanine, can be formed by oxidation of the C8-OH adduct radical, which in turn is the result of hydration of the guanine radical cation (guanine•+) in double-stranded DNA (Cooke et al., 2003; Kasai, Yamaizumi, Berger, & Cadet, 1992). The guanine radical cation is formed by elimination of OH– from the C4-OH adduct radical of guanine. Additional products of oxidatively damaged DNA bases have been reviewed in detail by Cooke et al. (2003).

As a result of oxidative damage, mitochondrial as well as nuclear DNA may undergo strand breaks, mutations, or deletions (Kregel & Zhang, 2007) with detrimental effects. Unless repaired or eliminated, oxidative lesions of DNA can lead to aberrant cellular processes, including uncontrolled cell proliferation or DNA damage–induced apoptosis (Evans, Dizdaroglu, & Cooke, 2004; Grishko et al., 2003; Kil, Huh, Lee, & Park, 2006; Kregel & Zhang, 2007). Indeed, many cancers have been linked to mutations in specific genes or to reduced DNA repair capability (Cooke et al., 2003). It is, therefore, crucial to rapidly remove oxidative lesions in DNA, and most organisms are equipped with multiple redundant repair mechanisms to ensure the integrity of mitochondrial and nuclear genomes.

Elimination of oxidatively damaged bases from DNA is accomplished by two main types of activities—base excision repair and nuclear excision repair—for the removal of single lesions or lesion-containing nucleotides, respectively (Cooke et al., 2003). Multiple enzymes are responsible for the repair of lesions related to 8-hydroxy-guanine, depending on whether the damage occurs to guanine within double-stranded DNA or to an unincorporated nucleotide, and for correction of misincorporated bases opposite 8-hydroxy-guanine.

By degrading free 8-hydroxy-deoxyguanosine triphosphate, MutT homologue 1 (MTH1) prevents the incorporation of this damaged base into DNA (Hayakawa, Taketomi, Sakumi, Kuwano, & Sekiguchi, 1995). The enzymes 8-oxoguanine glycosylase 1 and 8-oxoguanine glycosylase 2 are responsible for removing 8-hydroxy-guanine paired to cytosine or adenosine, respectively, via a glycolytic mechanism (Boiteux & Radicella, 2000; Bruner, Norman, & Verdine, 2000; David-Cordonnier, Boiteux, & O'Neill, 2001; Hazra, Izumi, Maidt, Floyd, & Mitra, 1998). Other enzymes, including MutY homologue, MTH1, and elements of the mismatch repair system, MutS, along with proliferating cell nuclear antigen are also involved in the removal of bases misincorporated opposite 8-hydroxy-guanine (Boldogh et al., 2001; Cooke et al., 2003; Gu et al., 2002; Mazurek, Berardini, & Fishel, 2002). The repair of some of the other oxidative DNA lesions has not been as clearly elucidated, although additional proteins involved in repair of oxidatively damaged DNA have been identified (Cooke et al., 2003).

Despite the previously mentioned repair mechanisms, oxidative damage to DNA increases with age and in certain disease states such as malignancies, the risk of which also increases with age. This may be the result of reduced DNA repair capability as well as increased oxidative stress during aging; alteration or functional attenuation of DNA repair enzymes has been associated with the many cancers (Cooke et al., 2003). An age-related increase in DNA oxidation markers, such as 8-hydroxy-deoxyguanosine, has been well documented for a wide range of ages in mitochondrial and nuclear DNA (Hagen et al., 2004; Hamilton et al., 2001; Miquel et al., 1980; Muller et al., 2007; Rattan, Siboska, Wikmar, Clark, & Woolley, 1995; Sohal, Ku, Agarwal, Forster, & Lal, 1994).

Mitochondrial DNA is postulated to harbor greater oxidative damage compared to nuclear DNA not only because of its proximity to mitochondrial reactive oxygen species but also because of a less efficient DNA repair system (Kregel & Zhang, 2007; Muller et al., 2007). Oxidative damage to mitochondrial DNA may lead to mitochondrial dysfunction, resulting in generation of more reactive oxygen species and less adenosine triphosphate, leading to another cycle of oxidative damage to mitochondria and an even greater production of reactive oxygen species (Balaban et al., 2005), eventually culminating in self-propagated, severe mitochondrial dysfunction. Further support of the mitochondrial theory of aging comes from a recent study in fruit flies demonstrating that mitochondria from older flies have significantly greater "swirls," or morphological changes in mitochondrial cristae, in response to oxidative stress compared to younger flies and that mutants selected for increased swirl formation have a shorter life span (Balaban et al., 2005; Walker & Benzer, 2004). In summary, all aerobic organisms suffer from oxidative damage to DNA; however, elaborate repair mechanisms have evolved, and repair capacity appears to be directly correlated to life span.

Lipid Peroxidation

Cellular membranes containing polyunsaturated fatty acids are extremely susceptible to oxidative damage. Initiation of oxidative damage on a phospholipid molecule can lead to a self-propagating chain of oxidative events until termination products such as 4-hydroxy-2-nonenol (HNE), malondialdehyde (MDA), or F2-isoprostanes are formed. Such chain reactions can be minimized by the antioxidant vitamin E. Alterations to cellular membranes can result in "leaky" membranes dysregulating active transport or lead to structural modifications. Oxidatively damaged membranes can release lipid peroxidation products such as 4-hydroxy-2-nonenal (4-HNE) and malonyldialdehyde (MDA) that are considered toxic to cells. Aging and a number of age-related pathologies have been associated with an increased accumulation of 4-HNE and MDA, both extensively studied markers of lipid peroxidation (Lee et al., 1999; Oxenkrug & Requintina, 2003; Poon, Calabrese, Scapagnini, & Butterfield, 2004; Wozniak, Drewa, Wozniak, & Schachtschabel, 2004). Both 4-HNE and MDA are capable of forming adducts with free amino acids and proteins and may facilitate formation of cross-links between two proteins or peptides. An age-associated increase has also been demonstrated for F2 isoprentanes; this increase was attenuated by caloric restriction, an intervention known to extend life span (Ward et al., 2005). Most oxidation products of lipids cannot be repaired, and such damaged lipids, therefore, need to be removed and then replaced.

Protein Oxidation and Proteolysis

Proteins are now recognized as critical targets of intracellular oxidative damage (Stadtman, 2001), and an increase in free radical–mediated damage to cellular proteins has been associated with aging (Berlett & Stadtman, 1997; Levine & Stadtman, 2001) and a number of age-related disorders (Markesbury, 1997). In addition to losing their designated function, oxidatively damaged proteins can cause further damage unless repaired or eliminated from the cells. The consequences of protein oxidation and the reaction products formed when proteins are exposed to a variety of reactive oxygen and nitrogen species have been extensively studied, and a number of reaction products of protein oxidation have been well characterized (Berlett & Stadtman, 1997; Davies & Delsignore, 1987; Davies, Delsignore, & Lin, 1987; Garrison, Jayko, & Bennett, 1962). The hydroxyl radical (•OH) and H_2O_2, along with O_2, $O_2{\bullet}^-$ and $HO{\bullet}_2$, can lead to oxidation of amino acid side chains, formation of protein–protein covalent cross-links, and protein fragmentation due to oxidation of the peptide backbone, as described in greater detail later in this chapter (Berlett & Stadtman, 1997; Davies, Lin, & Pacifici, 1987; Dean et al., 1997; Stadtman, 2001).

The sulfur-containing amino acids cysteine and methionine are highly susceptible to oxidative damage. In fact, oxidation of these amino acids has been postulated to serve as a first line of antioxidant defense against damaging free radicals, as some of the damage to the sulfur-containing amino acids can be enzymatically reversed (Berlett & Stadtman, 1997; Chao, Ma, & Stadtman, 1997; Levine, Mosoni, Berlett, & Stadtman, 1996). Oxidation of cysteine results in the formation of intra- or intermolecular disulfides leading to possible aggregation of proteins or peptides, while methionine oxidation forms primarily methionine sulfoxide. The formation of disulfide bridges can be reversed by protein disulfide isomerases; methionine sulfoxide reductase can reverse this oxidation process in free methionines, and a similar but distinct enzyme, peptide methionine sulfoxide reductase, can reduce oxidized methionine residues in peptides and proteins (Berlett & Stadtman, 1997; Chao et al., 1997; Grune et al., 1997; Levine et al., 1996). Other oxidation products of cysteine and methionine cannot be repaired enzymatically and must be eliminated from cells.

Aromatic amino acids can be readily oxidized by different reactive oxygen species, leading to the formation of various hydroxy derivatives (Berlett & Stadtman, 1997; Davies, Delsignore et al., 1987; Grune et al., 1997). Oxidation of several other amino acids, such as lysine, arginine, proline, or threonine residues, may yield carbonyl derivatives that are often used as markers to measure the extent of protein oxidation. As mentioned earlier, oxidation of amino acid side chains can also mediate polypeptide chain fragmentation (Berlett & Stadtman, 1997; Davies & Delsignore, 1987; Davies, Delsignore, et al., 1987; Davies, Lin, et al., 1987; Grune et al., 1997). Often the withdrawal of a hydrogen atom from an amino acid residue generates a carbon-centered radical that in turn can initiate downstream reactions that lead to protein fragmentation by peptide bond cleavage, giving rise to peptide fragments with derivatized terminal amino acids. Interaction between two carbon-centered radicals can form protein cross-links (Berlett & Stadtman, 1997; Grune et al., 1997). Another major consequence of protein oxidation is the formation of large protein aggregates that are often toxic to cells if allowed to accumulate (Berlett & Stadtman, 1997; Davies & Delsignore, 1987; Davies, Lin, et al., 1987; Grune et al., 1997; Sitte, Huber, et al., 2000; Sitte, Merker, Von Zglinicki, Davies, & Grune, 2000; Sitte, Merker, Von Zglinicki, Grune, & Davies, 2000). These aggregates can result from noncovalent interactions among oxidized amino acid residues or formation of covalent cross-links such as the disulfide cross-link and the 2,2′-biphenyl cross-link formed by two tyrosyl radicals (Berlett & Stadtman, 1997; Grune et al., 1997; Friguet, Stadtman, & Swezda, 1994; Friguet & Swezda, 1997; Giuilivi & Davies, 1993, 1994; Levine et al., 1996; Shringarpure, Grune, Sitte, & Davies, 2000). Oxidative modification frequently results in increased surface hydrophobicity as a result of partial unfolding of proteins (Chao et al., 1997; Pacifici, Kono, & Davies, 1993), and proteins with increased hydrophobicity can interact with each other via hydrophobic interactions. Cross-links between proteins can also be generated by products of lipid peroxidation that act as natural protein cross-linkers (Shringarpure et al., 2000).

Unless eliminated from cells, oxidized proteins tend to form large aggregates, eventually leading to the formation of ceroid bodies or inclusion bodies in the cytoplasm or lipofuscin entrapped within lysosomes. Accumulation of oxidized protein aggregates can affect cell viability as seen in a number of age-related and neurodegenerative disorders. Unlike oxidative damage to DNA, which can be directly repaired by highly efficient enzymes, most forms of oxidative protein damage cannot be reversed, and oxidatively damaged proteins must be eliminated from cells to avoid the formation of insoluble aggregates.

It is now well recognized that oxidative modification of proteins makes them susceptible to proteolysis (Davies & Delsignore, 1987; Davies, Delsignore, et al., 1987; Davies, Lin, et al., 1987; Giulivi & Davies, 1993, 1994; Grune & Davies, 1997; Grune, Reinheckel, & Davies, 1996; Grune, Reinheckel, Joshi, & Davies, 1995; Grune et al., 1997; Pacifici et al., 1993; Rivett, 1985) and that exposure of cells to different forms of mild oxidative stress significantly increases the intracellular degradation of both short-lived and long-lived proteins (Grune & Davies, 1997; Grune et al., 1995, 1996). By preventing the formation of large aggregates or potentially toxic fragments with derivatized terminal amino acids, intracellular proteases responsible for the selective degradation of oxidized proteins function as efficient damage removal and repair systems. In eukaryotic cells, the proteasome is the site for degradation of most soluble intracellular proteins.

A vast majority of short-lived regulatory cell proteins as well as most abnormal proteins are degraded by the proteasome. Several studies have demonstrated that the proteasome is responsible primarily for selective proteolysis of oxidatively damaged proteins as seen by results of proteasome immunoprecipitation, treatment of cells with antisense oligonucleotides to essential proteasome subunits, and proteasome inhibitor profiles (Grune et al., 1995, 1996, 1997). These studies, as well as inhibitor profiles for the degradation of oxidized proteins, indicate that the proteasome is responsible for about 70% to 80% of the reactive oxygen species–induced increase in cellular protein degradation (Grune & Davies, 1997; Grune et al., 1995, 1996; Pacifici et al., 1993).

In young, healthy cells, the occurrence of oxidized proteins is maintained at a low level by efficient proteolysis; however, oxidized as well as ubiquitinylated proteins accumulate intracellularly in a number of age-related pathologies (Berlett & Stadtman, 1997; Levine & Stadtman, 2001; Markesbury, 1997; Mori, Kondo, & Ihara, 1987; Stadtman, 2001; Uchida, Szweda, Chae, & Stadtman, 1993), demonstrating either increased oxidative damage, reduced antioxidant capacity and efficiency of repair systems, or both with age. An increase in markers of protein oxidative damage has been associated with age in gerbils, humans, rats, as well as mice (reviewed in Grune, Shringarpure, Sitte, & Davies, 2001). Oxidatively damaged, cross-linked proteins may eventually be encapsulated by the lysosomes, forming insoluble, fluorescent aggregates called lipofuscin (Grune et al., 2001). Ceroid, inclusion bodies, and lipofuscin are all terms for age-related, yellow-brown pigments with a characteristic autofluorescence that is known to accumulate with aging postmitotic cells (Sitte, Huber, et al., 2000; Sitte, Merker, Von Zglinicki, Davies, et al., 2000; Sitte, Merker, Von Zglinicki, Grune, et al., 2000). A number of protein oxidation markers, such as protein carbonyls and lipid peroxidation products like 4-hydroxynonenal, have been detected in these intracellular particles or age-related pigments (Friguet et al., 1994; Friguet & Swezda, 1997; Shringarpure et al., 2000; Sitte, Huber, et al., 2000; Sitte, Merker, Von Zglinicki, Davies, et al., 2000; Sitte, Merker, Von Zglinicki, Grune, et al., 2000).

During aging or in the presence of certain age-related disorders, insoluble aggregates of oxidized proteins or specific proteins prone to aggregation can severely inhibit the proteasome, causing further accumulation of damaged proteins, eventually leading to cell death. There is substantial evidence documenting the cross-linking action of two abundant lipid-peroxidation products, 4-hydroxynonenal and malondialdehyde (Friguet et al., 1994; Friguet & Swezda, 1997; Shringarpure et al., 2000).

It is believed that protein aggregation arises from interactions of nonnative, partially folded conformations, as those often exhibited by oxidized proteins. The final forms of these aggregates usually have a well-defined fibrillar nature and are termed as "amyloid" on the basis of their properties of birefringence and selective dye affinities, specifically affinity for Congo red. Some examples of amyloid-forming proteins or proteins prone to aggregation associated with different diseases include the amyloid-beta peptide, which accumulates in Alzheimer's disease; variant transthyretin in hereditary systemic amyloidosis; serum amyloid A in reactive amyloidosis associated with chronic inflammatory disease; low-density lipoprotein in atherosclerotic lesions; and pancreatic amylin in diabetes.

In conclusion, early removal of oxidatively damaged or denatured proteins is crucial in order to avoid the formation of large insoluble aggregates. The proteasome represents the major cytosolic protease responsible for eliminating such damaged proteins, and most oxidized protein degradation is believed to be carried out by the 20S proteasome without the requirement for ubiquitin conjugation (Shringarpure, Grune, Mehlhase, & Davies, 2003). Nevertheless, correlative evidence suggests that oxidized proteins accumulate with age, and oxidative damage of specific proteins may be involved in certain age-related pathologies.

Summary and Discussion

The free radical theory of aging, initially proposed in the 1950s, has gradually garnered many adherents and has become a major aging theory. It is now well established that free radicals are generated in vivo as by-products of a number of physiological processes, the most prominent being mitochondrial electron transport. Although most organisms are equipped with several mechanisms of antioxidant defenses, including small molecules to quench free radicals and enzymes that convert free radicals to less reactive molecules, oxidative damage to cellular macromolecules cannot be avoided and increases further with age. Several mechanisms have evolved to directly repair certain damaged macromolecules or to eliminate oxidized macromolecules from the cells. These defense and repair mechanisms, although effective in young, healthy cells, become less effective with age, possibly because of an increased oxidative burden or an inhibition of the repair/removal systems. Support for the free radical theory of aging comes from a plethora of evidence demonstrating increased accumulation of oxidized DNA, proteins, and lipids in association with age and certain age-related disorders. Evidence exists for generalized increase in oxidized proteins as well as for oxidative modification of specific proteins in certain disease states.

Direct evidence demonstrating a shortening of life span with increased oxidative stress is, however, very limited. A few studies in model organisms, such as *Drosophila melanogaster,* have shown that overexpression of certain antioxidant enzymes can extend life span, although other enzymes may not be as effective in modifying life span. Besides, these results have not been unequivocal, and further studies are warranted to conclusively test the effects of increased antioxidant capacity on extension of life span in multiple species. Thus, a mounting body of evidence unequivocally supports the correlation between accumulation of increased oxidative damage to macromolecules with age in support of the free radical theory of aging; however, evidence to demonstrate a causal relationship between oxidative stress and aging remains rather weak and warrants further rigorous investigation.

References

Balaban, R. S., Nemoto, S., & Finkel, T. (2005). Mitochondria, oxidants, and aging. *Cell, 120,* 483–495.

Berlett, B. S., & Stadtman, E. R. (1997). Protein oxidation in aging disease and oxidative stress. *Journal of Biological Chemistry, 272,* 20313–20316.

Boiteux, S., & Radicella, J. P. (2000). The human OGG1 gene: Structure, functions, and its implication in the process of carcinogenesis. *Archives of Biochemistry and Biophysics, 377,* 1–8.

Boldogh, I., Milligan, D., Lee, M. S., Bassett, H., Lloyd, R. S., & McCullough, A. K. (2001). hMYH cell cycle-dependent expression, subcellular localization and association with replication foci: Evidence suggesting replication-coupled repair of adenine:8-oxoguanine mispairs. *Nucleic Acids Research, 29,* 2802–2809.

Breen, A. P., & Murphy, J. A. (1995). Reactions of oxyl radicals with DNA. *Free Radical Biology and Medicine, 18,* 1033–1077.

Bruner, S. D., Norman, D. P., & Verdine, G. L. (2000). Structural basis for recognition and repair of the endogenous mutagen 8-oxoguanine in DNA. *Nature (London), 403,* 859–866.

Chance, B., Sies, H., & Boveris, A. (1979). Hydroperoxide metabolism in mammalian organs. *Physiological Reviews, 59,* 527–605.

Chao, C., Ma, Y., & Stadtman, E. R. (1997). Modification of protein surface hydrophobicity and methionine oxidation by oxidative systems. *Proceedings of the National Academy of Sciences of the United States of America, 94,* 2969–2974.

Commoner, B., Townsend, J., & Pake, G. E. (1954). Free radicals in biological materials. *Nature, 174,* 689–691.

Cooke, M. S., Evans, M. D., Dizdaroglu, M., & Lunec, J. (2003). Oxidative DNA damage: Mechanisms, mutation, and disease. *FASEB Journal,* 17, 1195–1214.

Cutler, R. (2005). Oxidative stress profiling. Part I. Its potential importance in optimization of human health. *Annals of the New York Academy of Sciences, 1055,* 93–135.

David-Cordonnier, M. H., Boiteux, S., & O'Neill, P. (2001). Efficiency of excision of 8-oxoguanine within DNA clustered damage by XRS5 nuclear extracts and purified human OGG1 protein. *Biochemistry, 40,* 11811–11818.

Davies, K. J. (1995). Oxidative stress: The paradox of aerobic life. *Biochemical Society Symposium, s61,* 1–31.

Davies, K. J. A., & Delsignore, M. E. (1987). Protein damage and degradation by oxygen radicals: III. Modification of secondary and tertiary structure. *Journal of Biological Chemistry, 262,* 9908–9913.

Davies, K. J. A., Delsignore, M. E., & Lin, S. W. (1987). Protein damage and degradation by oxygen radicals: II. Modification of amino acids. *Journal of Biological Chemistry, 262,* 9902–9907.

Davies, K. J. A., Lin, S. W., & Pacifici, R. E.. (1987). Protein damage and degradation by oxygen radicals: IV. Degradation of denatured protein. *Journal of Biological Chemistry, 262,* 9914–9920.

Dean, R. T., Fu, S., Stocker, R., & Davies, M. J.. (1997). Biochemistry and pathology of radical-mediated protein oxidation. *Biochemical Journal, 324,* 1–18.

de Grey, A. D. (1997). A proposed refinement of the mitochondrial free radical theory of aging. *BioEssays, 19,* 161–167.

de Grey, A. D. (2002). The reductive hotspot hypothesis of mammalian aging: Membrane metabolism magnifies mutant mitochondrial mischief. *European Journal of Biochemistry, 269,* 2003–2009.

Deng, H.-X., Hentati, A., Tainer, J. A., Iqbal, Z., Cayabyab, A., Hung, W. Y., et al.(1993). Amyotrophic lateral sclerosis and structural defects in Cu,Zn superoxide dismutase. *Science, 261,* 1047–1051.

Dionisi, O., Galeotti, T., Terranova, T., & Azzi, A. (1975). Superoxide radicals and hydrogen peroxide formation in mitochondria from normal and neoplastic tissues. *Biochimica and Biophysica Acta, 403,* 292–301.

Dizdaroglu, M. (1992). Oxidative damage to DNA in mammalian chromatin. *Mutation Research, 275,* 331–342.

Dizdaroglu, M., Holwitt, E., Hagan, M. P., & Blakely, W. F. (1986). Formation of cytosine glycol and 5,6-dihydroxycytosine in deoxyribonucleic acid on treatment with osmium tetroxide. *Biochemical Journal, 235,* 531–536.

Drew, B., & Leeuwenburgh, C. (2002). Aging and the role of reactive nitrogen species. *Annals of the New York Academy of Sciences, 959,* 66–81.

Evans, M. D., Dizdaroglu, M., & Cooke, M. S. (2004). Oxidative DNA damage and disease: Induction, repair, and significance. *Mutation Research, 567,* 1–61.

Friguet, B., Stadtman, E. R., & Swezda, L. I. (1994). Modification of glucose-6-phosphate dehydrogenase by 4-hydroxynonenal: Formation of cross-linked protein that inhibits the multicatalytic protease. *Journal of Biological Chemistry, 269,* 21639–21643.

Friguet, B., & Swezda, L. I. (1997). Inhibition of multicatalytic proteinase (proteasome) by 4-hydroxynonenal cross-linked protein. *FEBS Letters, 405,* 21–25.

Garrison, W. M., Jayko, M. E., & Bennett, W. (1962). Radiation-induced oxidation of protein in aqueous solution. *Radiation Research, 16,* 487–502.

Giuilivi, C., & Davies, K. J. A. (1993). Dityrosine and tyrosine oxidation products are endogenous markers for selective proteolysis of oxidatively modified red blood cell hemoglobin by (the 19S) proteasome. *Journal of Biological Chemistry, 268,* 8752–8759.

Giuilivi, C., & Davies, K. J. A. (1994). Dityrosine: A marker for oxidatively modified proteins and selective proteolysis. *Methods in Enzymology: Oxygen Radicals in Biological Systems, Part C., 233,* 363–371.

Grishko, V., Pastukh, V., Solodushko, V., Gillespie, M., Azuma, J., & Schaffer, S. (2003). Apoptotic cascade initiated by angiotensin II in neonatal cardiomyocytes: Role of DNA damage. *American Journal of Physiology: Heart and Circulatory Physiology, 285,* H2364–H2372.

Grune, T., & Davies, K. J. A. (1997). Breakdown of oxidized proteins as a part of secondary antioxidant defenses in mammalian cells. *BioFactors, 6,* 165–172.

Grune, T., Reinheckel, T., & Davies, K. J. (1996). Degradation of oxidized proteins in K562 human hematopoietic cells by proteasome. *Journal of Biological Chemistry, 271,* 15504–15509.

Grune, T., Reinheckel, T., & Davies, K. J. (1997). Degradation of oxidized proteins in mammalian cells. *FASEB Journal, 11,* 526–534.

Grune, T., Reinheckel, T., Joshi, M., & Davies, K. J. (1995). Proteolysis in cultured liver epithelial cells during oxidative stress: Role of the multicatalytic proteinase complex, proteasome. *Journal of Biological Chemistry, 270,* 2344–2351.

Grune, T., Shringarpure, R., Sitte, N., & Davies, K. (2001). Age-related changes in protein oxidation and proteolysis in mammalian cells. *Journal of Gerontology: Biological Sciences, 56,* B459–B467.

Gu, Y., Parker, A., Wilson, T. M., Bai, H., Chang, D. Y., & Lu, A. L. (2002). Human MutY homolog, a DNA glycosylase involved in base excision repair physically and functionally interacts with mismatch repair proteins human MutS homolog2/human MutS homolog 6. *Journal of Biological Chemistry, 277,* 11135–11142.

Hagen, J. L, Krause, D. J., Baker D. J., Fu, M. H., Tarnopolsky, M. A., & Hepple, R. T. (2004). Skeletal muscle aging in F344BN F1-hybrid rats: I. Mitochondrial dysfunction contributes to the age-associated reduction in VO2 max. *Journal of Gerontology: Biological Sciences, 59,* 1099–1110.

Hamilton, M. L., Van Remmen, H., Drake, J. A., Yang, H., Guo, Z. M., Kewitt, K., et al. (2001). Does oxidative damage to DNA increase with age? *Proceedings of the National Academy of Sciences of the United States of America, 98,* 10469–10474.

Harman, D. (1956). Aging: A theory based on free radical and radiation chemistry. *Journal of Gerontology, 2,* 298–300.

Harman, D. (1972). The biologic clock: The mitochondria? *Journal of the American Geriatrics Society, 20,* 145–147.

Harman, D. (1992). Free radical theory of aging. *Mutation Research, 275,* 257–266.

Harman, D. (2006). Free radical theory of aging: An update. Increasing the functional life span. *Annals of the New York Academy of Sciences, 1067,* 10–21.

Hayakawa, H., Taketomi, A., Sakumi, K., Kuwano, M., & Sekiguchi, M. (1995). Generation and elimination of 8-oxo-7,8-dihydro-2-deoxyguanosine 5 triphosphate, a mutagenic substrate for DNA synthesis, in human cells. *Biochemistry, 34,* 89–95.

Hazra, T. K., Izumi, T., Maidt, L., Floyd, R. A., & Mitra, S. (1998). The presence of two distinct 8-oxoguanine repair enzymes in human cells: Their potential complementary roles in preventing mutation. *Nucleic Acids Research, 26,* 5116–5122.

Huang, T. T., Carlson, E. J., Gillespie, A. M., Shi, Y., & Epstein, C. J. (2000). Ubiquitous overexpression of CuZn superoxide dismutase does not extend life span. *Journal of Gerontology, 55,* B5–B9.

Kasai, H., Yamaizumi, Z., Berger, M., & Cadet, J. (1992). Photosensitized formation of 7, 8-dihydro-8-oxo-2 deoxyguanosine (8-hydroxy-2 deoxyguanosine) in DNA by riboflavin: A non-singlet oxygen mediated reaction. *Journal of the American Chemical Society, 114,* 9692–9694.

Kenny, P., & Commoner, B. (1969). Transitory free radicals in irradiated animal tissues. *Nature, 223,* 1229–1233.

Kil, I. S., Huh, T. L., Lee, Y. S., & Park, J. W. (2006). Regulation of replicative senescence by NADP-dependent isocitrate dehydrogenase. *Free Radical Biology and Medicine, 40,* 110–119.

Kirkwood, T. B., & Rose, M. R. (1991). Evolution of senescence: Late survival sacrificed for reproduction. *Philosophical Transactions of the Royal Society of London. Series B, Biological Sciences, 332,* 15–24.

Kregel, K. C., & Zhang, H. J. (2007). An integrated view of oxidative stress in aging: Basic mechanisms, functional effects, and pathological considerations. *American Journal of Physiology: Regulatory, Integrative and Comparative Physiology, 292,* R18–R36.

Laboissiere, M. C., Sturley, S. L., & Raines, R. T.. (1995). The essential function of protein-disulfide isomerase is to unscramble non-native disulfide bonds. *Journal of Biological Chemistry, 270,* 28006–28009.

Lee, H. C., Lim, M. L. R., Lu, C. Y., Liu, V. W. S., Fahn, H. J., Zhang, C., et al. (1999). Concurrent increase of oxidative DNA damage and lipid peroxidation together with mitochondrial DNA mutation in human lung tissues during aging—smoking enhances oxidative stress on the aged tissues. *Archives of Biochemistry and Biophysics, 362,* 309–316.

Levine, R. L., Mosoni, L., Berlett, B. S., & Stadtman, E. R. (1996). Methionine residues as endogenous antioxidants in proteins. *Proceedings of the National Academy of Sciences of the United States of America,* 93, 15036–15040.

Levine, R. L., & Stadtman, E. R. (2001). Oxidative modification of proteins during aging. *Experimental Gerontology, 36,* 1495–502.

Li, W. G., Miller, F. J., Zhang, H. J., Spitz, D. R., Oberley, L. W., & Weintraub, N. L. (2001). H_2O_2-induced O_2-production by a non-phagocytic NAD(P)H oxidase causes oxidant injury. *Journal of Biological Chemistry, 276,* 29251–29256.

Markesbury, W. R. (1997). Oxidative stress hypothesis in Alzheimer's disease. *Free Radical Biology and Medicine, 23,* 134–147.

Mazurek, A., Berardini, M., & Fishel, R. (2002). Activation of human MutS homologs by 8-oxo-guanine DNA damage. *Journal of Biological Chemistry, 277,* 8260–8266.

McCord, J. M., & Fridovich, I. (1969). Superoxide dismutase: An enzymic function for erythrocuperin (hemocuperin). *Journal of Biological Chemistry, 244,* 6049–6055.

Miller, R. A. (1999). Kleemeier award lecture: Are there genes for aging? *Journal of Gerontology: Biological Sciences, 54,* B297–B307.

Miquel, J., Economos, A. C., Fleming, J., & Johnson, J. E., Jr. (1980). Mitochondrial role in cell aging. *Experimental Gerontology, 15,* 575–591.

Mori, H., Kondo, J., & Ihara, Y. (1987). Ubiquitin is a component of paired helical filaments in Alzheimer's disease. *Science 235, 4796,* 1641–1644.

Morley, A. (1995). The somatic mutation theory of ageing. *Mutation Research, 338,* 19–23.

Muller, F. L., Lustgarten, M. S., Jang, Y., Richardson, A., & Van Remmen, H. (2007). Trends in oxidative aging theories. *Free Radical Biology and Medicine, 43,* 477–503.

Nowak, D. (1990). Hydrogen peroxide release from human polymorphonuclear leukocytes measured with horseradish peroxidase and o-dianisidine: Effect of various stimulators and cytochalasin B. *Biochimica and Biophysica Acta, 49,* 353–362.

Orr, W. C., & Sohal, R. S. (1993). Effects of Cu-Zn superoxide dismutase overexpression on life span and resistance to oxidative stress in transgenic *Drosophila melanogaster. Archives of Biochemistry and Biophysics, 301,* 34–40.

Orr, W. C., & Sohal, R. S. (1994). Extension of life span by overexpression of superoxide dismutase and catalase in *Drosophila melanogaster. Science, 263,* 1128–1130.

Oxenkrug, G. F., & Requintina, P. J. (2003). Mating attenuates aging-associated increase of lipid peroxidation activity in C57BL/6J mice. *Annals of the New York Academy of Sciences, 993,* 161–167.

Pacifici, R. E., Kono, Y., & Davies, K. J. (1993). Hydrophobicity as the signal for selective degradation of hydroxyl radical-modified hemoglobin by the multicatalytic proteinase complex, proteasome. *Journal of Biological Chemistry, 268,* 15405–15411.

Phillips, J. P., Campbell, S. D., Michaud, D., Charbonneau, M., & Hilliker, A. J. (1989). Null mutation of copper/zinc superoxide dismutase in *Drosophila* confers hypersensitivity to paraquat and reduced longevity. *Proceedings of the National Academy of Sciences of the United States of America, 86,* 2761–2765.

Poon, H. F., Calabrese, V., Scapagnini, G., & Butterfield, D. A. (2004). Free radicals and brain aging. *Clinics in Geriatric Medicine, 20,* 329–359.

Radi, R., Turrens, J. F., Chang, L. Y., Bush K. M., Crapo, J. D., & Freeman B. A. (1991). Detection of catalase in rat heart mitochondria. *Journal of Biological Chemistry, 266,* 22028–22034.

Rattan, S., Siboska, G. E., Wikmar, F. P., Clark, B. F. C., & Woolley, P. (1995). Levels of oxidative DNA damage product 8-hydroxy-2-deoxyguanosine in human serum increases with age. *Medical Science Research, 23,* 469–470.

Reveillaud, I., Niedzwiecki, A., Bensch, K. G., & Fleming, J. E. (1991). Expression of bovine superoxide dismutase in drosophila melanogaster augments resistance to oxidative stress. *Molecular Cell Biology, 11,* 632–640.

Richter, C., Park, J. W., & Ames, B. N. (1988). Normal oxidative damage to mitochondria and nuclear DNA is extensive. *Proceedings of the National Academy of Sciences of the United States of America, 85,* 6465–6467.

Ricklefs, R. E. (1998). Evolutionary theories of aging: Confirmation of a fundamental prediction, with implications for the genetic basis and evolution of life span. *American Naturalist, 152,* 24–44.

Rieger, J. M., Shah, A. R., & Gidday, J. M. (2002). Ischemia-reperfusion injury of retinal endothelium by cycloxygenase- and xanthine oxidase-derived superoxide. *Experimental Eye Research, 74,* 493–501.

Rivett, A. J. (1985). Purification of a liver alkaline protease which degrades oxidatively modified glutamine synthetase: Characterization as a high molecular weight cysteine protease. *Journal of Biological Chemistry, 260,* 12600–12606.

Schrader, M., & Fahimi, H. D. (2004). Mammalian peroxisomes and reactive oxygen species. *Histochemistry and Cell Biology, 122,* 383–393.

Seto, N. O. L., Hayashi, S., & Tener, G. M. (1990). Overexpression of Cu-Zn superoxide dismutase in *Drosophila* does not affect life span. *Proceedings of the National Academy of Sciences of the United States of America, 218,* 348–353.

Shringarpure, R., Grune, T., Mehlhase, J., & Davies, K. J. (2003). Ubiquitin conjugation is not required for the degradation of oxidized proteins by proteasome. *Journal of Biological Chemistry, 278,* 311–318.

Shringarpure, R., Grune, T., Sitte, N., & Davies, K. J. (2000). 4-Hydroxynonenal-modified amyloid-beta peptide inhibits the proteasome: Possible importance in Alzheimer's disease. *Cell & Molecular Life Sciences, 57,* 1802–1808.

Sitte, N., Huber, M., Grune, T., Ladhoff, A., Doecke, W. D., & Von Zglinicki, T., et al. (2000). Proteasome inhibition by lipofuscin/ceroid during postmitotic aging of fibroblasts. *FASEB Journal, 14,* 1490–1498.

Sitte, N., Merker, K., Von Zglinicki, T., Davies, K. J., & Grune, T. (2000). Protein oxidation and degradation during cellular senescence of human BJ fibroblasts: Part II—Aging of nondividing cells. *FASEB Journal, 14,* 2503–2510.

Sitte, N., Merker, K., Von Zglinicki, T., Grune, T., & Davies, K. J. (2000). Protein oxidation and degradation during cellular senescence of human BJ fibroblasts: Part I—Effects of proliferative senescence. *FASEB Journal, 14,* 2495–2502.

Sohal, R. (2002). Oxidative stress hypothesis of aging. *Free Radical Biology and Medicine, 33,* 573–574.

Sohal, R. S., Ku, H. H., Agarwal, S., Forster, M. J., & Lal, H. (1994). Oxidative damage, mitochondrial oxidant generation and antioxidant defenses during aging and in response to food restriction in the mouse. *Mechanisms of Ageing and Development, 74,* 121–133.

Sohal, R. S., Mockett, R. J., & Orr, W. C. (2002). Mechanisms of aging: An appraisal of the oxidative stress hypothesis. *Free Radical Biology and Medicine, 33,* 575–586.

Sohal, R. S., & Weindruch, R. (1996). Oxidative stress, caloric restriction, and aging. *Science, 273,* 59–63.

Stadtman, E. R. (2001). Protein oxidation in aging and age-related diseases. *Annals of the New York Academy of Sciences, 928,* 22–38.

Stavely, B. E., Phillips, J. P., & Hilliker, A. J. (1990). Phenotypic consequences of copper/zinc superoxide dismutase overexpression in *Drosophila melanogaster. Genome, 33,* 867–872.

Steenken, S. (1987). Addition-elimination paths in electrontransfer reactions between radicals and molecules. *Journal of the Chemical Society. Faraday Transactions. I, 83,* 113–124

Sun, J., Folk, D., Bradley, T. J., & Tower, J. (2002). Induced overexpression of mitochondrial Mn-superoxide dismutase extends life span of adult *Drosophila melanogaster. Genetics, 161,* 661–672.

Sun, J., & Tower, J. (1999). FLP recombinase-mediated induction of Cu/Zn-superoxide dismutase transgene expression can extend life span of adult drosophila melanogaster flies. *Molecular Cell Biology, 19,* 216–228

Teoule, R. (1987). Radiation-induced DNA damage and its repair. *International Journal of Radiation Biology and Related Studies in Physics and Chemistry and Medicine, 51,* 573–589.

Uchida, K., Szweda, L. I., Chae, H. Z., & Stadtman, E. R. (1993). Immunochemical detection of 4-hydroxynonenal protein adducts in oxidized hepatocytes. *Proceedings of the National Academy of Sciences of the United States of America, 90,* 8742–8746.

Wagner, J. R. (1994). Analysis of oxidative cytosine products in DNA exposed to ionizing radiation. *Journal of Chemical Physics, 91,* 1280–1286.

Wagner, J. R., Van Lier, J. E., Berger, M., & Cadet, J. (1994). Thymidine hydroperoxides: Structural assignments, conformational features and thermal decomposition in water. *Journal of the American Chemical Society, 116,* 2235–2242.

Walker, D. W., & Benzer, S. (2004). Mitochondrial swirls induced by oxygen stress and in *Drosophila* mutant hyperswirl. *Proceedings of the National Academy of Sciences of the United States of America, 101,* 10290–10295.

Ward, W. F., Qi, W., Van Remmen, H., Zackart, W. E., Roberts, L. J., & Richardson, A. (2005). Effects of age and caloric restriction on lipid peroxidation: Measurement of oxidative stress by F_2-isoprostane levels. *Journal of Gerontology: Biological Sciences, 60,* 847–851.

Wood, W. B. (1998). Aging of *C. elegans:* Mosaics and mechanisms. *Cell, 95,* 147–150.

Wozniak, A., Drewa, G., Wozniak, B., & Schachtschabel, D. O. (2004). Activity of antioxidant enzymes and concentration of lipid peroxidation products in selected tissues of mice of different ages, both healthy and melanoma bearing. *Zeitschrift für Gerontologie und Geriatrie, 37,* 184–189.

Zangar, R. C., Davydov, D. R., & Verma, S. (2004). Mechanisms that regulate production of reactive oxygen species by cytochrome P450. *Toxicology and Applied Pharmacology, 199,* 316–331.

Psychological Theories of Aging

14 Convoys of Social Relations: An Interdisciplinary Approach

Toni C. Antonucci
Kira S. Birditt
Hiroko Akiyama

The convoy model of social relations provides a theoretical base to describe, explain, and understand the pervasive influence of social relations on health and well-being. It underscores the importance of individual development, a life span perspective, and the role of situational or contextual experiences over the life course. An additional goal of the convoy model is to organize, in a coherent and consistent manner, the major components of social relations—that is, social networks, social support, and satisfaction with support (Antonucci, 1985, 1986, 1990, 2001; Kahn, 1979; Kahn & Antonucci, 1980). In this chapter, we summarize the major tenets of the original model and present empirical evidence concerning various aspects of the model. With increasingly higher-quality data available, it has become possible to identify and confirm specific aspects of the model empirically. We summarize a select portion here. Finally, we briefly outline theoretical developments over the years, specifically identifying additions to and extensions of the model, influenced both by the accumulating evidence and by an increasingly sophisticated perspective of developmental science (Cairns, Elder, & Costello, 1996). In sum, we utilize this chapter to provide a brief history of the model, a presentation of recent developments, and a summary of empirical evidence now available.

The Original Convoy Model

The term "convoy" was first used by the anthropologist David Plath (1980) to refer to a cohort of people, or "consociates," with whom the children he was observing in Japan grew up and matured. He described a special closeness that involved supportive interactions that included both positive and negative feedback. He noted that these consociates or convoy members provided the feedback needed to successfully meet developmental challenges. The term "convoy" is used in the convoy model to describe the close social relationships that surround the individual and, under normal conditions, provide a protective, secure base for personal development and exploration. The model suggests that one's convoy is shaped by personal (e.g., age, gender, race, and personality) and situational (e.g., social roles, expectations, norms, and demands) characteristics that influence the support relations experienced by the individual. Those objective characteristics of the convoy are most often termed as network structure. Network structure or social networks describe the members of the network by their structural characteristics (e.g., the number of people in or the size of a network; their age, gender, and relationship to the target individual; the number of years known; geographic proximity; and contact frequency). The network is the skeleton or structure that provides a foundation from which more subjective aspects of social relations can develop. Thus, large networks indicate that there are many people who might provide support. In this way, the structural characteristics do influence support relationships. However, it is clear that just having a large number of people who might provide support does not in any way guarantee that they will actually provide social support. Social support has been variously defined but basically refers to the provision or receipt of something perceived to be needed by the provider, the recipient, or both.

While the convoy model assumes that all people need social relations, it does not assume that everyone needs the same amount or the same type of support. What one needs is influenced by personal and situational characteristics and is likely to vary considerably. Kahn and Antonucci (1980) identified three types of social support or support exchanges: aid, affect, and affirmation. Although researchers have identified additional types of support or used different terminologies (e.g., Cohen & Willis, 1985; House, Kahn, McLeod, & Williams, 1985), these three terms generally encompass all known types of support. Aid refers to tangible assistance, which may include concrete help, such as money or sick care, or less tangible but equally important assistance, such as information and advice. Affect refers to emotional support and can be the type reserved for close and significant others, such as the love and care that one shares with spouse, children, and parents, or it can refer to a less intense type of affect, such as the fondness or affection one might feel toward a close friend or less close family member. Finally, affirmation is the intangible communication to another convoy member that members share or respect the same values, goals, and aspirations. Delineating the different types of support is a useful tool for obtaining some uniformity in definition and explanation concerning social support.

Kahn and Antonucci (1980) also recognized that neither the objective characteristics of the social network nor the more carefully delineated descriptions of social support capture all the critical characteristics of social relations. Also important is the degree to which the support is evaluated as satisfactory or dissatisfactory. To fully capture the nature of social relations, they argued, it is necessary to identify the descriptive as well as the interpretative nature of social relations. Thus, one might carefully and successfully—and even completely—describe the social network and the social support that is exchanged, but it is also necessary to include the individual's personal assessment of his or her experience. One of the important elements of this interdisciplinary model is that it recognizes that while objective characteristics may influence the subjective interpretation of an event, they rarely fully predict interpretation of support received. A simple example will make this point clear. While one must be married (a structural social network characteristic) to be supported by one's spouse (e.g., give or receive aid, affect, or affection), being married does not guarantee that one will receive support. Similarly, the receipt of support from one's spouse does not guarantee that one will be satisfied with the support received (e.g., too much or too little aid, affection, and so on).

The convoy model suggests that it is important to understand social relations because of their far-reaching effects on health and well-being. These effects are both psychological and physical. We provide several illustrative examples here. Early theoretical and empirical research documented the effects of social relations on psychological or mental health. It was hypothesized that social relations were more psychological than physical and, therefore, would affect psychological or mental health, that is, depression, life satisfaction, or happiness (Antonucci, Fuhrer, & Dartigues, 1997; Fratiglioni, Wang, Ericsson, Maytan, & Winblad, 2000) rather than physical health. However, the convoy model suggests that social relations influence both psychological and physical health. Evidence has increasingly supported this claim with empirical research documenting the effect of social relations on physical health and mortality (e.g., Berkman & Syme, 1979; Valliant, Meyer, Mukamal, & Soldz, 1998). It has been established cross-sectionally, in our own data as well as in other data sets, that personal and situational characteristics of social relations are associated with health and well-being. We turn next to a select consideration of the empirical evidence.

Empirical Evidence: The Influence of Personal and Situational Characteristics on Social Relations

Early empirical studies explored the effect of personal characteristics on social relations. The Supports of the Elderly Study (Antonucci & Akiyama, 1987a, 1987b), a national representative sample of people over 50, documented a number of age and gender differences in the structure of social networks. For example, older people had network members who were older, and younger people had younger networks. However, there were no age differences in the size of support networks, and people 65 to 74 had more friends in their networks than any other age-group. On the other hand, the examination of the provision and receipt of support suggested a different pattern. While younger people reported providing more support than older people, there were few age differences in the amount or type of support received. There were consistent gender differences in structure of support with men and women reporting more women in their networks and women reporting both giving and receiving more support than men. Women had larger networks and received support from a number of people, while men had smaller networks and usually received support from their wives. Interestingly, in an analysis of only married people with at least one child, the well-being of both men and women were more affected by support received (e.g., feels they can confide in and are reassured and respected) than by the network structural characteristics (e.g., size of network contact frequency and so on). Of special note is the fact that this finding was stronger for wives than for husbands (Antonucci & Akiyama, 1987a).

A larger, more recently conducted study, the Social Relations and Health Across the Life Course Study (Antonucci & Akiyama, 1994), provides some confirmation as well as additional details. This study involved face-to-face interviews of a community-dwelling regionally representative sample of individuals 8 to 93 years of age in 1992 from the metropolitan Detroit area. In this larger study, age, gender, race, and socioeconomic status (SES) were associated with social relations. This study is particularly important because of the full age range (8 to 93 years of age), a rarity in survey research. It allows for an examination of parallel findings at different stages over the life course. We summarize the relevant findings from this study here.

Beginning with a study of age and race, Ajrouch, Antonucci, and Janevic (2001) found that age and race individually and interactively were associated with social network structure. Older people had smaller networks that consist mostly of family members. They also reported less contact with and less proximal network members than younger people. On the other hand, while there were no racial differences in network proximity, African Americans had smaller, more family-oriented networks that they saw more frequently. Race differences in network characteristics tended to decrease with age.

In a related study, Ajrouch, Blandon, and Antonucci (2005) investigated gender differences in the adult portion of this same sample (ages 40 to 93). In analyses controlling for marital status and health, they found that men and women reported networks that were different in several significant respects, especially when SES was considered. Older men had older networks than younger men, and professional men had networks that were less geographically close than skilled workers. On the other hand, older women had smaller networks that were also older, lived farther away, and were in less frequent contact than younger women. Professional women had older networks with more friends than did women who were homemakers. Ajrouch et al. (2005) also found that people with less education had younger network members in midlife but that older women with less education did not have younger members than older women with more education. For both men and women, people with more education had larger networks overall, but there were no education differences in the number of people to whom men and women felt closest.

Although still limited, it seems clear that these findings suggest the importance of personal characteristics (i.e., age, gender, race, and SES) in determining the types of social relations people have. One additional set of results adds a comparison of variations in social relationships by personal factors across cultures. Antonucci, Akiyama, and Takahashi (2004) examined social networks according to age and gender in the previously mentioned Detroit area sample of people from 8 to 93 years of age and compared them with parallel data available from a study conducted in Yokahama, Japan, a city chosen because of its similarity to Detroit in population and industrial composition. They examined three levels of close relationships: close, very close, and closest. Using seven age-groups (8 to 12, 13 to 19, 20 to 39, 40 to 59, 60 to 69, 70 to 79, and 80 to 93), analyses indicated significant age differences in all close relationships. These can generally be described as curvilinear with middle-aged people in both countries overall reporting the most people in their network and both younger and older people reporting stable or slightly fewer people in their network. Also consistent across the two countries was a significant gender difference in very close relationships. Women reported more very close relationships than did men.

Research has considered the role of situational characteristics in social relationships as well. In this respect, culture or country differences represent important situational characteristics. Takahashi, Ohara, Antonucci, and Akiyama (2002) conducted comparative analyses on the sample described previously. They examined similarities and differences in close relationships considering not structural characteristics of the convoy members but rather characteristics of social support relationships, that is, whether they were affective, instrumental, or conflictual. The findings are especially useful in identifying similarities and differences between the two countries. Most interesting is the degree to which the findings did not support conventional wisdom concerning culture differences. Thus, despite the Japanese reputation for being a collective culture, Americans reported much higher positive affect toward their close relations than did the Japanese, but they also reported higher negative affect scores. Overall, Americans were much less likely to differentiate among relationships, providing generally high scores for spouse, child, other family, and friend. This was not true of the Japanese, who were more likely to distinctly differentiate their level of affect by relationship type. Interestingly, while Americans' affective scores were generally negatively correlated with conflict scores (females: –.31; men: –.27), this was much less true among the Japanese (females: –.02; men: –.09), suggesting a different overall conceptualization of the nature of social relationships. As this brief summary suggests, some findings are actually contrary to what might have been predicted on the basis of notions of East/West or collectivism/individualism. Takahashi et al. (2002) conclude that there are situational or cultural differences in social relations but that culture does not distinguish all relationships, nor can these relationships be easily or stereotypically categorized.

Positive and Negative Social Relations

In the original formulation of the model (Antonucci, 1985; Kahn & Antonucci, 1980), it was noted that while social relations have pervasively positive effects on individuals, social relations could have negative effects. Empirical evidence has been accumulating regarding negative relationships and indicates that the majority of relationships include at least a little negativity and/or conflict. Relationships that are very close may also have many irritating qualities (e.g., unsolicited advice and criticisms). Indeed, Luescher and Pillemer (1998) and Suitor, Pillemer, Keeton, and Robinson (1996) have introduced the concept of ambivalence in close relationships. This term signifies that relationships can be both positive and negative even with the same people. They argue that ambivalence is more frequent among close family relationships since individuals are less likely to terminate such relationships as one might with less close relatives or friends. In the same vein, Smith and Goodnow (1999) found that unasked-for support and unsolicited advice was perceived negatively among both younger and older people. Interestingly, the reason for this negative perception was the implication of incompetence. Hence, even when not overtly negative, support provision can have negative effects.

The convoy model clearly recognizes the potential for social interactions to be negative and to have negative effects. People can behave badly, they can provide negative feedback, and they can both withhold love and affection as well as engage in more direct and purposefully hurtful behaviors, such as hostility and dismissiveness. Evidence is increasingly available to document such exchanges as well as their negative outcomes.

Empirical Evidence: Negative Interactions

In a detailed examination of negative interactions, Akiyama, Antonucci, Takahashi, and Langfahl (2003) considered both positive and negative interactions among people aged 13 to 93 in the Social Relations and Health Across the Life Course studies using both U.S. and Japanese data. They found that self-reports of negative interactions with parents, child, and best friend but not spouse decreased with age. They noted that decreased contact frequency appeared to account for some of the decline in negative interactions, which may explain why there was no reduction in negative spousal interactions.

Empirical Evidence: Influence of Social Relations on Health

The evidence accumulating in support of the convoy model has come from a variety of perspectives. We provide several in the following pages. We begin with a series of studies that examined effects of social relations on health among people of varying personal and situational characteristics. Antonucci, Ajrouch, and Janevic (2002) found that social relations affected the health of middle-aged men and women differently, depending on both the support exchanged and their education. People of lower education, in general, are less healthy, and their networks were smaller. On the other hand, men but not women with less education who had larger networks and felt that their children would provide them with emotional, financial, and sick care were as healthy as men with higher levels of education. This finding is unique for several reasons. First, it supports the convoy model in that it shows that even among people who might otherwise be considered vulnerable (e.g., those with less education), social relations may provide a form of protection against the increased health risks common in this group. Also of importance is the documentation that these associations are differentially influenced by personal characteristics, as in this case of the effect being evident for men but not women.

Extending this exploration of the effect of social relations on health, Janevic, Ajrouch, Merline, Akiyama, and Antonucci (2000) compared older (aged 60 to 93) adults in the United States and Japan. They examined between-country differences in the association of illness with social relations and considered network structure, social support, and negative relations. Only one country difference emerged. In Japan, women with physical illness reported receiving more financial help from children than did women who were not ill. Overall, women who were ill reported less sick care from their spouse than men who were ill. Ill women in both countries were also more likely to report negative relations with their children than were women who were not ill. The findings of Janevic et al. suggest that social relations influence health but that the association varies by gender. Also interesting is the fact that, at least in this situation, gender appears to have more influence on the association between health and social relations than culture.

In a study including both quantitative and qualitative data, Lansford, Antonucci, Akiyama, and Takahashi (2005) examined the effect of social relations on depressed affect among individuals ages 13 to 93 using both survey and focus group data from the United States and Japan. They found, consistently across the two countries, that having a mother, spouse, and best friend was related to lower levels of depressed affect.

Further demonstrating that relationships can have both positive and negative effects, Antonucci, Lansford, and Akiyama (2001) showed that among older married adults (60 to 91 years old), women were more depressed than men if they did not have a best friend whom they felt they could confide in. However, women who did have a confidant showed lower levels of depression, in fact, levels comparable to those expressed by older men. Two interesting points can be made here. Men and women seem to be differently affected by their relationships and to seek and benefit from different types of relationships. Perhaps even more interesting, women's normally universally higher (than men's) levels of depressive symptoms can be offset by these relationships, and the gender difference in depression has been shown to decrease with age (Akiyama & Antonucci, 2002).

At the same time, women seem to be more vulnerable to the tensions or demand characteristics of their relationships. Antonucci, Akiyama, and Lansford (1998) studied older married adults and found that while women generally had more close relationships than did men, they were less happy the more close relationships they named. Antonucci et al. speculated that women feel more responsible for their close relations and are more sensitive to the needs and demands of their close social ties. Indeed, people are more likely to confide in women and expect support from women than men.

A number of relevant studies have been conducted in other countries. Using the French prospective PAQUID longitudinal study of aging, Antonucci et al. (1997) examined the effect of social relations on mental health. They found that both the structural characteristics of the social network and the quality of their social support significantly affected mental health as indicated by levels of depressive symptomatology. However, examined separately, social support had a much greater effect on mental health than did support network.

One unique study examined the effect of social relations on mental health in four countries. Antonucci et al. (2002) considered large representative samples of older people in the United States, Japan, France, and Germany. They examined how men and women experienced resource deficits and how social relations affected their ability to cope with these deficits. As one might expect, older women experienced more resource deficits (widowhood, illness, and financial strain) than older men. Among women in France and Japan but not men in any country, quality of social relations offsets the potentially negative effects of resource deficits. In all countries, more deficits and more negative social interactions were associated with higher levels of depressive symptomatology. These findings again suggest that gender may trump culture in defining the most important influences on many convoy characteristics.

Profiles of Relationships

A recent series of papers provides a unique approach to understanding social relations. Profile analyses permits the identification of the most common clusters of relationship characteristics or structures. Insight into the adaptiveness of these clusters can be assessed by the degree to which each is associated with well-being. Analyses on data from the United States as well as other countries allow a consideration of the consistency of these clusters and their effects in different cultural settings. These studies are briefly summarized here.

Using a national representative sample of older adults (60 and older) Fiori, Antonucci, and Cortina (2006) replicated the early work of Litwin (2001) on network profiles in Israel. Litwin identified four network types that he labeled diverse, family, friends, and restricted. These four were clearly replicated by Fiori et al. in their U.S. sample. However, they identified two types of restricted networks: one that could best be described as a nonfamily network and the other as a nonfriend network. As might be predicted, in both studies the restricted networks, especially the nonfriends network in the United States, were associated with higher levels of depressive symptomatology, while the diverse network was associated with the lowest levels. Fiori et al. also examined the degree to which the association between clusters and well-being was modified by the different network configurations. They found that the vulnerability evident among people with few family members in their networks was partially mediated by the presence of friendships but that the reverse was not true. Also of special interest is their finding that the quality of relationships significantly influenced the effect of network type on mental health.

Since the spousal relationship is perhaps the most intimate of all relationships, some questions have arisen about whether individuals could adjust to having a poor spousal relationship. In an examination of social relations profiles among married people 22 to 79 years of age, Birditt and Antonucci (2007) found that among people with same-sex best friends, having two high-quality relationships was associated with higher levels of well-being regardless of whether one of those involved relationships with a spouse. On the other hand, among people without a best friend, the quality of the relationship with a spouse was particularly and uniquely related to well-being. These findings question the exclusive importance of spousal relationship quality while at the same time identifying the degree to which it can be uniquely critical for well-being.

Profiles or clusters of relationships were also examined in a series of very similar studies in the United States, Japan, and Germany, and they offer some unique insights about cultural similarities and differences. Fiori, Antonucci, and Akiyama (2008) examined exactly parallel data from the United States and Japan. First, the same four common network types were identified: diverse, friend focused, family focused, and restricted. However, further specification of the distinctions in the two countries is also of interest. In the United States, the most prevalent type of network was the diverse/extensive type. Although this type does exist in Japan, it was much less prevalent. While both countries had family-focused network types, in Japan this was the most frequent type of network and consisted predominantly of very close family ties. On the other hand, in the United States, there was a family-focused network that was characterized predominantly by negative relations. Similarly, in Japan there was only one restricted type of network, while in the United States there were two. Both countries demonstrated a structurally restricted type of network that was characterized as small, with little contact among network members but also low negativity. The second restricted type in the United States was a functionally restricted type and characterized by both low positive and high negative support relations. Finally, there was one unique Japanese network type that could be described as married and distal. It was moderately common and consisted largely of men who were better educated and married but had a relatively small proportion of close network members in addition to their wives. It is speculated that they are typical Japanese workers in an urban area who commute a long distance, work long hours, and spend little time in the community in which they live.

Fiori et al. (2008) found expected associations between networks and well-being. Diverse networks were associated with better mental health, while restricted networks were associated with poorer mental health. However, this was true only in the United States. In Japan, there was no association between network type and mental health. Since the profiles in the two countries had many points of similarity, it is especially interesting to contemplate the lack of a significant association with mental health in Japan. Herein appears to be a deep-seated cultural difference that requires explanation.

The second set of comparisons capitalized on the availability of very similar data from the Berlin Aging Study (BASE) and also combined both structure and quality measures of social relations (Fiori, Smith, & Antonucci, 2007). They identified six network types similar to but also slightly different from those reported previously. These are diverse supported, family focused, friend focused supported, friend focused unsupported, restricted nonfriends unsatisfied, and restricted nonfamily unsupported. While the actual clusters are similar, their distribution in the population is somewhat different, perhaps reflecting the devastating effect of World War II on this city's population demographics. The clusters were also differentially associated with well-being. Individuals in the restricted networks had relatively high levels of depressive symptoms, but people with friend-focused-supported networks also had relatively high levels of depressive symptoms. Those with diverse and family-supported networks had relatively high levels of well-being and low levels of depressive symptoms, but once again a counterintuitive finding emerged indicating that friend-focused unsupported networks were also associated with better well-being. These findings underline the importance of considering both structure and quality of relationships. They suggest that there are similarities and differences in the links between network social relations profiles and well-being.

Modifications to the Convoy Model

Empirical evidence and theoretical questions have inspired several modifications of the convoy model. We discuss two of these: (a) the inclusion of stress and the role of social relations as a buffer and (b) the social relations/self-efficacy model, which considers possible mechanisms through which social relations affect health and well-being.

Stress

An important adaptation to the convoy model involved including the role of social relationships in the buffering of stress. Both social relations and stress are potential mediators of the relationship between personal and situational characteristics and mental health. For illustrative purposes, we have double-lined an example of mediation in the model that follows. In the original model, personal characteristics are hypothesized to influence social relations, in turn affecting mental health and thus reducing or even accounting fully for the direct effect of personal characteristics on mental health. In the modified model, the stress-buffering role of social relations is also included as indicated by the Social Relations × Stress interaction term illustrated in Figure 14.1. A significant path of this predictor on mental health indicates that the negative impact of stress is smaller for people with stronger social support. Of particular importance is how social relations might help the individual cope with specific stressful life events and daily hassles. Stress includes life events, such as moving to a new residence and the death of a close family member, as well as daily hassles, including minor irritations that occur in daily life, such as worries about being caught in a traffic jam or losing your keys. Social relationships may buffer or exacerbate the effects of stress on well-being. For example, the detrimental effects of the loss of a spouse may be buffered by emotional support received from friends. These effects can be consistent or inconsistent over time and can lead to accumulating negative or positive effects. The stress-buffering model is not new—however, the modified convoy model integrates mediation and buffering effects, allowing the empirical test of both these mechanisms simultaneously. Tests of this modified model are currently under way and do appear promising.

Support/Efficacy Model

The support/efficacy model was first outlined by Antonucci and Jackson (1987) to describe a possible mechanism through which social relations affect health and well-being. It was developed from the related literatures on social control, self-efficacy, and mastery (Gecas, 1989; Lachman & Weaver, 1998; Ross & Sastry, 1999). Self-efficacy, the belief that one can master a situation and produce positive outcomes, exemplifies the positive effects often associated with social support. For example, classic research by Bandura and colleagues (1977, 1986; Taylor, Bandura, et al., 1985) found that supportive wives were able to improve their husbands' sense of efficacy and hence recovery from myocardial infarction. Bisconti and Bergeman (1999) showed that perceived control, which is related to self-efficacy, can mediate the support–health relationship. These findings indicate that self-efficacy may be one of the mechanisms through which social support affects health.

It is suggested that social support influences health by conveying support to the target person, both contemporaneously and longitudinally, in turn enhancing the individual's feelings of self-efficacy. Higher levels of self-efficacy are associated with better health. Under optimal conditions, close network members provide support and hence efficacy enhancement. Of course, the opposite could also be true, and close supportive others could actually undermine the individual's efficacy and negatively influence health and well-being. Data have been accumulating in support of the support/efficacy model (Eizenman, Nesselroade, Featherman, & Rowe, 1997; Lang, Featherman, & Nesselroade, 1997). However, additional tests of the model are under way and should provide greater clarity and specificity. We hypothesize, for example, that certain types of relationships between an individual and his or her core network members are more likely than other types to enhance or disparage efficacy, consequently positively or negatively affecting the focal person's health and psychological well-being. The support/efficacy relationship is both idiosyncratic or specific to a certain event and cumulative or longitudinal, developing over time and both within and across relationships. Figure 14.2 illustrates this hypothesized ongoing association

Although it is unlikely that the support/efficacy model explains all of the association between social relations and health, it certainly may explain one significant pathway through which social relations influence health and well-being.

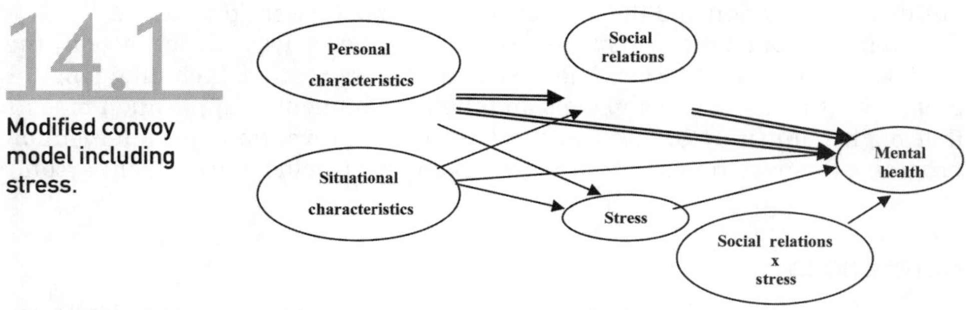

14.1

Modified convoy model including stress.

14.2

Illustrative longitudinal convoy model with mediating effect of self-efficacy.

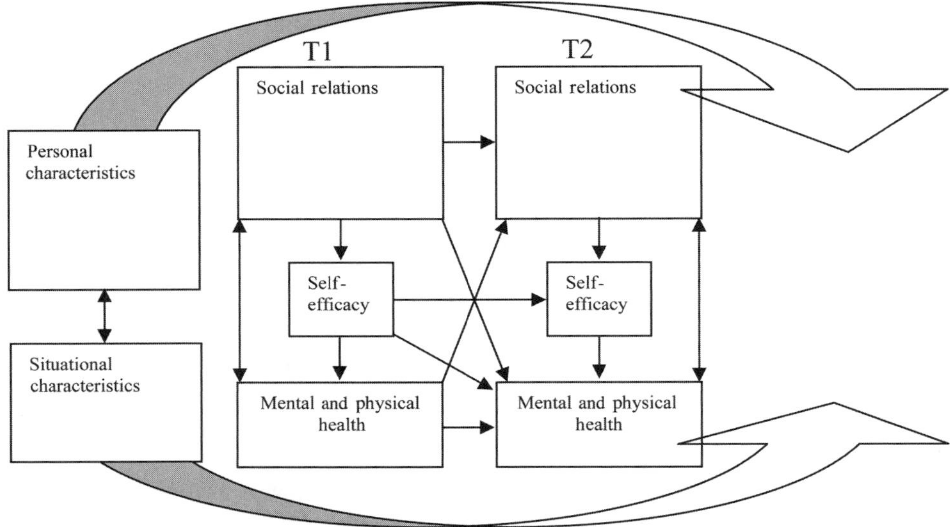

Summary and Conclusions

The early research on social relations was in a relative state of disarray, with poor conceptual definitions, little empirical evidence, and few theoretical explorations of the hypothesized associations. This chapter describes the convoy model of social relations, a life span, developmental, and cumulative perspective on both the antecedent and the consequent factors associated with social relations. The theory suggests that individuals are shaped by both personal and situational characteristics and that social relations consist of structural or network characteristics, exchanges of support, and satisfaction with the support received. Considerable evidence addressing each part of the model was presented and documents an overwhelming support for the model. Finally, recent modifications to the convoy model, including the addition of the social relations/stress-buffering association and the support/efficacy model, were presented.

There is abundant evidence in support of the convoy model in both the original and modified forms. Additional challenges remain, including longitudinal assessments of these models and the development of application models that might ultimately be used in the creation of prevention and intervention programs that would maximize the health and well-being of the older person.

References

Ajrouch, K. J., Antonucci, T. C., & Janevic, M. R. (2001). Social networks among Blacks and Whites: The interaction between race and age. *Journal of Gerontology: Social Sciences, 56,* S112–S118.

Ajrouch, K. J., Blandon, A. Y., & Antonucci, T. C. (2005). Social networks among men and women: The effects of age and socioeconomic status. *Journal of Gerontology: Social Sciences, 60,* 311–317.

Akiyama, H., & Antonucci, T. C., (2002). Gender differences in depressive symptoms: Insights from a life span perspective on life stages and social networks. In J. A. Levy & B. A. Pescosolido (Eds.), *Social networks and health* (Vol. 8, pp. 345–360). Boston, MA: Elsevier Science.

Akiyama, H., Antonucci, T. C., Takahashi, K., & Langfahl, E. S. (2003). Negative interactions in close relationships across the lifespan. *Journal of Gerontology: Social Sciences, 58,* 70–79.

Antonucci, T. C. (1985). Personal characteristics, social support, and social behavior. In R. H. Binstock & E. Shanas (Eds.), *Handbook of aging and the social sciences* (2nd ed., pp. 94–128). New York: Van Nostrand Reinhold.

Antonucci, T. C. (1986). Hierarchical mapping technique. *Generations, 10*(4), 10–12.

Antonucci, T. C. (1990). Social supports and social relationships. In R. H. Binstock & L. K. George (Eds.), *The handbook of aging and the social sciences* (3rd ed., pp. 205–226). San Diego, CA: Academic Press.

Antonucci, T. C. (2001). Social relations: An examination of social networks, social support, and sense of control. In J. E. Birren & K. W. Schaie (Eds.), *Handbook of the psychology of aging* (pp. 427–253). San Diego, CA: Academic Press.

Antonucci, T. C., Ajrouch, K. J., & Janevic, M. R. (2002). The effect of social relations on the education-health link in men and women aged 40 and over. *Social Science and Medicine, 56,* 949–960.

Antonucci, T. C., & Akiyama, H. (1987a). An examination of sex differences in social support among older men and women. *Sex Roles, 17,* 737–749.

Antonucci, T. C., & Akiyama, H. (1987b). Social networks in adult life and a preliminary examination of the convoy model. *Journal of Gerontology, 42,* 519–527.

Antonucci, T. C., & Akiyama, H. (1994). Convoys of attachment and social relations in children, adolescents, and adults. In K. Hurrelmann & F. Nestmann (Eds.), *Social networks and social support in childhood and adolescence* (pp. 37–52). Berlin: Aldine de Gruyter.

Antonucci, T. C., Akiyama, H., & Lansford, J. E. (1998). Negative effects of close social relations. *Family Relations, 47,* 379–384.

Antonucci, T., Akiyama, H., & Takahashi, K. (2004). Attachment and close relationships across the life span. *Attachment and Human Development, 64,* 353–370.

Antonucci, T. C., Fuhrer, R., & Dartigues, J. F. (1997). Social relations and depressive symptomatology in a sample of community-dwelling French older adults. *Psychology & Aging, 12,* 189–195.

Antonucci, T. C., & Jackson, J. S. (1987). Social support, interpersonal efficacy and health. In L. L. Carstensen & B. A. Edelstein (Eds.), *Handbook of clinical gerontology* (pp. 291–311). New York: Pergamon Press.

Antonucci, T. C., Lansford, J. E., & Akiyama, H. (2001). The impact of positive and negative aspects of marital relationships and friendships on well-being of older adults. *Applied Developmental Science, 5,* 68–75.

Antonucci, T. C., Lansford, J. E., Akiyama, H., Smith, J., Baltes, M. M., Takahashi, K., et al. (2002). Differences between men and women in social relations, resource deficits, and depressive symptomatology during later life in four nations. *Journal of Social Issues, 58,* 767–783.

Bandura, A. (1986). *Social foundations of thought and action: A social-cognitive theory*. Englewood Cliffs, NJ: Prentice-Hall.

Bandura, A., Adams, N. E., & Beyer, J. (1977). Cognitive processes mediating behavioral change. *Journal of Personality & Social Psychology, 35,* 25–139.

Berkman, L. F., & Syme, S. L. (1979). Social networks, host resistance, and mortality: A nine-year follow-up study of Alameda County residents. *American Journal of Epidemiology, 109,* 186–204.

Birditt, K. S., & Antonucci, T. C. (2007). Relationship quality profiles and well-being among married adults. *Journal of Family Psychology, 21,* 595–604.

Bisconti, T. L., & Bergeman, C. S. (1999). Perceived social control as a mediator of the relationships among social support, psychological well-being, and perceived health. *The Gerontologist, 39,* 94–103.

Cairns, R. B., Elder, G. H., & Costello, E. J. (1996). *Developmental science.* New York: Cambridge University Press.

Cohen, S., & Willis, T. A. (1985). Stress, social support, and the buffering hypothesis. *Psychological Bulletin, 98,* 310–357.

Eizenman, D. R., Nesselroade, J. R., Featherman, D. L., & Rowe, J. (1997). Intraindividual variability in perceived control in a older sample: The MacArthur successful aging studies. *Psychology & Aging, 12*(3), 489–502.

Fiori, K. L., Antonucci, T. C., & Akiyama, H. (2008). Profiles of social relations among older adults: A cross-cultural approach. *Ageing & Society, 28,* 203–231.

Fiori, K. L., Antonucci, T. C., & Cortina, K. (2006). Social network typologies and mental health among older adults. *Journal of Gerontology: Social Sciences, 61,* 25–32.

Fiori, K. L., Smith, J., & Antonucci, T. C. (2007). Social network types among older adults: A multidimensional approach. *Journal of Gerontology: Social Sciences, 62,* 322–330.

Fratiglioni, L., Wang, H., Ericsson, K., Maytan, M., & Winblad, B. (2000). Influence of social network on occurrence of dementia: A community-based longitudinal study. *Lancet, 355,* 1315–1319.

Gecas, V. (1989). The social psychology of self-efficacy. *Annual Review of Sociology, 15,* 291–316.

House, J. S., Kahn, R. L., McLeod, J. D., & Williams, D. (1985). Measures and concepts of social support. In S. Cohen & S. L. Syme (Eds.), *Social support and health* (pp. 83–108). San Diego, CA: Academic Press.

Janevic, M. R., Ajrouch, K. J., Merline, A., Akiyama, H., & Antonucci, T. C. (2000). The social relations-physical health connection: A comparison of elderly samples from the United States and Japan. *Journal of Health Psychology, 5,* 413–429.

Kahn, R. L. (1979). Aging and social support. In M. W. Riley (Ed.), *Aging from birth to death: Interdisciplinary perspectives* (pp. 72–92). Boulder, CO: Westview Press.

Kahn, R. L., & Antonucci, T. C. (1980). Conveys over the life course: Attachment, roles and social support. In B. P. Baltes & O. G. Brim (Eds.), *Life-span development and behavior* (Vol. 3, pp. 253–286). New York: Academic Press.

Lachman, M. E., & Weaver, S. L. (1998). The sense of control as a moderator of social class differences in health and well-being. *Journal of Personality and Social Psychology, 74,* 763–773.

Lang, F. R., Featherman, D. L., & Nesselroade, J. R. (1997). Social self-efficacy and short-term variability in social relationships: The MacArthur successful aging studies. *Psychology & Aging, 12,* 657–666.

Lansford, J. E., Antonucci, T. C., Akiyama, H., & Takahashi, K. (2005). A quantitative and qualitative approach to social relationships and well-being in the United States and Japan. *Journal of Comparative Family Studies, 36,* 1–22.

Litwin, H. (2001). Social network type and morale in old age. *The Gerontologist, 41,* 516–524.

Luescher, K., & Pillemer, K. (1998). Intergenerational ambivalence: A new approach to the study of parent child relations in later life. *Journal of Marriage and the Family, 60,* 413–425.

Plath, D. (1980). *Long engagements: Maturity in modern Japan*. Stanford, CA: Stanford University Press.

Ross, C. E., & Sastry, J. (1999). The sense of personal control: Social-structural causes and emotional consequences. In C. S. Aneshensel (Ed.), *Handbook of sociology of mental health* (pp. 369–394). New York: Kluwer Academic/Plenum Publishers.

Smith, J., & Goodnow, J. J. (1999). Unasked-for support and unsolicited advice: Age and the quality of social experience. *Psychology & Aging, 14,* 108–121.

Suitor, J. J., Pillemer, K. A., Keeton, S., & Robinson, J. (1996). Aged parents and aging children: Determinants of relationship quality. In R. Blieszner & V. H. Bedford (Eds.), *Handbook of aging and the family* (pp. 223–242). Westport, CT: Greenwood Press.

Takahashi, K., Ohara, N., Antonucci, T. C., & Akiyama, H. (2002). Commonalities and differences in close relationships among the Americans and Japanese: A comparison by the individualism/collectivism concept. *International Journal of Behavioral Development, 26,* 453–465.

Taylor, C. B., Bandura, A., Ewart, C. K., Miller, N. H., & DeBusk, R. F. (1985). Exercise testing to enhance wives' confidence in their husbands' cardiac capability soon after clinically uncomplicated acute myocardial infarction. *American Journal of Cardiology, 55,* 635–638.

Valliant, G. E., Meyer, S. E., Mukamal, K., & Soldz, S. (1998). Are social supports in late midlife a cause or a result of successful physical aging? *Psychological Medicine, 28,* 1159–1168.

Theoretical Perspectives on Social Context, Cognition, and Aging

15

Fredda Blanchard-Fields
Antje Kalinauskas

The majority of past research on cognitive changes and aging has provided compelling documentation of losses in cognitive abilities as we grow older (e.g., Zacks, Hasher, & Li, 2000). The question is whether these findings reflect a complete picture of how cognitive functioning changes across the latter half of the life span. In other words, do they accurately reflect the full potential of older adults' abilities and knowledge? A very different picture of aging emerges when cognitive functioning is placed in a socioemotional context. In fact, positive gains in cognitive functioning across adulthood have become increasingly more evident as research examines the role that pragmatic and socioemotional context plays as it interacts with cognitive performance. For example, along with cognitive decline, researchers also find that emotional processing, social expertise, and emotion regulation remain intact and may even demonstrate growth across the latter half of the life span (Blanchard-Fields, 2007; Carstensen & Mikels, 2005; Hess, 2005).

These findings highlight the importance of the functional dynamics of everyday cognitive behavior. Functional dynamics involve abilities and knowledge necessary to effectively adapt to the demands and opportunities that individuals are confronted with on an everyday basis (Blanchard-Fields, 2007). In order to understand the functional dynamics of cognitive functioning, one must take into consideration how life experiences, social interactions, beliefs, and emotions influence motivational goals for processing information in daily life. As individuals grow older, processing goals change, and what may seem like a deficit at one level can also be viewed as adaptive at another level. For example, a processing goal that has received much theoretical attention in the aging literature is reflected in the positivity effect (Carstensen, Mikels, & Mather, 2006). This effect involves a selective processing priority for positive over negative information on the part of older adults. Given that older adults tend to avoid negative information, examining such recall could underestimate an older adult's capacity. If, on the other hand, the focus is on neutral or more positive information, a more positive picture of an older adult's memory could be observed. In fact, in memory experiments, older adults recall and recognize more positive images and neutral images over negative ones in comparison with young adults (Charles, Mather, & Carstensen, 2003, experiment 1), and they show better performance in a working-memory task for positive emotional stimuli in comparison to negative emotional stimuli (Mikels, Larkin, Reuter-Lorenz, & Carstensen, 2005).

What becomes particularly evident in findings such as these is that although certain basic cognitive mechanisms decline, such as episodic memory or speed of processing, older adults may also possess social knowledge and abilities that allow them to function quite effectively, particularly when cognition is examined in a social context. In other words, cognitive decline in basic mechanisms does not necessarily translate into how older adults process information in an everyday social context. One avenue of research exemplifying this perspective focuses on age-related differences in the way adults process information in a social context and subsequently make social judgments. It is in this domain that older adults are able to draw on an accumulated wealth of social knowledge and adaptive strategies when confronted with situations requiring judgment and decision making. The goal of this chapter is to consider the impact of contextual factors on social judgments in older adulthood by identifying developmental mechanisms and contexts that determine when older adults' social judgments are optimal or adaptive and when they are not.

Age Differences in Social Judgments

There have been a growing number of studies examining age differences in social judgment accuracy. A typical finding suggests that older adults rely on heuristic processing when making social judgments, rendering them more susceptible to predispositions when making judgments (Chen & Blanchard-Fields, 2000; Hess, McGee, Woodburn, & Bolstad, 1998). For example, older adults tend to rely more on easily accessible knowledge structures when forming impressions (Hess &

Follet, 1994; Hess et al., 1998), to rely on stereotypes when making source attributions (Mather, Johnson, & De Leonardis, 1999), to be more susceptible to easily accessible information when making social judgments (Jacoby, 1999), and to exhibit an increased tendency toward making dispositional inferences when making causal attributions, such as laying blame on one individual for a negative outcome without considering extenuating circumstances (Blanchard-Fields, 1996, 1999).

In a number of studies, we consistently find that older adults tend to make more dispositional attributions than young adults (Blanchard-Fields, 1994, 1996; Blanchard-Fields, Baldi, & Stein, 1999; Blanchard-Fields & Horhota, 2005; Mienaltowski & Blanchard-Fields, 2005). For example, older adults attribute more blame for undesirable outcomes to characters involved in an ambiguous interpersonal conflict situation than young adults do without considering extenuating or exacerbating situational information (Blanchard-Fields, 1994, 1996; Blanchard-Fields et al., 1999). In addition, older adults are more likely to demonstrate judgmental biases in correspondence bias paradigms (see Blanchard-Fields & Horhota, 2005; Mienaltowski & Blanchard-Fields, 2005) and when detecting deceit (Stanley & Blanchard-Fields, 2008).

At first blush, evidence in the social cognitive literature suggests that reduced processing capacity and foreclosed thinking styles (as measured by the construct need for closure; Kruglanski & Webster, 1996) may account for the fact that older adults too often rely on easily accessible trait-based information in making social judgments as opposed to engaging in more elaborative and analytical processing (Hess, 1999; Hess, Waters, & Bolstad, 2000). Mainstream research on social cognition demonstrates that elaborative and deliberative social judgments depend on concurrent cognitive demand. For example, when under high cognitive load, individuals tend to rely on initial dispositional inferences while ignoring compelling situational causes (the correspondence bias) when making causal attributions (Gilbert & Malone, 1995), or they overweigh the most salient explanation (situational or dispositional) at the expense of less salient explanations (Trope & Gaunt, 2000). This suggests a cognitive mechanism accounting for older adults' reliance on heuristic processing when making judgments. If capacity limitations result in such biases in young adults, it stands to reason that older adults who have reduced processing capacity may be predisposed to rely even more on highly accessible social information and not deliberate on situational details.

For example, we found that in contrast to young adults, older adults' social judgments, such as indicating what a prison sentence should be for a target that committed a crime, were more influenced by false information exacerbating or extenuating the crime despite the fact that this information was explicitly labeled as false and they were instructed to ignore this information (Chen & Blanchard-Fields, 2000). According to social cognitive theory, individuals automatically process rapidly presented false information as true at first and then subsequently correct this initial processing bias. The latter process takes cognitive effort. Thus, it could be that older adults do not correct their initial processing of false information as true (or false) given limited cognitive capacity. In line with this assumption, a cognitive load was imposed on young adults to also deny them the cognitive capacity needed to correct the immediate processing. In turn, they performed similarly to older adults (i.e., in this condition, they too were unable to ignore the false information). We found similar findings when we imposed time constraint in making social judgments (Chen & Blanchard-Fields, 1997).

However, social cognitive research also suggests that individual differences in the content of relevant social schemas (beliefs, values, social rules, and so on) are activated when making causal attributions about particular problem situations (Bargh, 1989; Fazio, Sanbonmatsu, Powell, & Kardes, 1986; Gilbert & Malone, 1995; Krull, 1993). In other words, individuals differ in the extent to which the content of specific situations will trigger such social schemas relevant to their social judgments. Thus, regardless of age, individuals differ in the extent to which their beliefs are relevant to how a person should behave in particular social situations. If these beliefs are violated, a dispositional bias in causal explanations can result (Blanchard-Fields & Hertzog, 2000).

Consider the following example:

> *Allen had been dating Barbara for over a year. At Barbara's suggestion, they moved in together. Everybody kept asking when they were getting married. Allen found it extremely uncomfortable to live with Barbara and not be married to her. Even though Barbara disagreed, Allen kept bringing up the issue of marriage. Eventually, they broke up.*

If a person believes that "you should live together before you are married," then that person would not stop to consider situational information (such as peer pressure from the family) and blame Allen for the relationship breakup. According to social cognitive perspectives on causal attributions, the consideration of such situational factors requires more elaborative processing (Gilbert & Malone, 1995). In our research, we repeatedly find that older adults are more likely to attribute the cause of negative outcomes, such as the end of the relationship, to personal characteristics of the main character and blame him or her for the breakup (Blanchard-Fields, 1999). However, when we examined social beliefs related to the content of the story vignettes, such as the one illustrated previously, we found that age differences in social beliefs and values relevant to our vignette conflict situations accounted for age differences in causal attribution biases. Furthermore, cognitive functioning did not account for these age differences, suggesting that social mechanisms such as beliefs were the prepotent factors influencing when a social judgment bias occurs.

In essence, individuals who held traditional beliefs about romance (e.g., regarding whether to live with someone before marrying) were more likely to blame individuals whose behavior violated those beliefs, such as nontraditional characters like Barbara. Conversely, individuals who held nontraditional beliefs (e.g., living together before marriage) were more likely to blame traditional characters (e.g., Allen). This research demonstrates that different social contexts evoke differential beliefs and values that underlie one's judgments. In turn, the inhibition of deliberative processing should occur when a core belief of the rater is violated by the behavior of the actor. Thus, age differences in blame and/or dispositional attributions should arise when persons of different ages have different patterns of values and beliefs that will be primed by each vignette, resulting in age differences in the activation of analytic or heuristic modes of processing. By this account, age differences can be understood on the basis of generational differences in belief content rather than normative decline in information processing capacity or efficiency. In support of this, Horhota and Blanchard-Fields (2006) found that personal beliefs strongly held by older adults guide their judgments of others' attitudes more so than they do for young adults' judgments of others. More specifically, they found that personal beliefs predicted the correspondence bias in older adults but not in young adults.

Traditional beliefs also influence people's ability to take different perspectives in relationship conflicts, such as the Allen and Barbara scenario. Stange and Blanchard-Fields (2006) asked participants to take either the perspective of the woman, the man, or an objective adviser and investigated the effect of this perspective taking on attributions of blame. Age differences in blame disappeared for the partner whose perspective was not taken—everybody blamed the partner whose perspective was not taken. However, in contrast to young adults, older adults still blamed the person whose perspective they took, and this tendency was magnified in those individuals holding traditional family beliefs. This study suggests that age differences can be altered through instructions of perspective taking—but it is easier to encourage people to blame others more than to make them blame others less. And again, beliefs make it more difficult for individuals to put themselves in someone else's shoes.

The research reviewed thus far here highlights the importance of the socioemotional context. When beliefs are violated, it invokes an emotional reaction. It may be the case that this affective response influences when dispositional tendencies occur. However, there is a need for a more direct assessment of the role emotions play on age differences in social judgments. In a recent study, Mienaltowski and Blanchard-Fields (2005) induced positive, negative, and neutral moods in young and older participants. Participants then completed an attitude-attribution task in which they were asked to identify a target essay writer's true attitude toward a social issue. Within the attitude-attribution task, participants read an essay that was either in favor of or opposed to capital punishment. Participants were told that the essay writer was not free to choose the position endorsed in the essay. Past research suggests that in young adults, positive mood induces heuristic processing (and an increase in the correspondence bias) and negative mood induces more analytic processing (a reduction in the correspondence bias). This was replicated in young adults. However, for older adults, the opposite was true. A positive mood decreased the correspondence bias in older adults, whereas a negative mood increased this bias. Furthermore, again, individual differences in cognitive capacity (i.e., working memory) did not account for age- or mood-related effects. It appears that older adults are more likely than young adults to focus on emotion regulation when confronted with negative emotions, thus taxing their cognitive resources to deliberate on the situational information.

Finally, social context and beliefs are also implicated in other research that finds that a dispositional attribution tendency on the part of older adults is eliminated when the situation highlights the plausibility of extenuating explanations for the event. When the perceptual salience of the situational forces was accentuated, it did not encourage older adults to pay attention to situational information. However, when a social motivational explanation for the behavior was emphasized, it impacted older adults' explanations for the behavior (Blanchard-Fields & Horhota, 2005). In this case, it appears that although older adults may be prone to biased or misinformed social judgments in some situations, these biases can be eliminated when older adults access and use social knowledge structures related to beliefs as well as knowledge of social motivational components of how individuals behave.

In sum, we find that under certain conditions (e.g., when extensive use of cognitive capacities such as executive control or inhibitory control is required), cognitive mechanisms explain why older adults ignore other relevant sources of information and resort to more heuristic processing when making social judgments. Accordingly, in these situations, reducing cognitive load in older adults in order to free up cognitive resources, such as allowing more time to process information (Chen & Blanchard-Fields, 1997) or inducing a positive mood (Mienaltowski & Blanchard-Fields, 2005), attenuates social judgment biases.

We have also identified social mechanisms that account for age differences in social judgment biases: age differences in the content of social knowledge and social belief systems. In this case, individuals at any age will not engage in elaborative social cognitive processing when actors in social contexts violate strongly held beliefs about appropriate ways to behave in social situations. Accordingly, we find that age differences in social norms and rules regarding appropriate behaviors (in particular, the violation of social rules) account for age differences in causal attributions in the type of social vignettes we have examined in our research. Other social mechanisms involve the presentation of situational information that is relevant to older adults' beliefs regarding ways to approach social situations (e.g., the plausibility of situational pressure; Blanchard-Fields & Horhota, 2006). In this case, social judgment biases are also reduced.

However, what is not addressed in the previously mentioned social mechanism explanation of social judgment biases is whether a dispositional inference is truly a "bias" across situations. For example, in the case of the correspondence bias (underestimating the influence of situational information in favor of a rapid dispositional inference), one also needs to determine if the situational information is relevant or makes a difference in evaluating the particular social context. If it does, then, indeed, the situational information needs to be taken into account in one's assessment of the situation. However, if the situation information is deemed irrelevant to the context, initial dispositional attributions may be sufficient to evaluate the situation. In this set of circumstances, older adults may draw on accumulated experiences and strategies for evaluating social situations, in other words, a form of social expertise. This involves well-instantiated belief systems or knowledge about how individuals typically behave and react in social situations. At this point, it may be deemed unnecessary to consider situational information further given their extensive experience in dealing with the vicissitudes of daily life. In essence, applying a social expertise perspective suggests that it is not necessarily appropriate to adjust one's initial judgments, especially if you do not have the appropriate information to warrant an adjustment. It may be the case that older adults, with increasing levels of social expertise, know when *not* to deliberate over the situation given that a sufficient amount of information is not available to render a definitive judgment. We address this supposition in the next section.

Social Expertise, Aging, and Social Judgments

As illustrated here, older adults rely more on dispositional judgments than young adults. This corresponds with research suggesting that older adults may also have more social expertise in the domain of dispositional judgments than young adults do. Hess and colleagues provided participants with trait information that was more or less diagnostic for an underlying trait (Hess & Auman, 2001; Hess, Bolstad, Woodburn, & Auman, 1999; Hess & Pullen, 1994; Leclerc & Hess, 2007). Trait diagnosticity refers to the different implications of positive and negative behaviors in diagnosing an underlying trait. For instance, negative behaviors, such as lying, are seen as better cues, that is, more diagnostic cues for the underlying trait of honesty, than positive behaviors, such as telling the truth. Hess and his colleagues have demonstrated that older adults are more likely to make judgments corresponding to the trait implications of a behavioral description than young adults. Moreover, older adults are more likely to differentially adjust their initial ratings, depending on the trait diagnosticity of the behavior than young adults (Hess & Auman, 2001; Hess et al., 1999, Hess & Pullen, 1994; Leclerc & Hess, 2007). These findings suggest that older adults' social expertise in the use of trait diagnosticity contributes to more accurate dispositional judgments than young adults'. In other words, this is a case where relying on dispositional information can be adaptive.

Another adaptive influence that social expertise has on dispositional judgments may be in the ability of older adults to recognize the limits of their own knowledge as well as the knowledge presented to them. For instance, in situations when trait-related information is inconsistent with initial impressions of an individual, making an "accurate" social judgment may not simply involve correcting or updating a dispositional judgment to fit the new situational information. Rather, accurate judgments may involve the recognition that sufficient information is lacking to make a definitive statement about someone's trait (e.g., friendliness). The growing social expertise in older adults may be reflected in their ability to understand when their knowledge base is limited.

In support of this, Stange and Blanchard-Fields (2008a) found that older adults changed their impressions of a target's friendliness less than young adults did when they were provided with inconsistent information regarding the target actor's friendliness. In this study, an initial piece of information portrayed friendly or nonfriendly behavior of an actor when listening to an individual talk about his or her problems. This was followed by a second piece of information that extenuated the behavior through situational information (e.g., in the case of an unfriendly listener, additional information maintained that the listener had a long and trying day and had a headache and so on). In this scenario, young adults corrected their initial attributions with the situational information more than older adults did. However, young adults' corrections were so extreme that they basically discounted the first piece of information. In contrast, older adults' ratings tended to be less extreme than young adults, suggesting that they did not disregard the first piece of information but rather integrated both parts. In other words, older adults embraced the uncertainty created through the presentation of conflicting pieces of information by refraining from extreme judgments. It may be the case that in some situations, such as the one illustrated previously, young adults overuse situational correction and, accordingly, may be less able than older adults to appropriately gauge the amount of correction necessary. Overall, young adults may lack the social expertise necessary to recognize the limits of their knowledge. This would be in accordance with theories on postformal development suggesting that an adequate management of the uncertainty involved in complex life situations develops well into older adulthood (Blanchard-Fields, 1986; Commons, Richards, & Armon, 1984; Perry, 1970).

Together, these findings suggest that older adults' social judgment processes may be adaptive in contexts that require the weighing of dispositional information as well as the acknowledgment and management of uncertainty of social judgment situations. Refraining from extreme judgments when information is contradictory may be a result of extended experience with different social experiences and tasks. In general, social expertise will be found in tasks and situations in which older adults have more experience than young adults do. In this case, the main criterion for social expertise is the degree to which a social judgment is adaptive with respect to the particular situation one is encountering. However, what is missing at this point is an important validation to determine when social judgments are adaptive. In other words, what are the outcomes of social judgments?

Outcomes of Social Judgments: Why Do Social Judgments Matter?

How are social judgments related to everyday life functioning? When are social judgments adaptive? In our research, we have identified conditions under which older adults' social judgments are less than optimal and conditions under which older adults' judgment tendencies reflect adaptive functioning. As indicated earlier, conditions where older adults' performance is compromised correspond well to situations where basic mechanisms that decline with age are necessary for accurate judgments. An illustrative example is observed in a study in which we demonstrated that the accuracy of social judgments can have important implications for interpersonal functioning, as in the ability to detect deceit in others (Stanley & Blanchard-Fields, 2008). We found that older adults are less accurate in detecting whether someone is lying about a criminal or opinion question. In part, older adults' lower deceit detection judgments were attributed to the fact that emotion recognition ability (i.e., a form of pattern recognition in identifying emotions in others) is lower in older adults in comparison to young adults. In addition, there were social mechanisms operating. Older adults exhibited a truth bias and expected most people to be honest. Whereas this may be true in the majority of interactions, again, there may be contexts such as deceit detection judgments in which this general heuristic may not be adaptive.

The issue of adaptivity of social judgments is a key issue if we are attempting to go beyond simple social psychological models that rely on cognitive mechanisms and suggest that older adults' performance is inferior and biased in comparison to young adults. We are in the process of examining adaptive outcomes of social judgment in a number of different domains. Although at this stage our research in this area is very preliminary, there are interesting implications as to when older adults rely on dispositional attributional tendencies (or so-called biases) and how they lead to adaptive behavior. For instance, in one recent study we investigated the relationship between social judgments and reactions to one's own personal problems (Stange & Blanchard-Fields, 2008c).

When interviewed about recent personal problems that they experienced, older adults attributed less blame to themselves and others close to them when asked to describe what caused the problem. In this case, older adults seemed to make less dispositional judgments (in this case, blame judgments) than young adults. Why would it be adaptive for older adults not to blame themselves and close others for their own problems? We found that, regardless of age, individuals who blamed others for their family problems experienced more anger and confronted others more often than those who did not attribute the cause of their own problems to others. There is growing recognition that anger is a particularly toxic emotion for older adults (Blanchard-Fields, 2007; Consedine, Magai, & Bonanno, 2002). This suggests that by avoiding the tendency to blame one's own family members for causing a problem, older adults may protect themselves against the experience of anger. Given this potentially positive outcome, this study highlights the importance of investigating the adaptive value of social judgments. Whereas older adults may be comfortable blaming others in fictitious vignette scenarios, they may not do so in highly self-relevant contexts that potentially arouse high levels of anger. However, this research is in its beginning state. More research is needed to study outcomes of social judgments, such as anger and problem-solving strategies.

In some cases, there may be no age differences in the adaptive value of judgments. In a recent study, we examined individual differences in the quality of advice to a fictitious relationship conflict, such as the Allen and Barbara scenario. When asked what advice they would offer to the couple, some individuals presented extremely one-sided or negative perspectives in the advice they gave, whereas others demonstrated a positive, optimistic orientation toward the well-being of others that included an emphasis on the "common good" (see Sternberg, 1998). We called this quality "benevolence" of the advice. Individuals who perceived the conflict as simultaneously caused by both partners (i.e., interactive attributions) showed more benevolence in their advice to the couple than individuals with less interactive attributions, such as blaming one character or another (Stange & Blanchard-Fields, 2008b). This suggests that a general orientation toward interactive perceptions or attributions of behavior may be an important individual difference variable that has adaptive value in both young and older adults.

Together, these studies provide first evidence for the importance of attributions for different everyday life task outcomes, such as how to prevent one from succumbing to deceit or a scam, effective problem solving, and giving advice to others. An interesting route for future studies is to move beyond social judgments to decision making. How do attributions influence decision making in both young and older adults?

A Theoretical Model for Judgments in Social Context

In the previously mentioned review of our program of research, we have argued for two main points. First, whether social judgment processes rely on heuristic processing (e.g., dispositional or blame inferences) or more deliberative situational adjustments of initial judgments (e.g., correcting a dispositional inference to include situational constraints) depends on a confluence of factors that include the social context and person characteristics. Second, whether the outcome of a social judgment is adaptive or nonadaptive is not determined solely by whether heuristic or deliberative judgment processes are engaged. For example, in past social cognitive research, findings suggest that when an individual ignores situational information and relies on heuristic processes that lead to dispositional attributions, this reflects a bias in thinking (e.g., the correspondence bias). In contrast, we argue that we need to examine further whether such "biases" in reasoning or judgments lead to adaptive or nonadaptive outcomes. If it leads to an adaptive outcome (e.g., effective problem solving or avoiding anger), doubt is cast on whether the initial dispositional inference should be labeled a "bias." Instead, we turn our attention away from categorizing initial dispositional inferences as biased or not. Instead, we argue from a contextual approach that one must consider the joint effects of the social judgment process, the social context, and person factors in order to determine conditions under which the consequences of one's social judgment are adaptive or nonadaptive.

Figure 15.1 illustrates this approach. In the first set of factors, we list the antecedents and correlates of social judgment processes. On the one hand, individuals are intrinsically made up of personal characteristics or factors such as cognitive ability, personality traits and dispositions, levels of social expertise, and belief systems. On the other hand, the presenting problem consists of two major extrinsic contextual factors. First, the social content of the situation determines how relevant and important the situation is to the individual. This includes the degree to which the situation is relevant to one's self-concept, activates social and processing goals, and poses challenges to effective self-

15.1

A theoretical model for judgments in social context.

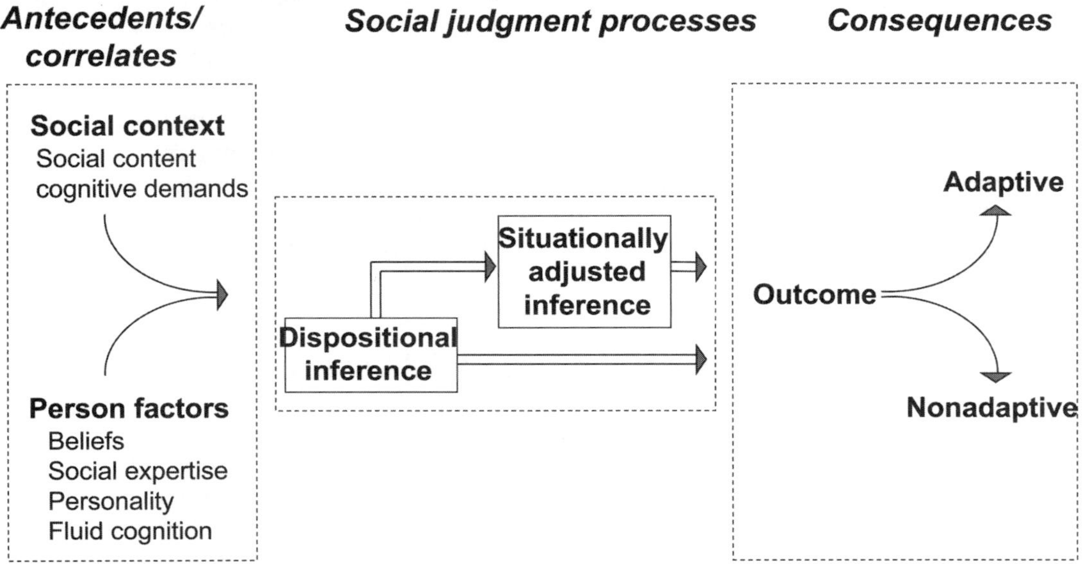

regulation. Second, the presenting problem situation can vary in the cognitive demands or cognitive load placed on the individual.

Together, these antecedents and correlates help determine when an individual will rely on the two social judgment processes depicted in the second set of factors in our model: an initial dispositional inference or a situational adjustment of that inference. Most social psychological models focus on the social judgment process level of our model. When considering antecedent factors, they are interested mainly in the degree to which one factor, cognitive load, influences when an individual does or does not correct an initial dispositional attribution given extenuating or exacerbating situational information. However, in our model, cognitive demand is only one influential factor and may not be the most important one. Instead, we argue that resource limitations may operate in conjunction with other eliciting antecedent conditions, such as violation of beliefs or social expertise, to produce a reliance on dispositional inferences.

Finally, a relatively understudied component of our model indicates whether a chosen social judgment process is adaptive or nonadaptive. This is the gold standard as to whether a social judgment such as a dispositional inference is "biased" or is simply contextually adaptive. In other words, a dispositional inference may rely on limited information but result in an adaptive assessment of a situation in which one must act. We are not the first to establish the notion that such heuristic judgments are adaptive. For example, Gigerenzer and colleagues (Gigerenzer, Todd, & the ABC Research Group, 2000) have advocated that "fast-and-frugal" judgments are quite adaptive in the context of daily living. Despite the fact that individuals tend to use less information (e.g., are more frugal in their use of information and rely on dispositional inferences), they are also just as accurate in the quality and outcome of their decision.

Thus far, our program of research has examined specific components of our model, in particular the relationship between antecedents/correlates and social judgment processes. For example, we have demonstrated that situations requiring a high cognitive demand lead to dispositional inferences. Similarly, we suggest that social expertise, such as embracing uncertainty in a situation, can also lead to less correction of initial dispositional inferences. Finally, a third mechanism, violation of one's beliefs, can also lead to a reliance on dispositional attributions, such as blaming tendencies. Although all these factors may lead to a reliance on dispositional inferences, they may also lead to differential outcome adaptivity. Reliance on dispositional inferences solely because one does not have the cognitive capacity to deliberate on situational constraints could indeed result in inaccurate judgments or decisions that have unfavorable outcomes. This is particularly illustrative when a judge orders the jury to ignore incriminating information presented in a court of law. In this case, reduced executive control and inhibitory processes may impair accurate judgments. However, when social judgments are based on social expertise, where the dispositional judgment is determined by accumulated social knowledge about how individuals operate in certain situations, the snap judgment could result in an adaptive outcome. This is illustrated in our example of trait diagnosticity or embracing uncertainty when making judgments about others. In this case, whether or not there is a cognitive load becomes immaterial. Given that social expertise entails a well-instantiated and easily accessible social knowledge structure to draw from, cognitive effort is not the determining factor. In such situations, social expertise can serve as a buffer against the negative effects of cognitive decline as we grow older.

Future Directions

In this chapter, we have outlined a model of studying adaptive social judgments across the life span. Our research in the area of adaptivity is still in its early stages. However, initial findings suggest that there are no uniform consequences of heuristic versus deliberate processing. We hope to convince the reader that older adults' performance on social judgment tasks not only is a reflection of their cognitive decline and social rigidity but reflects adaptive value as well. However, in order to do so, further research is needed to refine our operationalizations of outcomes, adaptivity, and social expertise. In the final section, we address these issues by outlining several areas for future investigation.

First, it is important to further identify a larger repertoire of outcomes of social judgments. What are some of the key domains of functioning we need to look at when considering consequences of social judgments? A first candidate is health and quality-of-life issues in older adulthood. One area essential to quality of life is relationship satisfaction or positive interpersonal functioning. Studies show that relationship satisfaction is highly related to positive and accurate perceptions and interpretations of the actions of one's partner (Blanchard-Fields & Cooper, 2003). However, the majority of these studies rely on self-report measures of satisfaction and well-being. Criteria for effective social judgments can be further extended to more objective measures of well-being, such as physiological outcome variables related to stress (e.g., diurnal cortisol patterns).

Second, judgments are closely related to decision-making outcomes. For instance, if you perceive a person as trustworthy, how will this influence your choice about buying a product from him or her? Although there is a multitude of research examining criteria and information one needs to make a good decision, the role of social judgments is relatively ignored. This has numerous implications for older adults when making economic decisions, for consumer behavior, for health decisions, and for advance directives, among others. For example, if the antecedent factors include time constraints (which increases cognitive load), older adults may be more susceptible to snap judgments and fall prey to a scam. When older adults rely on their social expertise, the deliberative or heuristic nature of the judgment process will not necessarily compromise the adaptivity of the outcome.

Second, it is important to better define criteria for adaptiveness. How can biases be distinguished from adaptive functioning? For example, relying on stereotypes may be adaptive in some ways (e.g., providing a quick judgment with useful but limited information). However, in other situations, it may lead to biased judgments by obscuring important information that needs to be considered to have an accurate perception of an individual. In addition, research shows that young and older adults have different processing goals (Carstensen et al., 2006; Hoppmann, Coats, & Blanchard-Fields, 2007), rendering different outcomes adaptive for people of different age groups. For instance, when blaming individuals who are socially close, the emotional costs are high, motivating older adults to avoid such snap dispositional judgments. One potential avenue for future research is to study processing goals in conjunction with social judgment processes.

Third, the concept of social expertise is theoretically not well developed and is vague. Several issues need to be addressed by future research to make the concept fruitful for empirical research. We need to first describe more precisely what constitutes social expertise. In which areas of social cognitive functioning do we find social expertise? How is expert social performance different from novice performance? In what way is expert performance superior to novice performance?

Finally, by taking a life span perspective, we need to identify mechanisms that lead to the development of expertise. One model of expertise in fundamental questions of life is the Berlin Wisdom Paradigm (Baltes & Smith, 1990; Baltes & Staudinger, 2000). Baltes and colleagues identify conditions that lead to the development of expertise in fundamental questions of life, such as general person-related factors, expertise-specific factors, and facilitative experiential contexts. Which factors contribute to the development of social expertise? Which age-related factors can facilitate the development of social expertise (see Staudinger, 1999)? Are there some age-related factors that can hinder the expression of social expertise? In a recent study, Stange and Blanchard-Fields (2008b) measured life knowledge expressed in advice giving for relationship conflicts. There was no overall effect of age on level of life knowledge. However, in high performers, older adults demonstrated higher levels of knowledge than young adults. In contrast, among low performers, young adults outperformed older adults. They found that among low performers, a lack of cognitive resources as well as measures of social rigidity (traditional family values and personal need for structure) predicted low levels of knowledge. These findings illustrate that social expertise may develop with age in some adults. However, age-related factors, such as decline in cognitive resources as well as increasing social rigidity, may hinder the expression of life knowledge. This study points to the importance of studying different trajectories of social expertise development. Along these lines, theories of life span development suggest that age per se does not explain developmental outcomes in adulthood very well (see Baltes, 1987, 1997). In our model, we identified social expertise as a person-related factor. However, future research needs to incorporate the dynamic change of social expertise across the life span and how it differentially impacts social judgments.

Conclusion

In this chapter, we outlined both conditions in which older adults' social judgments are more accurate and circumstances in which their judgments are less than optimal. Specifically, we tried to highlight the importance of expertise in older adults' functioning. In laboratory-based tasks that require decontextualized social judgments under conditions of time constraint, young adults will outperform older adults in terms of the accuracy of their judgments. However, in ill-defined real-life contexts, older adults may exhibit social expertise that allows them to make more appropriate judgments compared to young adults. These conditions include trait diagnosticity and embracing uncertainty.

We presented a theoretical model incorporating the confluence of factors that are involved in such social judgment processes. We believe that this approach can help examine the interactive influence of a processing resource view with a social contextual view of age differences in social judgments and their outcomes and, perhaps, other kinds of social information processing as well.

References

Baltes, P. B. (1987). Theoretical propositions of life-span developmental psychology: On the dynamics between growth and decline. *Developmental Psychology, 23,* 611–626.

Baltes, P. B. (1997). On the incomplete architecture of human ontogeny: Selection, optimization, and compensation as foundation of developmental theory. *American Psychologist, 52,* 366–380.

Baltes, P. B., & Smith, J. (1990). Toward a psychology of wisdom and its ontogenesis. In R. J. Sternberg (Ed.), *Wisdom: Its nature, origins, and development* (pp. 87–120). Cambridge: Cambridge University Press.

Baltes, P. B., & Staudinger, U. M. (2000). Wisdom: A meta-heuristic (pragmatic) to orchestrate mind and virtue toward excellence. *American Psychologist, 55,* 122–136.

Bargh, J. A. (1989). Conditional automaticity: Varieties of automatic influence in social perception and cognition. In J. S. Uleman & J. A. Bargh (Eds.), *Unintended thought* (pp. 3–51). New York: Guilford.

Blanchard-Fields, F. (1986). Reasoning on social dilemmas varying in emotional saliency: An adult developmental perspective. *Psychology and Aging, 1,* 325–333.

Blanchard-Fields, F. (1994). Age differences in causal attributions from an adult developmental perspective. *Journal of Gerontology, 49,* 43–51.

Blanchard-Fields, F. (1996). Causal attributions across the adult life span: The influence of social schemas, life context, and domain specificity. *Applied Cognitive Psychology, 10,* S137–S146.

Blanchard-Fields, F. (1999). Social schematicity and causal attributions. In T. M. Hess & F. Blanchard-Fields (Eds.), *Social cognition and aging* (pp. 219–236). San Diego, CA: Academic Press.

Blanchard-Fields, F. (2007). Everyday problem solving and emotion: An adult developmental perspective. *Current Directions in Psychological Science, 16,* 26–31.

Blanchard-Fields, F., Baldi, R., & Stein, R. (1999). Age relevance and context effects on attributions across the adult lifespan. *International Journal of Behavioural Development, 23,* 665–683.

Blanchard-Fields, F., & Cooper, C. (2003). Social cognition and social relationships. In F. Lang & K. Fingerman (Eds.), *Personal relationships across the lifespan* (pp. 268–289). New York: Cambridge University Press.

Blanchard-Fields, F., & Hertzog, C. (2000). Age differences in schematicity. In U. von Hecker, S. Dutke, & G. Sedak (Eds.), *Processes of generative mental representation and psychological adaptation* (pp. 1–24). Dordrecht: Kluwer.

Blanchard-Fields, F., & Horhota, M. (2005). Age differences in the correspondence bias: When a plausible explanation matters. *Journal of Gerontology: Social Sciences, 60,* 259–267.

Blanchard-Fields, F., & Horhota, M. (2006). How can the study of aging inform research on social cognition? *Social Cognition, 24,* 207–217.

Carstensen, L. L., & Mikels, J. A. (2005). At the intersection of emotion and cognition: Aging and the positivity effect. *Current Directions in Psychological Science, 14,* 117–121.

Carstensen, L. L., Mikels, J. A., & Mather, M. (2006). Aging and the intersection of cognition, motivation, and emotion. In J. E. Birren & K. W. Schaie (Eds.), *Handbook of the psychology of aging* (pp. 343–362). San Diego, CA: Academic Press.

Charles, S. T., Mather, M., & Carstensen, L. L. (2003). Aging and emotional memory: The forgettable nature of negative images for older adults. *Journal of Experimental Psychology: General, 132,* 310–324.

Chen, Y., & Blanchard-Fields, F. (1997). Age differences in stages of attributional processing. *Psychology and Aging, 12,* 694–703.

Chen, Y., & Blanchard-Fields, F. (2000). Unwanted thought: Age differences in the correction of social judgments. *Psychology and Aging, 15,* 475–482.

Commons, M. L., Richards, F. A., & Armon, C. (1984). *Beyond formal operations.* New York: Praeger.

Consedine, N. S., Magai, C., & Bonanno, G. A. (2002). Moderators of the emotion inhibition-health relationship: A review and research agenda. *Review of General Psychology, 6,* 204–228.

Fazio, R. H., Sanbonmatsu, D. M., Powell, M. C., & Kardes, F. R. (1986). On the automatic activation of attitudes. *Journal of Personality and Social Psychology, 50,* 229–238.

Gigerenzer, G. W., Todd, P. M., & the ABC Research Group. (2000). *Simple heuristics that make us smart.* Oxford: Oxford University Press.

Gilbert, D. T., & Malone, P. S. (1995). The correspondence bias. *Psychological Bulletin, 117,* 21–38.

Hess, T. M. (1999). Cognitive and knowledge-based influences on social representations. In T. M. Hess & F. Blanchard-Fields (Eds.), *Social cognition and aging* (pp. 237–263). San Diego, CA: Academic Press.

Hess, T. M. (2005). Memory and aging in context. *Psychological Bulletin, 131,* 383–406.

Hess, T. M., & Auman, C. (2001). Aging and social expertise: The impact of trait-diagnostic information on impressions of others. *Psychology and Aging, 16,* 497–510.

Hess, T. M., Bolstad, C. A., Woodburn, S. M., & Auman, C. (1999). Trait diagnosticity versus behavioral consistency as determinants of impression change in adulthood. *Psychology and Aging, 14,* 77–89.

Hess, T. M., & Follett, K. J. (1994). Adult age differences in the use of schematic and episodic information in making social judgments. *Aging, Neuropsychology, and Cognition, 1,* 54–66.

Hess, T. M., McGee, K. A., Woodburn, S. M., & Bolstad, C. A. (1998). Age-related priming effects in social judgments. *Psychology and Aging, 13,* 127–137.

Hess, T. M., & Pullen, S. M. (1994). Adult age differences in impression change processes. *Psychology and Aging, 9,* 237–250.

Hess, T. M., Waters, S. J., & Bolstad, C. A. (2000). Motivational and cognitive influences on affective priming in adulthood. *Journal of Gerontology: Social Sciences, 55,* P193–P204.

Hoppmann, C., Coats, A. H., & Blanchard-Fields, F. (2007). Examining the link between age-related goals and problem-solving strategy use. *Aging, Neuropsychology, and Cognition, 15,* 401–423.

Horhota, M., & Blanchard-Fields, F. (2006). Do beliefs and attributional complexity influence age differences in the correspondence bias? *Social Cognition, 24,* 310–337.

Jacoby, L. L. (1999). Deceiving the elderly: Effects of accessibility bias in cued recall performance. *Cognitive Neuropsychology, 16,* 417–436.

Kruglanski, A. W., & Webster, D. M. (1996). Motivated closing of the mind: "Seizing" and "freezing." *Psychological Review, 103,* 263–283.

Krull, D. S. (1993). Does the gist change the mill? The effect of the perceiver's inferential goal on the process of social inference. *Personality and Social Psychology Bulletin, 19,* 340–348.

Leclerc, C. M., & Hess, T. M. (2007). Age differences in the bases for social judgments: Tests of a social expertise perspective. *Experimental Aging Research, 33,* 95–120.

Mather, M., Johnson, M. K., & De Leonardis, D. M. (1999). Stereotype reliance in source monitoring: Age differences and neuropsychological test correlates. *Cognitive Neuropsychology, 16,* 437–458.

Mienaltowski, A., & Blanchard-Fields, F. (2005). The differential effects of mood on age differences in the correspondence bias. *Psychology and Aging, 20,* 589–600.

Mikels, J. A., Larkin, G. R., Reuter-Lorenz, P. A., & Carstensen, L. L. (2005). Divergent trajectories in the aging mind: Changes in working memory for affective versus visual information with age. *Psychology and Aging, 20,* 542–553.

Perry, W. (1970). *Forms of intellectual and ethical development in the college years.* New York: Holt, Rinehart and Winston.

Stange, A., & Blanchard-Fields, F. (2006, November). *Perspective taking and age-differences in causal attributions.* Paper presented at the Gerontological Society of America Conference, Dallas, TX.

Stange, A., & Blanchard-Fields, F. (2008a). *Correcting dispositional attributions in the face of uncertainty.* Manuscript submitted for publication.

Stange, A., & Blanchard-Fields, F. (2008b, April). *Giving wise advice—The relation between benevolence and life knowledge.* Poster presented at the 2008 Cognitive Aging Conference, Atlanta, GA.

Stange, A., & Blanchard-Fields, F. (2008c). *Causal attributions and everyday problem solving: How what you perceive becomes what you feel and do.* Manuscript in preparation.

Stanley, J. T., & Blanchard-Fields, F. (2008). Challenges older adults face in detecting deceit: The role of emotion recognition. *Psychology and Aging, 23,* 24–32.

Staudinger, U. M. (1999). Older and wiser? Integrating results from a psychological approach to the study of wisdom. *International Journal of Behavioral Development, 23,* 641–664.

Sternberg, R. J. (1998). A balance theory of wisdom. *Review of General Psychology, 2,* 347–365.

Trope, Y., & Gaunt, R. (2000). Processing alternative explanations of behavior: Correction or integration? *Journal of Personality and Social Psychology, 79,* 344–354.

Zacks, R. T., Hasher, L., & Li, K. Z. H. (2000). Human memory. In F. I. M. Craik & T. A. Salthouse (Eds.), *The handbook of aging and cognition* (pp. 293–357). Mahwah, NJ: Lawrence Erlbaum Associates.

16 Dynamic Integration Theory: Emotion, Cognition, and Equilibrium in Later Life

Gisela Labouvie-Vief

Over the past few decades, there has been substantial growth in research on the developmental course of emotions in adulthood and aging. In interpreting this body of research, two divergent points of views are currently proposed. On the one hand, some authors argue that aging is related to an increase in emotional well-being that is thought to be the result of general improvements in emotion regulation (e.g., Carstensen, Isaacowitz, & Charles, 1999). On the other hand, much evidence suggests that older adults' ability to process affective information is frequently compromised, especially when impairments of cognitive functions become increasingly evident (e.g., Labouvie-Vief, 2003; Labouvie-Vief & Marquez, 2004).

This work was supported by NIA grant AG09203 and Swiss National Foundation grant 100013–113857 to Gisela Labouvie-Vief.

In this chapter, I outline a theoretical integration of these two perspectives: dynamic integration theory (DIT), which suggests that the relationship between cognition and emotion is inherently dynamic. Emotion regulation is seen not as a trait like ability but as a dynamic response to challenges that for a given individual, depending on circumstances, can vary from mastery to breakdown. However, DIT proposes that this dynamic range is characteristic of individuals but changes with general developmental and more situational conditions. These changes are related to variations in the set point that determines if the individual responds with mastery or breakdown.

The core of DIT (see Labouvie-Vief & Marquez, 2004) has been influenced by Piaget's (1981) view of affect and invokes the equilibrium-maintaining interplay of automatic emotional processes on the one hand and conscious, computationally complex cognitive and executive processes (often tied to complex linguistic and symbolic processes) in the regulation of arousal on the other. Brent (1978) referred to this relationship as a trade-off of conceptual complexity for organic tension. On that view, the ability to manage high levels of arousal or tension requires higher-order conscious control processes that maintain arousal within tolerable limits and even, as in the model of Lawton and Nahemow (1973), seek out a certain level of tension. However, if the efficiency of these higher-order processes is suboptimal, individuals engage in compensatory strategies the primary aim of which is to maintain hedonic tone and organismic equilibrium. They do so, however, by falling back on a lower level of cognitive complexity.

I present this theory in three sections. First, I briefly discuss currently existing interpretations of emotions in adulthood and later life as well as the way in which they address problems of equilibrium regulation. Second, I extend this discussion to a life span developmental context and propose a theory of the dynamic interaction of developmental, situational, and individual difference-related mechanisms that result in more and less effective ways of regulating equilibrium. Third, I follow this theoretical section with a selected empirical review of studies that support this mechanism and suggest that it provides a broad integration of the literature on adult emotion regulation in development and aging generally.

Cognition, Emotion, and Views of Emotion Regulation in Later Life: Some Questions

One class of current theories of emotion regulation in later life tend to begin with what Mroczek and Kolarz (1998) called the paradox of well-being: despite the losses of health, cognition, and social functioning in later life, older individuals in general report high levels of well-being and positive emotions. Thus, despite the various losses, older individuals develop compensatory strategies that protect them from being emotionally overwhelmed and even may foster highly adaptive ways that preserve their emotional balance and guarantee the kind of well-being that Erikson (1985) referred to as integrity. In this section, I briefly summarize some of the models that talk about such strategies. I then raise some questions these models leave unanswered.

Adaptive Aging and Compensation

Of a handful of current theories of emotion regulation in later life, a particularly popular one is Carstensen's (e.g., Carstensen et al., 1999) social-emotional selectivity theory (SSC), which states that changes in aging individuals' emotion regulation processes are initiated by the perception that time is shortened. As they become aware of the limitations of time, they experience a change in goals, deemphasizing those that are related to the pursuit of knowledge and information gathering. Instead, according to Carstensen, they concentrate on emotion-related goals. In particular, to maximize their emotional well-being, they reduce their social networks, trimming more distant contacts and concentrating instead on closer, more intimate relationships.

In support of SSC, Carstensen and collaborators (for review, see Charles & Carstensen, 1997) point to the fact that older individuals tend to report good levels of well-being and positive affect especially if they are healthy (Kunzmann, Little, & Smith, 2000), that they display less physiological reactivity than young adults in many tasks, and that, generally, they appear to process positive information preferentially. While they also report changes in size of social networks and trimming those to closer contacts, it is not clear that time limitations are in fact related to improved emotion regulation (Kessler & Staudinger, 2007).

Brandtstädter (2008) also addresses the apparent paradox of how elders, in the face of decline, manage to maintain good self-concepts and well-being. This author proposes that this resilience can be accomplished by a shift from an assimilative to an accommodative mode of self-regulation. Assimilation, in this context, involves strategies that attempt to maintain self-aspects that were desired in the past. For example, in the face of physical decline, individuals may multiply their efforts to maintain physical or interpersonal attractiveness or, in the face of intellectual restrictions, strategies to maintain their accustomed-to level of energy and competence.

Accommodation, in contrast, involves adjustments to self-representations that are aimed at buffering the experience of loss. Realizing that our resources are failing, we may rearrange our values and rescale our goals, generally adjusting our aspirations in such a way that they fit with the given situation. In addition, we may immunize ourselves from the full experience of losses by palliative interpretations that put negative experiences in a positive light and so forth. Research by Brandtstädter and his colleagues suggests that this shift in strategy results in the recovery and maintenance of a positive view of self and adaptive personal development in later life (for review, see Brandstädter, 2008).

Both theories, as indicated, show substantial support, but they also leave questions open. Their focus on goal changes and adjustments remains highly metatheoretical and inferential in focusing on high-level intentional processes. As a result, they lack a detailed analysis of the bottom-up mechanisms involved. Just how do certain experiences of loss produce adaptive changes? How is it possible, in the face of cognitive (as well as other) losses that are implicated in emotion regulation, that individuals transform these losses into adaptive changes? Do *all* individuals achieve such adaptive gains, or are there important individual differences? Are the presumed gains in adaptive capacity absolute or rather relative given the losses? And in just *what ways* are they adaptive? For example, both Carstensen and Brandtstädter cite primarily hedonic criteria—the maintenance of positive affect and a sense of well-being. But what are the possible losses that individuals may need to accept in order to maintain a level of well-being? In particular, is this adaptation achieved at the cost of an overall reduction of complexity, whether in contextual breadth or general level of functioning (see Labouvie-Vief, 1981, 1982)? In short, what are the trade-offs individuals make to ensure well-being?

How aspects of hedonic tone and complexity of functioning are coordinated is a problem addressed by models of homeostatic regulation and equilibrium systems (Brent, 1978). Such systems always are adapted in a relative, not absolute, sense since they involve a range over which adaptive functioning can be maintained. If that range is exceeded, deterioration and even breakdown of functioning can result. A research project that quite dramatically illustrates this relationship between adaptation and its limits is a study by Lindenberger, Marsiske, and Baltes (2000), who studied how young and old individuals maintain balance in walking as they are concurrently engaged in the performance of a memory task. Postural stability requires the continuous coordination and integration of visual, proprioceptive, and vestibular sensory information as well as their coordination with corresponding muscle movements—a task that requires a high level of resources. Thus, it should be rather difficult to coordinate the maintenance of postural stability while simultaneously walking with a second resource-demanding task, such as a memory task—especially for older adults whose executive resources already are challenged. Indeed, Lindenberger et al. (2000) found that younger individuals were quite able to continue attending to the memory task while simultaneously walking. Older adults, however, needed to focus their attention nearly exclusively on maintaining balance. Hence, relinquishing one activity (memorizing) for one that is more vital (maintaining balance) is especially important for the elderly.

Baltes's (1997) work was performed in the framework of the theory of selection, optimization, and compensation (SOC). According to SOC, older individuals, when confronted with declining resources, can engage in a process of selection in which existing goals are reevaluated and individuals select those that are most important and realistic, given a particular level of resources. Note that the trade-off here can function in a way that is highly automatic and does not involve high-level inferential functioning. Maintaining balance is a crucial, absolutely vital goal, and restricting one's attention away from too much complexity and toward one's security is a dynamic adjustment that happens automatically through the participation of emotions. Thus, satisfying the crucial goal of bodily safety is adaptive in one sense, yet at the same time it also involves a sacrifice of complexity.

Equilibrium as Coregulation of Competence and Hedonic Tone

Although Baltes's project on maintaining physical balance has not directly addressed emotional mechanisms, it seems safe to assume that maintaining balance involves a range of emotions, from feeling safe and competent to fear of falling. The work thus shows how feeling-related hedonic processes interact with the complexity of behavior that is possible. Thus, the question is raised of what trade-off is involved: what losses in complexity are required to ensure necessary gains in actual physical safety (see also Labouvie-Vief, 1981, 1982).

This dialectic of gains and losses harkens back to a distinction often made by developmental psychologists who have concerned themselves with self-processes and ego processes. Is the self oriented primarily toward hedonic criteria, or is the interest rather in complexity, differentiation, and self-actualization (Helson & Wink, 1987; Labouvie-Vief & Medler, 2002; Loevinger, 1976; Ryff, 1989)? What compromise is struck between the two is, in essence, a problem of homeostasis and equilibrium maintenance.

A theory that has specifically addressed this trade-off dialectic between complexity and hedonic criteria was proposed more than 30 years ago by Lawton and Nahemow (1973). These authors invoked Harry Helson's (1964) concept of adaptation level (AL), which proposed that individuals' preferred level of stimulation changes as a function of experience. At a given AL, stimulation is experienced as neutral or comfortable. It permits experiences of well-being and positive feelings and adaptive behavior.

The AL principle was extended by Wohlwill (1966), who suggested that the AL functions through a principle of optimization. "According to this theory, stimuli that deviate *in either direction* from the adaptation level are experienced with positive affect up to a limiting point. Beyond the adaptation level, positive affect then decreases and again becomes negative as the stimulus increases or decreases further beyond the adaptation level" (Lawton & Nahemow, 1973, p. 660).

Lawton and Nahemow (1973) further extended this model to include the relationship between AL and complexity. Accordingly, comfort and adaptive behavior depend on both the individual's competence and the complexity of the environment. The higher the competences, the higher the level of stimulation and the wider the range of contexts (i.e., more complex the environment) over which comfort and adaptive behavior can be maintained. On the other hand, if the demands of the environment exceed the competence level corresponding to an AL, negative emotions and maladaptive behavior result. This general relationship implies a quite automatic way in which AL and individual complexity are coregulated. Thus, if competencies decline, the tolerance for stimulation declines as well, and well-being can be maintained by lowering environmental demands. Adaptation is quite automatically guaranteed yet by scaling down levels of complexity.

Lawton and Nahemow's (1973) model is congruent with the general view (e.g., Ekman & Davidson, 1994) that a core function of emotion systems is that of well-automated homeostatic regulation in the service of survival-relevant goals. To point to the automaticity of this process is not to say that adaptation in later life needs to be oriented toward self-preservative needs *only*. Rather, theorists often invoke a Maslovian hierarchical arrangement according to which needs of physical self-preservation take precedence over others that are more complex, such a consciously rearranging one's goals and searching for meaning and self-realization. According to that view, the quite direct and bodily experience of a shifting equilibrium is likely to signal vulnerabilities that, depending on individuals' capacities, can initiate more or less complex psychological decision mechanisms and ways of adapting. Yet it is a frequent assumption that those more complex processes are initiated, in a cascade process, by direct equilibrium changes at the level of bodily experience, of "the feeling of what happens" (Damasio, 1999). Jung (1931), for example, believed that such changes in equilibrium around mid-life define a bifurcation point: a "loss" of cognitive control that can initiate a surge and liberation of emotional resources—or else a flooding with unaccustomed-to and terrifying feelings (see also Erikson, 1985; Pascual-Leone, 2000).

Dynamic Equilibrium Regulation in Development and Aging

Lawton and Nahemow's (1973) model of the coregulation of hedonic tone and levels of complexity is highly compatible with theories of development, such as those stimulated by Freud (1957) and Piaget (1981), who proposed a dialectic between automatic and conscious regulation. Basic to such theories is the assertion that the development of complex cognitive and representational processes serves the function of widening the range of situations over which individuals can maintain equilibrium. More recent research on neurobiological and neurohormonal processes provides further evidence of the involvement of cognition in the regulation of organismic states. How do cognitions, representations, and symbolic processes perform such regulatory function, and how is that function affected by transitions in development?

Emotion, Cognition, and Equilibrium

The notion that development begins in the primacy of automatic, sensoriaffective experiences but gradually constructs more powerful cognitively based modes of regulation is basic to most major theories of development. Freud's theory of the tension between id-based primary processes and ego-based secondary processes is a case in point, as is Piaget's (1981) of the relationship of direct sensoriaffective experience on the one hand and the capacity of representation and symbolization to modify and extend those on the other.

Dynamic integration theory was most directly inspired by Piaget's theory, which placed the development of intellectual functions directly in the context of biological functioning. Yet apart from highly metatheoretical discussions (e.g., Piaget, 1971), the resulting view of intelligence did not discuss the specific mechanisms involved. Nevertheless, his research method was closely modeled on assumptions about the functioning of equilibrium systems, and, in fact, his analysis of children's cognitive performance directly follows the structure of such models. Equilibrium systems (e.g., Brent, 1978; Carver & Schaier, 2002) are able to protect themselves from too strong variations of some accustomed-to level of functioning (an AL or set point). They do so by a system of dynamic processes that compensate for variations within the system. This restorative and conservative process is possible as long as a certain set point is not exceeded—that is, if no too-critical discrepancy from this set point is registered. In that case, the systems initiate activities that dampen out variations from this set point through negative feedback. On the other hand, if deviations are extreme, the system's capacity for self-restoration fails, and the system can reach a breakdown point (see Brent, 1978).

As an example, take the child who cannot conserve quantity in the familiar problem of the cylinder or "sausage" that is rolled out to become longer but thinner (see Chapman, 1988). As long as variations of width and length from the original display are relatively minor, the child can maintain identity across variations of width and length by making relatively automatic compensations. The system thus functions as a feedback-reducing or negative feedback system that gates out variations within the critical range so that equality of the volume can be maintained. If that range is exceeded, in turn, a breakdown point is reached: the child's judgment becomes disequilibrated, changing from "same" to "different"—even though the increases in one dimension have been compensated for by corresponding decreases in the other dimension.

Emotion-Regulative Function of Representation

Although the example of the conservation of volume is not particularly emotional and does not involve high levels of arousal, Piaget (1981) suggested that his analysis of equilibria–disequilibria applied to emotions as well. His assertion that the development of higher-order schemas and concepts serves regulatory functions thus was quite implicit, but other researchers have concerned themselves more directly with how concepts and symbols affect the regulation of emotional states. For example, Luria (1982) measured motor tremor of the hand while individuals spoke of or drew situations with arousing emotional content. The results indicated that without symbolization, the arousal measured in this way was strongly reduced when individuals symbolized the respective events. Heinz Werner (1957), in his organismic developmental theory, also proposed that symbolization directly alters organismic states, permitting individuals to develop more "distance" from sensory, imaginative, and affective experience.

Recent research has begun to explore neurobiological mechanisms related to the regulatory function of symbolization. Although cognitive representation and affective processes reflect, in part, systems with different processing routes (based on prefrontal mechanisms and amygdala, respectively) (Damasio, 1999; LeDoux & Phelps, 2000), these systems interact in the regulation of emotion. This interaction involves the inhibitory action of the dorsal and lateral regions of the prefrontal cortical areas that down-regulate amygdala activation. Such down-regulation is evident when symbolization processes, such as language, produce activation in specific lateral and dorsal regions of the prefrontal cortex, an activation that in turn parallels decreased activation in emotional areas, such as the amygdala (Hariri, Bookheimer, & Mazziotta, 2000; Schore, 1994; see also Lieberman et al., 2007).

Importantly, this prefrontal–amygdala system appears to display negative feedback properties, as inhibitory regulative capacity appears to be dependent on degree of activation. Just as in Lawton and Nahemow's (1973) notion of the coregulation of AL and complexity, good regulation functions at levels that are slightly elevated but breaks down once a certain level of activation is exceeded (e.g., Eysenck, 1976; McEwen & Sapolsky, 1995; Metcalfe & Mischel, 1999). On one hand, the resulting overactivation causes a shift in which processing bypasses prefrontal mechanisms and creates highly automatic responding (LeDoux & Phelps, 2000; Metcalfe & Mischel, 1999). On the other hand, this system is integrated with the neurohormonal system since efficacy of negative feedback/down-regulation involves the interaction between the prefrontal–amygdala axis and levels of circulating glucocorticoids (e.g., de Kloet, Oitzl, & Joëls, 1999; Lupien, Maheu, Tu, Fiocco, & Schramek, 2007). Glucocorticoids are essential in regulating the organism's homeostasis to stress, but the effectiveness of regulation varies with the saturation of glucocorticoids: at relatively low levels, superior attention and cognitive performance result, but at even higher levels, memory and cognitive functioning are impaired. If these high levels are sustained over long time periods, they can even cause architectural and functional impairments, disturbing the equilibrium-regulating function of the prefrontal–amygdala system (Jay et al., 2004).

Cognitive Development and Expanding Equilibria

The previously discussed feedback-based analysis indicates that effective regulation depends on moderate levels of activation but deteriorates if stimulation increases beyond a set point. However, Piaget's (1971) work anticipated much recent thinking in dynamic and complex systems by asserting that living systems' activity is not just reactive and restorative. Rather, they can shift into a state that is oriented not toward stability but toward novelty and change. At such junctures, they move into regimes of instability ("disequilibration").

Important features of the widening of disequilibration are negative emotions and stress as individuals give up accustomed-to ways of being and begin a process of differentiation. Piaget's research of children beginning to deliberately differentiate and experiment is one example. On the emotional arena, newborns' tolerance for high levels of stimulation is limited and evokes distress. But over time, infants actively engage with more complex, dynamic, and intense stimulation and as a consequence reset their tension thresholds (Sroufe, 1996). Harter (1998) observed parallel processes in adolescents' coordination of positive and negative affect. She showed that cognitive growth can initiate a period of heightened negative affect as adolescents' advances in differentiation and complexity raise their awareness of conflicts between different self-attributes (e.g. "fun loving" versus "depressed"). At first, this awareness produces confusion and increased negative emotions, but eventually such opposites are quite comfortably integrated—for example, by noting that at different times or in different contexts, different self-aspects are highlighted.

More generally, with increasing capacities for reflection and self–other differentiation, individuals are capable of managing/accommodating experiences that are of higher complexity, more tension of opposites, and so on. In this way, emotions evolve into complex systems of emotion–cognition linkages (Lewis, 2005). Thus, periods of instability during transitions can reflect processes of "positive disintegration" (Dabrowski, 1970) that pave the way for new and more powerful organizations to emerge. In fact, in line with the notion that moderate deviations from equilibrium enhance cognitive and cortical functioning, Schore (1994) has argued that temporary periods of heightened negativity permit the internalization of standards and a rewiring of cortical circuits supporting self-regulation. In a similar fashion, studies show that throughout the first part of the life span, the contribution of prefrontal cortical processes increases, a process that continues well into adulthood (Eshel, Nelson, Blair, Pine, & Ernst, 2007).

Differentiation, Integration . . . or Fragmentation

Transitions to higher levels of complexity following periods of differentiation and "crisis" (Erikson, 1985) are a possible but by far not an automatic and necessary result of differentiation and disequilibrium. Rather, the process of integration itself is subject to homeostatic feedback mechanisms that act on trajectories themselves (Brent, 1978). The capacity for integration itself requires a developmental context that is well regulated: increases in complexity are highly constrained by the system's current capacity. What is too surprising becomes a source of threat to integrity and a shift to self-protection and negative feedback functioning. Hence, the equation of structure and self-organization with equilibrium processes does not imply that systems are static but means that change needs to be provided in a well-regulated fashion to ensure a balance between openness and closure and between stability and change. Such a balance between stability and change ensures "intelligible change, which does not transform things beyond recognition at one stroke, and which always preserves invariance in certain respects" (Piaget, 1971, p. 20). As a result, failures of integration are likely to be consequences of developmental contexts that do not protect from overactivation—a proposal that is inherent in the Eriksonian (1985) view of crises that bifurcate developmental trajectories at transition points as well as related views of attachment theory (Bowlby, 1973).

Emotional Regulation in Adulthood and Aging

Do similar expansions of the capacity to maintain equilibrium continue past adolescence and into late life? My colleagues and I investigated such transformations in individuals ages 10 to 80 and older (Labouvie-Vief, Chiodo, Goguen, Diehl, & Orwoll, 1995; Labouvie-Vief, DeVoe, & Bulka, 1989). We coded participants' descriptions of their emotions and their selves into qualitative levels of differing cognitive–affective complexity. We assessed valence contrasts and other indices of complexity and differentiation, such as self–other differentiation and the capacity to reflect on and mentalize emotions.

Findings showed that from adolescence to middle adulthood, individuals acquired more conscious insight into aspects of emotions that previously were unconscious, gained clearer differentiation of self from others, and blended distinct emotions, especially ones involving positive and negative contrasts (e.g., a mixture of joy and sadness) within the *same* representational event. These developments allowed many (but not all) adults to carve out a renewed sense of self that was complex, was historically situated, and entailed a more distinct sense of their individuality.

These results confirmed our expectation that significant growth in affective complexity continues through middle adulthood. However, they also contained surprises, even disappointments: not only did growth abate in late middle adulthood, but a significant decline occurred thereafter. These findings highlight the role of middle-aged adults as the carriers of complex knowledge integrating mind and emotion (Labouvie-Vief, 1994) but suggest that problems with regulation of emotions occur with aging. In retrospect, this is not astonishing given the dependence of emotion regulation on intact prefrontal–limbic functioning. Recent research suggests that of the aging changes affecting the brain, the most important are declines in prefrontal and hippocampal functioning (Raz 2004; Raz & Rodrigue, 2006), both structures that support complex cognitive activity. These losses may be partially offset or masked if individuals have already developed successful regulation strategies or if the tasks under consideration do not require a high level of complexity. However, their eventual effect is to create regulation vulnerabilities. Labouvie-Vief and Marquez (2004) propose that these vulnerabilities can result in a degradation of complexity—a general mechanism already suggested by Lawton and Nahemow (1973). I turn to a selected review of such forms of degradation and the mechanisms involved next.

Dynamic Integration in Aging: A Brief Empirical Review

Degradation of complexity can be viewed as a quasi-regressive movement in which individuals are no longer able to function at highest levels of complexity but fall back on lower levels (see also Fischer & Bidell, 2006). On the most general level, degradation of complexity results from the increased level of emotional activation caused by the disturbance in the regulatory function of the prefrontal–limbic axis (e.g., Eysenck, 1976; Metcalfe & Mischel, 1999). This mechanism applies to all periods of the life span when individuals are exposed (e.g., experimentally) to restrictions of cognitive resources but becomes particularly important in late life. However, whether this disturbance results in reduced functioning itself depends on the mechanisms of dynamic regulation of equilibrium. Under conditions of mild and transient disruption, it may even be related to positive consequences, but under severe and prolonged conditions, effects should be less positive.

An author who has concerned himself with the possible positive consequences of this shift was Jung (1931), who suggested long ago that middle to late adulthood can bring a liberation of unconscious processes. Whereas childhood and the earlier portions of the life span force individuals to become entrenched in societal rules and institutions and to overcontrol part of their inner potentials, midlife can bring freeing of the world of feelings. Indeed, Jung suggested that midlife becomes a crucial pivoting point in the life span that brings a turn away from preoccupations with the outer world and a "centroversion" toward the inner world (see Labouvie-Vief, 1994). Hence, it affords a unique opportunity for deeper levels of individuation. Nevertheless, it is evident that not all adults experience such a liberation of the inner world as they grow older. In her pathbreaking work, Bernice Neugarten (Neugarten, Havighurst, & Tobin, 1968) some 40 years ago already showed that only *some* older individuals are able to achieve higher levels of integration, while others become more highly defended or even appear to disintegrate. More recent research also suggests that the changing equilibrium between prefrontal control and automatic emotions can bring both felicitous and problematic consequences.

Benefits of Increased Automaticity

One sign of this inward shift is a general way in which individuals' relationship to information becomes restructured. For the young adult, information is seen as an outer given that one attempts to reproduce in a literal way. In contrast, middle and older adults turn more to the landscape of human motivations and intentions. Hence, they may become experts at the processing of information relating to subjective processes and inner dynamics. Although this symbolic processing style can result in deficits on the literal level, they may imply a richer psychological texture.

This shift from a more text-dependent mode to one that is more interpretive and subjective was shown in a series of studies (for review, see Jepson & Labouvie-Vief, 1992) about individuals' rendition and interpretation of narratives. For example, in one study young, middle-aged, and old adults were asked to respond to a series of fable-like stories. The young adults produced detailed, almost verbatim reproductions of the tales. But the older adults were concerned primarily with general meanings that were symbolic, moral, and inner psychological, such as "a lot of times things that appear to be situations outside ourselves are really things that we need to be conquering inside. But we have to have the outside confrontation to find out who we are and what we're made of" (Jepson & Labouvie-Vief, 1992, p. 130).

Research also suggests that older individuals' functioning is enhanced if experimental situations call on this inner orientation. Thus, several studies have noted that typical age differences between young and old adults on tasks of cognitive processing become diminished (for review, see Hess, 2005) or even disappear when older individuals can work with information that not only has direct implications for the self, but also carries moral or interpersonal implications (Rahhal, May, & Hasher, 2002). In fact, some research (Blanchard-Fields, 1977) reports that under some conditions, older adults excel in problem solving that permits them to draw on their accumulated experience.

The powerful effects of emotional facilitation for elders is consistent with the dynamic view proposed in this chapter. Yet it could also be interpreted differently as indicating that older individuals are more *dependent* on the emotional activation that produces this facilitation effect. Without it, the burden of processing is fully placed on the effortful conscious processing system. A widely known example in the memory literature is the superiority of free recall over recognition of stimuli. Here recognition is supported by external activation (i.e., making stimuli available), whereas free recall depends solely on internal generation (Craik, 2002). Age differences in memory performance are typically larger for recall than for recognition, suggesting that older adults have difficulties in providing vivid representations in the absence of external activation. Thus, at low and suboptimal levels of activation, age differences are probably more obvious than at optimal levels of activation. This interpretation is, in fact, important in the research to be discussed next, that related to emotional reactivity.

Problems Associated With Heightened Levels of Arousal

One prediction of DIT is that older individuals, whose systems are more easily activated, should be more easily overactivated than their more resilient younger counterparts. With respect to physiological (especially cardiac reactivity), research does not give a clear answer. Some studies suggest that older individuals are less easily aroused (for reviews, see Labouvie-Vief, Lumley, Jain, & Heinze, 2003). However, most of the experiments supporting this view deal with autobiographical accounts, which, by their very nature, depend on a high degree of control over the material processed—thus, they also involve internal generation of stimuli. In situations that are truly reactive and that involve high activation, such as those related to highly relevant life events (Kunzmann & Grühn, 2005) or social-emotional problems (Uchino, Holt-Lunstad, Bloor, & Campo, 2005), older individuals are much more easily dysregulated. Thus, overstimulation becomes a more severe conflict for the elderly.

In fact, DIT predicts that highly activating situations create escalating levels of arousal in older adults more easily that in younger ones—a prediction in line with the "glucocorticoid cascade hypothesis" (Sapolsky, Krey, & McEwen, 1986), which states that older organisms readily initiate a stress response but "are dramatically impaired in their capacity to repair it" (p. 285). In a similar fashion, we (Wurm, Labouvie-Vief, Aycock, Rebucal, & Koch, 2004) confirmed our prediction that older adults have difficulties processing high-arousing material in a study using an emotional Stroop task. In this task, individuals were asked to name the color of low-, medium-, and high-arousing emotional words presented in different colors as fast as possible. Findings showed no differences in response latencies between low- and high-arousing words for young adults, but for older adults, response latencies for high-arousing words were significantly elevated over low- and medium-arousing words. These results indicate that older individuals may have a problem inhibiting high arousal.

Evidence for older adults' difficulties with highly arousing words has also been obtained by Grühn, who found that high arousal interfered with effective processing in older but not younger adults (Grühn, Scheibe, & Baltes, in press; Grühn, Smith, & Baltes, 2005). This interpretation is also supported by a dramatic age differences in memorability scores for individual pictures and their associated arousal levels (Grühn & Scheibe, in press): for young adults, there was no significant correlation, but older adults showed a small but consistent and significant negative relation between memorability and arousal. Thus, older adults remembered high-arousing pictures (regardless of their valence) less well than low-arousing pictures, suggesting a processing deficit for highly arousing materials. Similar negative relationships between arousal and effectiveness of cognitive performance have been found by other authors as well (e.g., Bäckman & Molander, 1991; Eisdorfer, 1968) who have also reported on older adults' vulnerability to overactivation.

Problems of overactivation would be expected to be especially severe in individuals who already suffer from misregulation that exacerbate the effects of momentary stimulation. Deptula, Singh, and Pomora (1993) related the memory performance of young and elderly adults with their self-reports of anxiety, depression, and withdrawal tendency. Results indicated that for the young, the relationships were positive though nonsignificant, whereas for the elderly, higher scores on these dimensions had a significantly negative relationship with memory performance. Somewhat relatedly, we (Labouvie-Vief, Slater, & Jain, 2007) found that emotional Stroop performance was significantly related to attachment anxiety in the elderly but entirely unaffected by attachment in young adults.

All these findings support the prediction of DIT that, with advancing age, the capacity to integrate a sense of well-being and high levels of complexity should be strongly impaired—congruent with Lawton and Nahemow's (1973) work. To operationalize variations in integration in our own longitudinal research on self- and emotion development from preadolescence to late life, we (see Labouvie-Vief & Medler, 2002) drew on Heinz Werner's (1957) distinction of different forms of coordination. Integration, according to Werner, also presupposes differentiation, whereas integration without differentiation implies globality, but differentiation without integration implies fragmentation.

Accordingly, we defined an integrated group by high scores on both complexity and overall positive hedonic tone. These individuals displayed the most positive developmental outcomes. They scored high in positive but low in negative affect yet were comfortable acknowledging negativity. They reported high well-being, empathy, and health and a secure relationship style. They displayed high tolerance of ambiguity and openness to affect exploration. In contrast, the *dysregulated* (low complexity, low optimization) pattern was the diametric opposite with extremely low scores on all these variables except negative affect.

The *self-protective* (low differentiation, high optimization) and the *complex* (high differentiation, low optimization) displayed more mixed patterns that were nevertheless fairly coherent. Compared with the complex, the self-protective scored low in negative affect, but the two groups were similar in positive affect, relationship security, and health. However, the self-protective also placed less emphasis on personal growth than the complex, and they scored higher on conformity, denial, and repression but very low on doubt and depression—as well as empathy. This pattern suggests that the self-protective tend to dampen negative affect, whereas the complex amplify it.

The distribution of the patterns showed significant increases in integration from adolescence and early adulthood to middle adulthood. Only about 14% of the 10–30 age-group was classified as integrated compared to 43% each of the middle aged and elderly. In contrast, self-protective individuals were most likely to be elders (57%), compared to 17% of the young and 26% of the middle aged. Complex individuals were most strongly presented in the young (35%) and middle adult (47%) groups but were significantly less represented in the elderly (18%). For those classified as dysregulated, a significantly higher concentration was in the young (44%) as opposed to middle (30%) and old (26%).

Thus, our research agrees with studies showing high levels of negativity in youth and adolescence but adds that this likely reflects a developmental transition in which integration remains difficult. In contrast, we interpret the dramatic increases in the more simplifying, self-protective style of elders as a movement that is initiated by increasing vulnerability in regulating homeostatic processes, including emotions. Indeed, our research and that of others (see Diehl, Hastings, & Stanton, 2001; Helson & Soto, 2005; Labouvie-Vief, Diehl, Jain, & Zhang, 2007; Labouvie-Vief, Grühn, & Mouras, in press) suggests that high complexity puts elders at risk, as challenges to integrative capacity induce a more global style.

Conclusion

In sum, DIT states that as a result of increased automaticity of functioning, emotion regulation in later life may present a picture of bifurcation with possible positive consequences but also with increasing difficulty dealing with high-arousing situations. Eventually, this will encourage a pattern of increasing self-protectiveness and avoidance of complex situations. However, such shifts toward increased vulnerability not only are dependent on increasing age but will also be particularly likely under conditions of (a) resource limitations, (b) high levels of activation (i.e., arousal), or (c) low levels of socioemotional resources. Especially older adults with their low cognitive resources are found to be vulnerable to such conditions.

The proposed bifurcation of patterns in older adults is in line with our general homeostatic model. It also adds support to important theories of aging. Thus, Erikson (1985) already suggested that experiences of increased vulnerability in later life initiate a change in equilibrium that brings to the fore the core conflictual theme of integrity versus constriction or even despair in later life. Similarly, Jung (1931) has suggested that a decline of cognitive control can initiate a surge of emotional resources that can lead to a more positive reorganization in which a more mellow, integrated, and wise pattern of adaptation emerges (see also Pascual-Leone, 2000). The theoretical and empirical work here reported suggests that these changes may be initiated by a profound reorganization in the regulation of emotions as the involvement in different brain structures changes from young to late adulthood.

References

Bäckman, L., & Molander, B. (1991). On the generalizability of the age-related decline in coping with high-arousal conditions in a precision sport: Replication and extension. *Journal of Gerontology, 46,* 79–81.

Baltes, P. B. (1997). On the incomplete architecture of human ontogeny: Selection, optimization, and compensation as foundation of developmental theory. *American Psychologist, 52,* 366–380.

Blanchard-Fields, F. (1977). Everyday problem solving and emotion: An adult developmental perspective. *Current Directions in Psychological Science, 16,* 26–31.

Bowlby, J. (1973). *Attachment and loss: Vol. 2. Separation.* New York: Basic Books.

Brent, S. B. (1978). Motivation, steady state, and structural development: A general model of psychological homeostasis. *Motivation and Emotion, 2,* 299–332.

Carstensen, L. L., Isaacowitz, D. M., & Charles, S. T. (1999). Taking time seriously: A theory of socioemotional selectivity. *American Psychologist, 54,* 165–181.

Carver, C. S., & Schaier, M. F. (2002). Control processes and self-organization as complementary principles underlying behavior. *Personality and Social Psychology Review, 6,* 304–315.

Chapman, M. (1988). *Constructive evolution: Origins and development of Piaget's thought.* Cambridge: Cambridge University Press.

Charles, S. T., & Carstensen, L. L. (1977). Emotion regulation and aging. In J. L. Gross (Ed.), *Handbook of emotion regulation* (pp. 307–327). New York: Guilford.

Craik, F. I. M. (2002). Human memory and aging. In L. Bäckman & C. von Hofsten (Eds.), *Psychology at the turn of the millennium: Vol. 1. Cognitive, biological, and health perspectives* (pp. 261–280). Hove: Psychology Press.

Dabrowski, K. (1970) *Mental growth through positive disintegration.* London: Gryf.

Damasio, A. (1999). *The feeling of what happens: Body and emotion in the making of consciousness.* New York: Harcourt.

de Kloet, E. R., Oitzl, M. S., & Joëls, M. (1999). Stress and cognition: Are corticosteroids good or bad guys? *Trends in Neurosciences, 22,* 422–426.

Deptula, D., Singh, R., & Pomara, N. (1993). Aging, emotional states, and memory. *American Journal of Psychiatry, 150,* 429–434.

Diehl, M., Hastings, C. T., & Stanton, J. M. (2001). Self-concept differentiation across the adult life span. *Psychology and Aging, 16,* 643–654.

Eisdorfer, C. (1968). Arousal and performance: Experiments in verbal learning and a tentative theory. In G. A. Talland (Ed.), *Human aging and behavior: Recent advances in research and the theory* (pp. 189–216). New York: Academic Press.

Ekman, P., & Davidson, R. J. (1994). *The nature of emotion: Fundamental questions.* Oxford: Oxford University Press.

Erikson, E. H. (1985). *The life cycle completed: A review.* New York: Norton.

Eshel, N., Nelson, E. E., Blair, R. J., Pine, D. S., & Ernst, M. (2007). Neural substrates of choice selection in adults and adolescents: Development of the ventrolateral prefrontal and anterior cingulate cortices. *Neuropsychologia, 25,* 1270–1279.

Eysenck, M. W. (1976). Arousal, learning, and memory. *Psychological Bulletin, 83,* 389–404.

Fischer, K. W., & Bidell, T. R. (2006). Dynamic development of action and thought. In R. M. Lerner & W. Damon (Eds.), *Handbook of child psychology: Vol. 1. Theoretical models of human development* (6th ed., pp. 313–399). Hoboken, NJ: Wiley.

Freud, S. (1957). The id and the ego. In J. Rickman (Ed.), *A general selection of the works of Sigmund Freud* (pp. 310–235). Garden City, NY: Doubleday. (Original work published 1923)

Grühn, D., & Scheibe, S. (in press). Age-related differences in valence and arousal ratings of pictures from the International Affective Picture System (IAPS): Do ratings become more extreme with age? *Behavior Research Methods.*

Grühn, D., Scheibe, S., & Baltes, P. B. (in press). Reduced negativity effect in older adults' memory for emotional pictures: The heterogeneity-homogeneity list paradigm. *Psychology and Aging.*

Grühn, D., Smith, J., & Baltes, P. B. (2005). No aging bias favoring memory for positive material: Evidence from a heterogeneity-homogeneity list paradigm using emotionally toned words. *Psychology and Aging, 20,* 579–588.

Hariri, A. R., Bookheimer, S. Y., & Mazziotta, J. C. (2000). Modulating emotional responses: Effects of a neocortical network on the limbic system. *NeuroReport, 11,* 43–48.

Harter, S. (1998). The development of self-representations. In W. Damon & N. Eisenberg (Eds.), *Handbook of child psychology: Vol 3. Social, emotional, and personality development* (5th ed., pp. 553–557). Hoboken, NJ: Wiley.

Helson, H. (1964). *Adaptation level theory.* New York: Harper & Row.

Helson, R., & Soto, C. J. (2005). Up and down in middle age: Monotonic and nonmonotonic changes in roles, status, and personality. *Journal of Personality and Social Psychology, 89,* 194–204.

Helson, R., & Wink, P. (1987). Two conceptions of maturity examined in the findings of a longitudinal study. *Journal of Personality and Social Psychology, 53,* 531–541.

Hess, T. M. (2005). Memory and aging in context. *Psychological Bulletin, 131,* 383–406.

Jay, T. M., Rocher, C., Hotte, M., Naudon, L., Gurden, H., & Spedding, M. (2004). Plasticity at hippocampal to prefrontal cortex synapses is impaired by loss of dopamine and stress: Importance for psychiatric diseases. *Neurotoxicity Research, 6,* 233–244.

Jepson, K., & Labouvie-Vief, G. (1992). Symbolic processing in the elderly. In J. Sinnott & R. West (Eds.), *Everyday memory in later life* (pp. 124–137). Hillsdale, NJ: Lawrence Erlbaum Associates.

Jung, C. J. (1931). The stages of life. In J. Campbell (Ed.), *The portable Jung* (Trans. R. F. C. Hull, pp. 3–22). New York: Viking Press.

Kessler, E. M., & Staudinger, U. (2007). Intergenerational potential: Effects of social interaction between older adults and adolescents. *Psychology and Aging, 22*(4), 690–704.

Kunzmann, U., & Grühn, D. (2005). Age differences in emotional reactivity: The sample case of sadness. *Psychology and Aging, 20,* 47–59.

Kunzmann, U., Little, T. D., & Smith, J. (2000). Is age-related stability of subjective well-being a paradox? Cross-sectional and longitudinal evidence from the Berlin Aging Study. *Psychology and Aging, 15,* 511–526.

Labouvie-Vief, G. (1981). Re-active and pro-active aspects of constructivism: A life-span model. In R. M. Lerner & N. A. Busch-Rossnagel (Eds.), *Individuals as producers of their development: A life-span perspective* (pp. 197–230). New York: Academic Press.

Labouvie-Vief, G. (1982). Growth and aging in life-span perspective. *Human Development, 25,* 65–88.

Labouvie-Vief, G. (1994). *Psyche and Eros: Mind and gender in the life course.* New York: Cambridge University Press.

Labouvie-Vief, G. (2003). Dynamic integration: Affect, cognition, and the self in adulthood. *Current Directions in Psychological Science, 12,* 201–206.

Labouvie-Vief, G., Chiodo, L. M., Goguen, L. A., Diehl, M., & Orwoll, L. (1995). Representations of self across the life span. *Psychology and Aging, 10,* 404–415.

Labouvie-Vief, G., DeVoe, M., & Bulka, D. (1989). Speaking about feelings: Conceptions of emotion across the life span. *Psychology and Aging, 4,* 425–437.

Labouvie-Vief, G., Diehl, M., Jain, E., & Zhang, F. (2007). The relationship between changes in affect optimization and complexity: A further examination. *Psychology and Aging, 22*(4), 738–751.

Labouvie-Vief, G., Grühn, D., & Mouras, H. (in press). Dynamic emotion-cognition interactions in adult development: Arousal, stress, and the processing of affect. In H. B. Bosworth & C. Hertzog (Eds.), *Cognition in aging: Methodologies and applications.* Washington, DC: American Psychological Association.

Labouvie-Vief, G., Lumley, M. A., Jain, E., & Heinze, H. (2003). Age and gender differences in cardiac reactivity and subjective emotion responses to emotional autobiographical memories. *Emotion, 3,* 115–126.

Labouvie-Vief, G., & Marquez, M. G. (2004). Dynamic integration: Affect optimization and differentiation in development. In D. Y. Dai & R. J. Sternberg (Eds.), *Motivation, emotion, and cognition: Integrative perspectives on intellectual functioning and development* (pp. 237–272). Mahwah, NJ: Lawrence Erlbaum Associates.

Labouvie-Vief, G., & Medler, M. (2002). Affect optimization and affect complexity: Modes and styles of regulation in adulthood. *Psychology and Aging, 17,* 571–587.

Labouvie-Vief, G., Slater, J., & Jain, E. (2007). *Affective processing as a function of age and attachment style.* Manuscript submitted for publication.

Lawton, M. P., & Nahemow, L. (1973). Ecology and the aging process. In C. Eisdorfer & M. P. Lawton (Eds.), *The psychology of adult development and aging* (pp. 619–674). Washington, DC: American Psychological Association.

LeDoux, J. E., & Phelps, E. A. (2000). Emotional networks in the brain. In M. Lewis & J. M. Haviland-Jones (Eds.), *Handbook of emotions* (2nd ed., pp. 157–172). New York: Guilford.

Lewis, M. D. (2005). Bridging emotion theory and neurobiology through dynamic systems modeling. *Behavioral and Brain Sciences, 28,* 169–245.

Lieberman, M. D., Eisenberger, N. I., Crockett, M. J., Tom, S. M., Pfiefer, J. H., & Way, B. M. (2007). Putting feelings into words: Affect labeling disrupts amygdala activity in response to affective stimuli. *Psychological Science, 18,* 421–428.

Lindenberger, U., Marsiske, M., & Baltes, P. B. (2000). Memorizing while walking: Increase in dual-task costs from young adulthood to old age. *Psychology and Aging, 15,* 417–436.

Loevinger, J. (1976). *Ego development.* San Francisco: Jossey-Bass.

Lupien, S. J., Maheu, F., Tu, M., Fiocco, A., & Schramek, T. E. (2007). The effects of stress and stress hormones on human cognition: Implications for the field of brain and cognition. *Brain and Cognition, 65*(3), 209–237.

Luria, A. R. (1982). *Language and cognition.* New York: Wiley.

McEwen, B. S., & Sapolsky, R. M. (1995). Stress and cognitive function. *Current Opinion in Neurobiology, 5,* 205–216.

Metcalfe, J., & Mischel, W. (1999). A hot/cool-system analysis of delay of gratification: Dynamics of willpower. *Psychological Review, 106,* 3–19.

Mroczek, D. K., & Kolarz, C. M. (1998). The effect of age on positive and negative affect: A developmental perspective on happiness. *Journal of Personality and Social Psychology, 75,* 1333–1349.

Neugarten, B. I., Havighurst, R. J., & Tobin, S. S. (1968). Personality and patterns of aging. In B. I. Neugarten (Ed.), *Middle age and aging* (pp. 173–177). Chicago: University of Chicago Press.

Pascual-Leone, J. (2000). Mental attention, conscious, and the progressive emergence of wisdom. *Journal of Adult Development, 7,* 241–254.

Piaget, J. (1971). *Biology and knowledge.* Chicago: University of Chicago Press.

Piaget, J. (1981). *Intelligence and affectivity: Their relationship during child development* (T. A. Brown & C. E. Kaegi, Trans.). Oxford: Annual Reviews.

Rahhal, T. A., May, C. P., & Hasher, L. (2002). Truth and character: Sources that older adults can remember. *Psychological Science, 13,* 101–105.

Raz, N. (2004). The aging brain observed in vivo: differential changes and their modifiers. In R. Cabeza, L. Nyberg, & D. C. Park (Eds.), *Cognitive neuroscience of aging: Linking cognitive and cerebral aging* (pp. 17–55). New York: Oxford University Press.

Raz, N., & Rodrigue, K. M. (2006). Differential aging of the brain: Patterns, cognitive correlates and modifiers. *Neuroscience and Biobehavioral Reviews, 30,* 730–748.

Ryff, C. D. (1989). Happiness is everything, or is it? Explorations on the meaning of psychological well-being. *Journal of Personality & Social Psychology, 57,* 1069–1081.

Sapolsky, R. M., Krey, L. C., & McEwen, B. S. (1986). The neuroendocrinology of stress and aging: The clucocorticoid cascade hypothesis. *Endocrine Reviews, 7,* 284–301.

Schore, A. N. (1994). *Affect regulation and the origin of the self: The neurobiology of emotional development.* Hillsdale, NJ: Lawrence Erlbaum Associates.

Sroufe, L. A. (1996). *Emotional development: The organization of emotional life in the early years.* New York: Cambridge University Press.

Uchino, B. N., Holt-Lunstad, J., Bloor, L. E., & Campo, R. A. (2005). Aging and cardiovascular reactivity to stress: Longitudinal evidence for changes in stress reactivity. *Psychology and Aging, 20,* 134–143.

Werner, H. (1957). *Comparative psychology of mental development.* Oxford: International University Press.

Wohlwill, J. F. (1966). The physical environment: A problem for a psychology of stimulation. *Journal of Social Issues, 22,* 29–38.

Wurm, L. H., Labouvie-Vief, G., Aycock, J., Rebucal, K. A., & Koch, H. E. (2004). Performance in auditory and visual emotional Stroop tasks: A comparison of older and younger adults. *Psychology and Aging, 19,* 523–535.

17 Cognitive Plasticity

Sherry L. Willis
K. Warner Schaie
Mike Martin

The traditional approach to the study of cognition has been to focus on normative age-related changes in intelligence across the life span. In old age, the focus has been on age-related decline. This approach views intelligence as a set of stable traits within the individual, thus allowing long-term predictions of normative gain and decline across the life span (Cattell, 1963; Schaie, 2005; Terman, 1916; Thurstone, 1938). Most of the empirical studies have focused on describing normative or average change in intellectual abilities rather than on examining the full range of interindividual or intraindividual variability that might occur as a function of experimental manipulations, interventions, nonnormative life

This research was supported by grants from the National Institute on Aging to Sherry L. Willis (R37024102) and K. Warner Schaie (R37 AG08055) and support from the Swiss National Science Foundation to Mike Martin (SNSF-100013-103525).

events, or sociocultural change. Likewise, earlier neuroscience approaches assume that neural development came to completion in early life with little plasticity occurring in adulthood (Buonomano & Merzenich, 1998). Currently, it has been recognized that cognitive change in adulthood can be multidirectional, including gain and maintenance as well as decline.

This chapter focuses on issues of plasticity in adult cognition that are of current interest for both neuroscience and psychological theories of adult development and aging (Kramer, Bherer, Colcombe, Dong, & Greenough, 2004). We begin with a consideration of variations in the definition of plasticity in current use in both developmental psychology and neuropsychology and of related concepts such as neural plasticity, neural reserve, and cognitive reserve (Baltes, 1987; Stern, 2007). We embed our discussion of the concept of plasticity within a life span developmental theoretical perspective. Several key questions are then identified that should be addressed by a theory of cognitive plasticity in adulthood, and we discuss constructs and issues related to each question. We also briefly discuss the adequacy of current cognitive theories in addressing these questions.

Cognitive Plasticity: Construct and Theory

Life Span Developmental Theory and Cognitive Plasticity

The concept of plasticity is closely linked to life span theory's conception of development as a process of lifelong adaptation (Baltes, Lindenberger, & Staudinger, 2006; Thomae, 1979). Life span theory maintains that development is modifiable or plastic at all phases of development; however, there are constraints and limits on developmental plasticity, and these constraints and limits vary by period of development. A major goal of life span developmental research has been to examine the range and limits of plasticity at various phases of the life span. With respect to cognition, adaptation involves the interplay between assimilating the environment to existing forms of thought and accommodating one's thought to the environment. Development is conceptualized as multidimensional, multidirectional, and multifunctional (Baltes, 1987). Cognition would then be expected to involve multiple dimensions or levels rather than a single global approach to general intelligence (i.e., *g*). The multidirectionality of development implies that there will be both growth (gains) and decrement (losses) at any developmental stage, although with advanced aging the losses may outweigh the gains. Various abilities or cognitive processes would then be expected to vary in their developmental trajectories with some exhibiting positive or negative linear trends and others exhibiting nonlinear trends.

If development in general and cognition in particular are to be studied in terms of adaptivity (rather than static traits), then intraindividual processes that foster cognitive adaptation must be explained. That is, it needs to be specified why there are interindividual differences in intraindividual adaptation and plasticity. Theories of developmental regulation or adaptation may be one way to approach this issue. For instance, the SOC theory advocated by focuses on three mechanisms (selection, optimization, and compensation) for adaptation or the regulation of one's resources (including cognitive capacity) throughout development. *Selection* involves the individual's choice or election to focus on adaptation and optimization in certain areas and as a result to limit one's focus in other areas. Selection may involve an emphasis on cognition or the selection of specific cognitive domains (e.g., expertise) as a focus of adaptation. The theory posits that in old age there may be increasing restriction in the selection of domains because of age-related loss in the range of adaptive potential. *Optimization* involves maximization (e.g., gaining expertise) of one's performance and potential in selected areas; optimization may be an important mechanism for the building of reserve for future use. *Compensation* becomes operative when specific behavioral capacities are lost or one's capacity in an area drops below the threshold for adequate functioning. Compensation may result in acquisition of new behaviors or bodies of knowledge or reallocation of resources. Thus, the SOC model suggests specific behaviors to explain plasticity across the life span.

In addition to the study of plasticity at the level of the individual, the biocultural constructive perspective within the life span approach emphasizes that developmental adaptivity and plasticity may also be observed on a number of different and interacting levels (i.e., from the neurobiological to the behavioral and the sociocultural) and on different time scales ranging from momentary microgenesis over life span development to phylogenetic evolution (Baltes, 1997; Li, 2003; see also Willis & Schaie, 2006). This approach situates plasticity within a larger evolutionary framework of development. Three propositions in this perspective specify the interaction between neurobiological and sociocultural influences on adaptivity and plasticity: evolutionary selection processes most strongly influence development in early life; with increasing age, behavioral plasticity depends on ever-increasing cultural resources because of a smaller degree of neuronal plasticity; however, the beneficial effect of increasing cultural resources is diminished in old age because of a decline in neurobiological functions.

Cognitive Plasticity

Cognitive plasticity has often been defined in terms of the individual's latent cognitive potential under specific contextual conditions. Specifically, plasticity has been defined in terms of the capacity to acquire cognitive skills (Jones et al., 2006; Mercado, 2008). Cognitive skills are here defined as the abilities that an organism can improve through practice or observational learning and that involve judgment or processing beyond perceptual motor skills. The definition of cognitive plasticity usually involves a contrast between the individual's current average level of performance under normative conditions and one's latent potential.

Several aspects of the definition of cognitive plasticity should be noted. First, cognitive plasticity deals with *intraindividual* potential, the range of plasticity within an individual (Baltes & Lindenberger, 1988). While interindividual differences in intraindividual plasticity are often studied, plasticity focuses on intraindividual change or potential. Second, the *context* within which cognitive plasticity is studied needs to be specified. In most studies, cognitive plasticity has been examined within an experimental or intervention context.

The individual's average level of cognitive functioning in normative, everyday experience is then contrasted with the range of plasticity exhibited under experimental or training conditions. Specification of the contextual conditions under which plasticity is studied is critical since the range of plasticity manifested will vary on the basis of such factors as the duration, intensity, or instructional procedures used in the intervention. Third, cognitive plasticity has generally been studied within a short *time frame*. Most training studies range from one session to, at most, several months in length. Hence, the range of plasticity exhibited may also be constrained by the temporal length or intensity of the intervention. It should be noted that early in the study of cognitive plasticity within the field of cognitive aging, plasticity was assessed almost exclusively with behavioral measures. However, recently, there is increasing interest both in the conceptual relationship between cognitive plasticity and neural plasticity and in experimental studies that examine cortical changes occurring concurrently with the behavioral training or intervention efforts (Jaeggi, Buschkuehl, Jonides, & Perrig, 2008; Westerberg & Klingberg, 2007).

Cognitive Reserve

In the study of cognitive aging within neuropsychology, there has been considerable interest in the capability of the individual to continue to function at an adequate cognitive level when there have been neural deficits or pathology. Stern and colleagues (Stern, 2002, 2007) have proposed applying the concept of cognitive reserve to the study of this phenomenon. A distinction is made between passive and active reserve. *Passive reserve* is defined in terms of the amount of neuropathology that can be sustained before reaching a threshold for clinical expression. This model presupposes that there is a critical threshold of brain reserve capacity such that clinical or functional deficits become evident once brain reserve capacity is diminished beyond this threshold.

Active cognitive reserve, by contrast, is based on the premise that the brain may actively attempt to cope with and compensate for deficits by using alternative preexisting cognitive processes or by enlisting compensatory approaches (Stern, 2007). Rather than positing that brains of individuals with high levels of cognitive reserve are anatomically different than those of individuals with less reserve, the cognitive reserve hypothesis proposes that the high-functioning individuals process tasks in a more efficient manner. Individuals with higher cognitive reserve, therefore, are believed to be more successful at coping with the same amount of neuropathology. Two types of neural mechanisms underlie cognitive reserve: (a) *neural reserve* involves using brain networks or cognitive paradigms that are more efficient and flexible. Neural reserve is a normal process used by both healthy individuals coping with task demands and by individuals with brain damage, (b) *neural compensation* refers to adopting new compensatory brain networks because pathology has impacted those that are normally used.

In earlier writing, Stern (2002) differentiated between reserve as the ability to optimize or maximize normal performance and compensation, an attempt to maximize performance in the face of brain damage by using brain structures or networks not engaged when the brain is not damaged. There is variability in cognitive reserve—both variability between individuals and variability within individuals (intraindividual) across time. Variability in cognitive reserve can stem from genetic differences and also from life experiences, such as education, occupation, or leisure activities. Cognitive reserve is implicated not only in the emergence of a clinical condition but also in the rate and magnitude of recovery of function from brain injury. Cognitive reserve is a malleable entity the level of which at any point in time is dependent on summation of life experiences and exposures; thus, cognitive reserve can be enhanced by relevant purposeful activities.

These perspectives of cognitive plasticity within the life span approach and cognitive reserve within neuropsychology share a number of similarities. First, both approaches emphasize that the individual is an *active* agent of the development of reserve and in compensatory efforts. Stern differentiates between passive and active reserve, while the life span perspective sees the individual as a codirector of one's development and adaptation. Both acknowledge individual differences and variability in reserve. Likewise, multiple antecedents or correlates of reserve are enumerated in both perspectives. Both approaches acknowledge that there are limits or constraints to reserve or plasticity. At the same time, both approaches view reserve as malleable and suggest that there are opportunities for the enhancement of reserve. While the life span approach has utilized experimental and intervention techniques to study the range of plasticity and reserve at various developmental periods, the Stern approach has focused more on descriptive examples of cognitive reserve. Developmental differences in the range of plasticity across the life span are a major concern of life span theory, while Stern's cognitive reserve focuses primarily on old age and/or response to brain injury or neuropathology.

Conceptualization of Cognitive Plasticity: Key Questions

In this chapter, we discuss five broad issues or questions that we consider to be central to any theory or conceptual framework for the study of cognitive plasticity. The first question focuses on the various levels (brain, behavior, and society/culture) at which plasticity has been or needs to be examined. We consider the conceptualization of plasticity at each level, the types and range of plasticity at each level, the key concepts and issues driving research at each level, and the relationship or interplay between plasticity at various levels. The second question focuses on the temporal durability of cognitive plasticity. Both short-term and long-term conceptions of plasticity are discussed, and the adaptivity of plasticity at short-term versus long-term intervals is considered. The third question focuses on the processes or mechanisms for achieving plasticity. Processes associated with the three levels of plasticity identified in question one are discussed. Of interest are commonalities in processes or mechanisms among the levels of plasticity. The fourth question briefly considers some issues related to developmental differences in plasticity. We consider issues such as sensitive periods for plasticity, developmental differences in asymptote and range of plasticity, utilization of different abilities or processes at different developmental periods, and developmental differences in environmental demands. A number of methodological issues arise in relation to the previous four questions. In a final question, then, we address issues of the appropriate design and methods for study of various levels of plasticity, short-term versus long-term plasticity, and developmental differences in plasticity.

Levels of Plasticity

In this section, we consider three different levels at which cognitive plasticity occurs and that need to be considered in any comprehensive conceptualization of plasticity. We begin with discussion of plasticity in the brain, and then proceed to discuss cognitive plasticity at the behavioral and finally at the sociocultural levels.

Brain

Neural Plasticity

Both brain structure (morphology) and brain function have been studied in relation to cognitive plasticity (Kramer et al., 2004; Mercado, 2008; Raz, 2000). While the concept of neural plasticity has been closely related to the concept of cognitive plasticity, the exact relation (or even directionality of the relation) between the two concepts has not been fully explicated. It has been assumed that neural plasticity contributes to or underlies cognitive plasticity; however, Stern's concept of cognitive reserve would suggest that cognitive reserve can exist even when neural plasticity has been compromised. Neural plasticity refers to the capacity of neural circuits to change in response to fluctuations in neural or glial activity (Kemperman, Gast, & Gage, 2002) and is associated with changes in synaptic connections between neurons, addition of new neurons (neurogenesis), increased myelinization of axons, or change in the size or shape of a neuron. Neural organization and hence plasticity can occur at multiple levels—from molecules and synapses to cortical maps and large-scale neural networks (Buonomano & Merzenich, 1998; Garlick, 2002).

Neural plasticity has usually been studied through the neuroimaging methods of positron emission tomography (PET) and functional magnetic resonance imaging (fMRI). As Poldrack (2000) suggests, our conception and current understanding of neural plasticity may be at least partly a function of these methods used to study the concept. In fact, PET and fMRI techniques provide indirect measures of synaptic activity by examining brain function via measurement of blood oxygenation and blood flow. Hence, our current knowledge of neural plasticity is focused primarily at the level of changes in synaptic activity and cortical maps. Thus, our understanding of the interrelation or interaction between various levels of neural organization and cognitive plasticity is limited. Or, as Kramer et al. (2004) stated, "There is a gap in our knowledge with regard to identifying global changes in the brain" (p. 941). For example, there is limited understanding at present of the relation between synaptic activity as represented in functional imaging signals and the lower levels (e.g., biophysical and molecular) of neural organization. Likewise, current understanding of the relation between brain function as represented in synaptic activity and brain structure or morphology is limited (Poldrack, 2000). While much of the research on neural plasticity has come from functional imaging techniques, there is also some research based on size of brain structure. For example, significant relations between white matter lesions, cerebral atrophy, and low levels of education were found in a sample of nondemented community-dwelling elders (Koga et al., 2002).

With regard to brain function, PET and fMRI research has resulted in at least two tentative general findings (Kramer et al., 2004); alternative explanations are now offered for each finding. First, findings indicate that older adults show lower levels of activation in a wide variety of tasks and brain regions. While one explanation of reduced activation holds that aging is associated with loss of neural resources, another explanation is that neural resources are available but not adequately recruited. Instruction in strategy use, for example, has been shown to reduce underrecruitment (Logan, Sanders, Snyder, Morris, & Buckner, 2002).

A second general finding is that older adults exhibit nonselective recruitment of brain regions (Kramer et al., 2004). Older adults, compared to young adults, show recruitment of different brain regions in addition to those activated in younger adults. This observation of bilateral activation has led to the hemispheric asymmetry reduction in older adults (HAROLD) model of neurocognitive aging (Cabeza, 2002; Hayes & Cabeza, 2008). The model suggests that cortical activity tends to be less lateralized in older than younger adults. There is current debate as to whether additional activity observed in older adults is compensatory or a marker of cortical decline. There is contradictory evidence whether older adults who perform better on a task show bilateral recruitment; some studies report this finding, while other studies do not. A limitation in examining this phenomenon has been that MRI studies use indirect measures of activation that depend on the relative activation compared to activation in surrounding areas. Thus, smaller brain structures would suggest different activation patterns even when the active structures are similar. Another limitation is that most studies have been comparisons across different subjects; future research needs to examine intraindividual changes in performance–brain activation patterns across various tasks, across longer developmental periods, and within training conditions (Kramer et al., 2004).

Neural Plasticity: Availability, Reconfigurability, and Customizability

To integrate the existing conceptual approaches and to explain the empirical findings, Mercado (2008) has recently argued that three key processes impact cortical modules and thus indirectly neural and cognitive plasticity: availability, reconfigurability, and customizability. Each process may vary between and within individuals, and the interplay between these processes may explain why there is no simple relation between any single indicator of plasticity and plasticity in complex abilities and intellectual functioning. In addition, Mercado attempts to integrate three factors previously associated with intellectual capacity (brain size, prefontral cortex, and neural speed or efficiency; Deary, 2000).

Availability refers to the number and diversity of cortical modules that are available for differentiating stimulus representations (Mercado, 2008). Larger brain regions provide room for more complex circuitry, more dendritic expansion, more synapses, thicker myelin, more neurons, and larger neurons—all of which increase functional capacity. Brain size limits the maximum number and diversity of cortical modules and constrains cortical organization (Jerison, 2002). Prior explanations of the fact that bigger brains are related to cognitive capacity have focused on amount of additional cortical tissue or the overall computational power as estimated by the number of neurons or synapses. In contrast, Mercado suggests that the amount of tissue and neurons is less critical than the manner in which circuits within the tissue are organized; it is the resolving power that determines capacity rather than general information processing capacity. Environmental domains, furthermore, are believed to increase the diversity of cortical modules available (Kahn & Krubitzer, 2002).

Second, *reconfigurability* refers to the brain's ability to flexibly develop new configurations of cortical modules and to switch rapidly between them as a function of task demands (Crone, Donohue, Honomichi, Wendelken, & Bunge, 2006; Mercado, 2008). This refers to the flexibility in using the same modules for different cognitive tasks and even within tasks as one progresses in learning increasingly better ways to perform the task. In fact, different brain regions serve different roles at different stages of cognitive skill learning (Crone et al., 2006; Doeller, Opitz, Krick, Mecklinger, & Reith, 2006; Pauli et al., 1994; Poldrack, Prabhakaran, Seger, & Gabrieli, 1999). The involvement of any particular subset of brain regions in cognitive skill acquisition depends on task difficulty, an individual's level of expertise, and the particular task being performed. In addition, the specific set of cortical regions that become active during acquisition may depend on the specific strategies used. In addition, there are clear indications that as people age they tend to recruit neural circuits differently than they did as younger adults (HAROLD; Cabeza, 2002) and that it might actually be adaptive to use different neural circuits across task trials to perform well in the same cognitive task (Reichle, Carpenter, & Just, 2000). Reconfigurability is associated with maintenance and control of representations; of particular relevance, then, are the frontal lobes, which are considered the seat of cognitive control, supporting capacity through flexible coordination of decision processes and memory.

Third, *customizability* refers to the brain's capacity to dynamically adjust the selectivity of cortical modules based on experience (Mercado, 2008). That is, the degree to which repeated experience in turn shapes the structure of the brain to perform well-learned tasks more efficiently or more accurately. Thus, plasticity on the level of the brain presumes that specialized cortical modules throughout the brain can be used in a variety of combinations (and somewhat interchangeably) to enable the acquisition and performance of cognitive skills. Variability in cognitive plasticity across individuals of different ages also reflects variability in their capacity to reconfigure cortical modules. Evidence indicating that individuals with greater intellectual capacity may be able to configure their neural circuits more flexibly has come primarily from electroencephalographic studies in humans (Jausovec & Jausovec, 2000; Thatcher, North, & Biver, 2005).

Mercado differentiates between the older concept of neural *efficiency* and neural *plasticity* or customizability. The assumption critical to the neural efficiency model was that differences in efficiency accounted for variability in cognitive capacity. Faster brains that could process information more efficiently should have greater capacity. Mercado (2008) argues that the focus on neural efficiency has receded and has been replaced by the role of neural plasticity in relation to behavioral flexibility. According to Mercado, neural plasticity involves not only making connections stronger and more efficient but also enhancing the ability to reallocate and retune circuits. Neural plasticity may determine how quickly an individual can adapt to new situations. Different abilities require different connections across circuits; neural plasticity guided by experience establishes the patterns of connection. Different levels of neural plasticity across individuals could impact the number and complexity of neural connections—this could then affect processing speed and neural efficiency. The number and diversity of cortical circuits engaged during learning can change as a function of experience.

A major question regarding neural plasticity is the issue of how experience or cognitive stimulations impacts the brain and enhances brain functioning. Kramer et al. (2004) have suggested two alternative hypotheses regarding the relationship between cognitive stimulation including training and plasticity in neural structure and function. On the one hand, enhanced neuronal structure and brain function may occur as a result of additional environmental stimulation and play a protective function against neuronal degradation (Fillit et al., 2002). Alternatively, enhanced neuronal networks fostered through cognitive experiences may delay cognitive decline even in the face of morphological and functional deterioration in the aging brain; the later hypothesis seems congruent with Stern's (2007) concept of cognitive reserve.

A major question focuses on the directionality of the relation between cognitively stimulating activities and brain reserve: to what degree do education or other forms of cognitive reserve represent initial brain capacity versus to what degree does brain capacity reflect the effects of cognitive stimulation? Experimental studies with animals in which cognitive stimulation is manipulated provide one design for examining the directionality of relations between neural plasticity and cognitive stimulation (Kemperman, Kuhn, & Gage, 1997; Kramer et al., 2004). In animal research, neurons and synapses and also glial cells that permit and enhance neuronal function have been shown to be altered though cognitive stimulation, with greater effects in young animals but also occurring albeit more slowly in mature animals. Neurogenesis associated with cognitive stimulation has been found in the hippocampus of animals and humans both in young and in old age (Eriksson et al., 1998). Some support for neurogenesis in other cerebral cortical has been reported but is debatable.

There are a number of important questions regarding the relation between neural and cognitive plasticity that have not been fully answered (Kramer et al., 2004). Does cognitive experience at earlier ages affect the potential for neurogenesis at later ages that might provide reserve capacity? How long do newly generated hippocampal neurons in adults survive? Is their longevity dependent on continued environmental stimulation? Are there enough newly generated neurons at a given time to contribute to improved behavioral performance? How are these new neurons integrated morphologically and functionally with the existing neural networks?

The concepts of availability, reconfiguration, and customization are complemented by the cortical "disconnection" hypothesis (Hayes & Cabeza, 2008; O'Sullivan et al., 2001). Cortical disconnection is hypothesized to lead to a loss of functional integration of neurocognitive networks. A plausible anatomical substrate for functional disconnection is disruption of the white matter tracts that link the components of distributed cognitive networks. The capacity of a brain region such as the prefrontal cortex to become activated may not be attenuated by age; rather, the coordination of the whole neural response is impaired, implying a loss of functional connectivity. However, functional imaging techniques provide only indirect evidence of cerebral disconnection and depend on the assumption of a linear relation between neural activity and hemodynamic response that may not hold in elderly subjects. In relation to plasticity, reorganization of large, distributed cognitive networks is likely to depend on integrity of white matter tracts.

Just as there are multiple types of plasticity at the neural level, there are also multiple types of cognitive abilities/processes at the behavioral level. The interplay between different neural levels of plasticity and various cognitive abilities is an important area of inquiry. For example, there may be differential effects with regard to declarative (conscious, explicit memory) versus nondeclarative memory (not dependent on conscious processes, such as skill learning). A challenge is presented by the fact that different types of memory may involve very different underlying neural mechanisms. While declarative explicit memory relies on the medial temporal lobe (hippocampus), nondeclarative memory is not dependent on the medial temporal lobe and may be associated with different neural substrates depending on the nature of the task. For example, individuals learning a finger-tapping sequence consciously engage very different sets of brain regions than individuals learning the same sequence implicitly (nondeclarative memory), even though the behavioral demands of the task are identical (Grafton, Hazeltine, & Ivry, 1995; Poldrack, 2000).

Based on the what we have stated so far with respect to neural plasticity, we take the position throughout the rest of this chapter that it is important to go beyond a single-indicator approach to plasticity. That is, any theory about plasticity needs to explain the limiting conditions of (a) existing structures (e.g., the brain), (b) specialized substructures (e.g., particular circuitry used in the brain), (c) potential adaptation in the recruitment of substructures to manage higher-order tasks (e.g., flexibility in recruiting different networks to achieve the same result), and (d) potential change in structures and recruitment due to environmental stimulation.

Behavior Plasticity

Cognitive plasticity has been examined at multiple behavioral levels, just as neural plasticity involves multiple levels. Cognitive training research has focused on cognitive processes (e.g., processing speed and inhibition; Ball et al., 2002; Jones et al., 2006), primary mental abilities (e.g., inductive reasoning, spatial orientation, and episodic memory; Schaie & Willis, 1986), higher-order cognitive constructs (e.g., fluid intelligence and executive functioning; Jaegii et al., 2008), and global cognition involving multiple cognitive domains (Fried et al., 2004). In addition, the impact of noncognitive interventions (e.g., exercise and nutrition; Colcombe & Kramer, 2003) on cognition has been examined.

Most behavioral cognitive interventions have focused on processes and abilities previously shown in longitudinal research to exhibit relatively early age-related decline or to be associated with cognitive impairment. Thus, interventions have focused on fluid and process-based abilities (reasoning, speed, working memory, and executive functioning). There has been a parallel between the abilities targeted for training and the brain areas and structures of interest. The greatest atrophy in cortical volume has generally been reported for the prefrontal regions and somewhat smaller atrophy for the temporal and parietal areas. Executive control, fluid abilities, and some memory processes that have been the target of intervention are supported by prefrontal and temporal regions of the brain.

Indices of Plasticity at the Behavioral Level

Earlier in this chapter, we noted that cognitive plasticity has most commonly been conceptualized as an individual's latent cognitive potential or the individual's cognitive capacity under certain specified conditions. Hence, observable indicators or behavioral indices of cognitive plasticity are needed. For a number of cognitive researchers (Harlow, 1959; Thorndike, 1911), key behavioral indicators of intellectual capacity include the capacity to learn a cognitive skill, the rate at which the skill is learned, and the highest performance (asymptote) reached (Zimprich, Rast, & Martin, 2008).

Life span theorists (Baltes, 1987) have identified three levels of performance that provide a profile of an individual's plasticity. *Baseline performance* indicates the individual's initial status (level) of performance on cognitive tasks without intervention or support. *Baseline plasticity* refers to the extended range of possible performance (performance improvement) when additional resources are provided. For example, this form of plasticity has been examined shortly after participants are taught memory strategies, such as the method of loci. This level of plasticity involves brief instruction in a strategy or the provision of a cognitive resource but little or no practice in use of the strategy. *Developmental reserve capacity* or *developmental plasticity* refers to the further range of performance improvement that occurs as a result of the opportunity or context within which cognitive resources can be fully activated (e.g., through extensive practice that optimizes strategy or cue utilization). Recent training research has compared the range of performance improvement under baseline plasticity versus developmental plasticity conditions. A greater range of plasticity was found under the developmental reserve plasticity condition (extended practice with the strategy or mnemonic) than the baseline plasticity condition in memory training research using the method of loci (Brehen, Li, Muller, von Oertzen, & Lindenberger, 2007; Jones et al., 2006). It was suggested that the greater range of plasticity shown in the developmental plasticity condition is due to information binding (Craik, 2006) involved in use of the method of loci strategy, that is, the formation of associations between novel words to be remembered and different loci in a certain sequence. Functional imaging during the various phases of the training study indicated that greater activation in the medial temporal lobe was found for participants who exhibited greater plasticity during the developmental reserve capacity phase; activation of the medial temporal lobe was hypothesized to be related to formation of associations and with information binding.

Cognitive Training and Behavioral Plasticity

The contexts in which behavioral cognitive plasticity have been most commonly studied has been the behavioral training studies that target those fluid- and process-based abilities that exhibit relatively early age-related decline (Kramer & Willis, 2003). Several criteria have been involved in evaluating the effectiveness of cognitive training, and these criteria are of interest in the study of cognitive plasticity (Ball et al., 2002).

Magnitude of performance improvement on the target ability of training for the intervention group in comparison to control groups has been the primary outcome of interest and thus an indicator of the range of cognitive plasticity that could be evoked under the intervention condition. A testing-the-limits condition has been used in some training studies to examine the asymptotic level of training improvement under increasingly demanding conditions. For example, in a series of memory training studies using the method of loci, asymptotic level was assessed by increasing the speed of word recall (Kliegl, Smith, & Baltes, 1989) or by engaging in dual tasks of walking and memory recall (Li, Lindenberger, Freund, & Baltes, 2001).

Although cognitive plasticity is concerned with change at the intraindividual level, most training studies have reported performance improvement or plasticity at the level of the group mean; hence, information on the proportion of individuals exhibiting reliable intraindividual change is obscured, as is the absolute range of plasticity and asymptotic levels attained. Given that plasticity is an intraindividual concept, comparison of the individual's performance after training with performance at earlier developmental periods prior to training would be optimal. However, longitudinal data on intraindividual change are rarely available. Comparison of asymptotic levels across age-groups is problematic given that the groups may differ on factors other than age that affect plasticity.

A second criterion in training studies has focused on the maintenance of training effects. It is argued that temporal durability of effects is required in order for training outcomes to be meaningful and of lasting benefit. Although the number of training studies examining long-term maintenance has been limited (Jones et al., 2006), temporal durability of training effects on primary mental abilities have been reported for 5 years within a clinical trial (Willis et al., 2006) and up to 14 years after training in smaller studies (Boron, Willis, & Schaie, 2007; Willis & Nesselroade, 1990).

A third criterion and one that is currently of particular interest focuses on training transfer. Until recently, most training studies have focused on a single cognitive process (verbal memory, inhibition) or primary ability (reasoning), and the original interest was in the magnitude of training effects and the asymptote achieved. However, there has been increasing interest in the breadth of transfer achieved. Near transfer has focused on demonstration of training effects to one or more indicators of the ability trained; there is consensus that training does result in near transfer. However, there is much less consensus or empirical evidence for far transfer, that is, demonstration of training effects on cognitive processes or abilities that are conceptually and empirically distinct from the cognitive target of training.

A major limitation to the study of transfer has been lack of consensus on how to define or assess varying levels of transfer. Definitions of transfer have varied from similarity of the stimuli used in assessment materials to similarity in strategies used in various cognitive measures to the requirement for assessment of transfer at the latent construct level, demonstrating common shared variance across various indicators. We discuss this further in the section on methods to examine plasticity.

The second (durability) and third (transfer) criteria discussed with regard to training studies are of interest with regard to the concept of cognitive plasticity. Although cognitive plasticity has been most commonly studied in the context of training studies, definitions of cognitive plasticity have not focused on issues of durability or transfer. Indeed, in studies of neural plasticity, increased activation is usually assessed for very limited time periods. Kramer et al. (2004) have alluded to issues of durability and transfer in the numeration of questions still to be addressed: how long do newly generated neurons survive; do new neurons remain functionally specialized, or do they become functionally generalized; and how are new neurons are integrated with existing neural networks?

Dose–response relations are a fourth issue in training research related to cognitive plasticity. The question is whether the range of plasticity varies with the length or intensity of the treatment. Most training studies have been relatively brief, and thus the dose–response issue has received limited attention. Several studies have shown an increased magnitude of effect (range of plasticity) with booster sessions that supplemented the initial intervention (Ball et al., 2002; Jaeggi et al., 2008; Willis et al., 2006). Some recent studies also suggest that there may be age differences in dose–response relations (Brehmer, Li, Müller, Oertzen, & Lindenberger, 2007; Jones et al., 2006).

Cognitive Plasticity in Dyads

Definitions of cognitive plasticity have typically focused on intraindividual change. However, recent research on collaborative cognition has examined the range of enhancement of cognitive performance–associated dyadic cognitive activity or problem solving. It is possible that collaborative cognition could be considered a form of baseline plasticity within Baltes's levels-of-plasticity approach. Collaboration with others provides resources for enhancing one's range of performance in a manner similar to use of cognitive strategies. It appears that the effects of cognitive collaboration may be positive and facilitative of elders' everyday cognitive performance on a variety of tasks (i.e., prose recall, wisdom-related advice giving, comprehension of printed materials, and route planning/everyday life management; Strough & Margrett, 2002). At the same time, positive effects appear to be facilitated by having familiar social partners (Gould, Kurzman, & Dixon, 1994), explicit collaborative instructions, and tasks that do not rely on immediate memory recall. In addition, further research conceptualizing individual plasticity as embedded within the spousal or intergenerational dyads may be helping to explain individual differences in plasticity (Martin & Wright, 2008).

Sociocultural Plasticity

Much of the conceptualization and empirical work on cognitive plasticity has focused on neural plasticity examined over very brief intervals or on performance enhancement in behavioral interventions that span days, weeks, or, at most, months. However, cognitive plasticity can also be considered at the phylogenetic or sociocultural level as included in the biocultural constructivist approach discussed previously (Li, 2003).

Cohort-sequential longitudinal studies comparing the level of cognitive functioning of different birth cohorts at the same chronological age have suggested a range of cognitive plasticity that equals or exceeds that found across the ontogeny of a single individual, on average (Schaie, 2005). For example, there has been an average increase in reasoning ability performance on the order of over 1.5 standard deviations when comparing the performance of the 1896 birth cohort to the 1973 cohort. While inductive reasoning exhibits the largest positive cohort trend, positive cohort trends have also been shown for some spatial orientation and perceptual speed tasks. In contrast, number ability has exhibited curvilinear cohort trends. Significant or "massive IQ gains" on the order of 5 to 25 points within a single generation have been reported by Flynn and known as the "Flynn effect" (Dickens & Flynn, 2001; Flynn, 1984, 2007). Flynn and colleagues have reported that the largest cohort differences in intellectual functioning have been found for what are commonly known as fluid abilities. Less or no cohort gains have been found for acculturated skills acquired through schooling and commonly known as crystallized intelligence.

From a life span perspective, the question arises whether the findings of massive IQ gains (Flynn effect) represent a phenomenon unique to a specific historical period and to the post–World War II cohort or whether they are indicative of a long-term societal or evolutionary change. When cohort differences are examined over a broader historical period and a wider range of cohorts, the phenomenon of cohort gain in intellectual performance becomes more complex than described by the Flynn effect (Schaie, 2005; Schaie, Willis, & Pennak, 2005). Both fluid and crystallized abilities have exhibited significant positive gains, particularly in the early 1900 birth cohorts. The magnitude of cohort gain appears to have been greater in the early 1900s than that cited for the post–World War II cohorts. In addition, positive, negative, and curvilinear cohort trends have been observed. Moreover, cohort trends vary for different abilities within the same historical period.

Those studying cognition from a broad coevolutionary perspective propose that advances in cognition as would be represented in cohort and generational effects are due primarily to an accumulation of cultural resources and knowledge across time. This perspective has been largely nondevelopmental. It is concerned primarily with secular trends in level of cognition but with little consideration of how culture impacts developmental change.

Dickens and Flynn (2001) and Flynn (2007) have proposed that individuals' environment is largely matched to their IQ level. Through a *multiplier effect,* an individual with a higher IQ either seeks or is selected for a more stimulating environment, leading to further increases in IQ. The impact of small environmental changes could result in significant IQ gain due to the multiplier effect. By a similar process, a social multiplier effect can occur if intellect increases by a small amount for many persons in a society and leads across time to further reciprocal interactions between ability and environment. Increase in a person's IQ is thus influenced not only by his or her environment but also by the social multiplier effects occurring for others with whom the person has contact. The question remains of what determines the domain of development or cognition that is impacted by culture and environment.

Drawing on Darwin's work, Flynn suggests that an *X factor* may determine those aspects of cognitive development that are impacted by the environment (Dickens & Flynn, 2001). The X factor need not be inherently related to the developmental domain impacted. For example, introduction of technology (e.g., use of menus or linear thinking) might increase public attention and use of computer-based or electronic devices, leading to increased inductive reasoning. In the Schaie (2005) model, the X factor is represented as a period effect.

In a related coevolutionary approach, Tomasello and others (Tomasello, 1999) have proposed mechanisms for social transmission of cultural knowledge. Humans have evolved forms of social cognition unique to humans that have enabled them not only to create new knowledge and skills but also, more important, to preserve and socially transmit these cultural resources to the next cohort/generation. Cultural learning thus involves both social transmission of cultural knowledge and resources developed by one person and also sociogenesis or collaborative learning and knowledge creation.

Time Frame: Short-Term and Long-Term Plasticity

The sampling of time will influence analysis and interpretation of intraindividual plasticity and variability (Martin & Hofer, 2004). Indeed, we might expect that different intervals will yield different patterns of plasticity and result from different influences on the individual. For example, we might consider sampling moment to moment (attentional lapses), within test (fatigue and practice), within session (fatigue, order effects, and motivation), within day (time-of-day effects), across days or weeks (environmental perturbations, physical health, and practice), or months or years (characteristic change trajectory). In many cases, short-term plasticity or change contains meaningful information about psychological processes of interest. In fact, there may be many different manifestations of short-term plasticity and several possible theoretical interpretations. For example, intraindividual short-term variability in functioning may be an early indicator of deficits (Schaie, 2000) or later-onset declines.

With respect to the differentiation–dedifferentiation (Li, 2002) or the "common cause" hypothesis, intraindividual short-term variability might be indicative of the structure of aging-related changes. Intraindividual short-term plasticity could also indicate adaptive behavior to cope with a stressful event or the limitations that go along with physical ailments. As an example, an increase in short-term intraindividual variability in extreme old age is not necessarily maladaptive. Maintaining low levels of variability in developmental outcomes such as well-being or health requires a high level of regulatory effort. If, however, individual energy levels are low (e.g., Fairclough, 2001), it might be maladaptive to invest energy in the stability of a particular outcome variable. Given limited resources, such efforts might affect functioning in other life domains, such as social activities. Instead, setting wider margins between a maximum and a minimum value for the variability of a particular outcome variable may reduce the effort required to balance functioning in both domains. As a consequence, within- and across-domain short-term intraindividual variability might increase, and this range of plasticity indicates a successful adaptation with respect to the outcome of well-being.

Theories of development that attempt to explain age-related changes within individuals need to consider specifications of which short- and long-term intraindividual change relations are theory relevant and to which time scales predictions apply (Schaie, 1989a, 1989b). In addition to specifying that there should be age-related changes in both explanatory concepts (e.g., in speed) and aging-related outcomes (i.e., fluid intelligence), it is possible to specify what longitudinal short- and long-term relations are to be expected or if the theory even applies to particular time frames of change. To illustrate this point, one may consider the fact that to solve a new cognitive task, it is most adaptive to quickly acquire or learn the required skills. Thus, high levels of plasticity are expected in individuals coping best with the environment. However, several studies have reported that larger variability in performance in the long term may be a predictor of individuals at risk for strong cognitive declines and even dementia. Thus, any theory of plasticity needs to specify the relevant time frames because the explanations and predictions for short-term plasticity may not be the same as those for long-term plasticity. In this context, hypotheses about within-person changes need to be formulated and tested separately from hypotheses about population mean changes (e.g., Zimprich & Martin, 2002).

So far, there is little research on systematic intraindividual aging-related short-term plasticity, that is, on the interaction between short-term intraindividual plasticity of explanatory parameters and intraindividual changes in other short-term developmental outcome parameters (e.g., Li, Aggen, Nesselroade, & Baltes, 2001; Nesselroade, 2001; Strauss, MacDonald, Hunter, Moll, & Hultsch, 2002). There is also very little research on the predictive value of short-term intraindividual plasticity on later short-term variability, long-term changes, or long-term outcomes. With adequate research designs, the examination of short-term intraindividual plasticity offers new possibilities for developmental research in many domains of psychological functioning. Results from these study designs may help answer questions about the generality versus specificity of plasticity and about age-related differences in the range of observable intraindividual short-term plasticity. In the long run, these designs might add to the specificity of theories and predictions and support the development of tools allowing the early detection of problematic development.

Processes and Mechanisms Associated With Plasticity

Traditionally, in the study of both brain and behavior, the focus has been primarily on distinct, relative narrow domains, such as regions of interest in the brain, localized areas of activation, and specific primary mental abilities. However, there is growing awareness that cognitive functioning either in brain or in behavior needs to be conceptualized as involving connectivity and networks or maps rather than isolated abilities and brain regions. Relating specific cognitive abilities to specific brain regions is overly simplistic. Likewise, the role of connectivity must be given greater attention in the study of activation and underrecruitment in functional imaging; activation in any region must be seen as determined partially by the capacity for connectivity across broad cortical maps. Research findings suggest that different brain regions serve different roles at different stages of cognitive skill learning. The involvement of any particular subset of brain regions in cognitive skill acquisition depends on task difficulty, an individual's level of expertise, and the particular tasks being performed. The specific set of cortical regions that become activated may depend on the specific strategies used. Finally, connectivity may be related to the concept of information binding (Brehen et al., 2007; Craik, 2006) of interest in cognitive training research. The increased range of plasticity shown in Baltes's developmental cognitive reserve condition has been attributed to information binding (i.e., extensive practice in use of cognitive strategies or cognitive resources); this extensive practice may involve strengthening of certain connections or perhaps reconfiguration or customization of connections.

Cognitive and neural connectivity also underlies the capacity for reconfiguration and customization. A broad network or map of cortical modules or cognitive abilities (representing connectivity) must exist for reconfiguration and customization to occur. Reconfiguration and customization are instances of a greater focus on flexibility and adaptability that characterize more recent approaches to the study of development and plasticity. A central feature of the concepts of compensation and active reserve is the individual's flexibility to use alternative cognitive processes or neural resources to adapt to pathology or functional deficits. Compensation represents the ability to reconfigure and customize one's cognitive resources in the face of new challenges.

Availability of neural structures (e.g., neurons, synapses, and cortical networks) appears to be a necessary but not sufficient condition for plasticity. As noted by Mercado (2008), larger brain regions, more neurons (neurogenesis), or more synapses in themselves may not result in greater plasticity. Rather, these factors provide the limiting conditions for increased larger cortical networks leading to greater functional capacity and resolving power. Likewise, neural efficiency or speed of processing per se may not be the most critical feature of plasticity. The critical feature in connectivity is not solely the presence of stronger and more efficient connections but also the specific capacity required for flexibility to reconfigure and customize connections and cortical maps. Different abilities require different connections across circuits; neural plasticity guided by experience establishes the patterns of connection.

It is becoming increasingly evident that there is a reciprocal rather than unidirectional relation between brain, experience, and behavior. Changes in the brain do not always lead in a unidirectional manner to changes in behavior. Experience and behavior also significantly impact changes in the brain. Enhanced neuronal structure and brain function may occur as a result of environmental stimulation. An important task for future research is further explication of how this reciprocity between brain, experience, and behavior functions.

Developmental Issues and Plasticity

Sensitive Periods in Development

"Critical" or sensitive periods have been of interest in both neural and behavioral development and have been closely associated with learning and cognition. Traditionally, the concept of "critical" or sensitive periods included the conditions that learning or plasticity occur over a short, sharply defined period in the life cycle and that this learning was subsequently irreversible (Thomas & Johnson, 2008). However, more recent findings suggest that critical periods may not necessarily be sharply timed or irreversible; thus, "sensitive periods" rather than "critical periods" is the more commonly used terminology. Moreover, there appear to be multiple sensitive periods within a specific domain. For example, within the auditory domain, there are different sensitivity periods for different facets of speech processing and for music perception.

Sensitivity or plasticity is reduced in lower-level systems before it is reduced in high-level cognitive systems (Huttenlocher, 2002; Thomas & Johnson, 2008). Synapses, the structures through which neurons communicate, are initially overproduced in the brain, and the environment selects which ones are retained to support function. The density of synapses has been considered to be one indicator of plasticity since experience can alter connective strength of synapses. Synaptic density function peaks at different times in different regions of the brain, with the prefrontal cortex (middle frontal gyrus) showing the latest peak in synaptic density; this region is associated with higher-level cognition.

Developmental Differences in Plasticity

A major question in current research on sensitive periods focuses on the explanatory mechanisms that may underlie reduction in plasticity across development (Thomas & Johnson, 2008). Three alternative explanations are (a) termination of plasticity due to maturation, (b) self-termination of learning, and (c) stabilization of constraints on plasticity (without a reduction in the underlying level of plasticity). The first alternative suggests that reduction in plasticity is due to changes in neurochemistry of a particular brain region, resulting in an increased rate of pruning of synapses and thus the "fossilization" of existing patterns of functional connectivity. The second and third explanations, in particular, may be of most interest with respect to cognitive plasticity in the later part of the life span. The second explanation argues that the process of learning itself can produce changes that may reduce plasticity in a system (Thomas & Johnson, 2006). Leaning could reduce plasticity in several ways. First, learning could lead to neurobiological changes that reduce plasticity. Alternatively, prior learning may place a heavy demand on the neural system's computational resources such that new learning would have to compete for these resources, thus limiting the potential for new learning. A third option is that prior experience or learning puts the neural system in a nonoptimal state for new learning—that is, additional time would be required to reconfigure the system, and thus new learning would take longer than if the prior learning or experience had not occurred. The third explanation suggests that there may not be an end to plasticity per se but that the potential for plasticity may be "hidden" because of certain constraining factors; these constraining factors become increasingly stable with development. This third explanation may be useful in understanding evidence for certain types of plasticity observed in adulthood. For example, connectivity between various sensory systems (tactile and visual) appears to dissipate significantly with age; however, when sighted persons are deprived of vision, there is a sudden and sharp increase in activation of the visual cortex during tactile perception. This activation suggests that some level of connectivity (plasticity) remains but is not activated until visual input is constrained.

Recent findings in research on second-language acquisition provides insight into several issues regarding developmental differences and similarities in cognitive plasticity across the life span (Birdsong, 2006). First, adults and young children appear to differ in how they acquire a second language. Young children generally acquire a second language through large amounts of exposure to the new language. In contrast, second-language learning in adults appears to be most efficient when they adopt explicit strategies for learning the language and when they are more responsive to feedback than children. As a result, adults often learn a second language at a faster pace than young children. Indeed, there appears to be little evidence for total loss of plasticity to acquire a second language in adulthood. However, the final level attained is generally lower the older the age of acquisition. Second-language acquisition also provides insight into the association of prior learning (first-language acquisition) on future plasticity. While early research suggested that different areas of the cortex were activated for a second language, recent research findings indicate that the higher the level of competence in the second language, the more likely that the same cortex areas will be activated as for one's first language. This suggests that certain brain areas have become optimized for processing language (perhaps during acquisition of the first language) and that increased proficiency in the second language tends to activate the same brain areas. Thus, subsequent plasticity may be tempered by the processing structures created by earlier learning. Earlier in this chapter, we also discussed plasticity in adulthood as involving reconfiguration and customization of neural networks (Mercado, 2008).

Plasticity in adulthood may also vary across the multiple subskills involved in a complex task, such as second-language acquisition, as a result of sensitivity or plasticity being reduced in lower-level systems before it is reduced in high-level cognitive systems (Huttenlocher, 2002). For example, there may be greater or earlier loss of plasticity in phonology than in lexical semantics. Thus, the older second-language learner may find acquisition of new vocabulary easier than acquiring new sounds or new grammar.

In summary, developmental differences in cognitive plasticity may not be solely or even primarily associated with maturational changes, such as loss or deterioration in basic neural structures or functions. Rather, prior learning and experience may play a critical role in determining both the range of cognitive plasticity later in the life span as well as the mechanisms involved. Prior learning may reduce the availability of neural computational resources or may reduce the flexibility of cortical networks required for new learning. In earlier sections of this chapter, the important role of reconfiguration and customization of cortical modules and networks for continued cognitive plasticity in adulthood was discussed (Mercado, 2008). An important area of future research would be to examine in greater detail, at both the neural and the behavioral level, the role and impact of prior learning and experience on subsequent cognitive plasticity.

Methodological Issues in the Study of Plasticity

To examine individual-level plasticity, research designs must be sensitive to all types of plasticity in order to identify patterns and magnitudes of plasticity within individuals. Given both systematic and stochastic sources of fluctuation in individual characteristics over short periods of time, such designs must also be sensitive to intraindividual variation (Nesselroade, 1991). Temporal sampling designs can take many forms. One such design, the measurement burst design (Nesselroade, 1991; Nesselroade & Schmidt-McCollam, 2000), utilizes intensive measurements over a short period in time and follow-up with further measurement burst sessions after longer intervals and permits a window on individual-level characteristics as well as long-term change. Obtaining multiple, closely spaced assessments at each wave allows local temporal smoothing of data for each individual by averaging across multiple assessments. The addition of multiple indicators at each assessment permits further improvements in the modeling of random error components in models that incorporate true change. By improving measurement precision through multiple assessments or multiple indicators, such designs will increase statistical power to detect cognitive change at both the individual and the aggregate sample level and permit greater understanding of intraindividual processes within and across different time intervals. Indeed, measurement burst designs incorporating multiple indicators would permit an optimal opportunity for evaluating systematic short-term fluctuation and change. A further consideration is the context in which measurements are obtained. Most temporal sampling designs are performed under random contextual backgrounds, but individual variation in performance can be evaluated against defined contexts as well—more akin to experimental paradigms (e.g., levels of stress and dual-processing tasks).

Analytically, different types of plasticity can be distinguished. Each type is related to different theoretical assumptions and explanations. Structural plasticity can be found on the level of changes in covariation patterns among variables across time. That is, the covariation patterns of different intellectual abilities within persons may change over time, suggesting that more or fewer factors are sufficient to explain observed behaviors. Empirically, Schaie, Maitland, Willis, and Intrieri (1998) investigated longitudinal measurement invariance of six primary mental abilities (inductive reasoning, spatial orientation, perceptual speed, numeric facility, verbal ability, and verbal recall) across a 7-year period in a sample of 984 individuals, disaggregated into six age-groups (32, 46, 53, 60, 67, and 76 years at first testing). They found some structural plasticity in the older age-groups suggesting that in fact the covariation patterns of abilities change in old age. Theoretically, it remains an open question as to how this finding can be explained. If fewer factors suffice to explain the structural relations in old age as the dedifferentiation hypothesis would suggest (e.g., Anstey, Hofer, & Luszcz, 2003; Ghisletta & Lindenberger, 2003;

Zelinsky & Lewis, 2003), this might be caused by an underlying third variable such as neurophysiological degradation, physical changes due to closeness to death, restricted environmental challenges stimulating the use of fewer abilities, or restriction in activities.

Mean level plasticity refers to the change in the quantity or amount of a cognitive ability over time. Although one might be interested in cognitive plasticity in individual persons, mean plasticity is usually examined using average (i.e., sample values of groups of) persons. This provides an estimate of the range of plasticity within normal development by comparing average with better than average performance. In fact, from empirical findings, accelerating decline at the transition from middle to late adulthood seems to be evident for some but not all cognitive abilities. The mean stability in middle age often reported might be still indicating plasticity, that is, to the degree the level of performance is maintained despite increases and changes in work and family demands (Martin & Mroczek, in press). That is, examining mean plasticity requires longitudinal data to determine the influence of environmental factors on cognitive development, the effects of chronic stressors on cognitive performance, the interaction between changes in different cognitive domains, and cohort differences between early and late middle age in the amount of cognitive performance change.

Differential plasticity refers to the potential changes in the consistency of individual differences in cognitive abilities across time. Conceptually, differential change implies that some individuals change to a larger (or smaller) amount than others, such that the rank order of individuals is different at different time points. Thus, differential plasticity indicates actual changes within individuals. As with the other types of plasticity, however, it should be noted that changes can be in the direction of increases, decreases, or stability. A strength of examining differential change is that relative change, that is, the degree to which individuals' cognitive performance changes in similar directions over time, is considered. However, from a low stability implying pronounced differential change, we do not know whether the sample of persons—let alone an individual person—increases or decreases in their cognitive ability level. Theoretically, differential plasticity would imply models assuming that different environmental or activity factors are actively shaping changes in cognitive performance; were these influences not differentially influencing intraindividual change, then only biologically or maturation-based changes that may be assumed to be more similar between persons could explain development.

Plasticity of variability refers to the fact that using correlations, we do not know whether variances change over time. That is, across time there might be perfect differential stability and no absolute change, but variances might increase or decrease (Preece, 1982). This would still be indicative of individual differences in plasticity, although both the mean level and the rank order of individuals might be perfectly preserved across time (cf. Hertzog & Dixon, 1996). Plasticity in variability would be needed to explain differential developments between an individual at risk for further and stronger declines and an individual repeatedly profiting from gains in performance because they are starting from high levels of performance. A better understanding of the processes leading to this dissociation of development could point to events or ages in the life course when persons respond particularly sensitive to even small improvements or declines in performance, thus setting the stage for a developmental trajectory of lifelong gains or lifelong losses in performance.

Plasticity in dimensionality of change refers to the fact that if changes in cognitive abilities are highly related, this would suggest one factor or, at least, very few factors responsible for the individual plasticity observed; this factor would explain a similarly large degree of cognitive plasticity in most individuals. This could occur in stable environmental conditions leading to very similar cognitive activations or when similar physiological processes are strongly influencing performance despite environmental variations between persons and over time.

Plasticity of intraindividual variability refers to the fact that there is now sufficient empirical evidence to establish that intraindividual variability is a substantial source of systematic performance variability between people, especially in adults (Martin & Hofer, 2004; Nesselroade, 2001). In fact, recent studies suggest that intraindividual variability may predict later cognitive difficulties in older age (e.g., Rabbitt, Osman, Moore, & Stollery, 2001; Schaie, 2000). Even within the middle adult age range, there seem to be substantial interindividual differences in intraindividual change in particular cognitive functions (Ghisletta, Nesselroade, Featherman, & Rowe, 2002; Zimprich & Martin, 2002). Willis and Schaie (1999), in their review of longitudinal data on cognition, point out that there are significant individual differences above and beyond differences depending on design (i.e., cross-sectional versus longitudinal) and length of longitudinal interval. This renders it meaningful to examine individual differences in plasticity in cognitive functioning across the life span. Once sufficient data on life span cognition are available, it can be established to which degree individual differences in plasticity might be due to (a) individual differences in usage and training, (b) individual differences in the interaction between environmental demands and age-related levels of performance, or (c) individual differences in resilience and compensatory processes that individuals apply to maintain a high level of everyday functioning (e.g., Freund & Baltes, 2002).

Summary and Conclusion

In this chapter, we have conceptualized human development as representing the individual's lifelong capacity for adaptation. Development is thus assumed to be modifiable or plastic during all phases of the life span. Cognitive plasticity represents the individual's latent cognitive potential for adaptation and change. However, there are constraints and limits on cognitive plasticity, and these constraints and limits may vary by developmental period. A major concern in the study of cognitive plasticity, therefore, is to examine the range and limits of plasticity at various phases of the life span.

Cognitive plasticity occurs and can be studied at multiple levels—neural, behavioral, and sociocultural. Within each level, cognitive plasticity can also be studied on various time scales, ranging from momentary or short term to life span development (long term) and, finally, beyond the individual to plasticity on an evolutionary or phylogenetic time scale. In addition, at each level of cognitive plasticity, there are mechanisms and processes associated with the nature of plasticity and with the range and limits of plasticity. Finally, there are developmental differences in plasticity (e.g., asymptote and mechanisms) across the life span. A comprehensive conceptualization or theory of cognitive plasticity would address each of these topics.

With regard to the levels at which cognitive plasticity can be studied, there is increasing evidence that the relation between levels is not solely unidirectional, from brain to behavior. Rather, there appear to be reciprocal relations between brain, experience, and behavior. Current neural structures (brain size, number of neurons, and synaptic density) do not totally determine cognitive behavior and potential. As Stern's concept of cognitive reserve suggests, cognitive potential can remain even when neural structure has been compromised. Neurogenesis can occur even in older humans and animals as a result of cognitively stimulating activities at the behavioral level. Enhanced neuronal structure may play a role in protecting against neuronal degradation. Likewise, experiences at the behavioral level shape the capacity of the brain both to reconfigure cortical modules and networks and to customize cortical modules as needed for various tasks. Efficient acquisition of new cognitive skills and behaviors in later life depends on reconfiguration and customization of cortical networks in the brain. Hence, reconfiguration and customization of cortical modules and networks represent critical mechanisms for brain plasticity.

The role of learning and experience in relation to cognitive plasticity is complex and can impact cognitive plasticity both positively and negatively. On the one hand, as discussed previously, cognitive stimulation at the behavioral level can lead to neurogenesis and desirable changes in the reconfiguration and customization of cortical modules and networks. These neural changes as a result of cognitive stimulation can occur in old age as well as earlier in the life span, although perhaps to a lesser degree in old age. On the other hand, prior learning and experience can place limits or constraints on future levels of plasticity. The role of prior learning experiences in limiting cognitive plasticity is particularly important in the later part of the life span. Research on sensitive periods suggests that prior learning and experiences may result in limitations on existing neural resources needed for the acquisition of new cognitive skills (i.e., plasticity). Additionally, prior learning and experience result in the establishment of cortical networks; these preexisting networks may make the reconfiguration and customization that is required for further plasticity more difficult and less efficient.

While there is increasing evidence that cognitive plasticity is possible during all developmental periods, constraints and limits on plasticity at each level become more evident with increasing age. At the neural level, there are constraints due to degradation of the neural structure (brain atrophy, number of neurons, and synaptic density). Likewise, there are constraints at the functional level in the brain. Flexibility in reconfiguration of cortical networks or in customization of cortical modules is reduced with advancing age. At the behavioral level, there appear to be constraints in terms of the asymptotic level of performance attainable with increasing age. Although cognitive interventions result in significant behavioral improvement, the highest level attained is lower for older adults compared to young adults. Likewise, efficiency of new skill acquisition appears to be compromised with age under conditions of "testing the limits." For example, increasing the speed at which older adults must perform or requiring the engagement in dual tasks compromises the performance of older adults to a greater extent than those younger in the life span.

Finally with regard to plasticity at the sociocultural level, Flynn suggests that there are significant cohort differences in the range of plasticity during different historical periods. The Flynn effect suggests that the period after World War II may have been particularly supportive of plasticity with regard to fluid abilities. The cohort-sequential studies of Schaie suggest that different historical periods have been associated with significant cohort gains in crystallized versus fluid intelligence. The bioconstructionist perspective suggests that increasing cultural resources are required for cognitive plasticity with age but that utilization of these cultural resources becomes less efficient with age.

Future development of theories of plasticity will require further articulation of the dynamic interplay between different levels of cognitive plasticity (brain, behavior, and society/culture). There is increasing evidence that a reciprocal relation exists between plasticity in brain and behavior. The bioconstructionist perspective suggests further that there is also reciprocity between individual and cultural plasticity. Mechanisms and processes associated with cognitive plasticity at each level have been identified. Future theoretical development as well as empirical research is now needed to understand how these mechanisms change and adapt as a function of age and of prior learning and experience. Further consideration of the relation and interaction between short-term and long-term cognitive plasticity would facilitate an understanding of how development and adaptation occurs across the life span. Under what conditions is short- or long-term plasticity adaptive?

Finally, it is important to note that cognitive plasticity should serve to facilitate successful adaptation (i.e., development) across the life span. Plasticity, although often defined in terms asymptotic levels, faster and more efficient cortical networks or behaviors, or cognitive training effects, must ultimately involve a consideration of the individual's own developmental goals and life choices. Cognitive plasticity provides the individual with increased resources for better self-regulation in goal pursuits and in dealing with the challenges and adversities associated with development and aging. It is important that future theoretical development on cognitive plasticity include consideration of these higher-order strivings or needs of the aging individual.

References

Anstey, K. J., Hofer, S. M., & Luszcz, M. A. (2003). Cross-sectional and longitudinal patterns of dedifferentiation in late-life cognitive and sensory function: The effects of age, ability, attrition, and occasion of measurement. *Journal of Experimental Psychology: General, 132,* 470–487.

Ball, K., Berch, D. B., Helmers, K. F., Jobe, J. B., Leveck, M. D., Marsiske, M., et al. (2002). Effects of cognitive training interventions with older adults. *Journal of the American Medical Association, 288,* 2271–2281.

Baltes, P. B. (1987). Theoretical propositions of life-span developmental psychology: On the dynamics between growth and decline. *Developmental Psychology, 23,* 611–626.

Baltes, P. B. (1997). On the incomplete architecture of human ontogeny: Selection, optimization, and compensation as foundation of developmental theory. *American Psychologist, 52,* 366–380.

Baltes, P. B., & Baltes, M. M. (1990). *Successful aging: Perspectives from the behavioral sciences.* New York: Cambridge University Press.

Baltes, P. B., & Lindenberger, U. (1988). On the range of cognitive plasticity in old age as a function of experience: 15 years of intervention research. *Behavior Therapy, 19,* 283–300.

Baltes, P. B., Lindenberger, U., & Staudinger, U. M. (2006). Life span theory in developmental psychology. In R. M. Lerner (Ed.), *Handbook of child psychology: Theoretical models of human development* (Vol. 1, 6th ed., pp. 569–664). New York: Wiley.

Birdsong, D. (2006). Age and second language acquisition and processing: A selective overview. *Language Learning, 56,* 9–49.

Boron, J., Willis, S. L., & Schaie, K. W. (2007). Cognitive training gain as a predictor of mental status. *Journal of Gerontology: Social Sciences, 62,* 45–53.

Brehen, Y., Li, S-C., Muller, V., von Oertzen, T., & Lindenberger, U. (2007). Memory plasticity across the life span: Uncovering children's latent potential. *Developmental Psychology, 43,* 465–478.

Brehmer, Y., Li, S-C., Müller, V., Oertzen, T., & Lindenberger, U. (2007). Memory plasticity across the lifespan: Uncovering children's latent potential. *Developmental Psychology, 43,* 465–478.

Buonomano, D. V., & Merzenich, M. M. (1998). Cortical plasticity: From synapses to maps. *Annual Review of Neuroscience, 21,* 149–186.

Cabeza, R. (2002). Hemispheric asymmetry reduction in older adults: The HAROLD model. *Psychology and Aging, 17,* 85–100.

Cattell, R. B. (1963). Theory of fluid and crystallized intelligence: A critical experiment. *Journal of Educational Psychology, 54,* 1–22.

Colcombe, S., & Kramer, A. F. (2003). Fitness effects on the cognitive function of older adults: A meta-analytic study. *Psychological Science, 14,* 125–130.

Craik, F. I. M. (2006). Remembering items and their contexts: Effects of aging and divided attention. In H. Zimmer, Z. Mecklinger, & U. Lindenberger (Eds.), *Binding in human memory: A neurocognitive perspective* (pp. 571–594). Oxford: Oxford University Press.

Crone, E. A., Donohue, S. E., Honomichi, R., Wendelken, C., & Bunge, S. A. (2006). Brain regions mediating flexible rule use during development. *Journal of Neuroscience, 26,* 11239–11247.

Deary, I. J. (2000). *Looking down on intelligence: From psychometrics to the brain.* Oxford, England: Oxford University Press.

Dickens, W. T., & Flynn, J. R. (2001). Heritability estimates versus large environmental effects: The IQ paradox resolved. *Psychological Review 108,* 346–369.

Doeller, C. F., Opitz, B., Krick, C. M., Mecklinger, A., & Reith, W. (2006). Differential hippocampal and prefrontal striatal contributions to instance-based and rule-based learning. *Neuroimage, 31*(4), 1802–1816.

Eriksson, P. S., Perfilieva, E., Bjork-Eriksson, T., Alborn, A. M., Nordborg, C., Peterson, D. A., et al. (1998). Neurogenesis in the adult human hippocampus. *Nature Medicine, 4,* 1313–1317.

Fairclough, S. H. (2001). Mental effort regulation and the functional impairment of the driver. In P. A. Hancock & P. A. Desmond (Eds.), *Stress, workload, and fatigue: Human factors in transportation* (pp. 479–502). Mahwah, NJ: Lawrence Erlbaum Associates.

Fillit, H. M., Butler, R. N., O'Connell, A. W., et al. (2002). Achieving and maintaining cognitive vitality with aging. *Mayo Clinic Proceedings, 77,* 681–696.

Flynn, J. R. (1984). The mean IQ of Americans: Massive gains, 1932 to 1978. *Psychological Bulletin, 95,* 29–51.

Flynn, J. R. (2007). *What is intelligence? Beyond the Flynn effect.* New York: Cambridge University Press.

Freund, A. M., & Baltes, P. B. (2002). The adaptiveness of selection, optimization, and compensation as strategies of life management: Evidence from a preference study on proverbs. *Journal of Gerontology: Social Sciences, 57,* P426–P434.

Fried, L. P., Carlson, M. C., Freedman, M., Frick, K. D., Glass, T. A., Hill, J., et al. (2004). A social model for health promotion for an aging population: Initial evidence on the Experience Corps model. *Journal of Urban Health, 81,* 64–87.

Garlick, D. (2002). Understanding the nature of the general factor of intelligence: The role of individual differences in neural plasticity as an explanatory mechanism. *Psychological Review, 109,* 116–136.

Ghisletta, P., & Lindenberger, U. (2003). Age-based structural dynamics between perceptual speed and knowledge in the Berlin Aging Study: Direct evidence for ability dedifferentiation in old age. *Psychology and Aging, 18,* 696–713.

Ghisletta, P., Nesselroade, J. R., Featherman, D. L., & Rowe, J. W. (2002). The structure, validity and predictive power of weekly intraindividual variability in health and activity measures. *Swiss Journal of Psychology, 61,* 73–83.

Gould, O., Kurzman, D., & Dixon, R. A. (1994). Communication during prose recall conversations by young and old dyads. *Discourse Processes, 17,* 149–165.

Grafton, S. T., Hazeltine, E., & Ivry, R. (1995). Functional mapping of sequence learning in normal humans. *Journal of Cognitive Neuroscience, 7,* 497–510.

Harlow, H. F. (1959). Learning set and error factor theory. In S. Koch (Ed.), *Psychology: A study of science* (Vol. 2, pp. 492–537). New York: McGraw-Hill.

Hayes, S. M., & Cabeza, R. (2008). Imaging aging: Present and future. In S. M. Hofer & D. F. Alwin (Eds.), *Handbook of cognitive aging: Interdisciplinary perspectives* (pp. 308–326). Los Angeles: Sage.

Hertzog, C., & Dixon, R. A. (1996). Methodological issues in research on cognition and aging. In F. Blanchard-Fields & T. M. Hess (Eds.), *Perspectives on cognitive change in adulthood and aging* (pp. 66–121). Boston: McGraw-Hill.

Huttenlocher, P. R. (2002). *Neural plasticity: The effects of the environment on the development of the cerebral cortex.* Cambridge, MA: Harvard University Press.

Jaeggi, S. M., Buschkuehl, M., Jonides, J., & Perrig, W. J. (2008). Improving fluid intelligence with training on working memory. *Proceedings of the National Academy of Sciences of the United States of America, 10,* 1–5.

Jausovec, N., & Jausovec, K. (2000). Differences in event-related and induced brain oscillations in the theta and alpha frequency bands related to human intelligence. *Neuroscience Letters, 293,* 191–194.

Jerison, H. J. (2002). On theory in comparative psychology. In R. J. Sternberg & J. C. Kaufman (Eds.), *The evolution of intelligence* (pp. 251–288). Mahwah, NJ: Lawrence Erlbaum Associates.

Jones, S., Nyberg, L., Sandblom, J., Stigsdotter Neely, A., Ingvar, M., Petersson, K., et al. (2006). Cognitive and neural plasticity in aging: General and task-specific limitations. *Neuroscience & Biobehavioral Reviews, 30,* 864–871.

Kahn, D. M., & Krubitzer, L. (2002). Massive cross-modal cortical plasticity and emergence of a new cortical area in developmentally blind mammals. *Proceedings of the National Academy of Sciences of the United States of America, 99*(17), 11429–11434.

Kemperman, G., Gast, D., & Gage, F. H. (2002). Neuroplasticity in old age: Sustained five-fold induction of hippocampal neurogenesis by long-term environmental enrichment. *Annals of Neurology, 52,* 135–143.

Kemperman, G., Kuhn, H. G., & Gage, F. (1997). More hippocampal neurons in adult mice living in an enriched environment. *Nature, 386,* 493–495.

Kliegl, R., Smith, J., & Baltes, P. B. (1989). Testing the limits and the study of adult age differences in cognitive plasticity of a mnemonic skill. *Developmental Psychology, 25,* 247–256.

Koga, H., Yuzuriha, R., Yao, H., et al. (2002). Quantitative MRI findings and cognitive impairment among community dwelling elderly subjects. *Journal of Neurology, Neurosurgery, and Psychiatry, 72,* 737–741.

Kramer, A. F., Bherer, L., Colcombe, S. J., Dong, W., & Greenough, W. T. (2004). Environmental influences on cognitive and brain plasticity during aging. *Journal of Gerontology: Medical Sciences, 59,* 940–957.

Kramer, A. F., & Willis, S. L. (2003). Cognitive plasticity and aging. In B. H. Ross (Ed.), *The psychology of learning and motivation: Advances in research and theory* (Vol. 43, pp. 267–302). Amsterdam: Academic Press.

Li, K. Z. H., Lindenberger, U., Freund, A. M., & Baltes, P. B. (2001). Walking while memorizing: A SOC study of age-related differences in compensatory behavior under dual-task conditions. *Psychological Science, 12,* 230–237.

Li, S-C. (2002). Connecting the many levels and facets of cognitive aging. *Current Directions in Psychological Science, 11,* 38–43.

Li, S-C. (2003). Biocultural orchestration of developmental plasticity across levels: The interplay of biology and culture in shaping the mind and behavior across the life span. *Psychological Bulletin, 129,* 171–194.

Li, S-C., Aggen, S. H., Nesselroade, J. R., & Baltes, P. B. (2001). Short-term fluctuations in elderly people's sensorimotor functioning predict text and spatial memory performance: The MacArthur Successful Aging Studies. *Gerontology, 47,* 100–116.

Lindenberger, U., & Baltes, P. B. (1995). Testing the limits of experimental stimulation: Two methods to explicate the role of learning in development. *Journal of Human Development 38,* 349–360.

Logan, J. M., Sanders, A. L., Snyder, A. Z., Morris, J. C., & Buckner, R. L. (2002). Under-recruitment and non-selective recruitment: Dissociable neural mechanisms associated with cognitive decline in older adults. *Neuron, 33,* 827–840.

Martin, M., & Hofer, S. M. (2004). Intraindividual variability, change, and aging: Conceptual and analytical issues. *Gerontology, 50,* 7–11.

Martin, M., & Mroczek, D. K. (in press). Are personality traits across the lifespan sensitive to environmental demands? *Journal of Adult Development.*

Martin, M., & Wright, M. (2008). Dyadic cognition in old age: Paradigms, findings, and directions. In S M. Hofer & D. F. Alwin (Eds.), *Handbook of cognitive aging: Interdisciplinary perspectives* (pp. 629–646). Los Angeles: Sage.

Mercado, E. (2008). Neural and cognitive plasticity: From maps to minds. *Psychological Bulletin, 134,* 109–137.

Neisser, U., Brodoo, G., Bouchard, T. J., Jr., Boykin, A.W., Brody, N., Ceci, S. J., et al., (1996). Intelligence: Knowns and unknowns. *American Psychologist, 41,* 77–101.

Nesselroade, J. R. (1991). The warp and the woof of the developmental fabric. In R. M. Downs & L. S. Liben (Eds.), *Visions of aesthetics, the environment & development: The legacy of Joachim F. Wohlwill* (pp. 213–240). Hillsdale, NJ: Lawrence Erlbaum Associates.

Nesselroade, J. R. (2001). Intraindividual variability in development within and between individuals. *European Psychologist, 6,* 187–193.

Nesselroade, J. R., & Schmidt-McCollam, K. M. (2000). Putting the process in developmental processes. *International Journal of Behavioral Development, 24,* 295–300.

O'Sullivan, M., Jones, D. K., Summers, P. E., Morris, R. G., Williams, S. C. R., & Markus, H. S. (2001). Evidence for cortical "disconnection" as a mechanisms of age-related cognitive decline. *Neurology, 57,* 632–638.

Pauli, P., Lutzemberger, W., Rau, H., Birbaumer, N., Rickard, T. C., Yaroush, R. A., et al. (1994). Brain potentials during mental arithmetic: Effects of extensive practice and problem difficulty. *Brain Research Cognitive Brain Research, 2*(1), 21–29.

Pedersen, N. L., & Lichtenstein, P. (1997). Biometric analyses of human abilities. In C. Cooper & V. Varma (Eds.), *Processes in individual differences* (pp. 125–147). London: Routledge.

Poldrack, R. A. (2000). Comments and controversies: Imaging brain plasticity: Conceptual and methodological issues—A theoretical review. *NeuroImage, 12,* 1–13.

Poldrack, R. A., Prabhakaran, V., Seger, C. A., & Gabrieli, J. D. (1999). Stiatal activation during acquisition of a cognitive skill. *Neuropsychology, 13*(4), 564–574.

Preece, P. F. (1982). The fan-spread hypothesis and the adjustment for initial differences between groups in uncontrolled studies. *Educational and Psychological Measurement, 42,* 759–762.

Rabbitt, P., Osman, P., Moore, B., & Stollery, B. (2001). There are stable individual differences in performance variability, both from moment to moment and from day to day. *Quarterly Journal of Experimental Psychology. A, Human Experimental Psychology, 54,* 981–1003.

Raz, N. (2000). Aging of the brain and its impact on cognitive performance: Integration of structural and functional findings. In F. I. Craik & T. A. Salthouse (Eds.), *Handbook of aging and cognition* (pp. 1–90). Mahwah, NJ: Lawrence Erlbaum Associates.

Reichle, E. D., Carpenter, P. A., & Just, M. A. (2000). The neural bases of strategy and skill in sentence-picture verification. *Cognitive Psychology, 40,* 261–295.

Sarter, M., Hasselmo, M. E., Bruno, J. P., & Givens, B. (2005). Unraveling the attentional functions of cortical cholinergic inputs: Interactions between signal-driven and cognitive modulation of signal detection. *Brain Research: Brain Research Reviews, 48,* 98–111.

Schaie, K. W. (1989a). The hazards of cognitive aging. *Gerontologist, 29,* 484–493.

Schaie, K. W. (1989b). Individual differences in rate of cognitive change. In V. L. Bengtson & K. W. Schaie (Eds.), *The course of later life: Research and reflections* (pp. 65–85). New York: Springer Publishing.

Schaie, K. W. (2000). The impact of longitudinal studies on understanding development from young adulthood to old age. *International Journal of Behavioral Development, 24,* 257–266.

Schaie, K. W. (2005). *Developmental influences on adult intelligence: The Seattle Longitudinal Study.* London: Oxford University Press.

Schaie, K. W., Maitland, S. B., Willis, S. L., & Intrieri, R. C. (1998). Longitudinal invariance of adult psychometric ability factor structures across 7 years. *Psychology and Aging, 13,* 8–20.

Schaie, K. W., & Willis, S. L., (1986). Can decline in adult intellectual functioning be reversed? *Developmental Psychology, 22,* 223–232.

Schaie, K. W., Willis, S. L., & Pennak, S. (2005). A historical framework for cohort differences in intelligence. *Research in Human Development 2,* 43–67.

Singley, M. K., & Anderson, J. R. (1998). *The transfer of cognitive skill.* Cambridge, MA: Harvard University Press

Spearman, C. (1904). "General intelligence," objectively determined and measured. *The American Journal of Psychology, 15,* 201–292.

Stern, Y. (2002). What is cognitive reserve? Theory and research application of the reserve concept. *Journal of the International Neuropsychological Society, 8,* 448–460.

Stern, Y. (Ed.). (2007). *Cognitive reserve: Theory and applications.* New York: Taylor & Francis.

Strauss, E., MacDonald, S. W., Hunter, M., Moll, A., & Hultsch, D. F. (2002). Intraindividual variability in cognitive performance in three groups of older adults: Cross-domain links to physical status and self-perceived affect and beliefs. *Journal of the International Neuropsychological Society, 8,* 893–906.

Strough, J., & Margrett, J. A. (2002). Introduction. Collaboration in later life. *International Journal of Behavior Development, 26,* 2–5.

Terman, L. M. (1916). *The measurement of intelligence.* Boston: Houghton.

Thatcher, R. W., North, D., & Biver, C. (2005). EEG and intelligence: Relations between EEG coherence, EEG phase delay and power. *Clinical Neurophysiology, 116,* 2129–2141.

Thomae, H. (Ed.). (1979). *The concept of development and life-span developmental psychology, Vol. II.* New York: Academic Press.

Thomas, M. S. C., & Johnson, M. H. (2006). The computational modeling of sensitive periods. *Developmental Psychobiology, 48,* 337–344.

Thomas, M. S. C., & Johnson, M. H. (2008). New advances in understanding sensitive periods in brain development. *Current Directions in Psychological Science, 17,* 1–5.

Thorndike, E. L. (1911). *Animal intelligence.* New York: Macmillan.

Thurstone, L. L. (1938). *The primary mental abilities.* Chicago: University of Chicago Press.

Tomasello, M. (1999). *The cultural origins of human cognition.* Cambridge, MA: Harvard University Press.

Westerberg, H., & Klingberg, T. (2007). Changes in cortical activity after training of working memory—A single subject analysis. *Physiology & Behavior, 92,* 186–192.

Willis, S. L., & Nesselroade, C. S. (1990). Long term effects of fluid ability training in old-old age. *Developmental Psychology, 26,* 905–910

Willis, S. L., & Schaie, K. W. (1999). Intellectual functioning in midlife. In S. L. Willis & J. D. Reid (Eds.), *Life in the middle* (pp. 234–247). San Diego, CA: Academic Press.

Willis, S. L., & Schaie, K. W. (2006). Cognitive functioning among the boomers. In S. K. Whitbourne & S. L. Willis (Eds.), *The baby boomers* (pp. 205–234). New York: Lawrence Erlbaum Associates.

Willis, S. L., Tennstedt, S. L., Marsiske, M., Ball, K., Elias, J., Koepke, K. M., et al. (2006). Long term effects of cognitive training on everyday functional outcomes in older adults. *Journal of the American Medical Association, 296,* 2805–2814.

Zelinsky, E. M., & Lewis, K. L. (2003). Adult age differences in multiple cognitive functions: Differentiation, dedifferentiation, or process-specific change? *Psychology and Aging, 18,* 727–745.

Zimprich, D., & Martin, M. (2002). Can longitudinal changes in processing speed explain longitudinal age changes in fluid intelligence? *Psychology and Aging, 17,* 690–695.

Zimprich, D., Rast, P., & Martin, M. (2008). Individual differences in verbal learning in old age. In S. M. Hofer & D. Alwin (Eds.), *Handbook on cognitive aging: Interdisciplinary perspectives* (pp. 224–243). Thousand Oaks, CA: Sage.

18 The Role of Cognitive Control in Older Adults' Emotional Well-Being

Nichole Kryla-Lighthall
Mara Mather

Recently, the focus in gerontology has expanded from trying to avoid age-related decline to also trying to promote optimal aging. One key component of optimal aging is maintaining or even enhancing emotional well-being over the life span (Baltes & Baltes 1990; Lawton, 2001; Rowe & Kahn, 1987). The traditional stereotype of old age depicts a period of inevitable and continuous loss, with decreased subjective well-being. However, although negative life events tend to become more frequent and cognitive function and health tend to decline as people get older, emotional well-being does not appear to be compromised by the aging process. In fact, accumulating evidence indicates that healthy emotional aging—characterized by an overall *enhancement* of emotional experience across the life span—is part of normal human development (see Carstensen, Mikels, & Mather, 2006; Charles & Carstensen, 2007; Diener, Suh, Lucas, & Smith, 1999).

Theories of aging must explain this phenomenon. How is it that older adults have such emotionally gratifying lives in the face of significant losses?

In this chapter, we attempt to explain the surprising robustness of emotional well-being in aging by integrating perspectives from cognition, emotion, and neuroscientific research. First, we review evidence that emotional well-being improves with age and discuss how age-related changes in goals motivate older adults to pursue emotionally gratifying experiences. Next, we present behavioral evidence that older adults use cognitive control to enhance their current emotional states. Then we use research findings from cognitive neuroscience to outline the requirements of implementing emotion regulation–focused strategies. We then evaluate older adults' capacity to exert cognitive control given the trajectory of cognitive and brain function in aging. Finally, we present findings indicating that older adults use cognitive resources to regulate emotion.

In this chapter, we argue that older adults use strategic control processes to achieve their emotional goals within the limitations of age-related changes to neural structures. The intersection of neurological function and affective goals in aging indicates that cognitive function—particularly executive function—is a critical factor in promoting emotional well-being in late life. Our theoretical framework emphasizes older adults' power in determining their own emotional destiny. Cognitive control allows people to direct attention and memory in ways that help satisfy emotional needs. Using cognitive control as an emotion regulation tool becomes increasingly useful with advancing age as emotional well-being takes on more importance to those with more limited futures.

Improvements in Emotional Experience With Age

Studies reveal that negative affect decreases and positive affect increases or remains stable over the life course (for reviews, see Carstensen, Isaacowitz, & Charles, 1999; Carstensen et al., 2006). From a clinical perspective, older adults have lower rates of subsyndromal depression, dysthymia, major depression, and anxiety disorders compared with younger adults (Bland, Orn, & Newman, 1988; George, Blazer, Winfield-Laird, Leaf, & Fischback, 1988; Jorm, 2000; Kobau, Safran, Zack, Moriarty, & Chapman, 2004; Weissman, Bruce, Leaf, Florio, & Holzer, 1991; Weissman, Leaf, Bruce, & Florio, 1988). This reduced prevalence of depression and anxiety among older adults signals a decrease in negative affect with age. One possibility is that emotional intensity decreases with age. Indeed, older adults show fewer physiological reactions than younger adults when reliving negative experiences (Levenson, Carstensen, Friesen, & Ekman, 1991) and less distress than younger adults after natural disasters (Phifer, 1990). Yet an overall reduction in experienced emotional intensity cannot explain the reduced rates of depression and anxiety in the aged, as the subjective experience of emotions does not decrease with age. Older adults report experiencing emotions with the same intensity as younger adults (Carstensen, Pasupathi, Mayr, & Nesselroade, 2000; Levenson et al., 1991; Magai, Consedine, Krivoshekova, Kudadjie-Gyamfi, & McPherson, 2006; Malatesta, Izard, Culver, & Nicolich, 1987; Mikels, Larkin, Reuter-Lorenz, & Cartensen, 2005; Tsai, Levenson, & Carstensen, 2000). One recent study even found that middle-aged and older adults had more intense subjective emotional experiences than younger adults, even though bodily responses to emotions were dampened in the two older groups (Burriss, Powell, & White, 2007). These studies underscore the importance of cognition in determining emotional experiences with age.

The enhanced sense of well-being among older adults reflects both decreased negative affect and increased positive affect. On a daily basis, older adults have fewer negative emotional experiences than younger adults (Carstensen et al., 2000; Gross et al., 1997; Mroczek & Kolarz, 1998), less negative affect (Diehl & Hay, 2007), and more positive affect (Mroczek & Kolarz, 1998) and are less likely to report any unhappiness in their lives (Ryff, 1989). Thus, in group comparisons, older people seem to have greater overall well-being than younger people. There is less consistency, however, on the trajectory of well-being across adulthood—some studies reveal improvement (Carstensen et al., 2000; Charles, Reynolds, & Gatz, 2001; Lawton, Kleban, & Dean, 1993; Kunzmann, Little, & Smith, 2000; Labouvie-Vief, Diehl, Jain, & Zhang, 2007; Magai, 2001; Mroczek & Kolarz, 1998; Schroots, 2003; Staudinger, Bluck, & Herzberg, 2003), and others stability (Costa, McCrae, & Zonderman, 1987; Diener & Diener, 1996; Stacey & Gatz, 1991) or even decline (Pinquart, 2001). For instance, a literature review by Magai (2001) lends support to the enhancement trajectory with findings of a reliable decrease in anger experiences with age, whereas Stacy and Gatz (1991) found stability in older adults' negative affect over 14 years.

The complexity of the age and well-being relationship may explain some of the inconsistency in the literature. For instance, some studies find an inverse curvilinear relationship with peak life satisfaction and emotional experience occurring in late adulthood and then declining somewhat in the oldest old (Mroczek, 2001; Mroczek & Spiro, 2005). Despite this overall pattern, adults in their 80s show levels of life satisfaction equal to adults in their 40s and higher than those in younger cohorts (Mroczek & Spiro, 2005), indicating that the emotional health of the elderly is well maintained. Other age-related variables, such as chronic illness, should be considered in determining how well-being may vary in adulthood. Controlling for health status can reverse negative relationships between age and emotion to reveal age-associated improvements to well-being (Kunzmann et al., 2000), yet not all studies finding age-related declines in well-being have evaluated the impact of health (see Pinquart, 2001).

As many emotion and aging studies have employed cross-sectional methods, it may be that emotional well-being is a characteristic of the current elderly population and not an effect of aging. However, a 23-year longitudinal study found decreases in negative affect across the life span in four different cohorts (Charles et al., 2001). Overall, these data indicate that, among healthy older adults, late life is a period characterized mostly by emotional health and well-being. In the next section, we review how older adults' successful maintenance of positive affect and reduction of negative affect may be related to changes in time perspective and a greater focus on regulating emotion as people get older.

Socioemotional Selectivity Theory and Prioritizing Well-Being

Socioemotional selectivity theory provides the foundation for the framework we outline here for understanding the trajectory of emotional well-being in adult development. According to the theory, the perception of time is a key element in determining human motivation (Carstensen et al., 1999; Lang & Carstensen, 2002). The theory posits that those who view their time remaining as unconstrained, such as younger adults, are motivated to invest in the future. Information-seeking goals are particularly salient to those who perceive time as unlimited because expanding one's knowledge increases the chance of success in the future. As adults get older, however, accruing knowledge for future payoffs becomes less relevant. Those in late life benefit more from pursuing goals that provide immediate gratification; emotional goals serve this purpose. By emphasizing emotional well-being in the present, older adults optimize the time they have remaining. Thus, socioemotional selectivity theory proposes that people are motivated to pursue knowledge-seeking goals in early adulthood and transition to focusing on emotion regulation goals as they age.

Research on social relationships across the life span supports the idea that emotional goals become more important with advancing age. Longitudinal data reveal that the amount of time spent with acquaintances and close friends declines during adulthood, while time spent with close family members—and one's sense of emotional closeness with these social partners—increases with age (Carstensen, 1992). These changes suggest that young adulthood is a time for learning which people make the best social partners. Over time, social partners who provide the least emotional gratification are "pruned" to derive more emotional gains from social relationships. Even the oldest old—who experience the most death-related loss of loved ones—actively select and maintain intimate social relationships from their remaining social networks (Lang & Carstensen, 1994). Thus, the reduction in number of personal relationships in older age appears to reflect the selection of social partners in the service of emotional goals. Further, when young adults' futures are constrained by time experimentally or by circumstances that influence time perspectives, such as political upheaval or terminal illness, their desire to spend time with social partners that support emotional goals increases (Carstensen & Fredrickson, 1998; Fung, Carstensen, & Lutz, 1999).

When describing their major life goals for the future, older adults emphasize goals that hold intrinsic meaning, such as creating meaningful relationships or contributing to society. Younger adults, on the other hand, describe life span goals that emphasize learning and taking on new challenges (Bauer & McAdams, 2004). Shifts in emotional goals with age are likewise represented by age differences in the qualities people expect in an ideal person. In their descriptions of an ideal person, middle-aged adults are more likely to include qualities such as being career oriented and enjoying life (i.e., productivity and pleasure), whereas those in old age are more likely to mention having a positive view about life and social relationships (i.e., enhancing feeling of life satisfaction; Ryff, 1989). This comparison supports the idea that active regulation of emotional experience—that is, putting a positive spin on one's life experiences—becomes more important with advancing age.

Evidence of a greater focus on active emotion regulation with age goes beyond the social relationships literature. Many studies reveal that older adults have superior emotion regulation skills than younger adults do (Carstensen et al., 2000; Gross et al., 1997; Lawton, Kleban, Rajagopal, & Dean, 1992; Magai et al., 2006; McConatha, Leone, & Armstrong, 1997; Mroczek, 2001). To enhance well-being, emotion regulation can be used to increase positive feelings (using up-regulation) or to decrease negative feelings (using down-regulation), and older adults demonstrate proficiency at both. For example, a recent study by Kliegel, Jäger, and Phillips (2007) shows that older people are more effective than younger people at "repairing" or down-regulating moods—restoring positive affect after a negative mood induction.

Older people are conscious of their emotion regulation ability, as they report greater control over their emotional states and mood stability than do younger people (Gross et al., 1997; Lawton et al., 1992). Older adults are more likely than younger adults to report controlling anger by using internal calming strategies (such as soothing oneself through self-talk; Phillips, Henry, Hosie, & Milne, 2006). In addition, older people report ruminating less about negative experiences (McConatha et al., 1997). Finally, from the coping literature, there are many studies demonstrating older adults experience less distress during difficult situations than do younger adults (see Charles & Carstensen, 2007). Thus, evidence indicates that individuals prioritize emotion regulation more as they age.

It may be argued that older adults report better emotion regulation in order to conform to social expectations. Yet older people are more effective at regulating anger than younger people even when social desirability is accounted for (Phillips et al., 2006). Along these lines, age-related emotion regulation gains lead to less intense negative emotions during interpersonal conflict (Birditt & Fingerman, 2003, 2005). Older adults are also capable of up-regulating emotions on command and show physiological profiles and subjective experience demonstrating they can enhance emotional experience as successfully as younger adults (Kunzmann, Kupperbusch, & Levenson, 2005). Taken together, this literature indicates that the ability to consciously shape emotional responses to suit regulation goals is as effective, if not more effective, with advancing age.

Positivity in Older Adults' Cognitive Processing

Cognition and emotions are inextricably linked—how we think influences how we feel and vice versa. For instance, cognitive processing can alter the quality of emotional experiences already in motion (Mauss, Cook, Cheng, & Gross, 2007; Ochsner & Gross, 2007; Pasupathi & Carstensen, 2003), effectively diminishing or intensifying those experiences. Given the power of cognition in determining emotional outcomes, goal-directed cognition has been proposed as a tool for modifying affective experiences (Carstensen et al., 2006; Isaacowitz, 2006; Mather & Carstensen, 2005; Mather & Knight, 2005). Focusing cognitive resources on emotional goals offers a way to feel positive in the present. Cognitive strategies can be used to focus on positive and suppress negative information in order to enhance emotional well-being, leading to a "positivity effect" in attention and memory (Carstensen & Mikels, 2005; Mather & Carstensen, 2005). We define the positivity effect as an age-by-valence interaction—such that a smaller proportion of older adults' memory or processing time is devoted to negative stimuli than for younger adults and a larger proportion is devoted to positive stimuli than for younger adults.

Indeed, numerous studies have revealed positivity effects in older adults' cognitive processing (for reviews, see Carstensen et al., 2006; Mather, 2006;

Mather & Carstensen, 2005). In particular, age-by-valence interactions are often found in memory studies (Charles, Mather, & Carstensen, 2003; Grady, Hongwanishkul, Keightley, Lee, & Hasher, 2007; Grühn, Scheibe, & Baltes, 2007; Kensinger, 2008; Knight, Maines, & Robinson, 2002; Leigland, Schulz, & Janowsky, 2004; Mather & Knight, 2005; Thomas & Hasher, 2006). Recent studies suggest that older adults' memory advantage for positive stimuli is specific to memory for the items themselves and does not extend to contextual details associated with the positive items (Kensinger, Garoff-Eaton, & Schacter, 2007; Kensinger, O'Brien, Swanberg, Garoff-Eaton, & Schacter, 2007).

As memory reconstruction is influenced by internal goals (Bahrick, Hall, & Berger, 1996; Brunot & Sanitioso, 2004), we expect that older people will remember the past positively, even at the expense of accuracy. Consistent with our hypothesis, older adults selectively distort their memories in ways that promote emotional well-being—remembering their life events, affect, and choices as more positive than they actually were (Kennedy, Mather, & Carstensen, 2004; Mather & Johnson, 2000; Ready, Weinberger, & Jones, 2007). Likewise, older adults' self-defining memories are more positive than those of younger adults (Singer, Rexhaj, & Baddeley, 2007). Further, even when older adults consider their personal memories to be highly negative, they report higher levels of positive feelings associated with such memories than do younger adults (Comblain, D'Argembeau, & Van der Linden, 2005). Remembering the past in a positive light does seem to enhance older adults' well-being, as their moods improve more than those of younger adults after reminiscing about their pasts (Cappeliez & O'Rouke, 2006; Kennedy et al., 2004; Pasupathi & Carstensen, 2003).

Selective attention can also be used to achieve emotion regulation goals by allowing people to focus on and subsequently process more positive than negative information. Studies using eye tracking to monitor the visual gaze of older and younger adults while they view emotional images reveal that older adults tend to look toward positive images and away from negative ones (Isaacowitz, Wadlinger, Goren, & Wilson, 2006a, 2006b; Knight et al., 2007) or show less of a negativity bias in their sustained attention than younger adults do (Rösler et al., 2005).

Declines in emotion detection abilities cannot explain the shift toward attending to more positive information with age. Studies find that older adults can detect and visually orient to emotionally arousing and negative stimuli as well as younger adults (Hahn, Carlson, Singer, & Gronlund, 2006; Knight et al., 2007; Mather & Knight, 2006; Rösler et al., 2005). Thus, it appears that when older adults detect negative stimuli, they employ attention strategies to reorient and focus on more positive information. These studies support the proposition that older people use visual attention to implement their chronically activated emotional goals, as selective attention allows them to focus on goal-consistent information and away from goal-irrelevant information.

Central to our cognitive control framework is the proposition that these age-associated shifts in cognitive processing are the result of shifts in goals, leading older adults to have chronically activated emotional goals, whereas younger adults are not usually focused on emotional goals. Thus, we predict that younger adults will show more of a positivity effect when something in the environment induces them to activate emotional goals. At least two studies support this prediction. Mather and Johnson (2000) found that when younger adults are instructed to focus on emotional aspects of their decision making, they remember their past decisions more positively. In this study, older adults also showed a positivity bias, but they did so with or without external emotional cues. In another study, older and younger nuns recalled autobiographical memories first reported 14 years prior (Kennedy et al., 2004). The nuns were assigned to one of three conditions: emotion focused, accuracy focused, or control. While accuracy-focused and younger control groups exhibited a negativity effect in memory processing, emotion-focused and older control groups showed similar patterns of positivity in memory processing. Like the results from the decision-making study, these research findings suggest that emotion regulation goals are chronically activated in older adults leading to more positive cognitive processing, whereas emotion regulation goals can be activated in younger adults if they are given the right cues.

Behavioral Evidence of a Cognitive Control Pathway to Well-Being

The findings presented so far suggest that older adults' path to emotional well-being in aging begins with a change in time perspectives. As perceived time remaining shrinks, older adults seek to satisfy their emotional goals by regulating their affect, and the positivity effect in cognitive processing is a result of their emotion regulation efforts (Charles & Carstensen, 2007; Carstensen et al., 2006; Mather, 2004). This section presents evidence that successful emotion regulation depends on older adults' active use of cognitive control strategies. That older adults use cognitive control to achieve well-being is supported by three lines of evidence: (a) older adults with better strategic processing abilities are more effective in regulating emotional states, (b) the presence of the positivity effect depends on cognitive processing constraints (i.e., positive bias occurs when circumstances allow for goal-directed processing), and (c) when cognitive resources are limited, older adults are more likely to exhibit a negativity bias.

Executive Processing Abilities

As stated earlier, focusing on emotional goals during information processing requires cognitive control. In order to feel positive in the face of negative information, several strategies can be implemented to direct affective outcomes. Gross (2001, 2002) outlines common strategies people use to down-regulate their affect when presented with negative material, including selecting a situation by its expected emotional outcome, modifying the emotional impact or meaning of a situation, focusing on select aspects of a situation, and altering an ongoing emotional response. All these methods of controlling emotions require self-initiated cognitive processing—in other words, executive functioning. As emotion regulation requires cognitive control, those with superior executive functioning should be better at achieving emotional goals through the use of cognitive control strategies. To test this proposition, Mather and Knight (2005) measured executive function (specifically self-initiated processing dependent on the prefrontal brain region) in older and younger adults to see if better cognitive control abilities predicted enhanced positivity in emotional memory processing. The executive function battery included measures to assess selective attention (Fan, McCandliss, Sommer, Raz, & Posner, 2002), working memory (Baddeley, Logie, & Nimmo-Smith, 1985), and the ability to refresh recently activated representations (Johnson, Mitchell, Raye, & Greene, 2004). The study revealed that, while older adults remembered more positive than negative information compared with younger adults overall, the older adults with the best performance on cognitive control tasks were the ones most likely to express the positivity effect. Further, those older adults with low cognitive control abilities had negatively biased memories. Some have proposed that older adults are more likely to "gate out" negative affect when they have low cognitive control abilities (e.g., Labouvie-Vief, 2005). On the contrary, this section indicates that those older people with the best cognitive control function are the most positively biased—remembering less negative and more positive information than their lower-functioning counterparts.

Indeed, the way that adults make choices with advancing age provides further support for the idea that high-functioning older adults use their executive processing resources to enhance well-being. A recent study by Mather, Knight, and McCaffrey (2005) found that, when deciding between two options, older adults with better performance on tasks measuring executive functioning made decisions based on alignable features (features comparable across choices) and had better memory accuracy for alignable features than for nonalignable features. Focusing on alignable features allows people to avoid regret (and thus negative affect) when making choices, as this decision strategy requires fewer trade-offs than whole-option comparisons (Luce, Bettman, & Payne, 1997). Younger adults with high executive functioning, on the other hand, were less likely to use feature-based comparisons. This makes sense given that avoiding regret is not a priority for the young. Conversely, older adults have a greater motivation to maintain well-being in the present than do younger adults; thus, we propose that cognitive control resources are increasingly allocated for enhancing emotional well-being with advancing age.

Cognitive Processing Constraints

Our cognitive control framework of aging and emotional well-being posits that older adults will experience emotional enhancement to the extent that they are capable of exerting cognitive control. We have provided evidence that older adults with better executive function are more successful at creating positive cognition via goal-directed processing. However, regulating emotions requires considerable cognitive effort, even for younger adults (Ochsner et al., 2004). Controlling emotions, whether attempting to amplify or decrease emotional experiences, requires increased neural activation in executive function regions of the brain including the prefrontal cortex. Given that the prefrontal cortex—which is largely responsible for self-initiated cognitive processing—deteriorates significantly with advancing age (Greenwood, 2000; West, 1996), regulating emotional states using effortful control strategies may be more resource demanding for older people than for younger people. Thus, older adults may need to compensate for age-related neural deficits by recruiting more cognitive resources in their emotion regulation efforts. Additionally, even in cognitively healthy young adults, control strategies can be utilized to service emotional goals only if processing circumstances allow (Muraven, Tice, & Baumeister, 1998; Wegner, Erber, & Zanakos, 1993). Therefore, we expect that the effectiveness of goal-directed processing will be inversely related to the amount of processing constraints present. In other words, older adults will be more successful in regulating emotions when they can devote considerable cognitive resources to regulation and less successful when they must split their attention between multiple tasks.

Mather and Knight's (2005) findings support this hypothesis, as they found a positivity effect in older adults' memory for pictures when participants were allowed to direct their full attention to picture viewing at encoding but a striking reversal to a negativity bias in older adults' memory when they had completed a concurrent goal-irrelevant task at encoding (monitoring sound patterns; see Figure 18.1). Thus, detracting from available cognitive resources appears to derail older adults' pursuit of emotional gratification through memory processing. This is not the case for young people, as those in the full-attention and divided-attention conditions both exhibited a negative bias in their picture memory. The younger adults' negativity in both conditions is not surprising given the lower priority of emotional well-being early in life. This study suggests that emotion regulation requires cognitive resources, and when processing constraints prohibit the use of effortful goal-related strategies, older adults cannot effectively enhance their well-being through cognitive control.

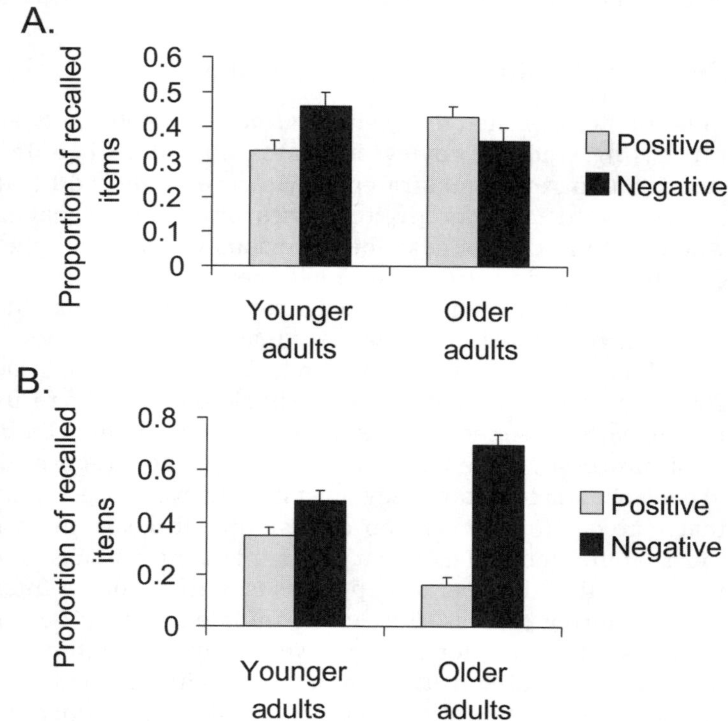

18.1

When participants could devote full attention to a picture slide show, a higher proportion of the pictures recalled later were positive among older adults than among younger adults (A). However, when distracted during the picture slide show, this positivity effect among older adults was reversed (B). Figure adapted with permission from Mather and Knight (2005).

Further support for this proposition comes from a study conducted by Knight et al. (2007) in which younger and old adults' visual attention for pairs of emotional and neutral scenes and faces was monitored using eye tracking. Visual gaze was monitored under either full- or divided-attention conditions. Similar to the memory findings of Mather and Knight (2005), older adults in the eye-tracking study showed a positivity bias in visual attention when they were allowed to devote full attention to the pictures but a negativity bias when they were forced to complete another goal-irrelevant task simultaneously. Thus, when cognitive resources are limited, older adults are not able to implement emotional goals effectively. Context can also limit access to cognitive resources. In another study, married couples reported on marital satisfaction in general (via mailed questionnaire) and under controlled conditions (in a lab while completing a conversation protocol; Henry, Berg, Smith, & Florsheim, 2007). Older married couples reported greater martial satisfaction than middle-aged couples in general, and the increase in satisfaction was explained by older adults' more positive perception of their spouses. In contrast, when couples were asked to evaluate their spouses' behavior during an experimentally controlled conversation in a lab (including an experimenter selected topic and regimented turn taking), there were no age differences in the number of negative characteristics attributed to spousal interactions. The laboratory experiment had more constraints than the overall evaluation of spousal satisfaction, and it is possible that this reduced older adults' ability to engage in regulatory processing when making emotional judgments about their partners. These studies suggest that well-being in the elderly is influenced by contextual demands on cognitive processing—only when situations allow for the implementation of control strategies can the well-being of older adults be enhanced by cognitive control.

Resource Limitation-Related Negativity

This chapter has cited many studies finding the positivity effect in older adults' processing, and the review indicates that older people control their processing using effortful strategies. However, older adults do not always have access to sufficient cognitive resources for emotional goal implementation (e.g., when multitasking as described previously). Interestingly, when older adults' cognitive resources are constrained, they sometimes show a negativity bias in information processing. Unlike older control participants, older adults in divided-attention conditions are negatively biased when processing emotional material in memory and visual attention tasks (Knight et al., 2007; Mather & Knight, 2005). This seems perplexing. Why should older adults focus on negative information *more* when their access to cognitive resources is limited? In his theory of ironic processes of mental control, Wegner (1994) proposes that when people try to control their cognition, they must initiate two processes: an operating process that searches for information consistent with goals and a monitoring process that searches for evidence that goal implementation has failed. Wegner's theory maintains that the operating process is more resource intensive than the failure monitoring process. Thus, if self-initiated control is used to create a desired mental state, encountering cognitive resource limitations can compromise the processing of goal-consistent information while allowing goal-inconsistent material (i.e., negative information) to get through. Applying this theory to our research, we expect that older adults' emotion regulation strategies can backfire as cognitive loads increase. Given this expectation, the observation that older adults show a negativity bias when they are distracted but not when they can devote their full attention to processing information is consistent with the notion that they are, in fact, attempting to implement emotional goals by using cognitive control strategies.

Neuroscientific Evidence of a Cognitive Control Pathway to Well-Being

Socioemotional selectivity theory has contributed greatly to our understanding of human development and the trajectory of emotional well-being throughout the life span. Elaborating on Carstensen's socioemotional selectivity theory, our cognitive control framework of aging and emotional well-being attempts to explain—from a neurocognitive perspective—*how* older adults direct their emotional states to align with their emotional goals using cognitive processing. Thus far, we have considered the behavioral evidence supporting the proposal that cognitive control influences well-being in the elderly, but we must also consider findings from cognitive neuroscience in order to determine if adults have the functional capacity to implement control strategies in late life. To accomplish this, we must determine the neurological functioning requirements for regulating emotions through controlled processing, and we must demonstrate that older adults have these functional resources intact.

Neurofunctional Requirements

Controlling emotions through cognitive processing requires the appraisal of affective information (Ochsner & Gross, 2004) and the alignment of cognition with emotional goals (Mather & Carstensen, 2005; Mather & Knight, 2005). These two criteria require cognitive processes dependent on the amygdala, prefrontal cortex, and the anterior cingulate (see Davidson, Jackson, & Kalin, 2000; Kim & Hamann, 2007; Knight & Mather, 2006; Ochsner & Gross, 2007).

The amygdala is responsible for appraising the affective quality of information (for review, see Lane & Nadel, 2000). This type of processing is often referred to as a "bottom-up" processing, as it is reactive and automatic (Ochsner & Gross, 2007). The amygdala is especially useful in detecting emotionally intense material (Anderson, Christoff, Panitz, De Rosa, & Gabrieli, 2003; Cunningham, Raye, & Johnson, 2005; Dolcos, LaBar, & Cabeza, 2005; Kensinger & Corkin, 2004) and providing rapid responses to emotional information (Grieve, Clark, Williams, Peduto, & Gordon, 2005; Mu, Xie, Wen, Weng, & Shuyun, 1999). The amygdala is necessary for implementing emotion regulation strategies because the affective value of information must be known before goal-directed processing can take place. For example, if you are watching a horror film but want to avoid feeling disgusted during the gruesome scenes, you can use distracting thoughts to reduce emotional engagement in those scenes. However, you must recognize when those gruesome scenes occur so that you can quickly initiate and terminate your emotion regulation strategy without missing too much of the movie.

As the amygdala activates early in emotion processing, (LeDoux, 2003), it can help determine when regulation strategies should be implemented.

In contrast, the prefrontal cortex and anterior cingulate cortex are considered "top-down" processing regions, as they are involved in higher-order cognition allowing for flexible, situation-dependent responses necessary in emotional control (for review, see Ochsner & Gross, 2007). The prefrontal cortex is responsible for executive function—coordinating sensory inputs, internal goals, and monitoring outputs—and is a critical region in the implementation of cognitive control (MacDonald, Cohen, Stenger, & Carter, 2000; Miller & Cohen, 2001). The lateral prefrontal cortex is involved in working memory function (Smith & Jonides, 1999), which is useful for keeping goal-consistent information in mind. Also important in emotional control is the medial region of the prefrontal cortex, which is thought to govern emotion regulation (including up- and down-regulation; Bonanno, Papa, Lalande, Westphal, & Coifman, 2004; Damasio, 1996). Accordingly, research suggests the prefrontal cortex modulates activity in the amygdala in a top-down manner (Berkowitz, Coplan, Reddy, & Gorman, 2007). For example, studies with younger adults have found that conscious use of emotion regulation strategies leads to enhanced brain activation in the lateral, particularly the dorsolateral, prefrontal cortex and decreased amygdala activation (Anderson et al., 2004; Beauregard, Le'vesque, & Bourgouin, 2001; MacDonald et al., 2000; Ochsner, Bunge, Gross, & Gabrieli, 2002). Thus, the prefrontal cortex appears to assist in emotion regulation by inhibiting automatic activation in the amygdala. As older adults are motivated to avoid negative feelings, we expect to see this same pattern of enhanced prefrontal activity and decreased amygdala activity when older adults encounter negative information.

The anterior cingulate has also been associated with emotional control (Botvinick, Braver, Barch, Carter, & Cohen, 2001; Knight & Mather, 2006; Ochsner et al., 2004; Ochsner & Gross, 2004). Specifically, this structure has been associated with implementing reappraisal strategies and monitoring emotion regulation efforts. For example, reappraising (reinterpreting) the emotional quality of a situation is linked with activation of the dorsal anterior cingulate cortex (see Ochsner & Gross, 2005). The anterior cingulate is also activated when people monitor the results of their control strategy for evidence of implementation failures (MacDonald et al., 2000). This region, like the prefrontal cortex, has been implicated in regulating activity in the amygdala (Beauregard et al., 2001). Finally, the proximity of the anterior cingulate to autonomic and endocrine regions suggests that this structure has the anatomical connections to evaluate and regulate emotional responses.

Aging and Emotion Regulation-Dependent Brain Function

As outlined in previous sections, we propose that older adults use control strategies, such as inhibiting negative information, refreshing goal-relevant information, and selectively rehearsing positive memories, to achieve their emotional goals. Yet such control processes typically decline with age (Grady, Springer, Hongwanishkul, McIntosh, & Winocur, 2006; Hedden & Gabrieli, 2004; Johnson & Raye, 2000; Knight & Mather, 2006; MacPherson, Phillips, & Della Sala, 2002; Prull, Gabrieli, & Bunge, 2000; Zacks, Hasher, & Li, 2000). In addition, the brain regions associated with initiating control processes face considerable decline with age. For example, the prefrontal cortex is subject to more atrophy than other brain regions (Coffey et al., 1992; Raz, 2000; Resnick, Pham, Kraut, Zonderman, & Davatzikos, 2003) with the lateral prefrontal cortex encountering the greatest decline of any prefrontal subregion (Tisserand et al., 2002). Furthermore, findings from positron-emission tomography reveal age-related declines in glucose metabolism in frontal brain regions (Mielke et al., 1998). Other emotion regulation structures also show pronounced deterioration with advancing age. Cross-sectional and longitudinal imaging data reveal significant brain atrophy in the anterior cingulate in older adults, even within a 4-year time span (Good et al., 2001; Resnick et al., 2003). On the other hand, the amygdala is well maintained in aging compared with most other brain regions (Grieve et al., 2005; Mather, 2004; Mu et al., 1999). Thus, age-related changes to emotion processing structures appear to negatively impact those responsible for emotion control while leaving the amygdala more or less intact.

Despite the age-associated decline in cognitive control abilities and emotion control–related neural structures, regulation of emotion and social behavior (associated with the frontal lobe) functions well in older age (for review, see Mather, 2004). Recent functional imaging research supports the idea that older adults spontaneously recruit additional cognitive resources to meet their processing needs and are more successful at achieving their cognitive goals when they do so. For instance, older adults' memory processing abilities are challenged when distractors are present, as inhibiting goal-irrelevant information becomes more difficult with age (Earles, Smith, & Park, 1994). Yet Gutchess et al. (2007) found that when high-functioning older adults complete a recognition task while distracted, they recruit unique neural regions and have better memory performance than do low-functioning elders. It seems that while older adults may experience significant age-related losses to cognitive control structures, they can compensate for their losses by exerting more cognitive effort.

In sum, evidence presented so far indicates that the primary affective appraisal structure (amygdala) remains stable while emotion control regions decline with age. Yet even with age-related deterioration to regulation structures, healthy older adults can promote their emotional well-being by recruiting additional cognitive resources to implement their regulation goals. Age differences in neural activation during emotion processing provide further support for this proposition.

Functional Evidence of Goal-Directed Emotion Processing in the Elderly

Older adults report experiencing negative emotions less frequently than do younger adults (Birditt, Fingerman, & Almeida, 2005; Carstensen et al., 2000; Diehl & Hay, 2007; Gross et al., 1997; Mroczek & Kolarz, 1998). These self-reports are supported by functional imaging studies finding that older adults have less brain activation in response to negative information than do younger adults (Mather et al., 2004; Samanez-Larkin et al., 2007). Older adults' reduced brain activation in response to negative information does not appear to reflect declines in emotion detection structures or function (see Knight & Mather, 2006), as the ability to detect emotionally arousing stimuli more quickly than other stimuli is preserved in older age (Hahn et al., 2006; Knight et al., 2007; Mather &

Knight, 2006). Instead, older adults' reduced brain activation for negative material is consistent with the notion that older people apply cognitive control when attempting to reduce negative emotional experiences. Our theoretical framework predicts that if older adults use cognitive control to achieve well-being, they may have amygdala responses equal to younger adults in early emotion processing but more reappraisals and inhibition of amygdala responses when the experienced affective information is negative. On the other hand, when older adults encounter positive information, other prefrontal regions responsible for maintaining information should be more active (such as dorsolateral prefrontal regions associated with working memory).

These predictions for negative stimuli are supported by functional resonance imaging (fMRI) experiments comparing brain activation in younger and older adults while they view faces with emotional and neutral expressions. Evidence from these studies indicates that age is associated with reduced amygdala activation in response to negative information (Fischer et al., 2005; Gunning-Dixon et al., 2003; Iidaka et al., 2002; Keightley, Chiew, Winocur, & Grady, 2007; Mather et al., 2004; Tessitore et al., 2005). Another study, using event-related potential recording (ERP), found that older age was related to an elimination of the negativity bias in brain activation frequently observed in younger adults (Wood & Kisley, 2006). In addition, fMRI studies find evidence that dampened amygdala response to negative material in older people coincides with an enhanced activation in the anterior cingulate cortex (Gunning-Dixon et al., 2003; Iidaka et al., 2002) and the prefrontal cortex (Fischer et al., 2005; Gunning-Dixon et al., 2003; Tessitore et al., 2005). Furthermore, a study that measured brain activity in response to positive and negative faces using ERP in 252 participants and fMRI in a subset of 80 of these participants found that activation in the medial prefrontal cortex during viewing of fearful faces increased with age, whereas activation in the same region during viewing of happy faces decreased with age (Williams et al., 2006). These imaging findings support our hypothesis that emotion regulation structures responsible for inhibiting or reappraising information will activate when older people encounter negative information but not positive information. In addition, Mather et al. (2004) found that older adults but not younger adults experienced greater amygdala activation in response to positive pictures compared to negative pictures. We interpret these findings as evidence that older adults use cognitive control to diminish their negative emotional experiences but not their positive emotional experiences.

While older adults may be grouped together for research purposes, they are by no means homogeneous. Widely variable experiences, health, and functioning lead to increased diversity in late life. As outlined previously, we predict that differences in cognitive function among older people will relate to variability in emotional well-being, as access to cognitive resources allows older people to direct information processing toward emotional goals. Behavioral evidence presented earlier demonstrated an enhanced positivity effect in older people with higher cognitive control abilities (Mather & Knight, 2005; Mather et al., 2005). Applied to the neural correlates of emotional control, we predict that older adults will enlist cognitive resources, supported by prefrontal regions, to down-regulate emotional experience when they are confronted with negative information. If this is the case, older adults' prefrontal function should predict their success at down-regulating negative affect. One research team has found that resting electrical activity in the left prefrontal cortex predicts emotion regulation abilities in younger and older adults (Jackson, Burghy, Hanna, Larson, & Davidson, 2000; Jackson et al., 2003). Notably, this investigation measured emotion regulation using a technique that minimized subject-expectancy effects (eyeblink startle responses), addressing the criticism that many studies on aging and emotion regulation use self-report to measure the use of regulation strategies. Taken together, the neuroscientific literature on aging and emotional control strongly indicates that cognitively healthy older adults can successfully regulate their emotions through the use of effortful processing strategies.

Closing Remarks

In conclusion, this chapter offers a theoretical framework for understanding the source of enhanced well-being in late life by integrating research from socioemotional and cognitive neuroscientific orientations. We build on Carstensen's socioemotional selectivity theory that argues that older adult's heightened awareness of time's value brings about an enhancement in motivation to find emotional gratification in life. Socioemotional selectivity theory focuses on the changes with goals seen as people's time perspective changes (the first box shown in Figure 18.2). Recent formulations of the theory have argued that older adults shift to focus relatively more on positive than negative information than younger adults do (Carstensen & Mikels, 2005; Charles & Carstensen, 2007) and that they avoid situations that are likely to be emotionally negative (Carstensen, Gross, & Fung, 1997; Charles & Carstensen, 2007), but these discussions of socioemotional selectivity theory have not focused much on the mechanisms of how the age differences in goals result in differences in emotional well-being. In this chapter, we outlined our account of how cognitive control plays a key role in implementing older adults' emotional goals, filling in some of the mechanisms represented by the middle box in Figure 18.2.

While we have focused primarily on the impact of cognitive control on well-being, research indicates that emotional status can affect cognitive status as well. Older adults who have a positive outlook about their cognitive abilities are more

18.2

In order for older adults' emotion-regulation goals to have an impact on what they attend to and remember, cognitive control mechanisms are necessary to implement the goals.

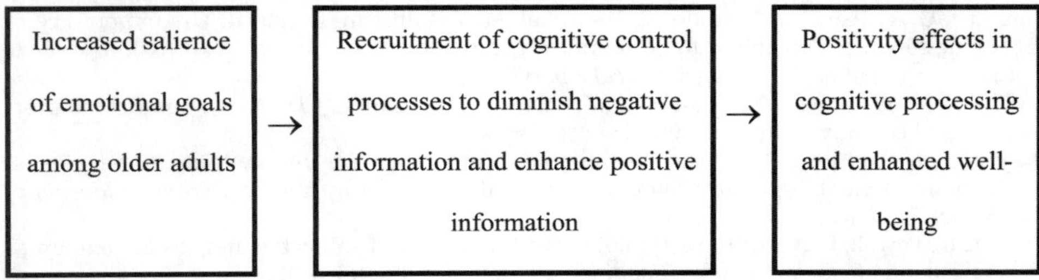

likely to set challenging goals for themselves and experience enhanced gratification from doing cognitive tasks (West, Thorn, & Bagwell, 2003). In addition, higher levels of emotional well-being predict more gradual decline in perceptual speed (Gerstorf, Lövdén, Röcke, Smith, & Lindenberger, 2007). Finally, maintaining a focus on emotional well-being can produce gains in physical health by reducing physiological symptoms of stress (Urry et al., 2006). Thus, it is likely that emotional well-being and cognitive function affect each other in a feedback loop wherein enhanced well-being leads to greater cognitive engagement and better health, in turn promoting greater life satisfaction (Rowe & Kahn, 1997). Our framework linking cognitive control and well-being reflects the changing tenor in the field of aging—from evitable decline to new opportunities.

References

Anderson, A. K. Christoff, K., Panitz, D., De Rosa, E., & Gabrieli, J. D. E. (2003). Neural correlates of the automatic processing of threat facial signals. *Journal of Neuroscience, 23,* 5627–5633.

Anderson, M. C., Ochsner, K. N., Kuhl, B., Cooper, J., Robertson, E., Gabrieli, S. W., et al. (2004). Neural systems underlying the suppression of unwanted memories. *Science, 303,* 232–235.

Baddeley, A., Logie, R., & Nimmo-Smith, I. (1985). Components of fluent reading. *Journal of Memory and Language, 24,* 119–131.

Bahrick, H. P., Hall, L. K., & Berger, S. A. (1996). Accuracy and distortion in memory for high school grades. *Psychological Science, 7,* 265–271.

Baltes, P. B., & Baltes, M. M. (1990). Psychological perspectives on successful aging: The model of selective optimization with compensation. In P. B. Baltes & M. M. Baltes (Eds.), *Successful aging: Perspectives from the behavioral sciences* (pp. 1–34). Cambridge: Cambridge University Press.

Bauer, J. J., & McAdams, D. P. (2004). Growth goals, maturity, and well-being. *Developmental Psychology, 40,* 114–127.

Beauregard, M., Le'vesque, J., & Bourgouin, P. (2001). Neural correlates of conscious self-regulation of emotion. *Journal of Neuroscience, 21,* RC165.

Berkowitz, R. L., Coplan, J. D., Reddy, D. P., & Gorman J. M. (2007). The human dimension: How the prefrontal cortex modulates the subcortical fear response. *Reviews in the Neurosciences,18,* 191–207.

Birditt, K. S., & Fingerman, K. L. (2003). Age and gender differences in adults' descriptions of emotional reactions to interpersonal problems. *Journal of Gerontology: Social Sciences, 58,* 237–245.

Birditt, K. S., & Fingerman, K. L. (2005). Do we get better at picking our battles? Age group differences in descriptions of behavioral reactions to interpersonal tensions. *Journal of Gerontology: Social Sciences, 60,* 121–128.

Birditt, K. S., Fingerman, K. L., & Almeida, D. M. (2005). Age differences in exposure and reactions to interpersonal tensions: A daily diary study. *Psychology and Aging, 20,* 330–340.

Bland, R. C., Orn, H., & Newman, S. C. (1988). Lifetime prevalence of psychiatric disorders in Edmonton. *Acta Psychiatrica Scandinavica, 77*(s338), 24–32.

Bonanno, G. A., Papa, A., Lalande, K., Westphal, M., & Coifman, K. (2004). The importance of being flexible: The ability to both enhance and suppress emotional expression predicts long-term adjustment. *Psychological Science, 15,* 482–487.

Botvinick, M. M., Braver, T. S., Barch, D. M., Carter, C. S., & Cohen, J. D. (2001). Conflict monitoring and cognitive control. *Psychological Review, 108,* 624–652.

Brunot, S., & Sanitioso, R. (2004). Motivational influence on the quality of memories: Recall of general autobiographical memories related to desired attributes. *European Journal of Social Psychology, 34,* 627–635.

Burriss, L., Powell, D. A., & White, J. (2007). Psychological and subjective indices of emotion as a function of age and gender. *Cognition and Emotion, 21,* 182–210.

Cappeliez, P., & O'Rourke, N. (2006). Empirical validation of a model of reminiscence and health in later life. *Journal of Gerontology: Social Sciences, 61,* 237–244.

Carstensen, L. L. (1992). Social and emotional patterns in adulthood: Support for socioemotional selectivity theory. *Psychology and Aging, 7,* 331–338.

Carstensen, L. L., & Fredrickson, B. L. (1998). Influence of HIV status and age on cognitive representations of others. *Health Psychology, 17,* 494–503.

Carstensen, L. L., Gross, J., & Fung, H. H. (1997). The social context of emotional experience. In K. W. Schaie & M. P. Lawton (Eds.), *Annual review of gerontology and geriatrics: Vol. 17. Focus on emotion and adult development* (pp. 325–352). New York: Springer Publishing.

Carstensen, L. L., Isaacowitz, D. M., & Charles, S. T. (1999). Taking time seriously: A theory of socioemotional selectivity. *American Psychologist, 54,* 165–181.

Carstensen, L. L., & Mikels, J. A. (2005). At the intersection of emotion and cognition: Aging and the positivity effect. *Current Directions in Psychological Science, 14,* 117–121.

Carstensen, L. L., Mikels, J. A., & Mather, M. (2006). Aging and the intersection of cognition, motivation, and emotion. In J. E. Birren & K. W. Schaie (Eds.), *Handbook of the psychology of aging* (6th ed., pp. 343–362). San Diego, CA: Academic Press.

Carstensen, L. L., Pasupathi, M., Mayr, U., & Nesselroade, J. R. (2000). Emotional experience in everyday life across the adult life span. *Journal of Personality and Social Psychology, 79,* 644–655.

Charles, S. T., & Carstensen, L. L. (2007). Emotion regulation in aging. In J. J. Gross (Ed.), *Handbook of emotion regulation* (pp. 307–327). New York: Guilford.

Charles, S. T., Mather, M., & Carstensen, L. L. (2003). Aging and emotional memory: The forgettable nature of negative images for older adults. *Journal of Experimental Psychology: General, 132,* 310–324.

Charles, S. T., Reynolds, C. A., & Gatz, M. (2001). Age-related differences and change in positive and negative affect over 23 years. *Journal of Personality and Social Psychology, 80,* 136–151.

Coffey, C. E., Wilkinson, W. E., Parashos, I. A., Soady, S. A., Sullivan, R. J., Patterson, L. J., et al. (1992). Quantitative cerebral anatomy of the aging human brain: A cross-sectional study using magnetic resonance imaging. *Neurology, 42,* 527–536.

Comblain, C., D'Argembeau, A., & Van der Linden, M. (2005). Phenomenal characteristics of autobiographical memories for emotional and neutral events in older and younger adults. *Experimental Aging Research, 31,* 173–189.

Costa, P. T., McCrae, R. R., & Zonderman, A. B. (1987). Environmental and dispositional influences on well-being: Longitudinal follow-up of an American national sample. *British Journal of Psychology, 78,* 299–306.

Cunningham, W. A., Raye, C. L., & Johnson, M. K. (2005). Neural correlates of evaluation associated with promotion and prevention regulatory focus. *Cognitive, Affective & Behavioral Neuroscience, 5,* 202–211.

Damasio, A. R. (1996). The somatic marker hypothesis and the possible functions of the prefrontal cortex. *Philosophical Transactions of the Royal Society of London. Series B, Biological Sciences, 351,* 1413–1420.

Davidson, R. J., Jackson, D. C., & Kalin, N. H. (2000). Emotion, plasticity, context, and regulation: Perspectives from affective neuroscience. *Psychological Bulletin, 126,* 890–909.

Diehl, M., & Hay, E. L. (2007). Contextualized self-representations in adulthood. *Journal of Personality, 75,* 1255–1284.

Diener, E., & Diener, C. (1996). Most people are happy. *Psychological Science, 7,* 181–185.

Diener, E., Suh, E. M., Lucas, R. E., & Smith, H. L. (1999). Subjective well-being: Three decades of progress. *Psychological Bulletin, 125,* 276–302.

Dolcos, F., LaBar, K. S., & Cabeza, R. (2005). Remembering one year later: Role of the amygdala and the medial temporal lobe memory system in retrieving emotional memories. *Proceedings of the National Academy of Sciences of the United States of America, 102,* 2626–2631.

Earles, J. L., Smith, A. D., & Park, D. C. (1994). Age differences in the effects of facilitating and distracting context on recall. *Aging & Cognition, 1,* 141–151.

Fan, J., McCandliss, B. D., Sommer, T., Raz, A., & Posner, M. I. (2002). Testing the efficiency and independence of attentional networks. *Journal of Cognitive Neuroscience, 14,* 340–347.

Fischer, H., Sandblom, J., Gavazzeni, J., Fransson, P., Wright, C. I., & Bäckman L. (2005). Age-differential patterns of brain activation during perception of angry faces. *Neuroscience Letters, 386,* 99–104.

Fung, H. H., Carstensen, L. L., & Lutz, A. M. (1999). Influence of time on social preferences: Implications for life-span development. *Psychology and Aging, 14,* 595–604.

George, L. K., Blazer, D. F., Winfield-Laird, I., Leaf, P. J., & Fischback, R. L. (1988). Psychiatric disorders and mental health service use in late-life: Evidence from the Epidemiologic Catchment Area Program. In J. Brody & G. Maddox (Eds.), *Epidemiology and aging* (pp. 189–219). New York: Springer Publishing.

Gerstorf, D., Lövdén, M., Röcke, C., Smith, J., & Lindenberger, U. (2007). Well-being affects changes in perceptual speed in advanced old age: Longitudinal evidence for a dynamic link. *Developmental Psychology, 43,* 705–718.

Good, C. D., Johnsrude, I. S., Ashburner, J., Henson, R. N., Friston, K. J., & Frackowiak, R. S. (2001). A voxel-based morphometric study of ageing in 465 normal adult human brains. *NeuroImage, 14,* 21–36.

Grady, C. L, Hongwanishkul, D., Keightley, M., Lee, W., & Hasher, L. (2007). The effect of age on memory for emotional faces. *Neuropsychology, 21,* 371–380.

Grady, C. L., Springer, M. V., Hongwanishkul, D., McIntosh, A. R., & Winocur, G. (2006). Age-related changes in brain activity across the adult lifespan. *Journal of Cognitive Neuroscience, 18,* 227–241.

Greenwood, P. M. (2000). The frontal aging hypothesis evaluated. *Journal of the International Neuropsychological Society, 6,* 705–726.

Grieve, S. M., Clark, C. R., Williams, L. M., Peduto, A. J., & Gordon, E. (2005). Preservation of limbic and paralimbic structures in aging. *Human Brain Mapping, 25,* 391–401.

Gross, J. J. (2001). Emotion regulation in adulthood: Timing is everything. *Current Directions in Psychological Science, 10,* 214–219.

Gross, J. J. (2002). Emotion regulation: Affective, cognitive, and social consequences. *Psychophysiology, 39,* 281–291.

Gross, J. J., Carstensen, L. L., Pasupathi, M., Tsai, J., Götestam Skorpen, C. G., & Hsu, A. Y. C. (1997). Emotion and aging: Experience, expression, and control. *Psychology and Aging, 12,* 590–599.

Grühn, D., Scheibe, S., & Baltes, P. B. (2007). Reduced negativity effect in older adults' memory for emotional pictures: The heterogeneity-homogeneity list paradigm. *Psychology and Aging, 22,* 644–649.

Gunning-Dixon, F. M., Gur, R. C., Perkins, A. C., Schroeder, L., Turner, T., Turetsky, B. I., et al. (2003). Aged-related differences in brain activation during emotional face processing. *Neurobiology of Aging, 24,* 285–295.

Gutchess, A. H., Hebrank, A., Sutton, B. P., Leshikar, E., Chee, M. W. L., Tan J. C., et al. (2007). Contextual interference in recognition memory with age. *NeuroImage, 35,* 1338–1347.

Hahn, S., Carlson, C., Singer, S., & Gronlund, S. D. (2006). Aging and visual search: Automatic and controlled attentional bias to threat faces. *Acta Psychologica, 123,* 312–336.

Hedden, T., & Gabrieli, J. D. E. (2004). Insights into the ageing mind: A view from cognitive neuroscience. *Nature Reviews: Neuroscience, 5,* 87–96.

Henry, N. J. M., Berg, C. A., Smith, T. W., & Florsheim, P. (2007). Positive and negative characteristics of marital interaction and their association with marital satisfaction in middle-aged and older couples. *Psychology and Aging, 22,* 428–441.

Iidaka, T., Okada, T., Murata, T., Omori, M., Kosaka, H., Sadato, N., et al. (2002). Age-related differences in the medial temporal lobe responses to emotional faces as revealed by fMRI. *Hippocampus, 12,* 352–362.

Isaacowitz, D. M. (2006). Motivated gaze: The view from the gazer. *Current Directions in Psychological Science, 15,* 68–72.

Isaacowitz, D. M., Wadlinger, H. A., Goren, D., & Wilson, H. R. (2006a). Is there an age-related positivity effect in visual attention? A comparison of two methodologies. *Emotion, 6,* 511–516.

Isaacowitz, D. M., Wadlinger, H. A., Goren, D., & Wilson, H. R. (2006b). Selective preference in visual fixation away from negative images in old age? An eye-tracking study. *Psychology and Aging, 21,* 40–48.

Jackson, D. C., Burghy, C. A., Hanna, A. J., Larson, C. L., & Davidson, R. J. (2000). Resting frontal and anterior temporal EEG asymmetry predicts ability to regulate negative emotion. *Psychophysiology, 37,* S50.

Jackson, D. C., Mueller, C. J., Dolski, I., Dalton, K. M., Nitschke, J. B., Urry, H. L., et al. (2003). Now you feel it, now you don't: Frontal brain electrical asymmetry and individual differences in emotion regulation. *Psychological Science, 14,* 612–617.

Johnson, M. K., Mitchell, K. J., Raye, C. L., & Greene, E. J. (2004). An age-related deficit in prefrontal cortical function associated with refreshing information. *Psychological Science, 15,* 127–132.

Johnson, M. K., & Raye, C. L. (2000). Cognitive and brain mechanisms of false memories and beliefs. In D. L. Schacter & E. Scarry (Eds.), *Memory, brain, and belief* (pp. 35–86). Cambridge, MA: Harvard University Press.

Jorm, A. F. (2000). Does old age reduce the risk of anxiety and depression? A review of epidemiological studies across the adult life span. *Psychological Medicine, 30,* 11–22. American Psychological Manual style Retrieved from http://people.ucsc.edu/%7Emather/pdffiles/MatherTsukubainpress.pdf

Keightley, M. L., Chiew, K. S., Winocur, G., & Grady, C. L. (2007). Age-related differences in brain activity underlying identification of emotional expressions in faces. *Social Cognitive and Affective Neuroscience, 2,* 292–302.

Kennedy, Q., Mather, M., & Carstensen, L. L. (2004). The role of motivation in the age-related positivity effect in autobiographical memory. *Psychological Science, 15,* 208–214.

Kensinger, E. A. (2008). Age differences in memory for arousing and nonarousing emotional words. *Journal of Gerontology: Social Sciences, 63,* P13–P18.

Kensinger, E. A., & Corkin, S. (2004). The effects of emotional content and aging on false memories. *Cognitive, Affective & Behavioral Neuroscience, 4,* 1–9.

Kensinger, E. A., Garoff-Eaton, R. J., & Schacter, D. L. (2007). Effects of emotion on memory specificity in young and older adults. *Journal of Gerontology: Social Sciences, 62,* 208–215.

Kensinger, E. A., O'Brien, J. L., Swanberg, K., Garoff-Eaton, R. J., & Schacter, D. L. (2007). The effects of emotional content on reality-monitoring performance in young and older adults. *Psychology and Aging, 22,* 752–764.

Kim, S. H., & Hamann, S. (2007). Neural correlates of positive and negative emotion regulation. *Journal of Cognitive Neuroscience, 19,* 776–798.

Kliegel, M., Jäger, T., & Phillips, L. H. (2007). Emotional development across adulthood: Differential age-related emotional reactivity and emotion regulation in a negative mood induction procedure. *International Journal of Aging and Human Development, 64,* 217–244.

Knight, B. G., Maines, M. L., & Robinson, G. S. (2002). The effects of sad mood on memory in older adults: A test of the mood congruence effect. *Psychology and Aging, 17,* 653–661.

Knight, M., & Mather, M. (2006). The affective neuroscience of aging and its implications for cognition. In T. Canli (Ed.), *Biology of personality and individual differences* (pp. 159–183). New York: Guilford.

Knight, M., Seymour, T. L., Gaunt, J. T., Baker, C. Nesmith, K., & Mather, M. (2007). Aging and goal-directed emotional attention: Distraction reverses emotional biases. *Emotion, 7,* 705–714.

Kobau, R., Safran, M. A., Zack, M. M., Moriarty, D. G., & Chapman, D. (2004). Sad, blue, or depressed days, health behaviors and health-related quality of life: Behavioral Risk Factor Surveillance System, 1995–2000. *Health Quality and Life Outcomes, 2,* 40.

Kunzmann, U., Kupperbusch, C. S., & Levenson, R. W. (2005). Behavioral inhibition and amplification during emotional arousal: A comparison of two age groups. *Psychology and Aging, 20,* 144–158.

Kunzmann, U., Little, T. D., & Smith, J. (2000). Is age-related stability of subjective well-being a paradox? Cross-sectional and longitudinal evidence from the Berlin Aging Study. *Psychology and Aging, 15,* 511–526.

Labouvie-Vief, G. (2005). Self-with-other representations and the organization of the self. *Journal of Research in Personality, 39,* 185–205.

Labouvie-Vief, G., Diehl, M., Jain, E., & Zhang, F. (2007). Six-year change in affect optimization and affect complexity across the adult life span: A further examination. *Psychology and Aging, 22,* 738–751.

Lane, R. D., & Nadel, L. (Eds.). (2000). *Cognitive neuroscience of emotion: Series in affective science.* New York: Oxford University Press.

Lang, F. R., & Carstensen, L. L. (1994). Close emotional relationships in late life: Further support for proactive aging in the social domain. *Psychology and Aging, 9,* 315–324.

Lang, F. R., & Carstensen, L. L. (2002). Time counts: Future time perspective, goals, and social relationships. *Psychology and Aging, 17,* 125–139.

Lawton, M. P. (2001). Emotion in later life. *Current Directions in Psychological Science, 10,* 120–123.

Lawton, M. P., Kleban, M. H., & Dean, J. (1993). Affect and age: Cross-sectional comparisons of structure and prevalence. *Psychology and Aging, 8,* 165–175.

Lawton, M. P., Kleban, M. H., Rajagopal, D., & Dean, J. (1992). Dimensions of affective experience in three age groups. *Psychology and Aging, 7,* 171–184.

LeDoux, J. (2003). The emotional brain, fear, and the amygdala. *Cellular and Molecular Neurobiology, 23,* 727–738.

Leigland, L. A., Schulz, L. E., & Janowsky, J. S. (2004). Age related changes in emotional memory. *Neurobiology of Aging, 25,* 1117–1124.

Levenson, R. W., Carstensen, L. L., Friesen, W. V., & Ekman, P. (1991). Emotion, physiology, and expression in old age. *Psychology and Aging, 6,* 28–35.

Luce, M. F., Bettman, J. R., & Payne, J. W. (1997). Choice processing in emotionally difficult decisions. *Journal of Experimental Psychology: Learning, Memory, and Cognition, 23,* 384–405.

MacDonald, A. W., III, Cohen, J. D., Stenger, V. A., & Carter, C. S. (2000). Dissociating the role of the dorsolateral prefrontal and anterior cingulate cortex in cognitive control. *Science, 288,* 1835–1838.

MacPherson, S. E., Phillips, L. H., & Della Sala, S. (2002). Age, executive function and social decision making: A dorsolateral prefrontal theory of cognitive aging. *Psychology and Aging, 17,* 598–609.

Magai, C. (2001). Emotions over the life span. In J. E. Birren & K. W. Schaie (Eds.), *Handbook of the psychology of aging* (5th ed., pp. 399–426). San Diego, CA: Academic Press.

Magai, C., Consedine, N. S., Krivoshekova, Y. S., Kudadjie-Gyamfi, E., & McPherson, R. (2006). Emotion experience and expression across the adult life span: Insights from a multimodal assessment study. *Psychology and Aging, 21,* 303–317.

Malatesta, C. Z., Izard, C. E., Culver, C., & Nicolich, M. (1987). Emotion communication skills in young, middle-aged, and older women. *Psychology and Aging, 2,* 193–203.

Mather, M. (2004). Aging and emotional memory. In D. Reisberg & P. Hertel (Eds.), *Memory and emotion* (pp. 272–307). New York: Oxford University Press.

Mather, M. (2006). Why memories may become more positive with age. In B. Uttl, N. Ohta, & A. L. Siegenthaler (Eds.), *Memory and emotion: Interdisciplinary perspectives* (pp. 135–159). Malden, MA: Blackwell.

Mather, M., Canli, T., English, T., Whitfield, S., Wais, P., Ochsner, K., et al. (2004). Amygdala responses to emotionally valenced stimuli in older and younger adults. *Psychological Science, 15,* 259–263.

Mather, M., & Carstensen, L. L. (2005). Aging and motivated cognition: The positivity effect in attention and memory. *Trends in Cognitive Sciences, 9,* 496–502.

Mather, M., & Johnson, M. K. (2000). Choice-supportive source monitoring: Do our decisions seem better to us as we age? *Psychology and Aging, 15,* 596–606.

Mather, M., & Knight, M. (2005). Goal-directed memory: The role of cognitive control in older adults' emotional memory. *Psychology and Aging, 20,* 554–570.

Mather, M., & Knight, M. R. (2006). Angry faces get noticed quickly: Threat detection is not impaired among older adults. *Journal of Gerontology: Social Sciences, 61,* 54–57.

Mather, M., Knight, M., & McCaffrey, M. (2005). The allure of the alignable: Younger and older adults' false memories of choice features. *Journal of Experimental Psychology: General, 134,* 38–51.

Mauss, I. B., Cook, C. L., Cheng, J. Y. J., & Gross, J. J. (2007). Individual differences in cognitive reappraisal: Experiential and physiological responses to an anger provocation. *International Journal of Psychophysiology, 66,* 116–124.

McConatha, J. T., Leone, F. M., & Armstrong, J. M. (1997). Emotional control in adulthood. *Psychological Reports, 80,* 499–507.

Mielke, R., Kessler, J., Szelies, B., Herholz, K., Wienhard, K., & Heiss, W. D. (1998). Normal and pathological aging—Findings of positron-emission-tomography. *Journal of Neural Transmission, 105,* 821–837.

Mikels, J. A., Larkin, G. R., Reuter-Lorenz, P. A., & Carstensen, L. L. (2005). Divergent trajectories in the aging mind: Changes in working memory for affective versus visual information with age. *Psychology and Aging, 20,* 542–553.

Miller, E. K., & Cohen, J. D. (2001). An integrative theory of prefrontal cortex function. *Annual Review of Neuroscience, 24,* 167–202.

Mroczek, D. K. (2001). Age and emotion in adulthood. *Current Directions in Psychological Science, 10,* 87–90.

Mroczek, D. K., & Kolarz, C. M. (1998). The effect of age on positive and negative affect: A developmental perspective on happiness. *Journal of Personality and Social Psychology, 75,* 1333–1349.

Mroczek, D. K., & Spiro, A., III. (2005). Change in life satisfaction during adulthood: Findings from the Veterans Affairs Normative Aging Study. *Journal of Personality and Social Psychology, 88,* 189–202.

Mu, Q., Xie, J., Wen, Z., Weng, Y., & Shuyun Z. A. (1999). A quantitative MR study of the hippocampal formation, the amygdala, and the temporal horn of the lateral ventricle in healthy subjects 40 to 90 years of age. *American Journal of Neuroradiology, 20,* 207–211.

Muraven, M., Tice, D. M., & Baumeister, R. F. (1998). Self-control as a limited resource: Regulatory depletion patterns. *Journal of Personality and Social Psychology, 74,* 774–789.

Ochsner, K. N., Bunge, S. A., Gross, J. J., & Gabrieli, J. D. E. (2002). Rethinking feelings: An fMRI study of the cognitive regulation of emotion. *Journal of Cognitive Neuroscience, 14,* 1215–1229.

Ochsner, K. N., & Gross, J. J. (2004). Thinking makes it so: A social cognitive neuroscience approach to emotion regulation. In R. F. Baumeister & K. D. Vohs (Eds.), *Handbook of self-regulation: Research, theory, and applications* (pp. 229–255). New York: Guilford.

Ochsner, K. N., & Gross, J. J. (2005). The cognitive control of emotion. *Trends in Cognitive Sciences, 9,* 242–249.

Ochsner, K. N., & Gross, J. J. (2007). The neural architecture of emotion regulation. In J. J. Gross (Ed.), *Handbook of emotion regulation* (pp. 87–109). New York: Guilford.

Ochsner, K. N., Ray, R. D., Cooper, J. C., Robertson, E. R., Chopra, S., Gabrieli, J. D., et al. (2004). For better or for worse: Neural systems supporting the cognitive down- and up-regulation of negative emotion. *NeuroImage, 23,* 483–499.

Pasupathi, M., & Carstensen, L. L. (2003). Age and emotional experience during mutual reminiscing. *Psychology and Aging, 18,* 430–442.

Phifer, J. F. (1990). Psychological distress and somatic symptoms after natural disaster: Differential vulnerability among older adults. *Psychology and Aging, 5,* 412–420.

Phillips, L. H., Henry, J. D., Hosie, J. A., & Milne, A. B. (2006). Age, anger regulation, and well-being. *Aging and Mental Health, 10,* 250–256.

Pinquart, M. (2001). Age differences in perceived positive affect, negative affect, and affect balance in middle and old age. *Journal of Happiness Studies, 2,* 375–405.

Prull, M. W., Gabrieli, J. D. E., & Bunge, S. A. (2000). Age-related changes in memory: A cognitive neuroscience perspective. In F. I. M. Craik & T. A. Salthouse (Eds.), *The handbook of aging and cognition* (2nd ed., pp. 91–153). Mahwah, NJ: Lawrence Erlbaum Associates.

Raz, N. (2000). Aging of the brain and its impact on cognitive performance: Integration of structural and functional findings. In F. I. M. Craik & T. A. Salthouse (Eds.), *The handbook of aging and cognition* (2nd ed., pp. 1–90). Mahwah, NJ: Lawrence Erlbaum Associates.

Ready, R. E., Weinberger, M. I., & Jones, K. M. (2007). How happy have you felt lately? Two diary studies of emotion recall in older and younger adults. *Cognition and Emotion, 21,* 728–757.

Resnick, S. M., Pham D. L., Kraut, M. A., Zonderman, A. B., & Davatzikos, C. (2003). Longitudinal magnetic resonance imaging studies of older adults: A shrinking brain. *Journal of Neuroscience, 23,* 3295–3301.

Rösler, A., Ulrich, C., Billino, J., Sterzer, P., Weidauer, S., Bernhardt, T., et al. (2005). Effects of arousing emotional scenes on the distribution of visuospatial attention: Changes with aging and early subcortical vascular dementia. *Journal of Neurological Sciences, 229–230,* 109–116.

Rowe, J. W., & Kahn, R. L. (1987). Human aging: Usual and successful. *Science, 237,* 143–149.

Rowe, J. W., & Kahn, R. L. (1997). Successful aging. *The Gerontologist, 37,* 433–440.

Ryff, C. D. (1989). In the eye of the beholder: Views of psychological well-being among middle-aged and older adults. *Psychology and Aging, 4,* 195–210.

Samanez-Larkin, G. R., Gibbs, S. E., Khanna, K., Nielsen, L., Carstensen, L. L., & Knutson, B. (2007). Anticipation of monetary gain but not loss in healthy older adults. *Nature Neuroscience, 10,* 787–791.

Schroots, J. J. F. (2003). Life-course dynamics: A research program in progress from The Netherlands. *European Psychologist, 8,* 192–199.

Singer, J., Rexhaj, B., & Baddeley, J. (2007). Older, wiser, and happier? Comparing older adults' and college students' self-defining memories. *Memory, 15,* 886–898.

Smith, E. E., & Jonides, J. (1999). Storage and executive processes in the frontal lobes. *Science, 283,* 1657–1661.

Stacey, C. A., & Gatz, M. (1991). Cross-sectional age differences and longitudinal change on the Bradburn Affect Balance Scale. *Journal of Gerontology, 46,* P76–P78.

Staudinger, U. M., Bluck, S., & Herzberg, P. Y. (2003). Looking back and looking ahead: Adult age differences in consistency of diachronous ratings of subjective well-being. *Psychology and Aging, 18,* 13–24.

Tessitore, A., Hariri, A. R., Fera, F., Smith, W. G., Das, S., Weinberger, D. R., et al. (2005). Functional changes in the activity of brain regions underlying emotion processing in the elderly. *Psychiatry Research: Neuroimaging, 139,* 9–18.

Thomas, R. C., & Hasher, L. (2006). The influence of emotional valence on age differences in early processing and memory. *Psychology and Aging, 21,* 821–825.

Tisserand, D. J., Pruessner, J. C., Sanz Arigita, E. J., van Boxtel, M. P., Evans, A. C., Jolles, J., et al. (2002) Regional frontal cortical volumes decrease differentially in aging: An MRI study to compare volumetric approaches and voxel-based morphometry. *NeuroImage, 17,* 657–669.

Tsai, J. L., Levenson, R. W., & Carstensen, L. L. (2000). Autonomic, subjective, and expressive responses to emotional films in older and younger Chinese Americans and European Americans. *Psychology and Aging, 15,* 684–693.

Urry, H. L., van Reekum, C. M., Johnstone, T., Kalin, N. H., Thurow, M. E., Schaefer, H. S., et al. (2006). Amygdala and ventromedial prefrontal cortex are inversely coupled during regulation of negative affect and predict the diurnal pattern of cortisol secretion among older adults. *Journal of Neuroscience, 26,* 4415–4425.

Wegner, D. M. (1994). Ironic processes of mental control. *Psychological Review, 101,* 34–52.

Wegner, D. M., Erber, R., & Zanakos, S. (1993). Ironic processes in the mental control of mood and mood-related thought. *Journal of Personality and Social Psychology, 65,* 1093–1104.

Weissman, M. M., Bruce, M. L., Leaf, P. J., Florio, L. P., & Holzer, C. (1991). Affective disorders. In L. N. Robins & D. A. Regier (Eds.), *Psychiatric disorders in America* (pp. 53–80). New York: Free Press.

Weissman, M. M., Leaf, P. J., Bruce, M. L., & Florio, L. (1988). The epidemiology of dysthymia in five communities: Rates, risks, co-morbidity, and treatment. *American Journal of Psychiatry, 145,* 815–819.

West, R. L. (1996). An application of prefrontal cortex function theory to cognitive aging. *Psychological Bulletin, 120,* 272–292.

West, R. L., Thorn, R. M., & Bagwell, D. K. (2003). Memory performance and beliefs as a function of goal setting and aging. *Psychology and Aging, 18,* 111–125.

Williams, L. M., Brown, K. J., Palmer, D., Liddell, B. J., Kemp, A. H., Olivieri, G., et al. (2006). The mellow years? Neural basis of improving emotional stability over age. *Journal of Neuroscience, 26,* 6422–6430.

Wood, S., & Kisley, M. A. (2006). The negativity bias is eliminated in older adults: Age-related reduction in event-related brain potentials associated with evaluative categorization. *Psychology and Aging, 21,* 815–820.

Zacks, R. T., Hasher, L., & Li, K. Z. H. (2000). Human memory. In F. I. M. Craik & T. A. Salthouse (Eds.), *The handbook of aging and cognition* (2nd ed., pp. 293–357). Mahwah, NJ: Lawrence Erlbaum Associates.

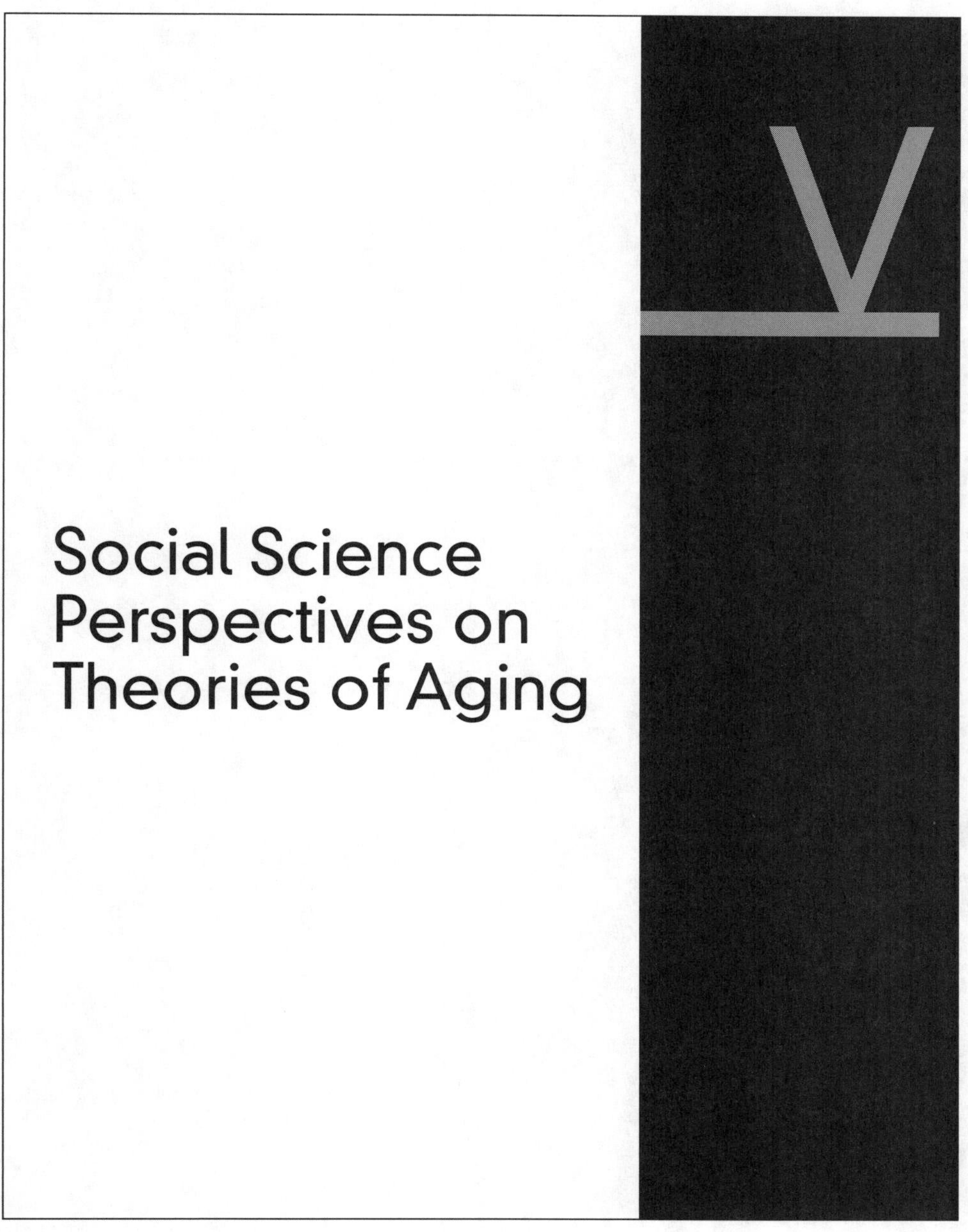

V

Social Science Perspectives on Theories of Aging

Toward an Integrative Theory of Social Gerontology

19

Scott A. Bass

This chapter provides a brief overview of trends in the sciences toward greater interdisciplinary research and the exploration of theoretical frameworks that seek to integrate previously disparate disciplinary perspectives. Using this as a background, the chapter examines the developments in the interdisciplinary field of gerontology and an emerging distinction between those scholars who are invested in disciplinary theories of aging and those who are associated with emerging theories in the interdisciplinary field of gerontology.

A vibrant literature has emerged among a subset of gerontology scholars in the area of social gerontology. Among social gerontologists, two major schools of thought have emerged each with deep philosophic roots. The first school to emerge is that of the critical gerontologists and the second school is that of the postmodernist gerontologists. Perspectives among each of the two schools are discussed.

The later portion of the chapter focuses on an integrative approach to a theoretical framework for social gerontology. Both the conceptual framework and specific elements are presented regarding an integrative theory in social gerontology.

Throughout the chapter, the term "interdisciplinary" is used frequently. While the gerontology literature distinguishes interdisciplinary inquiry from that which is multidisciplinary or cross-disciplinary, the term "interdisciplinary" used in this chapter explicitly refers to the contributions of two or more disciplines where the disciplinary boundaries are sufficiently muted and the plurality of contributions creates a synergistic nature of original insight (see Bass & Ferraro, 2000).

An Era of Interdisciplinary Research and Discovery

Interdisciplinary research and discovery has become the holy grail of the scientific establishment. With funding provided by the W. M. Keck Foundation, America's premier scientific societies were asked in 2003 to respond to a series of questions about the state of interdisciplinary research. Through the Futures Initiative supported by the Keck Foundation, the National Academy of Sciences, the National Academy of Engineering, and the Institute of Medicine's Committee on Science, Engineering, and Public Policy (COSEPUP) sought to explore the full potential of scientific research that crosses disciplinary boundaries. The initiative's purpose was to "stimulate new modes of inquiry and break down the conceptual and institutional barriers to interdisciplinary research that could yield significant benefits to science and society" (National Academy of Sciences, National Academy of Engineering, & Institute of Medicine [NAS et al.], 2005, p. ix).

To carry out the Futures Initiative, the participating organizations established the Committee on Facilitating Interdisciplinary Research to examine the current conditions that surround the support and development of interdisciplinary research. In 2005, as a result of the committee's efforts, the National Academies published a comprehensive report on the development of interdisciplinary research, aptly titled *Facilitating Interdisciplinary Research.*

The project, which involved the participation of luminaries from universities, government, and industry, pointed out that interdisciplinary research is far from something new but has been at the vanguard of investigation since the early origins of science. Critical advances in science have been made historically, where curious investigators have explored intellectual terrain that was well beyond their previous knowledge base. With ever greater and more complex horizons, great minds such as Isaac Newton or Louis Pasteur extended the reach of their disciplines to delve into questions that led to the emergence of whole new areas of understanding (NAS et al., 2005). Driven by curiosity, Leonardo da Vinci, Benjamin Franklin, and countless others embarked on projects that led to insights that could not have been conceived within a single disciplinary tradition.

Today, the same search for new knowledge finds scholars exploring subjects that cross the boundaries of any single discipline. Our understanding of the structure of DNA has engaged scientists from computer science, biology, medicine, mathematics, and information sciences, resulting in the development of a new field called bioinformatics. Studies at the scale of 1 micrometer that combine the tools of physics, chemistry, materials science, mechanical, and electrical engineering have created the field of nanotechnology. Research at the nanoscale has already resulted in numerous innovative applications to daily life, from fibers that resist staining to improved lines of cosmetics and pharmaceuticals. New doctoral programs have been created to respond to the need to train scientists in these fields. Other interdisciplinary fields, such as neuroscience, environmental science, photonics, and genomics—all merging and blending different sciences and subject areas—have also emerged as new doctoral programs at some of the leading research universities.

Defined by the National Academies (NAS, NAE, IOM, 2005), interdisciplinary research

> *is a mode of research by teams or individuals that integrates information, data, techniques, tools, perspectives, concepts, and/or theories from two or more disciplines or bodies of specialized knowledge to advance fundamental understanding or to solve problems whose solutions are beyond the scope of a single discipline or field of research practice. (p. 26)*

Gerontology and Interdisciplinarity

Predating many of the new technical scientific fields identified previously, studies in the interdisciplinary field of gerontology came into their own with the establishment of the Gerontological Society of America taking place in 1945. These pioneering scholars also established the *Journal of Gerontology,* which was first issued in 1946 (Achenbaum, 1995).

Gerontology sought to bridge the worlds of life sciences, medicine, and the social sciences in a comprehensive view of the aging individual within a larger societal context. Despite its more than 60-year history, gerontologists have been highly self-critical of the field's development as its own science (Bass, 2006; Bass & Ferraro, 2000; Bengtson, Parrott, & Burgess, 1996; Bengtson, Rice, & Johnson, 1999; Biggs, Lowenstein, & Hendricks, 2003; Birren & Bengtson, 1988; Ferraro, 2006; Hagestad & Dannefer, 2001; Katz, 1996; Longino, 2005; Maddox & Campbell, 1985; Marshall, 1999; Minkler, 1996; Moody, 1988; Myers, 1996; Phillipson, 1998; Walker, 1999). Lagging behind the swiftly evolving interdisciplinary fields in the natural sciences and engineering, gerontology has not produced its own widely shared methodologies or well-subscribed and accepted theories.

Unfortunately, gerontology has fallen prey for a variety of different reasons to its lack of advancement in shared methodologies and accepted theories. The National Academies note that interdisciplinary work in the social sciences has not advanced in the same way that it has in the natural sciences and engineering: "Social science research has not yet fully elucidated the complex social and intellectual processes that make for successful IDR [interdisciplinary research]" (NAS et al., 2005, p. 3). Indeed part of gerontology's problems reflect larger issues within the social sciences, the departments in which faculty reside, and their overall investment and engagement in interdisciplinary studies.

Emboldened with the notion of solving complex puzzles, the natural sciences, life sciences, and engineering have had financial support from foundations and government (e.g., the National Aeronautics and Space Administration, the

National Oceanic and Atmospheric Administration, the National Institute of Standards and Technology, the National Institutes of Health, the National Science Foundation, and the Department of Defense) to explore interdisciplinary issues of basic and applied science. New centers and institutes have been created to carry out this promising research as well as funding for graduate students in allied doctoral programs. The result has been a steady stream of investigators who have made significant strides outside the core discipline. This in turn has led to more stable and well-funded structures within the academy and industry. Success breeds more success with cadres of doctoral students attracted to these new cutting-edge, well-funded, and institutionally embraced initiatives.

This is not to say that these new fields have not had their challenges for faculty positions, space, start-up costs, laboratory equipment, support staff, and funding for graduate assistantships, but it is to acknowledge that the path to institutional recognition and support has been relatively swift and, in some universities, well supported with high visibility and significant recognition from campus leaders.

For the most part, developing fields in the social sciences have not had the same experience as these emerging science and engineering fields. Despite the intellectual connectedness between psychology, sociology, anthropology, economics, political science, and public policy (to name a few of the social science disciplines), the social science disciplines have for the most part remained their own territories with their own journals, societies, and organizations. Intradisciplinary exchanges have crystallized around several thematic areas, such as women's studies or Africana studies, that have further established their own academic programs and/or departments with the ability to confer tenure. However, in the core disciplines, intellectual exchanges that cross the disciplines remain topic specific with the weight of promotion and tenure for faculty focused on scholarship evidenced from contributions to the literature in the discipline's primary refereed journals.

In social science departments at many of America's leading research universities, it would be customary for a publication to have greater value for annual faculty merit review if placed in one of the discipline's premier journals as opposed to a contribution to a journal in an allied applied area. Take the discipline of economics, for example. An economist publishing in a respected environmental journal would, in most nationally ranked economics departments, be of less significance to the departmental annual review process than appearing in, say, the *American Economic Review* or similar journal. For the social scientist gerontologist in the United States, this poses a genuine challenge. For most junior faculty interested in gerontology, it would be unusual for senior faculty to recommend that they stray too far from the home discipline prior to tenure.

The exploration of a unified theory across the social sciences that bridges the components of individual, context, epoch, community, economy, policy, and society is a topic that commands minimal attention in the halls of the modern research university. A crying call for unification of the social sciences has not materialized in the way it has for, say, physicists—with efforts concentrated at unification of the fundamental laws that govern both atomic structures and the celestial bodies. While still exploring different theories, such as string theory, physicists since Einstein have struggled unsuccessfully toward the goal of one unifying theory of the universe. While a parallel attempt at unification across the social sciences would provide a unique approach to the understanding of human behavior and the environment, efforts at creating broad theoretical foundations have garnered insufficient interest in the existing well-established intellectual guilds of the social sciences.

Other examples of intellectual integration include buildings designed to provide offices and laboratories that mix faculty from different science and engineering disciplines in one location, such as Stanford's Bio-X Building (the James H. Clark Center). Facilities that serve such a purpose have become a sought-after commodity among a number of faculty in the sciences and engineering. Social scientists, however, seem more interested in segregated floors or buildings of scholars with similar affinity than voluntarily giving up their home department offices to deliberately mix with those of different disciplinary backgrounds. While this kind of location-based design to encourage scholarship across disciplines may be in the future, it would not be forefront among the demands for new space among most social science faculty.

Hence, those social scientists interested in gerontology face a number of cultural and employment-related obstacles in the full pursuit of their scholarship. They come from a culture where inquiry is more likely disciplinary based and many rewards are directed accordingly. As Achenbaum (1995) so carefully delineates in *Crossing Frontiers,* these institutional traditions are powerful cultural norms that must be carefully navigated by faculty whose promotion, merit, and tenure is determined by their departmental colleagues.

And so it goes, should we be surprised to learn, when all is said and done, that much of the theoretical development and research approaches in the social sciences have been a reflection of a single discipline? While gerontology claims to seek a broader perspective, it would be more common to find work that reflects a psychologist's perspective on aging, a sociologist's, an economist's, and so on where theories and methods derive from the core discipline and are applied to the study of the aged or their societal circumstances. On occasion, scholars from two or more disciplines may collaborate on a single work or on a collection of articles while discussing the subject within the confines of their disciplinary boundaries (i.e., multidisciplinary). The gerontologist is often a consumer of the different disciplinary approaches while resting safely within a disciplinary home. Always interested in gerontology but often limited in the ability to tarry too far from the academic unit and community where career rewards are administered, the gerontology scholar—and, as a result, his or her scholarship—is unquestionably influenced by the structure of the reward system of the university (Achenbaum, 1995; Bass, 2006; Bass & Ferraro, 2000).

On the other hand, there are those who read the gerontology literature anticipating a greater unification of theory and methodologies and find the material lacking. Frustrated with the single disciplinary point of view when approaching a broad field like gerontology, some gerontologists have criticized this literature as overly simplistic and unresponsive to the complexity associated with the field of gerontology (Hagestad & Dannefer, 2001). Yet, to be fair, many scholars studying issues associated with aging may not be attempting to write about gerontology per se but are writing about aging from their disciplinary perspective.

Distinguishing Between Gerontology and the Study of Aging

Let me develop this point a bit further and distinguish between gerontology and the study of aging. Gerontology is by definition a field that draws on many different disciplines and professions. It is enriched by the plurality of disciplinary perspectives blending into original concepts. Yet its academic infrastructure in the academy has not evolved sufficiently to support its full independence from its allied disciplines. Its federal and foundation support, while better than many areas, is quite modest when compared to some of the hot interdisciplinary science and engineering fields that have experienced greater infrastructure support in the university. A few universities have gerontology schools, centers, and departments that should be welcoming of interdisciplinary research, but they remain in the minority, with many universities organized by disciplinary or professional departments. Hence, we have an emerging conflict of turf, territory, and ideas where the traditional disciplines see the study of aging well within their sphere of control and at the same time a smaller group of gerontologists are seeking to shape the world from a more integrated vantage point.

There is a certain ironic duality; on the one hand, we have a field that is defined as interdisciplinary but in practice is dominated by research that is often evaluated for funding and acceptance by those from specific disciplinary frameworks. In fact, gerontology's very survival depends on support and funding from the core disciplinary departments. We have critics who complain that the research is dominated by single disciplinary paradigms, retarding the development of more sophisticated theory, but who at the same time acknowledge the environmental reality that faces faculty interested in the field. Thus, we have a field with investigators with certain intellectual aspirations living life as another. True interdisciplinary inquiry in gerontology for many scholars is something someone else should do, and the safest route is to study aging from within a discipline or two. For some, this safer route becomes the habit, and the gerontological imagination is displaced by the realities and rewards found in the disciplinary study of aging.

Nevertheless, there are voices from senior faculty, from newly minted PhDs in gerontology and from those whose departments are less dominated by a single discipline or profession. They are calling for academic work in gerontology—not the disciplinary study of aging. Worldwide, an emerging gerontological group has coalesced and is beginning to acknowledge the distinction that exists among disciplinary-based scholars of aging who are interested and read the gerontology literature and those who have the opportunity to practice it.

An interesting dilemma exists where the Gerontological Society of America (GSA) has long embraced the disciplinary study of aging, encouraged the multidisciplinary study of aging, and at the same time welcomed interdisciplinary gerontological thought. As an organization, it has tried to attract members from all disciplinary points of view affiliated with the study of aging. Nevertheless, many more members of the GSA are employed by a traditional department or profession than in gerontology and naturally have certain loyalties to that home base. As an effective membership organization, decisions are made by its voting members, many of whom are centrally involved with disciplinary-based research and, understandably, may even be reluctant to embrace interdisciplinary research. In such an arena where there is intellectual interest in gerontology but a significant constituency engaged in monodisciplinary research, one can understand how the field has been affected. Developments such as an interdisciplinary PhD in gerontology may bring some pause among GSA members, particularly when there is a PhD program in their own home disciplinary department where a graduate student, with possible financial support, could study and work with them. The PhD in gerontology is a new competitor and, unlike the interdisciplinary developments in the sciences, is often occurring in a playing field with far fewer resources.

For investigators or graduate students interested in a single disciplinary perspective about aging, they would likely find support and approval from their core disciplinary reference group inside and outside the university. The result is a situation of emerging tension that has yet to be fully articulated between gerontologists and those who approach the subject from a single disciplinary perspective about aging.

While this underlying structural difference is only beginning to be articulated, it is time that it is brought forward and discussed, for it may actually be restricting the intellectual development of the field. Instead of criticizing the field as one laced with oversimplistic microtheories from the core disciplines parading as gerontology, we need to better understand the situation and distinguish gerontology from aging studies.

The kinds of biting criticisms, intense debates, schools of thought, and precision of terms common in other fields, new or emerging, have been less evident within gerontology or among the membership of the GSA. Now is the time to encourage those kinds of scholarly (and civil) exchanges (Bass, 2007).

Why has such a peculiar situation emerged? Perhaps the explanation revolves around the desire for inclusion and membership, perhaps it is the marginality that individuals who are without a gerontology community at their home university feel perhaps it could be a concern for the vulnerability and survival of the field, or it could be all of these. For whatever reason, the desire to attract scholars and foster collegiality and a genuine sense of community has perhaps overridden the debates needed to shape the intellectual foundation. While collegiality has its place, gerontology has not come to terms with an appropriate relationship between the disciplinary study of aging and gerontology. It is interesting to note that the GSA has only recently included gerontology as one of the many fields from which to choose on its membership form. In an effort to embrace all who are interested in aging, the broader gerontological leadership may have inadvertently helped foster a muddling of the core ideas of the field. While building a supportive scholarly community with a viable membership financial base is important to a group of scholars seeking affiliation, identity, and collegiality, it also has its costs if that community is unable or unwilling to distinguish between the extension of theories and methods from the core disciplines and those that belong exclusively to an interdisciplinary gerontology.

The emergence of the PhD in gerontology is one important direction for the field to help delineate its distinctive components and unabashedly embrace gerontology in its own right. These doctoral students and PhD graduates have chosen gerontology as the area of study among many quality options available to them. They find the GSA the primary organization with which to affiliate and its journals the most prestigious in which to publish. They are part of a future that is interdisciplinary, more closely paralleling the developments in interdisciplinary areas of science and engineering. We need to embrace these pioneering students as central to the future of the field, for it is they who may be able to develop the research models and test novel theories reflective of the complexity expected of the field.

Social Gerontology

While acknowledging that there is and will continue to be major aging-related research done within a single disciplinary perspective, it is important to note that a smaller but growing number of scholars have staked out gerontological intellectual territory, drawing on traditions from multiple disciplines. These gerontologists, predominantly from the social sciences, are pushing the discourse and understanding of the social aspects of gerontology. Writing primarily to an audience interested in social gerontology, these scholars have developed a rich and fast-paced dialogue of fresh insights and perspectives into the complexity of the social aspects of gerontology. Often appearing as works in edited volumes but also publishing in books and journals, these writers are building a knowledge base and a set of intellectual traditions that defy any single discipline and must be considered wholly gerontological. These authors are developing a body of material that is advancing layer by layer, building on previous efforts. The discourse also has its disagreements, making the scholarly effort that much more vigorous and intense. The intensity has resulted in important distinctions and is cumulative regarding the dialogue and foundations being set. With passion and reason, we are now in the throes of the development of what can be considered the maturation of social gerontology.

For the most part, these social gerontology scholars have abandoned concerns over intellectual territory and sluggishness over the development of gerontology and have immersed themselves in arguments about the aging individual within a larger historical, political, social, cultural, and economic environment. Borrowing ideas from a range of disciplinary sources and, at times, creating their own nomenclature and insights along pathways that are occasionally completely original, these scholars are providing the elements for what will be the theoretical foundations of social gerontology.

In 2006, Ken Ferraro wrote in *The Gerontologist* about what he calls seven tenets of the gerontological imagination and asks if we are now at the tipping point where gerontology is arriving as its own discipline. To summarize, Ferraro identifies a series of tenets that help build the gerontological imagination. Playing off C. Wright Mills's classic work on the sociological imagination, Ferraro, like a number of others, are beginning to point the way toward gerontology as its own discipline and area of inquiry. Previous research has identified a series of principles that underlie what is gerontological. According to Ferraro, they include concepts such as (a) aging and causality—those items frequently attributed to age may not be age-related phenomena with gerontologists keeping a healthy skepticism for what is an age effect; (b) aging as multifaceted change—changes associated with growing older are not necessarily linearly associated with chronological age, with the process of aging being multidimensional in nature and involving changes touching on biopsychosocial influences; (c) genetic influences on aging—the individual genetic makeup has profound influences through the entire life course; (d) aging and heterogeneity—the diversity of the population is positively associated with aging; (e) aging and life course analysis—aging is not just for the old but occurs throughout the years, and this lifelong perspective helps understand later life; (f) aging is cumulative—similar to item e, advantages and disadvantages for individuals and groups accumulate over many years; and (g) aging and ageism—ageism remains a phenomenon that is part of modern society and may exist even among the aged themselves (Ferraro, 2006).

Paralleling Ferraro's article in the same journal issue, Alkema and Alley (2006) identify three unique gerontological theories and orienting frameworks: (a) a life course perspective, (b) cumulative advantage and disadvantage theory, and (c) ecological theories in aging. Alkema and Alley point out that in an earlier work, Morgan and Kunkel (1998) identify two foundational elements in gerontological research, including (a) time-related change at levels that vary from cells to society and (b) a recognition that these time-related changes interact, respond to, and influence changes on other levels and dimensions from various systems and events (Alkema & Alley, 2006). What Ferraro's essay, Alkema and Alley's article, and Morgan and Kunkel's book provide is a framework that covers all of gerontology—vast territory that is beginning to emerge with some consistency in perspective. The focus of this chapter, however, is on a narrower slice of gerontology that is aimed at thinking about the social aspects of gerontology.

Within this narrower slice of theoretical efforts focused on social aspects of gerontology, there have been numerous contributions that include a life course perspective, rational choice perspective, postmodernist theories, cumulative advantage/disadvantage theory, and exchange theories, among others. Allied with these conceptual efforts, at least two distinctive "schools of thought" have emerged among social gerontologists. By schools of thought, I refer to perspectives that have emerged from historical philosophic roots and are evident in the modern perspectives or theories. While there may be a variety of conceptual or theoretical frameworks within the two schools of thought, they are linked through these deeper ideological roots.

The underlying framework that connects the scholars associated with a particular perspective can be considered a school of thought where there are basic intellectual and philosophic positions embedded in the perspective and the associated theories. While there may be multiple schools of thought currently influencing social gerontology writing, I have been able to identify only two schools of thought that meet the definitional standard identified. It is up to others to make a case for other schools of thought that have emerged among the social gerontology perspectives, and there may be more, but this chapter discusses two. Across the two perspectives that are discussed, the reader will find fundamental underlying philosophic differences in perspective that make the debate rather dynamic and intense among scholars.

The Critical Gerontologists

This interest in writing about social gerontology has engaged both North American and European contributors and has been particularly active since the 1970s.

Some of the most frequently cited authors include W. Andrew Achenbaum, Jan Baars, Vern Bengtson, Simon Biggs, Toni Calasanti, Thomas Cole, Dale Dannefer, Carroll Estes, Kenneth Ferraro, Chris Gilleard, Anne-Marie Guillemard, Jon Hendricks, Paul Higgs, Martha Holstein, Jaber Gubrium, Stephen Katz, Martin Kohli, Charles Longino, Ariela Lowenstein, Victor Marshall, Meredith Minkler, H. R. (Rick) Moody, John Myles, Laura Katz Olson, Chris Phillipson, Larry Polivka, Jason Powell, the late Matilda and John Riley, K. Warner Schaie, Richard Settersten, and Alan Walker, to name a few of the major contributors. It should be noted that the strong theoretical and philosophic training in the preparation of European doctorates is evidenced in the literature and the intellectual leadership provided by contributors from the United Kingdom and Europe.

Among the different schools of thought that have emerged among the social gerontologists, the most prolific belongs to the "critical gerontologists," which is a broad categorization for those writing from the perspective of the political economy, the moral economy, feminist theory, cumulative advantage/disadvantage, or structured dependency of aging (Minkler & Estes, 1999). The writings of the critical gerontologists have sought to connect the disparate outcomes evidenced in the psychosocial and economic conditions in later life to the larger social forces, such as role of the state, governmental policy and programs, distribution of power, status, prejudice, the balance of risk between government, corporations and individuals, and the consequences of international globalization (Estes, 1999).

The critical gerontologists have deep theoretical roots that draw on the philosophies of Theodor Adorno, Walter Benjamin, Jürgen Habermas, Max Horkheimer, Herbert Marcuse, Erich Fromm, and, of course, Karl Marx. From roughly the years of 1923 through 1973, a group of loosely affiliated intellectuals who shared a similar perspective sought to expand on and revise the theories of Karl Marx. They became known as the Frankfurt school—as in a school of thought—linked to the Institute of Social Research at the University of Frankfurt, Germany. According to David Weininger (1995), "Their studies—which go under the name of 'Critical Theory'—were among the first which can be properly labeled interdisciplinary, encompassing insights from so many different areas," hence the appropriate name "critical gerontologists" for the modern contributors to a critical gerontology school of thought.

The Frankfurt school of critical theorists historically sought to draw on Marxist theory and reconcile it with the circumstances of the times through an examination of how individuals and institutions interact through a large-scale meta-analysis of modern society. Today's critical gerontologists have extended this meta-analysis of social systems and the consequences to the elderly.

According to Estes (1999), "Status, resources, and health of the elderly, and even the trajectory of the aging process itself, are conditioned by one's location in the social structure and the relations generated by the economic mode of production and the gendered division of labor" (p. 19). Critical gerontologists such as Minkler, Cole, and Moody have extended the political economy perspective to include cultural questions that relate to individuality and the experience of aging. A moral economy of aging is one that seeks deeper meaning and purpose in later life that is free from alienation and disinvestment (Minkler & Cole, 1999).

In particular, the critical gerontologists point out that developed nations have, in general, demonstrated declining financial commitment to the public good through social welfare while displacing this responsibility and risk to individuals and their families. It is argued that this erosion of the social contract between the government and its citizenry has altered the expectations of the role of the state in ensuring a quality of later life free from obligatory labor and uncertainty. The displacement of responsibility from the collective to the individual has created further inequity for the vulnerable aged and their families and has altered the notion of a collective society with overarching concerns for the human welfare for all. A vision of a moral and just society is one where there is interconnectedness between generations and classes with mutual responsibility for the security of one another. Further, it is believed that both wealthy and poor are enriched through better public health, stronger neighborhoods, and reduced fear of crime in a society where financial and health security are attainable for everyone.

The shifting nature of social responsibility of the nation-state has been an area of concern to critical gerontologists. They have pointed to the influences of international corporations and transnational policy bodies in a world of increased globalization (Estes & Phillipson, 2002). Institutions such as the World Bank, the International Monetary Fund, the Organization for Economic and Cooperative Development, and the World Trade Organization, all agencies that operate outside the realm of any single nation, are playing an increasing role in influencing the flow of resources and the political economy in which nation-states operate (Phillipson, 2006).

Critical gerontologists have highlighted the increasing interdependence between the developed nations and developing nations where companies and agencies that operate without borders are ever more common (Phillipson, 2003; Torres, 2006; Vincent, 2006). These organizations and companies ensure a steady flow of low-cost goods to consumers in the developed world. With relatively inexpensive goods coming from distant shores, any connection between laborer and consumer is completely lost. The consumer has no idea of what the implications might be to the laborer in a far-off land in exchange for the lower prices they enjoy in the homeland. The supply chain that provides parts and goods from the developing world has become increasingly sophisticated, buttressed by multinational companies and their subsidiaries with the capability to search out the lowest cost of production wherever it may be in order to maximize profit and offer consumables at the lowest prices. Americans have seen the consequences to the economies of local neighborhoods when companies shift their production from one region to another. The consequences for the transient nature of production to laborers in developing countries are no different—except it is ever more distant to the consumer.

Frequently, the labor supplied takes place in countries with little or no pension or social security system with individual earnings covering basic subsistence needs. The consequences of cheap labor, without a support system provided by the government or the corporation, have profound implications for the security and welfare of the laborer and his or her family as they age. In a world with increased life expectancy, where mobile corporations are willing to shift the location of production to the lowest and most productive cost labor pools, there is revealed a significant vulnerability to all workers and particularly to those who are older and without other means of financial support. The invisibility of the actual producer in a globalized society has further distanced the consumer from the laborer. When several different nations are sources of labor for the production and the distribution of goods, it makes it far more difficult for a single nation to protect both the consumer and the laborer. Not only have the critical gerontologists sought to analyze the changing milieu, but they have argued for a more comprehensive social compact within and between nation-states and their citizenry.

The Postmodernist Gerontologists

A second school of thought among social gerontologists has a more recent origin. Inspired by a different collection of earlier European thinkers, these social gerontologists would be classified as "postmodernists." Postmodernists draw on the works of philosophers such as Jean Baudrillard, Jacques Derrida, Michel Foucault, and Jean-François Lyotard (Gilleard & Higgs, 2000; Powell, 2006). While these French thinkers were influential in their own right, they were often critical of one another. Their careers, which spanned roughly the same time period of the 1960s–1990s, influenced many scholars in conceptualizing a postmodern approach in their analysis of contemporary society.

For the most part, the postmodernists were bound together by their critique of Marxists and their disciples. Lyotard, for example, was a strong critic of the grand narratives, popular among Marxists, and argued that postmodern societal frameworks are influenced by many "micronarratives." The postmodernists forged a direction in philosophy that was poststructuralist and deconstructionist in approach, reflecting a growing shift from an industrial economy to a service economy. These intellectuals, among others, took concepts of society that were formal and structural and substituted a view of society that was much more flexible, fluid, and alterable. In a postmodern society, they argue, the power of the state is diminished and reallocated to the hands of consumers. Nevertheless, while decentralized, consumer choice is impressionable and can be influenced by advertisement, social pressure, and sales (Bass, 2007; Powell, 2006).

Powell (2006) summarized the postmodern movement with six themes: (a) objective truth is unlikely or impossible to achieve—truth is variable, depending on situation and circumstance; (b) the components are what are most important rather than broad universal metaphors; (c) decentralized power and authority is preferable to the power held centrally, particularly at the level of the federal government; (d) there is a questioning of what is reality and truth; (e) individual choice dominates postmodern society, which is focused on individual consumption of goods and services; and (f) interest in conformity and universality is replaced with understanding of uniqueness and diversity.

Christopher Gilleard and Paul Higgs have written two books, *Cultures of Ageing* (2000) and *Contexts of Ageing* (2005), that serve as significant efforts of the postmodernists interested in social gerontology. Gilleard and Higgs explicitly critique many of the writings and positions taken by the critical gerontologists—be it structured dependency theory or the political or moral economy of aging positions. From the postmodernist view, the world has changed from an industrial economy with structured mass production to an economy focused on customized services and consumer choice (Bass, 2002). The changing nature of the economy and the availability of greater economic security in later life have fostered an epoch of sustained leisure time with sufficient personal resources that extend beyond bare subsistence. This postindustrial economy affords the individual significant choice in goods and services as part of its cultural terrain. With the changing nature of labor, individuals have far greater time for hobbies, travel, entertainment, personal enrichment, and material acquisition.

Drawn from earlier philosophic writings, Gilleard and Higgs see aging as a flexible time of opportunity and choice, highly influenced by a cultural reality of marketing and material consumption (Bass, 2007). The resulting individual choices often involve the acquisition of products and services of which some attempt to counter the aging process itself, encouraged by a society that glamorizes youth. These products can be in the form of food, vitamin supplements, cosmetics, pharmaceuticals, exercise programs, physical therapy, clothing, travel, plastic surgery, and bioengineered body parts.

Postmodernists point out that individuals have far greater choice among the available options in a culture the economy of which is dependent on consumer spending. As mentioned earlier and reflected by Gilleard and Higgs, in a postmodern world the structured role of the nation-state in affording universality is diminished, replaced by a malleable experience in later life shaped in a customized manner for the individual. Even the concept of community in contemporary society has a far broader meaning today than it would for the previous generation that took part in the industrial economy. Rather than thinking of community as a geographic group brought together by proximity, ethnic, or religious identity, for postmodernists it extends to collectives of individuals who share similar hobbies, beliefs, and interests and who have been brought together through associations or in virtual contexts (Gilleard & Higgs, 2005).

Central to the postmodernists is a desire to describe the changed and changing world, not as one would idealize it but as it appears today. The way we conceptualize the world around us has significant implications for how we think about the experience of aging. For the postmodernist gerontologists, the ideas of Marx and, by association, the ideas of the critical gerontologists are no longer relevant to this changed society. New frameworks and lenses are needed to understand and interpret the society in which we are living and aging.

Is There Common Ground?

The arguments surrounding the way we interpret the aging experience, the way we theorize about it, and, as a result of those theories, the way we carry out research constitute a crucial debate. By fostering debate, it sharpens the dialogue between camps; it improves the thinking within each group, recognizing the weaker points on which they stand; and it moves us forward as an intellectual community. Idea debates have been a cornerstone of scholarly exchanges over the centuries. Sometimes these disagreements have been uncivil and created deep rifts among influential thinkers and their students. In other instances, groups have broken off communication from a wider scholarly community and developed their own language and communication style that is digested by subscribers of that particular ideology, restricting the branch of the field to ideological proponents and adherents.

At this point, the arguments between the critical gerontologists and the postmodernist social gerontologists are relatively new, and the readership is a rather small but focused audience. The communication across groups has been direct but civil and respectful. The discourse has been universal and not destined exclusively for ideological proponents. In order to move the discourse along, between, and among social gerontologists, more opportunities are needed to expose a wider range of scholars to the nature of the debate. In addition, a broader readership is needed—particularly those who have been entrenched in a single social science disciplinary perspective.

Nevertheless, the critical gerontologists and postmodernist gerontologists appear to be reading each other's work. Alan Walker (2006), a critical gerontologist from the United Kingdom, defended the position of the political economy of aging by stating, "The social construction of old age showed that in important respects the risks associated with aging differ between social groups—class/occupation, gender, race, and so on—and that these differences are determined to a large extent prior to old age, and that this core message is as true today as it was nearly three decades ago" (p. 69).

On the one hand, the constituencies are responding to one another by defending their ideas and, at times, hardening positions. On the other hand, there is some recognition of the others' point of view. Walker (2006) goes on to say in the same article that "the relevance of this discussion of the theoretical basis of the social is that it provides a methodology for understanding the constant tension between structure and agency in everyday life, including over the life course, and thereby, a way to reconcile the critiques that political economy overemphasizes structure . . . and that life course and some culture perspectives overemphasize agency" (p. 76).

Here we have a bit of a concession, an effort to forge some common ground, by Walker. Indeed, there may be extremist positions emerging from each of the camps, and while the philosophic roots are divergent, there may be some broader understanding of social gerontology that can be generalized for wider audiences.

Toward an Integrative Theory of Social Gerontology

An integrative theory of social gerontology (Alkema & Alley, 2006) is one that draws on the elements that have emerged over the years and places them in context that is acceptable to a wide range of investigators. Rather than drawing on any single philosophy, an integrative theory of social gerontology blends the components, providing coherence to our understanding of the aging individual in contemporary society.

An integrative theory blends a macroperspective that examines the larger social, economic, environmental, cultural, and political contexts that influence human behavior and health with the microperspective and individual and family perspectives along the very same dimensions. How these macrostructures prioritize resource allocation and support an aging population and, as a result, how the individual responds to his or her own aging and that of others is critical to the framework. The contexts in which aging takes place change over different time periods, are influenced by major historical events, and vary among nations and geographic locations. The accrued advantages or disadvantages that take place over the life course must be considered in understanding the aging experience—experiences accumulate and influence later life abilities, access, resources, networks, choices, and actions.

Further, this multifaceted perspective in understanding the experience of aging acknowledges the influence of political power, which can be triggered by crisis, previous ideological positions, or the impact of mass movements. The use of political power and the resulting services or programs for the aged and their families hold significant consequences for older people.

A conceptual model of such an integrative theory that is reflective of the consequences of time, inclusive of culture, social position, economic circumstances, larger environmental forces, and individual attributes, poses a challenge to model and visualize. Clearly, from what has been described, a visual model of human developmental steps or stages is far too simplistic. Another visual representation of aging appearing in the literature involves overlapping circles in a kind of Venn diagram (e.g., Lowenstein, 2003; Treas & Passuth, 1988). Jon Hendricks (2003), in an influential chapter on structure and identity, has used a three-dimensional cube to describe personal resource dimensions. In another conceptualization, Hendricks used an atomic structure–type format that describes the influences on the individual—in this model, Hendricks does identify time–space considerations. Classical theorists, for the most part, have used sticks and arrows that show a sequence or progression in society or more sophisticated models that reveal an interaction between individual, family, the economy, the polity, and the law (Allen, 2005). Essentially, however, most of the models have been static and two dimensional.

The integrative theory of social gerontology, however, is not static but changes and shifts over time. The complicated three-dimensional structures of intertwined chemical strands in viruses seen at the molecular level and moving over time and space provide a much more appropriate visual image of the concept. Rather than lines and arrows, a cube, or interfacing spheres, the image may be more of a lattice, a three-dimensional web, or a network where the various elements are interactive with influences on each other at different moments in time.

Presented in Figure 19.1 is a conceptual work in progress and one for further discussion, with the vertical dimension reflecting time, accumulated experience, history, and events influencing the individual, located at the center. The four larger structural elements that hold the figure together reflect the economy, the polity, culture, and the collective. Each of the interacting components and supports represents the many different interactions that individuals have with different structures over time. In the model, not only do the four macrostructural elements interact with the individual and the individual with them, but the cross members represent the combinations of interactions that take place across and among the structural elements. Choice, as well as chance, can influence the different touchstones over time as the individual progresses through the structure over time.

In examining Figure 19.1, imagine looking upward through the inside of a radio tower while lying on the ground. Along each side, four large beams support the tower. Each beam is labeled, reflecting the major structural components influencing an individual's life course: culture, economics, the state, and the society. Each of the four structural beams is anchored in a block, reflecting the antecedent events of the past that carry over into the present and future.

19.1

An integrative theory of social gerontology.
A = family, religion, and cultural traditions and expectations
B = macro- and microeconomic circumstances and individual assets
C = public policy, health services and social support systems, and government programs
D = social constructs (e.g., status, power, and social stratification)
E = residual historical contexts
F = individual genetic, physiological, and psychological condition

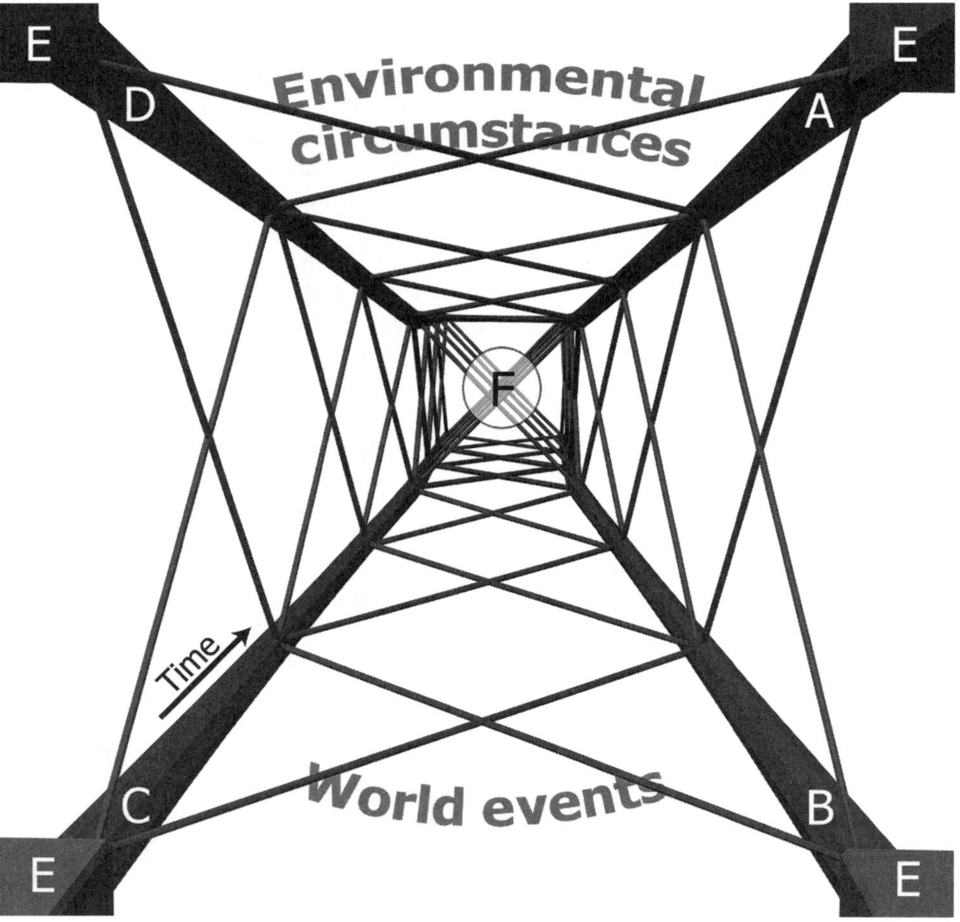

You will notice as you look up into the center of the tower that you are exploring the time dimension experienced for an individual and his or her cohort as he or she ages. Each of the different rungs near the top of the tower is layered one above each other with a circle in the middle. The layering reflects different points in time as one moves up the tower structure, and the circle in the middle represents the aging individual surrounded by his or her birth cohort.

Not only does the tower have the four main structural beams, but the beams have diagonal supports that are interconnected. This is to highlight the flow and interaction between and among the different social, economic, government, and cultural elements. In addition, cited as an inset is the larger environmental circumstances and world events that may dramatically affect the life experience and even the structural supports themselves.

More specifically, Figure 19.1 can be described as follows: item F in the circle reflects the individual with his or her individual genetic, physiological, and psychological condition along with his or her birth cohort suspended among the interacting structural components. The infrastructure surrounding the individual reflects the insights drawn from major disciplines of the social sciences, all of which have a cumulative effect on the aging individual and are critical to integrate in a comprehensive view of social gerontology. Over time, the individual moves up the tower structure, accumulating advantages and disadvantages accrued over the life course. The path and life course are fluid and river-like, with the individual and the larger cohort flowing up through Figure 19.1, interacting with the environment and world events, government, society, culture, and the economy over time. The entire tower structure is set in the broader environmental and world conditions, which may include the consequences of catastrophic natural events, such as storms, drought, floods, famines, fires, and earthquakes, as well as other significant world events, such as revolutions and wars. In addition, the broader environmental conditions may also include circumstances in the built environment that may have longer-term consequences for the individual. These conditions might include a residence located in a former toxic site, sanitation conditions, contaminated drinking water, air quality, exposure to lead or known carcinogens, radiation poisoning, and the like. The qualities of the air, water, soil, and the surrounding built environment have long-term consequences for the aging individual. Some of these larger environmental circumstances have immediate traumatic consequences for older individuals, while others are nearly invisible and accrue only over many years or decades.

Item A reflects family, culture, religion, and the traditions and expectations of that larger culture on the individual. Culture is not a static item. It evolves over time, and within different subpopulations, different expectations and norms exist. Cultural norms and messages can exist in the larger societal surroundings, and they can exist within a specific ethnic, religious, geographic, or self-defined community. The cultural messages conveyed sometimes can be subtle and at other times quite overt. Anthropologists often see the world through the lens of culture and its powerful consequences to mold and shape the human experience. Postmodernists as well attribute the role of culture and, in particular, the influence of consumerism on adult behavior and choice. Many times, the push for consumption in a capitalist society reflects images created by the popular media, often presenting the aspiration of youth as the ideal. Further, through advertising on billboards, radio, and television and in magazines and the press, marketing has fostered a demand for products among all segments of the population. Many times, these images encourage older consumers to seek goods and services that perpetuate a youthful image in contrast to natural and inevitable aging. Among social scientists, the task is to understand and describe both the micro- and the macrocultural norms surrounding the individual. At the same time, the individual may influence the cultural surrounding with new ideas, changes in traditions, and innovations in practices. In some cultures, working for pay into the twilight of one's life may be discouraged, where in others it might be encouraged. These powerful influences help shape the options under consideration for the aging individual.

Item B represents the macro- and microeconomic circumstances in which the individual or couple finds him- or herself. They may have grown up during an economic depression that has had a profound effect on how they save and spend income later in life. Individual savings may be significant, allowing for a retirement with economic security, or just the opposite, requiring labor until one can physically no longer work. Pensions, private or public, have a significant influence on options in later life. And as individual economic assets accrue over time, those who have had larger incomes or spent less of the income they earned may have accumulated more assets and are likely to be better off financially later in life. Nevertheless, the older individual is still subject to the uncertainties of the economy. A recession could reduce the value of a major asset such as a house, wipe out invested savings, or end or limit a private pension. And on a larger scale, inequality increases with age within cohorts, leaving some with an economic bounty and others with far less.

Item C represents the role of government and public or private support systems. This includes public policies, health services, government programs, and social support systems. Changes in public policies can have a direct effect on the quality of life of an older person. For example, a reduction in the coverage of a prescription drug may cause an elder to not use the drug as prescribed or, even worse, not take the medication at all. The type of health care coverage may influence the frequency with which an individual visits the doctor. As the model is fluid, the lack of health or dental care in one's youth may have significant implications for the older individual's physical condition. Social services may also vary by community, state, or nation with some communities providing extensive social supports to its citizens and others providing far less. The relationship between the availability of quality services, family and culture, and personal assets is linked in those settings where public support is limited. In these circumstances, either the private support system is available and leveraged through social networks or through purchase or it is not provided at all, putting the elder at risk.

Item D reflects the larger social constructs that surround the individual, such as status, power, social stratification. Individuals by birth may come from different social strata with varying degrees of influence and prestige. For some, mobility may be possible through education, but for many, mobility may be limited. One's social standing may be influenced by external prejudices associated with their religious affiliation, race, gender, disability, or nationality. These influences can cause individuals or communities of like-minded individuals to react to these circumstances by creating alternative mechanisms of reward and recognition in a larger world where they have encountered rejection, discomfort, and disharmony.

Item E is the residual historical context in which all the elements are anchored. Each of the items from A to D emerges from a past prior to an individual's birth and has an influence on the major structural elements and as a result has consequences for the individual.

Table 19.1 provides a more detailed description of some of the elements that are included under each of the items.

19.1 Examples of Items Found in Figure 19.1

A. Family, religion, and cultural traditions and expectations
   Nuclear and extended family beliefs, attitudes, and expectations
   Religious beliefs, traditions, and expectations
   Neighborhood traditions and expectations
   Virtual community expectations and pressures
   Media influences
   Marketing and advertising
   Arts, music, technology, and literary influences
   Ethics, morals, and norms

B. Macro- and microeconomic circumstances and individual assets
   National economy, wealth, debt, and balance of trade
   Globalization and international economic conditions
   Economic and tax incentives and disincentives
   Capitalization resources and market conditions
   Savings rate and interest rates
   Cost of essential goods/services: housing, food, health care, and transportation
   Labor market conditions and benefits
   Personal assets: income, property, investments, pension, health care insurance, life insurance, and savings
   Family and/or other financial support systems

C. Public policy, health services and social support systems, and government programs
   Economic security programs for disabled, infirm, and aged
   Medical, mental health and rehabilitation services
   Social support services for meals, bathing, toileting, dressing, and house cleaning
   Education
   Recreational programs
   Long-term care: institutional and home based
   Employment training programs
   Transportation services
   Subsidized housing
   Food/nutritional assistance
   Legal assistance programs
   Volunteer and social network programs
   Day care and senior center programs
   Self-help programs, services, and institutions
   Police, courts, and prisons

(Continued)

19.1 Examples of Items Found in Figure 19.1 (*continued*)

D. Social constructs
- Status
- Power
- Social stratification
- Authority and control
- Modernity and postmodernity
- Class
- Social behavior of groups
- Laws and formal and informal rules
- Discrimination, prejudice, and oppression
- Interaction within and across social systems
- Nation-states
- Corporate entities

E. Residual historical contexts
- Prior conditions
- Inherited circumstances
- Family, community, and nation historical situations
- Choices made prior to birth

F. Individual genetic, physiological, and psychological condition embedded among their birth cohort
- Race, gender, and age
- Physical attributes (e.g., height, weight, proportions, bone structure, and image)
- Disabilities and birth defects
- Genetics and individual biology
- Genetically associated ailments or propensity for disease
- Personality, identity, and character
- Mental health, sense of purpose, and meaning
- Health condition
- Aptitude and cognitive functions
- Coping mechanisms
- Maintenance, nutrition, hygiene, and care of the body
- Trauma, injury, and accidents
- Surgery and physical changes to the body
- Environmental circumstances and world events
  - War
  - Revolutions

(*Continued*)

19.1 Examples of Items Found in Figure 19.1 (*continued*)

Genocide

Epidemics

Economic depressions

Drought, floods, fires, earthquakes, storms, and tsunami

Famines and desertification

Quality of air, water, and soil

Sanitation

Toxins, carcinogens, metals, poisons, and radiation in food or the built environment

In the real world, the individual traverses over time facing complex interactions among different social, political, economic, and cultural forces, all embedded in the environmental milieu. The visual description is an attempt to integrate these many factors as they influence a person over time.

For example, let's explore the tower model for a case of a lower-income elder, aged 70, who was raised in a poor urban family. In this case, the older woman owns a house and lives independently in an ethnic neighborhood where she is able to walk to her church as well as the local shops to buy food and necessities. She has a high school education and has lived in the neighborhood most of her life. When she was a young woman, she and her husband did not have health insurance, and, among other things, she did not adequately take care of her teeth. She lost most of her teeth by age 55 and, in addition, now has a variety of chronic ailments. She is embarrassed to meet people because of the way she looks and finds that others have some difficulty understanding her diction.

One day, this older women finds a notice in her mailbox that the location of her home is in the path of major new highway construction. To move from the neighborhood where she has lived most of their adult life would be traumatic for her. Further, the small financial nest egg she is living on would be insufficient to cover the cost of a new home in a new neighborhood. Currently, she is a widow without children and is of limited means. She draws considerable support from the leadership of the local church with whom over the years she has grown very close.

The state is encouraging residents to move to a nearby neighborhood and will assist with relocation. To go shopping or return to her church from the relocated neighborhood, however, would require the use of a car. Unfortunately, she does not know how to drive, nor does she own a car, and for that matter, because of poor eyesight, she does not want to drive.

In this case, we have the interaction between the individual (F), his or her historical antecedents (E), the broader environment, his or her social standing (D), state policies (C), economic circumstances (B), and the cultural traditions found in an older neighborhood (A). To model such a set of exchanges necessitates a more dynamic and interactive visual model such as suggested in Figure 19.1.

Overarching Principles of a Theoretical Model of Social Gerontology

Building on the conceptual model detailed here, a series of overarching principles emerge that may help guide us as we seek to construct an integrated theory of social gerontology.

First, the individual is set in a larger sociopolitical environment. Individual options are highly influenced by the social structures that support them (see the literature by the critical gerontology theorists). The experiences encountered later in life are different for the individual with an adequate pension compared to the individual who has little or none; the same is true if health care is provided at low cost, if housing is affordable, and if there is a support system in place. There are multileveled influences from family, community, employer, state, federal government, and international economies that can significantly affect the possibilities and options available to older people. Even the ability to imagine possibilities can be shaped by these powerful external forces.

Unfortunately, we observe that these macrolevel influences have variable outcomes according to race, class, and gender (e.g., see Martin & Soldo, 1997). The influence of the underlying economic and social structure can shape life's chances and even life itself. Disciplines that would contribute significantly to this discourse include sociology, political science, public policy, and economics.

Second, these larger, often invisible macrolevel influences are dynamic and change over time and vary among nations. That is, the nature of labor, the economy, world events, and the public–private financial benefit systems will vary at different historical moments and in different locations. For example, the experience of an older Iraqi during wartime in 2007 is quite different than it will be for an older person in a less stressed part of the world.

An integrative theory is not a static one but recognizes the changes in circumstances depending on larger world events. Today, developed nations are in a postindustrial era of relative abundance driven by consumerism and materialism (e.g., see the literature by the postmodern theorists). Social security schemes and private pensions have provided large numbers of older people economic security and freedom from financial destitution as they age. Nevertheless, these schemes are vulnerable to changes in policy and approaches. Rather than centralized support systems from government and employers, pension schemes are increasingly dependent on individual savings that will vary significantly from individual to individual. Today's pension provision may be very different from tomorrow's. The underlying cultural and structural support system in China is different than in Sweden—and our theory must provide a framework in which both can be understood for its impact on the aged.

Our integrated theory acknowledges that circumstances change, macroinfluences change and evolve, and the circumstances in the developed world, what King and Calasanti call our preoccupation with the "Global North" (King & Calasanti, 2006, p. 139), are not universal truths or the primary perspective from which to understand the aging experience. Much of the world's aged, unfortunately, do not enjoy the privileges taken for granted in the Global North.

Disciplines that would be significant contributors to this theoretical area include political science, sociology, history, and anthropology.

Third, advantages and disadvantages accrue over the life course. An assumption of an integrative theory is that late life is but a point in time in an individual's life path and that to understand that experience requires an understanding of the accumulated experiences throughout the life course. For example, the advantages and disadvantages that may be accrued differentially by race, class, and gender identified previously are, in many circumstances, cumulative over time (for cumulative disadvantage theory, see Dannefer, 2006). The accrual of resources over time can be in the form of financial enhancement, status or reputation, social networks that have been built, influential alliances and associations that can assist, health and dental care, nutrition, education, and interactions with law enforcement, to name a few.

Like accumulated pocket change, the aggregation of these advantages and disadvantages add up over time and can influence the individual and the supports that will be there in later life. The cumulative consequences are not just destined to one individual but can carry forward across generations through inheritances, both financial and circumstantial. For the financially destitute locked in a cycle of poverty, the consequences are too often passed on to children and their children, where accumulated inequities transfer across generations. In considering the phenomenon of aging, the circumstances of the past and the legacy they leave—both good and bad—are carried into the range of options that can come into play as support is needed.

The aggregation of advantages and disadvantages extends beyond the social, economic, cultural, political, health, and educational systems but also are evident in the environment itself—be it the built or the natural environment. The impact of air, water, and soil quality can have significant adverse effects if the local environmental conditions have high levels of pollution, radiation, or toxicity. Weather, in the form of violent storms resulting in desertification or flooding or excess heat or cold, can also have long-term consequences for the aging individual and his or her health, as well as his or her ability to grow food, earn a living, or have adequate shelter. The built environment might contain lead, asbestos, mold, or other carcinogens unknown to the inhabitants. It might have inadequate sanitation or waste removal, improper treatment of garbage, or poor water quality of which the consequences might take many years to become manifest but surface as either an acute or a chronic health condition in later life. The built environment may house vermin or other organisms that can lead to adverse physical consequences. And the workplace may be another location that harbors long-term health risks. Many of these environmental hazards are more likely to affect those from poorer economic strata who may be less prepared to fight local polluters, have less flexibility to respond to shifts and changes in weather, and be more likely to live or work in neighborhoods with substandard housing.

Disciplines that would significantly contribute to this theoretical theme would be sociology, public health, epidemiology, anthropology, psychology, social work, economics, and geography.

Fourth, from an integrative social gerontological perspective, the psychological, social, cultural, and economic consequences of bodily changes are of interest. As the body inevitably changes through the aging process, how individuals respond and how society treats the aging individual are of concern (e.g., Gilliard & Higgs, 2000). For example, what would be the consequences of no longer being physically able to continue with paid employment? Leaving work may have profound impact on income, status, role, meaning, identity, and interpersonal relations in the home. Is there a cultural expectation to leave work even if the aging individual would like to continue with paid labor? To what extent does the individual, based on social pressures and/or marketing, seek to purchase cosmetic aides, physical aides, and alter his or her body through more radical means, such as surgery, to achieve a desired image? The aging body is a subject that social scientists are concerned with less from an organic physiological or medical perspective and from the point of view of the consequences and response to these changes as identified from the larger culture as well as from the individual's perspective.

The way a state plans for its care of the aged, finances its costs, and monitors its quality of care is another indicator of the society at large and its values. Much attention is paid in the gerontology literature to the issues associated with chronic care of the aged. The structures associated with the care, how it is financed, and who provides the care are examples of the kinds of analysis that would be relevant under this broader theoretical theme.

Disciplines that would contribute significantly to this area include psychology, anthropology, sociology, public policy, economics, and public heath.

Fifth, the influence of policy development in democratic societies is politically stratified. For social gerontologists, the desire for a rational merit-based decision-making process that would provide the necessary resources to the aged remains a goal, but the reality of the process is quite different. Robert Putnam (1976) argues that there is a stratification of those who influence public policy. There are those individuals in positions of influence who may have the power to make decisions and craft policies. They are surrounded by influential individuals who may be technical specialists, special constituencies, or representative of special interests whose agenda, values, and self-interests may be quite different from those in the gerontology community. However, the role of each influential individual in shaping a decision may be significant. In addition, but with less direct influence, there are activists who have an explicit and clearly defined view on a specific policy and make their voice heard through letters, campaigns, publications, the media, and public demonstration. Finally, with the least influence on a specific policy is the public and voters themselves.

Further, the policy process in a representative democracy is one where elected officials bring to their offices certain ideological belief systems. Sometimes these belief systems are stated while campaigning for office or in the positions of their party platforms. Other times these underlying values may be harder to determine, but they are there. In addition to the basic ideological and value perspectives, an elected official can be swayed on the basis of the positions of influential organizations and special interests. These special interests can provide the financial capital to run for office and/or deliver constituencies necessary for votes in elections, essential if the individual seeks to remain in a position of power or influence.

In considering an integrative theoretical framework, it is important to recognize that politics is an important component in shaping public policy and subsequent treatment for groups or individuals. Change in public policy can come about through crises (e.g., a catastrophic failure of a bridge), self-interests (e.g., an elected official with a disabled brother), or political power that can be obtained through a variety of mechanisms. For those without financial means, political capital may be earned by organizing large numbers of voting constituents. Change can come about through political pressure, confrontation, or persuasion. Unfortunately, rarely does change occur exclusively on the basis of objective information.

Disciplines that can contribute significantly to this area include public policy, history, and political science.

Sixth, there is a constant interaction between the individual and society, each influencing each other over time, creating multiple perspectives on phenomena and introducing the notion of chance. The relationship between the individual and social, economic, and political forces is dynamic. On the one hand, the individual is molded and shaped by the influences of policies, regulations, cultural norms, traditions, and expectations. On the other hand, these social and political norms evolve and change as a consequence of the influences of the citizenry. The exchanges are unordered and unpredictable with change coming about after multiple and repeated exchanges. The interaction and mutual exchange is fluid, organic, and of significance with neither party remaining the same over time.

Rather than being static, an integrative theory needs to evolve as external circumstances change. It is essential for a counterperspective to challenge the prevailing perspective on social gerontology as social and political structures change and adapt. Part of the theory itself is that it evolves and changes with the changing situation. For example, as increased globalization creates changes from what was historically "organized capitalism" to capitalism that is less centralized and "disorganized" or as society shifts from "simple" to "reflexive modernity" (Phillipson, 2006, p. 165), the conceptual model needs to be sufficiently adaptable to adjust and change to reflect the changing milieu. Presented in this chapter is the struggle for insight in the human aging experience that embraces complexity and anticipates dynamic change. Disagreement in interpreting these changes is fundamental to a successful social gerontology model and theory, as the ideas put forward demand rigorous debate prior to acceptance and, once accepted, are subject to further debate, as circumstances that have fostered the accepted position may now have evolved.

Finally, chance plays a role. Individuals matched by demographics, age, education, health, and experience can have distinctly different outcomes in later life by the sheer chance of being hired at Microsoft rather than Enron. In one case, the individual had been offered stock options that are valuable today, and the other did not. Luck, chance, and randomness are illusive factors that operate and must be understood and accepted as part of an integrative theory.

Disciplines that can contribute significantly to this theme include philosophy, psychology, and sociology.

Conclusion

Social gerontology, by definition, takes a comprehensive view that cuts across the social sciences. It is different from other disciplines of aging in that these fields are drawing from within the disciplinary paradigm. While discipline-based scholars are interested in understanding aging, they bring a different framework to the discussion than those who are navigating beyond their discipline and embarking on an interdisciplinary exploration of social gerontology. It is essential to articulate these differences so that there is both less confusion and greater coherence in the literature. The moment has arrived to encourage social gerontologists to develop conceptual frameworks, models, perspectives, and theories that span the social sciences and beyond. We are at the cusp of articulating what that theory is and how we conceptualize it. This is new intellectual territory and will require the efforts of social science pioneers. This chapter is intended to foster further discussion, encourage others to present alternative conceptualizations, and give voice and shape to a true integrative social gerontology.

References

Achenbaum, W. A. (1995). *Crossing frontiers: Gerontology emerges as a science.* New York: Cambridge University Press.

Alkema, G. E., & Alley, D. E. (2006). Gerontology's future: An integrative model for disciplinary advancement. *The Gerontologist, 46,* 574–582.

Allen, K. (2005). *Explorations in classical sociological theory: Seeing the social world.* Thousand Oaks, CA: Pine Forge Press.

Bass, S. A. (2002). The resurgence of gerontological scholarship. *The Gerontologist, 42,* 127–131.

Bass, S. A. (2006). Gerontological theory: The search for the holy grail. *The Gerontologist, 46,* 139–144.

Bass, S. A. (2007). The emergence of the golden age of social gerontology? *The Gerontologist, 47,* 406–412.

Bass, S. A., & Ferraro, K. F. (2000). Gerontology education in transition: Considering disciplinary and paradigmatic evolution. *The Gerontologist, 40,* 97–106.

Bengtson, V. L., Parrott, T. M., & Burgess, E. O. (1996). Progress and pitfalls in gerontological theorizing. *The Gerontologist, 36,* 768–772.

Bengtson, V. L., Rice, C. J., & Johnson, M. L. (1999). Are theories of aging important? Models and explanations in gerontology at the turn of the century. In V. L. Bengtson & K. W. Schaie (Eds.), *Handbook of theories of aging* (pp. 3–20). New York: Springer Publishing.

Biggs, S., Lowenstein, A., & Hendricks, J. (Eds.). (2003). *The need for theory: Critical approaches to social gerontology.* Amityville, NY: Baywood Publishing.

Birren, J. F., & Bengtson, V. L. (Eds.). (1988). *Emergent theories of aging.* New York: Springer Publishing.

Dannefer, D. (2006). Reciprocal co-optation: The relationship of critical theory and social gerontology. In J. Baars, D. Dannefer, C. Phillipson, & A. Walker (Eds.), *Aging, globalization and inequality: The new critical gerontology* (pp. 103–120). Amityville, NY: Baywood Publishing.

Estes, C. L. (1999). Critical gerontology and the new political economy of aging. In M. Minkler & C. L. Estes (Eds.), *Critical gerontology: Perspectives from political and moral economy* (pp. 17–35). Amityville, NY: Baywood Publishing.

Estes, C. L., & Phillipson, C. (2002). The globalization of capital, the welfare state and old age policy. *International Journal of Health Services, 32,* 279–297.

Ferraro, K. F. (2006). Imagining the disciplinary advancements of gerontology: Whither the tipping point? *The Gerontologist, 46,* 571–573.

Gilleard, C., & Higgs, P. (2000). *Cultures of ageing: Self, citizen, and the body.* Harlow: Prentice Hall.

Gilleard, C., & Higgs, P. (2005). *Contexts of ageing: Class, cohort and community.* Cambridge: Polity Press.

Hagestad, G. O., & Dannefer, D. (2001). Concepts and theories of aging: Beyond microfication in social science approaches. In R. H. Binstock & L. K. George (Eds.), *Handbook of aging and social sciences* (5th ed., pp. 3–21). San Diego, CA: Academic Press.

Hendricks, J. (2003). Structure and identity—Mind the gap: Toward a personal resource model of successful aging. In S. Biggs, A. Lowenstein, & J. Hendricks (Eds.), *The need for theory: Critical approaches to social gerontology* (pp. 63–90). Amityville, NY: Baywood Publishing.

Katz, S. N. (1996). *Disciplining old age: The formation of gerontological knowledge.* Charlottesville: University Press of Virginia.

King, N., & Calasanti, T. (2006). Empowering the old: Critical gerontology and anti-aging in a global context. In J. Baars, D. Dannefer, C. Phillipson, & A. Walker (Eds.), *Aging, globalization and inequality: The new critical gerontology* (pp. 139–157). Amityville, NY: Baywood Publishing.

Longino, C. F., Jr. (2005). Editorial: Exploring the connections: Theory and research. *Journal of Gerontology: Social Sciences, 60,* S172.

Lowenstein, A. (2003). Contemporary later life family transitions: Revisiting theoretical perspectives on aging and the family—Toward a family identity framework. In S. Biggs, A. Lowenstein, & J. Hendricks (Eds.), *The need for theory: Critical approaches to social gerontology* (pp. 105–125). Amityville, NY: Baywood Publishing.

Maddox, G. L., & Campbell, R. T. (1985). Scope, concepts, and methods in the study of aging. In E. Shanas & R. H. Binstock (Eds.), *Handbook of aging and social sciences* (2nd ed., pp. 3–28). New York: Van Nostrand Reinhold.

Marshall, V. (1999). Analyzing social theories of aging. In V. L. Bengtson & K. W. Schaie (Eds.), *Handbook of theories of aging* (pp. 434–455). New York: Springer Publishing.

Martin, L. G., & Soldo, B. J. (1997). *Differences in late life health in the United States.* Washington, DC: National Academies Press.

Minkler, M. (1996). Critical perspectives on ageing: New challenges for gerontology. *Ageing and Society, 16,* 467–487.

Minkler, M., & Cole, T. (1999). Political and moral economy: Getting to know one another. In M. Minkler & C. Estes (Eds.), *Critical gerontology: Perspectives from political and moral economy* (pp. 37–49.) Amityville, NY: Baywood Publishing.

Minkler, M., & Estes, C. L. (1999). *Critical gerontology: Perspectives from political and moral economy.* Amityville, NY: Baywood Publishing.

Moody, H. R. (1988). Toward a critical gerontology: The contribution of the humanities theories of aging. In J. Birren & V. L. Bengtson (Eds.), *Emergent theories of aging* (pp. 19–40). New York: Springer Publishing.

Morgan, L., & Kunkel, S. (1998). *Aging: The social context.* Thousand Oaks, CA: Pine Forge Press.

Myers, G. C. (1996). Aging and the social sciences: Research directions and unresolved issues. In R. H. Binstock & L. K. George (Eds.), *Handbook of aging and social sciences* (4th ed., pp. 1–11). San Diego, CA: Academic Press.

National Academy of Sciences, National Academy of Engineering, & Institute of Medicine, (2005). *Facilitating interdisciplinary research.* Washington, DC: National Academies Press.

Phillipson, C. (1998). *Reconstructing old age: New agendas in social theory and practice.* London: Sage.

Phillipson, C. (2003). Globalization and the reconstruction of old age: New challenges for critical gerontology. In S. Biggs, A. Lowenstein, & J. Hendricks (Eds.), *The need for theory: Critical approaches to social gerontology* (pp. 163–180). Amityville, NY: Baywood Publishing.

Phillipson, C. (2006). Aging and globalization: Issues for critical gerontology and political economy. In J. Barrs, D. Dannefer, C. Phillipson, & A. Walker (Eds.), *Aging globalization and inequality: The new critical gerontology* (pp. 43–58). Amityville, NY: Baywood Publishing.

Powell, J. L. (2006). *Social theory and aging.* Lanham, MD: Rowman & Littlefield.

Putnam R. D. (1976). *The comparative study of political elites.* Englewood Cliffs, NJ: Prentice Hall.

Torres, S. (2006). Culture, migration, inequality, and "periphery" in a globalized world: Challenges for ethno- and anthropogerontology. In J. Barrs, D. Dannefer, C. Phillipson, & A. Walker (Eds.), *Aging globalization and inequality: The new critical gerontology* (pp. 231–244). Amityville, NY: Baywood Publishing.

Treas, J., & Passuth, P. (1988). Age, aging, and the aged: The three sociologies. In E. Borgatta & K. S. Cook (Eds.), *The future of sociology* (pp. 394–417). Newbury Park, CA: Sage and the Pacific Sociological Association.

Vincent, J. (2006). Globalization and critical theory: Political economy of world population issues. In J. Barrs, D. Dannefer, C. Phillipson, & A. Walker (Eds.), *Aging globalization and inequality: The new critical gerontology* (pp. 245–271). Amityville, NY: Baywood Publishing.

Walker, A. (1999). Public policies and theories of aging: Constructing and reconstructing. In V. L. Bengtson & K. W. Schaie (Eds.), *Handbook of theories of aging: In honor of Jim Birren* (pp. 361–378). New York: Springer Publishing.

Walker, A. (2006). Reexamining the political economy of aging: Understanding the structure/agency tension. In J. Barrs, D. Dannefer, C. Phillipson, & A. Walker (Eds.), *Aging globalization and inequality: The new critical gerontology* (pp. 59–80). Amityville, NY: Baywood Publishing.

Weininger, D. (1995, March). [Review of the book *The Frankfurt school: Its history, theories, and political significance*]. Retrieved January 9, 2008, from http://www.bookwire.com/bbr/politics/frankfurt-school.html

Toward a Phenomenology of Aging

20

Charles F. Longino Jr.
Jason L. Powell

This chapter explores the theory of phenomenology and its relevance for aging studies. We begin by attempting to unravel the main conceptualizations of phenomenology and then look to see how it can be used in gerontological contexts. In particular, we assess the relevance of the aging body, aging identity, and the life course for pointing toward a general theory that can be defined as a "phenomenology of aging." Part of the context for realizing the potential of phenomenology is its dissection of meaning, not as fixed but as fluid (May & Powell, 2008) as found in the context of everyday life. Phenomenology provides a significant contribution to unlocking an understanding of what it means to be a human person situated within and across the life course. It can be used to reveal critical consciousness, understanding of personal identity, and social meanings. This chapter explores the contexts, examples, and situations within which the perspective can be illuminated.

The Lineage of Phenomenology: From Husserl to Schutz

Phenomenology was first developed by the German philosopher Edmund Husserl in the final decade of the 19th century. It involves the systematic investigation of consciousness, or, as he called it, the "science" of consciousness. Consciousness as an intentional process is composed of thinking, perceiving, feeling, remembering, imagining, and anticipating directed toward the world (Husserl, 1931). The objects of consciousness, these intentional acts, are the sources of all social realities (Sibeon, 2004). It is assumed that our experience of the world, including everything from our perception of objects through to social formulas, is constituted in and by consciousness (Powell, 2006).

Husserl's (1931) prose is difficult to penetrate, so his writings never gained a popular audience. His ideas are influential today largely because of his students. Several of Husserl's students continued his work on phenomenology, some taking it in new directions. Although Martin Heidegger is the best-known existential phenomenologist, Gabriel Marcel, Simone de Beauvoir, Maurice Merleau-Ponty, and Jean-Paul Sartre also participated in the movement in Europe.

Alfred Schutz (1932) brought phenomenology to the United States in the 1930s when he left Germany to avoid the Holocaust. Schutz's work finds several points of congeniality between that of Husserl and of another German theorist, Max Weber, whose theoretical writings were widely admired among American sociologists.

Weber is a social action theorist who looked at meanings in a social context, whereby situations are interpreted and meanings constructed and shared. His work laid the foundation for an "interpretive sociology," or what has been labeled as the sociology of understanding (Layder, 2004). The principle of interpretive sociology states that social theory can never be exclusively inductive and must always approach understanding human behavior as framed within a conceptual platform of ideal types (May & Williams, 2002). An ideal type is formed from characteristics and elements of the given phenomena, but it is not meant to correspond to all the characteristics of any particular case. Such a model includes the central idea that while individuals are thoroughly enmeshed in and influenced by social involvements, crucially they retain a subjective life. Weber's attention to theoretical interpretation stands as a principal source of interpretive sociology, trying to understand the meaning of a social action from the viewpoint of social actors.

Alfred Schutz had a great interest in using, extending, and criticizing Weber's work. In Weber's notion of ideal types, Schutz found a key to the epistemological and theoretical foundations of Weber's interpretive sociology that made possible a phenomenologically grounded analysis (May & Powell, 2008). Schutz applauded Weber's refusal to reduce his theoretical approach to positivism yet at the same time to allow the ideal–typical result to be tested for adequacy. However, Schutz also extended Weber, pointing out how interpretation was involved even in selecting an experience out of one's stream of experience. These reflective criticisms of Weber required Schutz to develop his own theory of meaning and action, engaging with Husserl's study of the consciousness of internal time (Ritzer, 2004).

Schutz influenced another generation of social theorists, led by Harold Garfinkel, Peter Berger, Thomas Luckmann, and Maurice Nathanson. They were his students at the New School of Social Research in New York City. The emphasis on the social construction of reality continues to resonate in sociology today. All of Husserl's intellectual descendants promoted descriptive studies of everyday life, uncovering the meaning beneath social forms and activities. Having examined briefly a few of the thoughts of Husserl and the lineage that traces back to him through his students, particularly Schutz and his students, let us turn to some of the key conceptual components of phenomenology.

What Is Phenomenology?

Alfred Schutz (1932) describes how we construct the objects and our knowledge of these objects that we take for granted in our everyday lives. The basic act of consciousness is a first-order typification: bringing together typical and enduring elements in the stream of experience, building up typical models of things and people, and thereby building a shared social world. Second-order typifications are constructed as rational models of the social world based on the first-order theories that actors offer to explain their own activities. Schutz talks about sociology as creating a world of rational puppets that we then manipulate to discover how people might act in the real world. Schutz's legacy led to a growing body of knowledge that can be called interpretive sociology (May & Powell, 2008). Two expressions of this approach have been called *reality constructionism* and *ethnomethodology*. Reality constructionism synthesizes Schutz's distillation of phenomenology and the corpus of classical sociological thought to account for the possibility of social reality (Berger & Luckmann, 1966). Ethnomethodology examines the means by which actors make ordinary life possible (Garfinkel, 1967; Garfinkel & Sacks, 1986). Reality constructionism and ethnomethodology are now recognized as among the established orientations in the various fields of social science (Ritzer, 2007). This continuing influence on contemporary sociology can be seen in the increased humanization of theoretical works (Layder, 2007). Phenomenological thought has influenced the work of postmodernist, poststructuralist, critical, and neofunctional theory (Ritzer, 1996). Notions such as constructionism, situationalism, and reflexivity that are at the core of phenomenology also provide the grounds for these recent formulations. For example, the premise of poststructuralism that language is socially constituted, thus denying the possibility of objective meaning, is clearly rooted in phenomenology. The procedure known as *deconstruction* essentially reverses the reification process highlighted in phenomenology (May & Powell, 2008). The argument that knowledge and reality do not exist apart from discourse is also clearly rooted in phenomenology (May & Williams, 2002). Postmodernism's emphasis on the representational world as reality constructor further exemplifies the phenomenological bent toward reflexivity. On the other hand, phenomenology has been used to reverse nihilistic excesses of postmodernism and poststructuralism. Phenomenology also finds room for a microsocial foundation focusing on the actor as a constructive agent in theories of "critical realism" (Layder, 2007). Henceforth, phenomenology advances the notion that human beings are creative agents in the construction of their social worlds.

While this is at the level of understanding, phenomenological concerns are also frequently researched in investigating social life by using qualitative methods (Ritzer, 1996). Phenomenologists have undertaken analyses of small groups, social situations, and organizations using face-to-face techniques of participant observation (May & Powell, 2008). In-depth interviewing to uncover the subject's orientations or older people's "lifeworlds" is also widely practiced in social gerontology (Gubrium, 1992). Such qualitative tools are used in phenomenological research either to yield insight into the microphysical dimensions of specific spheres of human life or to exhibit the constitutive activity of human consciousness (Gubrium & Holstein, 1995). By using phenomenology through its in-depth qualitative gathering of intimate human feelings and meanings, the microbased theory highlights how individuals apprehend the means by which phenomena, originating in human consciousness, come to be experienced as features of the social world.

Since phenomenology insists that society is a human construction, social science itself and its theories and methods are also constructions (Cicourel, 1973). Thus, phenomenology seeks to offer a corrective to the field's emphasis on positivist conceptualizations and research methods that may take for granted the very issues that phenomenologists find of interest. Phenomenology presents theoretical techniques and qualitative methods that illuminate the human meanings of social life.

The central task in phenomenology is to demonstrate the reciprocal interactions among the processes of human action and reality construction (Sibeon, 2004). Rather than contending that any aspect is a causal factor, phenomenology views all dimensions as constitutive of all others. Phenomenologists use the term *reflexivity* to characterize the way in which constituent dimensions serve as both foundation and consequence of all human projects (May & Williams, 2002). The task of phenomenology, then, is to make manifest, reflexively, the incessant tangle of action, situation, and reality in the various modes of *being in the world.*

Now let us examine how this process works. Phenomenology begins with an analysis of the *natural attitude.* This is understood as the way ordinary individuals participate in the world, taking its existence for granted, assuming its objectivity, and undertaking action projects as if they were predetermined (May & Williams, 2002). Language, culture, and common sense are experienced in the natural attitude as objective features of an external world that are learned by actors in the course of their lives.

Human beings are open to patterned social experience and strive toward meaningful involvement in a knowable world. They are characterized by a typifying mode of consciousness tending to classify sense data. In phenomenological terms, humans experience the world in terms of *typifications.* That is, people are exposed to the sights of their environments, including their own bodies and other people. They come to apprehend the categorical identity and *typified* meanings of each in terms of conventional linguistic forms. In a similar manner, people learn the formulas for doing common activities. These practical means of doing are called *recipes for action* (May & Williams, 2002).

Schutz distinguishes different sets of interests: topical (which focus attention on themes), interpretive (which confer meanings on experiences or objects), and motivational. Such interests often involve a subject, with more or less systematic interests, interacting with the world. From this interaction between subject and world, it becomes evident what is of relevance to an actor. These interests, interdependent on each other and conjoined with one's system of types or categories, constitute a *stock of knowledge* at hand. Schutz examines stock of knowledge in terms of its genesis and structure. He further explores the meaning of a person's biographical situation, including types and interests. For example, one's body and the ontological constraints of space and time prevent one from being at certain places at certain times or compel one to wait.

After a more general account of the *lifeworld* and its relation to the sciences, Schutz takes up the various stratifications of the lifeworld, such as provinces of meaning, temporal and spatial zones of reach, and social structure. Schutz comments on the components of one's stock of knowledge, including learned and nonlearned elements, interests, and types, and he traces the buildup of such a stock. He studied the social conditioning of one's subjective stock of knowledge and inquires about the social stock of knowledge of a group and different possible combinations of knowledge distribution (generalized and specialized).

Schutz (1932) considers how subjective knowledge becomes embodied in a social stock of knowledge and how the latter influences the former. He asserts that intention comes before action and that all actions are not necessarily intended. Intentions are rather to be related to the phase before action. The "disposition" of an individual is important for social action. It can be based on the locus of control and implies a person's ability or inability to cope with a situation, that is, to act. There seems to be a demand on some kind of internal locus of control.

Hence, typifications and recipes, once internalized, tend to settle beneath the level of full awareness. That is, they become *sedimented,* as do layers of rock. Thus, in the natural attitude, the foundations of actors' knowledge of meaning and action are obscured to the actors themselves (Berger & Luckmann, 1966). For example, actors assume that knowledge is objective and that all people reason in a like manner. Each actor assumes that every other actor knows what he or she knows of this world. All believe that they share common sense. However, each person's biography is unique, and each develops a relatively distinct stock of typifications and recipes for action. Therefore, interpretations may diverge. Everyday social interaction is replete with ways in which actors create feelings that common sense is shared, that mutual understanding is occurring, and that everything is all right.

Phenomenology emphasizes that humans live within an intersubjective world, yet they at best approximate shared realities. While a *paramount reality* is commonly experienced in this manner, particular realities or *finite provinces of meaning* are also constructed and experienced by diverse cultural, social, or occupational groupings (Layder, 2007).

Thus, typifications derived from common sense are internalized, becoming the tools that individual consciousness uses to constitute a lifeworld, the unified arena of human awareness and action. Common sense serves as an ever-present resource to assure actors that the reality that is projected from human subjectivity is an objective reality. Since all actors are involved in this intentional work, they sustain the collaborative effort to reify their projections and thereby reinforce the very frameworks that provide the construction tools.

Phenomenologists analyze the ordering of social reality and how the usage of certain forms of knowledge contributes to that ordering. It is posited that typified action and interaction become *habitualized* (Ritzer, 2007). Through sedimentation in layered consciousness, human authorship of habitualized conduct is obscured and the product externalized. As meaning-striving beings, humans create theoretical explanations and moral justifications in order to legitimate the habitualized conduct. Located in higher contexts of meaning, the conduct becomes objectified. When internalized by succeeding generations, the conduct is fully institutionalized and exerts compelling constraints over individual volition.

The reality that most people inhabit is constituted by these legitimations of habitualized conduct. Ranging from commonsense typifications of ordinary language to theological constructions to sophisticated philosophical, cosmological, and scientific conceptualizations, these legitimations compose the paramount reality of everyday life. Moreover, segmented modern life, with its proliferation of meaning-generating sectors, produces multiple realities, some in competition with each other for adherents. In the current marketplace of realities, consumers, to varying degrees, may select their legitimations as they select their occupation and, increasingly, their religion (Berger & Luckmann, 1966).

However, there are layers of knowledge within modern society that are seen as privileged, and breaking these layers down is a hard task given the truth claims behind what they say. Such truth claims are often backed up by science. The biomedical model has been a dominant narrative pertaining to individual behavior that microperspectives like phenomenology have found hard to challenge. In particular, the view that the aging body is essentially an issue of declining viability is the master narrative behind biomedicine. For phenomenologists, such views mask the subjectification processes that are central to understand how bodies are made and experienced.

Phenomenology and Aging

Within social theory phenomenology is an established mainstream paradigm. It guides most qualitative research focused on everyday life in the social sciences today (Gubrium & Holstein, 1995). Within gerontology, however, it has had a very limited impact. In this section, we wish to explore two contexts: the body under the medical gaze and the body as a basis of identity.

Aging and the Biomedical Gaze

In this discussion, the biomedical model is understood to have four components: (a) the mind and body are essentially different, and medicine is restricted to considerations related to the body; (b) the body can be understood as analogous to a machine; (c) medical answers are thought to be more reliable when they are founded on the basic sciences; and (d) thus biophysical answers are preferred to all others (Longino & Murphy, 1995). This model is reductionistic, and by focusing almost entirely on the body, it ignores the person that animates the body and the lifeworld that contextualizes the person.

The biomedical model has dominated the perceptions of old age in gerontology. As Powell and Longino (2002) pointed out, the medicalization of old age is not an objective scientific process but rather a series of policy struggles at local, national, and international levels. These struggles to define the nature of aging are between several *provinces of meaning,* such as old and potentially old people, their network of informal caregivers, the helping professionals of different types, entrepreneurs from family-run care homes to pharmaceutical companies of global reach, and finally the institutions of the state and the organization and distribution of resources through policy spaces (Biggs & Powell, 2001).

The biomedical model has consistently problematized "truths" about the declining viability of adult aging. As Arthur Frank (1990) notes, the biomedical model is a dominant force in popular culture:

> *Medicine does . . . occupy a paramount place among those institutions and practices by which the body is conceptualized, represented and responded to. At present our capacity to experience the body directly, or theorize it indirectly, is inextricably medicalized. (pp. 135–136)*

The somewhat hegemonic dominance of the biomedical model goes beyond negative discourses pertaining to aging; it has sought to reinvent itself as the "savior" of biological aging via the biotechnological advancements that foster reconstruction of the "body" to prevent, hide, or halt the aging process (Powell & Wahidin, 2007). As Biggs and Powell (2001) point out,

> *Established and emerging master narratives of biological decline on the one hand, and consumer agelessness on the other co-exist, talking to different populations and promoting contradictory, yet interrelated, narratives by which to age. They are contradictory in their relation to notions of autonomy and independence, and dependency on others, yet [they are] linked through the importance of techniques for maintenance, either via medicalized bodily control or through the adoption of "golden-age" lifestyles. (p. 97)*

Because of the reluctance of socially trained gerontologists to deal directly with the body and their tendency to hand off the subject matter to the health scientists and clinicians, the social study of age and the aging body has gained theoretical momentum only recently, in the past 20 years, on both sides of the Atlantic (Phillipson, 1998; Powell, 2006).

The body in its material form has been taken for granted, absented, or forgotten in gerontological literature (Powell & Wahidin, 2007) until the body begins to mechanically break down. Thus, the role of the body in gerontology has for some time focused on the failing body and the political response to that aging body.

In those parts of the medical establishment where care rather than regimen and control is most emphasized, particularly in nursing, there seems to be a deeper focus on the provision of care based on a rigorous emphasis on the patient's subjective experience (Benner, 1995). In these patient care contexts, substantial attention has been devoted to the ethical implications of various disease definitions. Specifically, the discussion also focuses on how language shapes the response to illness and how disease definitions and paradigmatic models impact communication between health professionals and patients (Rosenberg & Golden, 1992). Significant work on the phenomenology of disability has demonstrated how the *lived body* is experienced in altered form and how taken-for-granted routines are disrupted, invoking new action recipes (Toombs, 1995).

Nonconventional healing practices have also been examined. In this context, embodiment and the actor's subjective orientation reflexively interrelate with cultural imagery and discourse to transfigure the self (Csordas, 1997). Further, phenomenological work has suggested that emotions are best analyzed as interpretive processes embedded within experiential contexts (Ritzer, 1996). The focus on the lived body is a central concern for phenomenological gerontology:

> *The body may be preoperative, transitional, or postoperative; even "seeing" the body may not answer the question . . . what are the categories through which one sees? The moment on which one's staid and usual cultural perceptions fail . . . one cannot with surety read the body that one sees. (Bordo, 1993, p. 18)*

Thus, phenomenological gerontology seeks to offer a corrective to the seeming dominant emphasis on biomedical conceptualizations of aging; it excavates how we problematize aging at a surface level by digging underneath such surfaces to reveal meanings and a subjective sense of self that have been historically silenced by rigid biomedical models of aging and body. Hence, phenomenology presents theoretical techniques and qualitative methods that illuminate the human meanings of social life that brings to life issues associated with understanding the body.

Aging and Identity

Only in the past two decades has there been any sustained attempt to fuse together phenomenological concerns about aging bodies in order to foster a deeper understanding of aging identity (Gubrium & Holstein, 1995). Gubrium (1992) has investigated how aging is constituted in the consciousness of persons. The struggle for meaning when accompanied by chronic pain may be facilitated or impaired by constructs that permit the smoother processing of the experiences. Biggs (1999) makes the point that phenomenological work encourages caregivers of older people to gain empathic appreciation of their clients' life-worlds. Enhanced affiliation with them through the use of biographical narratives highlight their individuality and humanity.

Where does the story of the human body begin? What is in fact meant by the "body"? One can simply argue that the body is "present," "lived," "real," and "experienced." The body, in terms of its biology, is always in the process of becoming. Cells die, mutate, and regenerate. It can be argued from this proposition, then, that the body never finally becomes but is left as an unfinished project, in a state of transition. In reality, however, typifications of old bodies intertwine with masculinity, femininity, sexual orientation, and race, which serve to regulate and define the spaces that older people use.

Writing about phenomenology and the aging body poses a series of theoretical challenges relating to the issue of human embodiment, the body, and body image (Featherstone & Hepworth, 1993). The body, like parchment, is written on, inscribed by variables such as gender, age, sexual orientation, and ethnicity and by a series of inscriptions that are dependent on types of spaces and places. However, as Shilling (1993) argues, the more we know about our bodies, the more we are able to govern, modify, and question gender norms highlighting how gendered and ageist discourses serve to confine and define old bodies.

Although social gerontologists have only recently begun to conceptualize the body, old people themselves are clearly concerned about their changed physical appearance and how to come to terms with the changing conditions of their identity and lived bodies. Morris (1998) argues that consumer culture promotes this concern and then exploits it; consumer culture is preoccupied with perfect bodies as presented by the glamorous images of advertising. Consumer culture's emphasis on youthfulness and the body beautiful increasingly marginalizes the identity of older people in later life. Such images, therefore, do not help old people to see themselves as able actors within the world.

This discontinuity between the experience of living in an aging body and images of aging has been identified as an issue. One may feel oneself to be a different age than one looks, as though one is wearing a mask. Featherstone and Hepworth (1993) maintain that old age can be a mask that "conceals the essential identity of the person beneath" (p. 314). A person's appearance may change with age, and one's identity may not. It is thus possible to be surprised by one's own image. As counterpoint to the notion of the mask of old age, Biggs (1999) argues that people derive their sense of self-identity in old age from the achievements of the past and what remains to be accomplished in the future rather than from a set of stereotypical images of old age.

Unless they are ill, older people do not necessarily feel old. Researchers can study, without reflecting the experienced reality of aging, whether the subjects' lived bodies are ignored. Aging is an embodied and meaningful process.

Bryan Turner (1995) emphasizes several key processes that work on and within the body across time and space. The body has to be contexualized within its polymorphous state of positions within and between a number of different discourses: the biological and the social, the collective and the individual, and that of structure and agency. The next section advances a phenomenology of aging by incisively stating that we need to capture the use of biography in order to appreciate and understand individuals and cohort groups across the life course.

Toward a Phenomenology of Aging: Biography and the Life Course

The notion of biography is central to understanding people's meanings and experiences of mind and body relevant to the life course. Schutz employed the life course as a second-order analytical construct to understand different classes of experience from early to later life. Individuals make their own biographical histories across the life course. From the earliest age to old age, individuals create biographical narratives to create a sense of coherence and self-identity. The social worlds that individuals create are put together by categorized experiences. Categories take on an existence of their own for interpreting and constructing meaning. Both natural and social objects are interpretively constituted and as such are evolving "stocks of knowledge" (Schutz, 1972), the cornerstone of common frameworks for making sense of experiences. The interior mental processes of individuals and their self-identities dynamically collide and interact with social forces to produce and reproduce the forms of experience.

Schutz's notion of "biographical work" (Starr, 1983) is the means of embracing this dynamic interplay of subjective and objective social processes. By tracing an individual's life career trajectory, the concept of biography allows us to document the development of their unique configuration of personal powers, skills, and emotional-cognitive capacities as they emerge out of the interplay of social involvements and constraints. This is because the concept of biography refers to tracing specific individual's experiential trajectories across the life course and the unique social configurations in which they are enmeshed.

Birth cohorts, who move through their life courses together, may have an overlap in their stocks of knowledge that is contextualized by their shared historical experience. Intersubjectivity based on birth cohort is therefore possible. However, as Passuth and Bengtson (1988) remind us, a phenomenological understanding of cohort is not the same as that used by demographers. Lives are linked through education, work, consumption, and family in everyday life, and these linkages give cohort membership and their related stocks of knowledge special significance (Davila & Pearson 1994; Gubrium, 1992).

For example, phenomenological work with young children at one end of the life course examines how both family interactions and the practices of everyday life are related to the social construction of childhood (Davila & Pearson, 1994). It is revealed how the children's elemental typifications of family life and common sense are actualized through ordinary social interaction. Penetrating the inner world of children requires a level of sensitivity among researchers of aging that would allow them to view the subjects in their own terms, from the level and viewpoints of children themselves (Shehan, 1999). Such theoretical interrogation transcends scientific perspectives and seeks to give voice to the children's experience of their own worlds and relationships with others. In this sense, children's communicative and interactive competencies are respected and are not diminished by the drive toward just listening to adults (Shehan, 1999).

One could apply this example just as well to the other end of the life course. According to Encandela (1997), when we look at aging and the social construction of "pain," we can see the use of a phenomenological perspective. Encandela investigated the interrelationship of aging and trauma and found that it was constituted in the consciousness of members and helping agents. The struggle for meaning accompanied by chronic pain may be facilitated or constrained by the availability of constructs that permit the processing of the experiences. Members of cultures that stock typifications and recipes for skillfully managing pain may well be more likely than others to construct beneficial interpretations in the face of these challenges (Encandela, 1997). Phenomenology in this context encourages the professionals who work in the field of pain management with older people to gain an empathic appreciation of their clients' lifeworlds and enhanced affiliation with them through the use of biographical narratives that highlight their individuality and subjective sense of self (Biggs, 1999).

Subjective experience, in this sense, is an amalgam of several, often seemingly diverse sensitivities and operations. Such experiences impinge on the fluidity of the life course.

Settersten (1999) suggests that the study of the life course teaches us that it is open to historical contingency. Distinctive changes for subgroups in the life course cannot be understood without reference to biographical contexts. At the same time, Settersten claims that there has been scarce study of inter- and intracohort variation in the ways that sociohistorical circumstances relate to particular lives. Members of cohort groups react in unpredictable ways to historical contexts. The timing into expectable social roles can influence the ways in which they are experienced and alter expectable role entrances and exits in life zones such as work and employment. Similarly, subgroups of individuals may hold basic values of their generational cohort but hold a different outlook to their larger cohort, a process of "self-identity." Understanding the aging self in such terms enables us to appreciate the power and control dimensions of human conduct, especially as they apply to individual self-identity that is linked to the social world. Because individuals vary in terms of their biographically produced personal powers and capacities across age cohorts, it is important to recognize how these differences feed into and in turn are influenced by other social domains.

There is a long-standing tendency to reduce the social dimension of aging to a set of normative "stages" across the life course that are said to determine the experience of old age. Such approaches present old age as primarily a private experience of adaptation to inevitable physical and mental decline and preparation for death. This common understanding of aging is quite alienating, and people logically flee from this image of senility. A fixed standpoint of stages openly contradicts the phenomenological challenge set by Schutz.

At the same time, life course theory has begun to emphasize that old age is part of a lifelong developmental process. Life course ideas coalesced as a theoretical orientation on aging during the 1960s and 1970s. Bernice Neugarten (1974) wrote an influential essay marking a distinction between what has since become more commonly referred to as the "third age" and the "fourth age," the youthful years of retirement and the older ones, respectively. She referred to persons in these stages of later adult development as the young-old and the old-old. The young-old are like late middle-aged persons. They generally have good health, and they are about as active as they want to be. The old-old, however, tend to be widowed and are much more likely to be living dependently. Consequently, the concept of old age, with its attending miseries, was only pushed later into life by this reconceptualization. The first decade after workers retire seems like a second middle age, but the declining body remains an issue in the fourth age (Gilleard & Higgs, 2000; Laslett, 1991).

During the 1980s and 1990s, life course theory increased in sophistication as proponents addressed variations in the process of aging and recognized that the individual's life course is embedded in relationships with others (Elder, 2001).

Conclusion

Phenomenology is a movement in social science that illuminates an understanding of the relationship between states of individual consciousness and social life. As an approach within social gerontology, phenomenology seeks to reveal how human aging awareness is implicated in the production of social action, social situations, and social worlds. Phenomenology asks of us to note the misleading substantiality of social products and to avoid the pitfalls of reification.

It is inadequate for gerontologists to view older people only as "objects." Older people are "subjects" with sentient experience. Phenomenology focuses on the investigation of social products as humanly meaningful acts. The "meaning contexts" applied by the social gerontologist explicates the points of view of older actors. It also expresses their lifeworld. Phenomenological gerontology strives to reveal how actors construe themselves, all the while recognizing that they themselves are actors construing their subjects and themselves.

References

Benner, P. (1995). *Interpretive phenomenology: Embodiment, caring and ethics in health and illness.* Thousand Oaks, CA: Sage.

Berger, P. L., & Luckmann, T. (1966). *The social construction of reality: A treatise in the sociology of knowledge.* New York: Anchor Books.

Biggs, S. (1999). *The mature imagination.* Milton Keynes: Oxford University Press.

Biggs, S., & Powell, J. L. (2001). A Foucauldian analysis of old age and the power of social welfare. *Journal of Aging & Social Policy, 12,* 93–111.

Bordo, S. (1993). *Unbearable weight: Feminism, Western culture and the body.* Berkeley: University of California Press.

Cicourel, A. V. (1973). *Cognitive sociology: Language and meaning in social interaction.* Harmondsworth: Penguin.

Csordas, J. (1997). *Embodiment and experience: The existential ground of culture and self.* Cambridge: Cambridge University Press.

Davilla, R., & Pearson, C. (1994). Children's perspectives of the family: A phenomenological inquiry. *Human Studies, 17,* 325–341.

Elder, G. H., Jr. (2001). Life course. In G. L. Maddox (Ed.), *The encyclopedia of aging* (3rd ed., pp. 593–596). New York: Springer Publishing.

Encandela, J. (1997). Social construction of pain and aging: Individual artfulness within interpretive structures. *Symbolic Interaction, 20,* 251–273.

Featherstone, M., & Hepworth, M. (1993). Images in ageing. In J. Bond & P. Coleman (Eds.), *Ageing in society* (pp. 304–332). London: Sage.

Frank, A. (1990). Review article: Bringing bodies back in a decade. *Theory, Culture and Society, 7,* 131–162.

Garfinkel, H. (1967). *Studies in ethnomethodology.* Englewood Cliffs, NJ: Prentice Hall.

Garfinkel, H., & Sacks, H. (1986). On formal structures of practical actions. In H. Garfinkel (Ed.), *Ethnomethodological studies of work* (pp. 160–193). London: Routledge & Kegan Paul.

Gilleard, C., & Higgs, P. (2000). *Cultures of ageing.* London: Prentice Hall.

Gubrium, J. (1992). *Out of control: Family therapy and domestic disorder.* Newbury Park, CA: Sage.

Gubrium, J., & Holstein, J. (1995). *The active interview.* Newbury Park, CA: Sage.

Husserl, E. (1931). *Ideas: General introduction to pure phenomenology* (W. R. Boyce Gibson, Trans.). New York: Humanities Press.

Laslett, P. (1991). *A fresh map of life: The emergence of the third age.* Cambridge, MA: Harvard University Press.

Layder, D. (2004). *Social and personal identity.* London: Sage.

Layder, D. (2007). *Understanding social theory* (2nd ed.). London: Sage.

Longino, C. F., Jr., & Murphy, J. W. (1995). *The old age challenge to the biomedical model: Paradigm strain and health policy.* Amityville, NY: Baywood Publishing.

May, T., & Powell, J. (2008). *Situating social theory.* Milton Keynes: McGraw-Hill.

May, T., & Williams, M. (2002). *Knowing the social world.* Milton Keynes: Oxford University Press.

Morris, D. (1998). *The culture of pain.* Berkeley: University of California Press.

Neugarten, B. L. (1974). Age groups in American society and the rise of the young-old. *Annals of the American Academy of Political and Social Sciences, 415,* 187–198.

Passuth, P. M., & Bengtson, V. L. (1988). Sociological theories of aging: Current perspectives and future directions. In J. Birren & V. Bengtson (Eds.), *Emergent theories of aging* (pp. 333–355). New York: Springer Publishing.
Phillipson, C. (1998). *Reconstructing old age.* London: Sage
Powell, J. (2006). *Social theory and aging.* New York: Rowman & Littlefield.
Powell, J. L., & Longino, C. F. (2002). Postmodernism v modernism: Rethinking theoretical tensions in social gerontology. *Journal of Aging & Identity, 7,* 107–118.
Powell, J., & Wahidin, A. (2007). Understanding aging bodies: A postmodern dialogue. In J. Powell & T. Owen (Eds.), *Reconstructing postmodernism* (pp. 27–32). New York: Nova Science.
Ritzer, G. (1996). *Modern sociological theory.* New York: McGraw-Hill.
Ritzer, G. (2004). *The globalization of nothing.* Thousand Oaks, CA: Pine Forge Press.
Ritzer, G. (2007). *The McDonalization of society.* Thousand Oaks, CA: Pine Forge Press.
Rosenberg, C., & Golden, J. (Eds.). (1992). *Framing disease: Studies in cultural history.* New Brunswick, NJ: Rutgers University Press.
Schutz, A. (1932). *The phenomenology of the social world.* London: Heinemann.
Schutz, A. (1972). *The phenomenology of the social world* (G. Walsh & F. Lehnert, Trans.). London: Heinemann. (Original work published 1932).
Settersten, R. (1999). *Lives in place and time: The problems and promises of developmental science.* Amityville, NY: Baywood Publishing.
Shehan, L. (Ed.). (1999). *Through the eyes of the child: Revisioning children as active agents of family life.* Greenwich, CT: JAI Press.
Shilling, C. (1993). *The body and social theory.* London: Sage.
Sibeon, R. (2004). *Rethinking social theory.* London: Sage.
Starr, J. M. (1983). Toward a social phenomenology of aging: Studying the self process in biographical work. *International Journal of Aging and Human Development, 16,* 255–270.
Toombs, S. (1995). The lived experience of disability. *Human Studies, 18,* 9–23.
Turner, B. (1995). Ageing and identity. In M. Featherstone & A. Wernick (Eds.), *Images of ageing* (pp. 245–260). London: Routledge.

Theorizing the Life Course: New Twists in the Paths

21

Dale Dannefer
Jessica A. Kelley-Moore

As reflected in the title, this chapter is intended as a refinement and update of Dannefer and Uhlenberg's (1999) chapter titled "Paths of the Life Course" (hereafter referred to as *Paths*) published in the original *Handbook of Theories of Aging*. Since that time, interest in the life course perspective (hereafter LCP) has continued to flourish and expand. Its growth has been both substantive and methodological and is increasingly global in scope. Substantively, applications of the LCP now extend well beyond its original linkages to the domains of age and family to other substantive areas, including health and physical functioning (Ferraro & Kelley-Moore, 2003), work and education (Dupre 2007;

Acknowledgment: We would like to thank Peter Uhlenberg for comments on an earlier version of this paper. We also thank Antje Daub for research assistance and Sherri Brown, Melinda Laroco, and Mary Ellen Stone for editorial assistance.

Pallas & Booher-Jennings, 2006), happiness (Yang, 2008), and crime (Sampson & Laub, 2005). At the same time, there has been substantial growth in number of data sources, a lengthening of windows of observation, and an increase in the number of observation points. Combined with methodological and statistical advances, we are observing more extensive and refined forms of quantitative data analysis applied to life course processes and new applications of qualitative methods, developments that may help to address some of the conceptual and methodological problems identified by numerous commentators over the past decade (e.g., Alwin & Wray, 2005; Bass, 2007; Dannefer, 2002; Hagestad & Dannefer, 2001). At the same time, interest in the life course has become more international and global, with expanding attention to global considerations (Baars, Dannefer, Phillipson, & Walker, 2006; Dannefer, 2003) and new and increasingly diverse forms of attention to the life course across Europe and beyond (de Ribaupierre et al., in press; Gluckman & Hanson, 2006; Priestley, 2001; Widmer, Burton-Jeangros, Bergman, & Dannefer, in press).

As noted in *Paths,* the life course is a flourishing, eclectic field, and these recent developments speak to its continued liveliness and energy. At the same time, it continues to be a field that lacks conceptual organization, is largely undertheorized, and is often poorly applied in empirical studies. Thus, it remains a field characterized by a number of theoretical and methodological challenges.

This chapter offers a reconsideration of the issues raised and the conceptual framework presented in *Paths* as well as an analysis of new developments that have emerged in life course theory and research over the past decade. The chapter consists of three major sections. The first reviews the necessary required founding premises—*first principles*—that are required as a conceptual foundation for approaching the life course, principles that remain unevenly recognized in life course research. The second section identifies some key problems in life course analysis, some of which derive from the neglect of these principles. Although it is clear that real progress has been made in regard to some of the problems identified a decade ago, additional challenges have emerged or require renewed attention. In the final section, we propose a refinement of the typology of life course research and scholarship based on a more detailed examination of the *explananda* and *explanans* of life course theory.

Founding Premises of Life Course Theory: The Individual, the Social, and the Asymmetry of Agency

The first principles concern the nature of the (a) human individual and (b) the social dynamics within which human lives are embedded. The special significance of the dynamics of social interaction and structure are anchored in the unique physiological and developmental characteristics of humans and also in the asymmetrical dynamics of structure and agency.

The Human Organism

Space does not permit a full treatment of the distinctively human features of individual development that underlie all life course processes. Discussions of these well-established—albeit neglected—features of human growth and change are available elsewhere (Berger & Luckmann, 1967; Dannefer, 1999b, 2008; Montagu, 1989; Morss, 1996; Perry & Svalavitz, 2006; Rogoff, 2003). In brief, the potentials of the human brain and body for flexibility and environmental responsiveness are not merely options to be occasionally exercised by individual human actors, nor are they variables to be sometimes included in causal models of those of us who study human activity. Rather, they reflect essential constitutional requirements of the human organism for external structuring and direction and for relating to the world through agentic action. Because of these constitutional requirements, human *organisms* are fundamentally incapable of becoming human *beings* without participation in human *society*. Born premature, unformed, and utterly dependent (Berger & Luckmann, 1967; Gould, 1977; Montagu, 1989), the perceptions, tastes, and activity routines to which each individual becomes habituated are learned in social company, and the form that their humanity takes and the forms that their aging and life course structures take depend on the nature of the society in which they participate. In Barbara Rogoff's (2002, 2003) terms, human beings are *hardwired for flexibility*, and human development is *biologically cultural.*

Social Interaction

These conditions point to the uniquely potent and unavoidably necessary dependence of individual activity routines, life patterns, and age-related change on socially variable processes of social interaction. Social interaction is the mechanism through which the human *organism* is transformed both physically and mentally into a human *being* and through which the capability for agentic human action is generated and maintained. Interaction is crucial in the early years of the life course, but it also remains decisively important throughout adulthood (when it is often taken for granted and its effects are unrecognized). This has recently been shown through research using brain imaging techniques to document brain change and growth in adulthood in response to experience (Maguire et al., 2000). In adulthood no less than in childhood, the skills and routines of everyday life, the "knowledge" and "values" that one accepts as natural and the routines by which days extend into years, are sustained by the familiar and constantly reproduced rhythms of everyday life.

Social Structure

Social structure refers to the established and regularly reproduced social practices and rules that provide a sense of predictability and taken-for-grantedness in everyday life. Structures exist at numerous levels and in many forms, ranging from the institutionalized mechanisms for allocating roles and resources to the underlying cultural systems of language and aesthetics. Operating at these multiple levels, social structure organizes and constrains individual lives in the immediacy of the present at every moment. Of course, one need only compare patterns of aging in different historical periods or across cultures to recognize the profound significance of social structure on life course patterns and outcomes. Indeed, as is evident from historical variation in *chronologization* and in age awareness, age itself is a feature not primarily of individuals but of social structure. For each society at any given moment, age is culturally defined as part of the knowledge system of that society. But the effects of interaction and structure also can be witnessed at the level of analyzing individual lives, as when comparing two teenagers growing up in socioeconomically different family and neighborhood situations or the different aging trajectories experienced by two similarly frail older persons who are placed in institutional care settings of divergent quality.

Agentic Asymmetry

Human activity is generically *agentic.* It results from the externalization of conscious intentionality in action. Because the process of forming intentions and acting in the world typically occurs against the backdrop of a taken-for-granted social world to which the actor is habituated, the power and scope of agency is typically overestimated. It is important to recognize that each human being enters the world as a helpless and dependent infant who learns language and other cultural forms and practices from parents or others more advanced in development. Thus, human agency is always fundamentally organized and constrained by the perceptual and motivational systems deriving from such situated learning experiences (Dannefer, 1999a; Lave & Wenger, 1991; Marshall & Clarke, in press).

Beyond such experience, agency is also constrained by other forces operating from the beginning of the life course onward. Important epidemiologic work has demonstrated that health outcomes such as adult obesity that have heretofore been linked to lifetime health behaviors of individuals (e.g., sedentary lifestyle and food choice) are substantially set by the developmental environment during the pre- and postnatal period, a time when individual "choice" is developmentally impossible (Parsons, Power, & Manor, 2001; Symonds & Gardner, 2006). Hence, social structure precedes individual agency in human development and continues to frame the range of choices across the life course.

Founding Premises, Enduring Problems: Six Challenges for Life Course Studies

In this section, we consider six significant challenges confronting life course theory and research. Some of these derive from a lack of attention to the founding principles set forth previously and their implications (as discussed in *Paths*). Others have become clear more recently, as researchers have grappled with new issues of analysis and interpretation to accompany large new data sets and new analytical problems. The six issues, in the order we discuss them, are as follows: (a) cohort analysis and the neglect of intracohort inequality, (b) confounding life course processes and change, (c) the need for renewed attention to intercohort variation, (d) time 1 encapsulation, (e) confounding the relation between age and time, and (f) expanding putative role of choice.

Cohort Analysis and Intracohort Variability and Inequality

Initially, cohort analysis provided a key fulcrum to draw attention to the importance of context and a corrective to the strong assumptions of a universal or "natural" trajectory of human aging because it compelled recognition that patterns of aging are historically variable. The resultant focus on intercohort comparisons and differences inevitably led researchers to characterize each cohort in summative terms, typically relying on central tendency measures. While fruitful for many purposes, this practice had the unfortunate consequence of encouraging researchers to treat aging as a normal or normative process *within* each cohort (so that each cohort had a characteristic age pattern). This inclination toward normativity served to normalize age effects, thereby reproducing a tendency that has its roots in the traditional organismic model of aging and development (Dannefer, 1984; Lerner, 1986; Morss, 1990). Thus, while the analytical tactic of comparing cohorts demonstrated the *importance* of context, it also allowed cohorts to stand as virtually *coterminous* with context so that the role of social forces operating within each cohort (e.g., regulating heterogeneity and homogeneity) received little attention.

Intracohort stratification was recognized as important in some early research in the life course tradition, notably including Elder's (1974) classic work. Nevertheless, the phenomenon of cohort-level variability and the dynamics of diversity and inequality over the life course received relatively little attention until the late 1980s. As the pervasiveness of intra-age diversity and the robust processes of cumulative dis/advantage that lead to an increase in intracohort inequality over the life course of each successive cohort became recognized, the practice of analyzing life course trajectories in terms of central tendency characterizations has become complemented by a growing emphasis on cumulative dis/advantage processes within each cohort.

Thus, this problem is one of those in which clear progress has been made. Over the past decade, it has received substantial attention in several published volumes (Baars et al., 2006; Crystal & Shea, 2002; Daatland & Biggs, 2006; O'Rand & Henretta, 1999),and it has been the subject of several theoretical papers (e.g., Bass, 2007; Dannefer, 2003; Ferraro & Shippee, in press; Pallas & Booher-Jennings, 2006) and of a special issue of an international journal, *Swiss Journal of Sociology* (Widmer et al., in press). It has also been an increasing focus of research on the life course, age, and gerontology.

Confounding Social Change With the Role of Social Forces in Shaping the Life Course

From the beginning, cohort analysis and the LCP were conceptually linked to *social change* since change is a major reason that cohorts age differentially. Mortality and longevity, health and morbidity, and intelligence and wealth have all been clearly linked to changing social conditions. Thus, a linkage between social change and individual change has long been established as a dominant theme of the life course literature. This problem is closely tied to the first, since this linkage invited a focus on between-cohort comparisons rather than an examination of intracohort variation.

By comparing across cohorts, one could observe how social change and the resultant differences in social structure affected aging. As a result, studies of aging since that time have often given the cohort variable a privileged conceptual status. This can be seen in the frequent pairing of social and individual change (as in innumerable references to, e.g., "the changing person in the changing world") by both life course sociologists and psychologists (see, e.g., Elder, 1996; Hareven, 1977; Hogan, 1981). This emphasis implies the salience of social change for understanding individual aging, and it invites the implicit assumption that social forces matter only in the case of social change. Absent is the acknowledgment that even if no social change occurred, human aging is no less socially constituted through fundamental processes of social interaction and allocation described in the founding premises set forth previously (see also Dannefer, 2008). A similar point has been made by Sampson and Laub (1993), who note that "stability itself is quite compatible with a sociological perspective on the life course" (p. 12).

In contrast to this recognition of the universal involvement of social processes in the constitution of life course outcomes, researchers often treated each cohort as having a pattern derived from historical circumstance. Thus, if there were no large-scale changes in circumstances, these cohort-specific patterns would be essentially identical. Such a condition of stability is improbable in any case, so there has been scant need to tease out this implication. Under stable conditions, then, one could worry less about historical and social effects and perhaps could more justifiably treat age as the master independent variable without worrying unduly about the specific factors that produced the age-related outcomes.

Age–Period–Cohort "Identification": The Renewed Neglect of Intercohort Variability

Among the salutary effects of the initial discovery of cohort differences was the recognition of the need to follow individuals over time and the development of a number of large-scale, high-quality longitudinal data sets. Currently, many longitudinal studies are based on samples of single age cohorts or adjacent cohorts. This type of design avoids the life course fallacy (Riley, 1973) and allows researchers to account for certain early-life structural constraints or opportunities. Although this commitment to longitudinal data is welcome and needed, it brings its own challenges concerning age–period–cohort identification. Indeed, this is a problem that has been chronically overlooked in recent work.

Notably, without the ability to compare multiple birth cohorts, we are unable to determine whether change or stability with age is cohort specific or universal across cohorts. In other words, we are studying a process within a single cohort and generalizing to the population of all persons independent of cohort (Alwin, McCammon, Wray, & Rodgers, 2008; Riley, 1973; Riley, Johnson, & Foner, 1972). This, in effect, confuses intracohort variability with the theoretical maximum range of heterogeneity across cohorts. Such an approach entails one or more implicit assumptions to which no thoughtful analyst would subscribe, namely, that birth cohort does not matter or that organismic age-related decline becomes the primary vehicle of change in the second half of the life course. In both cases, there is a substantial lack of attention to the social structural and historical context within which individual lives are embedded.

Time 1 Encapsulation of Social Forces

An additional challenge to understanding the life course has been called the *time 1 problem.* Commenting on this, Hagestad and Dannefer (2001) note that in much life course research, social forces are "systematically considered at the initial observation period. When social-structural characteristics are considered only at Time 1, social structure at subsequent periods is unmeasured, and therefore treated as given" (p. 7). The effects of time 1 context are thus carried forward through time and assumed to manifest themselves as a characteristic of the individual in middle and late life. Thus, examination of the effects of social forces is limited to and encapsulated in the time 1 data collection period.

It is important to make this distinction in temporal context because early-life events or circumstances receive great emphasis. Elements of the social structure that are continuous or that occur later in the life course are external to the individual and influence opportunity structures in mid- to late life. Although the original trajectory was set much earlier, social structure (and interaction with it) may lead to turning points, changes, or even reversals, and indeed the stability of the original trajectory depends in large part on a stable and predictable set of social relations and institutions. The true test of the impact of early-life structural barriers or opportunities is whether we see differences in individuals (or between groups) over the life course. It is only through these divergent pathways that we can truly observe the "long arm" of social structure.

Confounding the Relationship Between Age and Time

Stability and change are common themes in analyses of the life course, and social scientists have long been interested in their correlates, predictors, and consequences over time. In response, the number and quality of panel studies have increased substantially in recent decades, as have the statistical methods for modeling change accurately. Gerontologists have long argued that age in itself is not predictive of change (Birren, 1988; Yates, 1991), yet, as noted in the discussion of intracohort variation, change in social, psychological, and health phenomena is often conceptualized and explained in a developmental framework as a normative age pattern (e.g., Baltes, 1979; Heckhausen, 2006; Wrosch & Freund, 2001).

It is important to exercise caution in attributing change to aging per se. While age-related processes and change may occur at numerous points in the life course, many transitions, changes, and even stability are actually time-based phenomena. This is a critical challenge for life course scholars because issues of time and timing are embedded in opportunity structures, macrosocial forces, and individual choices over the entire life course. As an illustration, Ferraro and Kelley-Moore (2003) demonstrated that accounting for the timing and duration of adulthood obesity and physical exercise helps explain the observed heterogeneity in physical function among midlife and older adults. Bengtson, Horlacher, Putney, and Silverstein (2008) separated age- and time-related change in religious activity by integrating historical and cohort trends in these attitudes and behaviors. With careful conceptualization and measurement, age- and time-based characteristics can be applied at the individual level or in combination with cohort and period effects.

Saving for retirement is an important illustration of a time-based process. Investments and other savings vehicles work on an accumulation framework, accruing value over time. Financial planners emphasize the need to invest "early and often," even demonstrating that moderate investment in young adulthood can yield greater returns than significant investment begun in midlife and continued longer. Lifelong wealth accumulation is based on the age one begins and the amount saved. Yet there are structural influences on that timing, including the length of one's training period, the amount of debt one has after the training period, type of job and salary, and other competing expenditures. Further, this time-based process can be overlaid on the life course such that the amount saved is greatly influenced by other events, such as marriage, childbearing, caregiving responsibilities, and one's health status.

There are three key implications associated with the potential confounding of time and age. First, relying on age to explain time-based phenomena ignores the first principles of life course theory discussed earlier. The timing and duration of phenomena are often driven by social structural and microinteractional forces, potentially leading to underconceptualization and/or poor measurement of early and midlife exposures as well as more temporally proximate compensation mechanisms. Second, separating age and time processes allows us to examine the symbolic constructions of age that are commonly overlaid on the life course, creating the perception that certain events or transitions are "early," "on time," or "late." If age is considered to be the primary vehicle of individual change or stability, then it deemphasizes the *meaning* of the change from the LCP. As we note in the third section of this chapter, the importance of symbolic constructions of age are already a woefully underconsidered area of life course inquiry, especially in North America. Finally, separating age and time processes allows us to consider and test empirically the potential interaction between the two. Early timing or late timing may not yield the same impact on the life course not only because of the social construction of age but also because of ontogenetic aging processes (e.g., the impact of age-related decrease in metabolism on attempts to lose weight).

Expanding Putative Role of Choice

The continued emphasis on individual choice-making warrants attention as a problem. In the study of action, choice is a problem to be analyzed, not an accomplishment to be asserted (Dannefer, 1999a; Marshall & Clarke, in press). Given the problematic epistemological and ontological status of "choice" in the wider social science literature (compared with concepts such as "hidden curriculum," "alienation," "social control," and so on), its remarkably unproblematic appearance in life course theory cannot be defended. What is almost always measured in such discussions is behavior, and it is simply *presumed* that behavior is based on choice. In such a usage of choice, the degree of constraints an individual feels and the differential levels of constraint that confront the individuals who have, for example, different health histories or who are differently located in opportunity structures are not analyzed. Nor is the degree to which perceptions and preferences are shaped by media-certified experts or by advertising.

Without a systematic analysis of the life circumstances and subjective experiences that lie behind the observed behavior, an appealing and culturally familiar image of a volitional and more or less autonomous individual obscures the analytical problem of the constraints within which choices are made and the constitutive role of social interaction and social structure in constructing "choice" in the first place.

Summary

In this section, we have presented a diverse range of theoretical and epistemological challenges in studying the life course. These problems are often overlooked, yet they must ultimately be confronted if life course scholarship is to avoid the microfication involved in individualized conceptual formulations and lay understandings and if the field of life course studies is to apprehend fully the potentials of sociological explanation. As an added step toward that end, it will be useful to clarify what life course scholarship seeks to explain and the kinds of explanations proffered. These are the tasks of the next section.

Types of Phenomena and Types of Explanation: The *Explanans and Explananda* of Life Course Theory

To develop a general perspective of work on the life course that encompasses the foregoing points, Dannefer and Uhlenberg (1999) created a matrix based on the cross classification of types of *explananda* and *explanans* within the life course literature. The original matrix comprised three analytically distinct levels of *explananda:* (a) the individual level (the structure of discrete human lives extended from birth to death and the characteristics of those lives), (b) the level of social aggregation (the *collective patterning* of individual life course structures in a population), and (c) the cultural or symbolic level—the *societal representation* of the life course in the socially shared stock of knowledge, including the nature of its socially recognized demarcations by life events and roles and the attendant meanings and norms. To avoid undue idealization, the third category needs to be expanded to include actual social structures, policies, and practices on which many of the representations of the life course are based (such as the legal use of age as an eligibility criterion).

Each of these levels contains important phenomena that require careful description and analysis. At the individual level, these include the identification of key transition points and trajectories, at the collective level is the aggregation of these individual-level characteristics in a population, and at the sociocultural level are the social structuring of age-graded roles and the definition and evaluation of specific ages and life stages in the context of a given social system (e.g., adolescence, old age).

The columns of the matrix were defined by two categories of *explanans,* or *explanation,* termed *personological* and *sociological.* The term *personological* is intended to refer to any kind of individual characteristic that is assumed to be stable and enduring and that is postulated to influence life course outcomes. This category includes characteristics that are inherently individual, such as dispositions as well as early-life contextual characteristics that become embedded in the individual and have enduring impact on the life course. The term *sociological,* by contrast, refers to social structural and interactional forces that operate continuously to shape life course processes or that are proximate to the time at which outcomes are measured. As discussed in the second section of this chapter, there are important conceptual and methodological distinctions between context in early life and context in later life.

The sociological/personological distinction signals a major conceptual divide that is reflected in citation patterns in different strands of the life course literature. For example, authoritative reviews of the field by Elder (1998, 2003, 2006) and George (1993), exemplars of a personological approach, do not usually cite those who tend to conceptualize the life course as a feature of social structure (e.g., Kohli, 1988, 2007; Meyer, 1986; Sorensen, 1986), whereas the latter do not cite those whose work is primarily personological (see, e.g., Kohli, 2007; Kohli & Woodward, 2001).

The matrix generated by cross classifying the *explananda* and *explanans* is presented in Figure 21.1. The categories of both typologies—*explanandum* and *explanans*—are quite broad. Both they and the cells that are generated by their cross classification warrant further refinement. Although a full elaboration of the matrix is a task that lies beyond the scope of this chapter, we illustrate how subtypes can be created within the categories. We then apply these subtypes of explanation to individual-level outcomes, which constitute the top row of the matrix (see Figure 21.2).

Personological explanations include at least four identifiable types of characteristics that are often proposed to explain subsequent life course outcomes: (a) personal choice; (b) inherent traits or other hardwired, evolutionarily selected "ontogenetic" characteristics; (c) presumably stable and enduring individual characteristics that are regarded as having been shaped by social context early in the life course (enduring tastes and predispositions and some aspects of personality); and (d) individual characteristics shaped by contextual factors associated with sociohistorical change and upheaval (with the Great Depression

21.1

Framework for classifying life course studies by outcome of interest and type of explanation.

Focus of explanation

(Explanans)

Life course outcome *(Explananda)*	**Personological**	**Sociological**
Individual	A	B
Population	C	D
Symbolic	E	F

21.2

Subclassification of explanations for life course outcomes

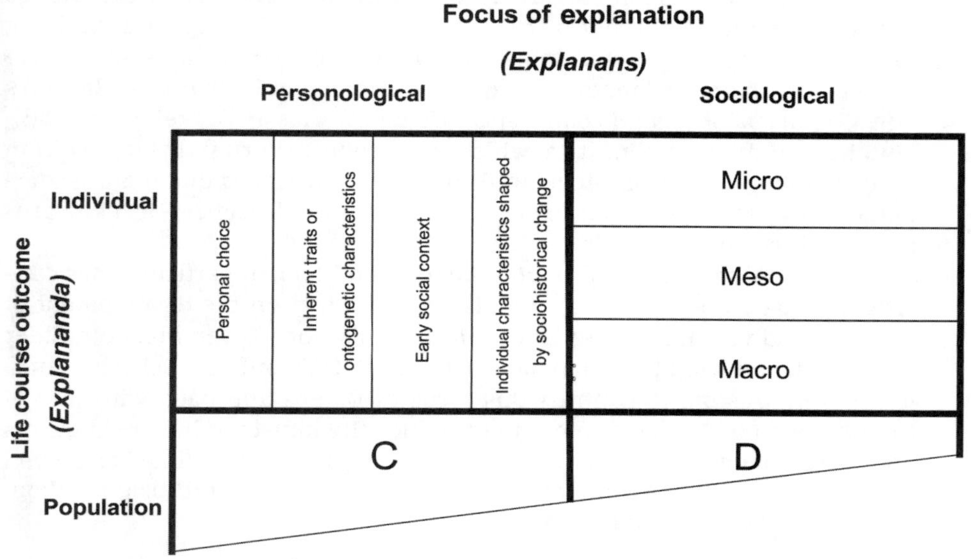

Focus of explanation
(Explanans)
Personological
Sociological
Individual
Life course outcome
(Explananda)
Personal choice
Inherent traits or ontogenetic characteristics
Early social context
Individual characteristics shaped by sociohistorical change
Micro
Meso
Macro
C
D
Population

as the prototypical example). With respect to *sociological* explanations, an obvious principle of subclassification is by system level: relevant studies have been conducted at macro-, meso-, and microlevels of analysis and are discussed in further detail later.

Cell A: Personological Explanations for Individual Outcomes

1. *Choice* (or synonymous terms such as *agency* or *decision making*). Choice is often invoked in discussions of the life course despite its problems (as described previously). In quantitative studies, choice is generally used to account for little more than the error term of an analytical model, and in narrative accounts of the life course it may be used quite uncritically. It is the deus ex machina that is brought in to account for unexplained variance. The frequency with which choice is mentioned as a factor to be considered is remarkable given its explanatory impotence (Dannefer, 1999a; Marshall & Clarke, in press). It is true that some detailed narrative studies of life history deconstruct individual choice-making as a reflective process occurring with an active consciousness (Gubrium, 1993; Matthews, 2002). In such cases, the process of deconstruction unavoidably brings context squarely into the "choice-making" process; hence, they may fit better in cell B.
2. *Inherent characteristics*. These include *traits* or other putatively inherent individual characteristics that can be discerned in some studies of life course outcomes within and beyond the field of life course studies. The diverse array of such permanent individual characteristics posited to have life

course outcomes includes alcoholism (e.g., Pandey, Roy, Zhang, & Xu, 2004), psychological invulnerability (Seifer & Sameroff, 1987), and reproductive strategies (Belsky, Steinberg, & Draper, 1991).

3. *Contextually formed characteristics. Personality* is an example of a characteristic that many scholars regard as forged on the basis of early experience in a social context, whether or not it is conceived as having an underlying inherent component. A well-known example of research that seeks to use personality as an explanatory factor for outcomes in later life is Clausen's (1993) analysis of *planful competence*. Using the classic Berkeley and Oakland human development data, which trace cohorts born in the 1920s from early childhood or adolescence until 1990, Clausen argues that planful competence—a personality characteristic formed by adolescence—is a key predictor of life course success.
4. *Sociohistorical change as a formative force.* Glen Elder, in particular, has consistently made the impact of sociohistorical context on the development of enduring individual characteristics central to his work. Given that both Elder and Clausen utilized the same databases of the Oakland and Berkeley studies, it is interesting to contrast this focus of Elder's approach with that of Clausen, who makes no attempt to introduce the impact of historical events and social change. The location of the life course in historical time has proven exceedingly fruitful in generating findings, hypotheses, and insights about the impact of circumstances on the life course.

As noted previously, however, it is important to consider how context is being utilized. In Elder's work, it is primarily as part of the prior experience of individuals, experiences that are carried forward through time within the individual. For example, early-life deprivation during the Depression was certainly a contextual factor, but its "effects" found in the 1980s are assumed to be carried forward in time largely through the effects of that early experience on the person. How those early experiences led individuals to occupy particular locations in social structure later on and the effects of temporally proximal social structures on the observed outcomes or the impact of temporally proximal economic circumstances or policy developments are not measured. This is a precise example of time 1 encapsulation described earlier in this chapter.

Cell B: Sociological Explanations for Individual Outcomes

Let us turn attention to cell B, which contains explanations of individual-level outcomes in terms of proximal or immediate aspects of social context. As noted, examples of such explanations can readily be found at the micro-, meso-, and macrolevels.

The microlevel considers studies that utilize ethnographic methods to explain the immediate dynamics of interaction and their relevance to individual characteristics, including the diagnosis and labeling of individuals and their management by social systems. Applications of labeling theory and of interactional analyses more generally to account for age-related outcomes fall into this cell (e.g., Dannefer, 2008; Holstein & Gubrium, 2000). The power of social forces in constituting individual outcomes can be most directly seen when observing their effects "close up" at the level of experience and face-to-face interaction.

The mesolevel considers studies that attempt to explain individual outcomes as a consequence of organizational dynamics—whether the organization is the workplace, the school, the neighborhood, or the mental hospital. With regard to schools, an especially clear example is provided; these also belong here, as do studies that focus on the effects on individuals of tournament-like (Lucas, 1999) and other organizational mobility processes (e.g., Rosenbaum, 1978, 1984; Sorensen, 1986). The power of self-fulfilling prophecies to create cycles of cumulative advantage for some individuals and disadvantage for others (Dannefer, 1987, 2003; O'Rand, 1996) has been observed in virtually all organizational settings—work, military, higher education, and prisons as well as schools, where it was first described and theorized (Buckley, 1967; Lemert, 1975; Rosenthal & Jacobson, 1968). Another important example of mesolevel forces is provided by the growing line of inquiry on community and neighborhood influences on well-being across the life course. Depending on its characteristics, neighborhoods can serve as buffers or exacerbators for physical health (Schootman et al., 2006), mental health (Ross, 2000), and even identity (Rosel, 2003).

The macrolevel includes at least two broad kinds of *explanans:* the effects of national-level policies (e.g., the consequences of welfare state provisions, including age-graded eligibility rules) and other macroforces, such as globalization and economic trends.

The second type of *explanans* at the macrolevel are structural variables, such as occupational position, education or other indicators related to social class, and race, ethnicity, and gender—characteristics that have explanatory power at a general level of social organization. Even if these categories are measured at the individual level (e.g., an individual's race), it is the ascribed status and social meaning of those categories that are consequential because it reflects the macrostructural hierarchy. For example, insurance status is an individual-level characteristic, but its implications for accessing health care are actually rooted in the broader political and economic structure. As Kelley-Moore and Ferraro (2004) demonstrate, racial disparities in late-life physical function are influenced by both socioeconomic status and lifelong social selection processes, both of which are individual-level indicators of the macrostructural forces that create opportunities and barriers over the life course. The social gradient manifests in individuals, leading to the widely observed patterns of inequality between socially defined groups. Or, as described in chapter 22 in this volume, social inequality "gets under the skin." Thus, scientists must carefully consider the inclusion and interpretation of individual-level variables to avoid mistakenly attributing them to personological explanations.

Because it has considered the effects of temporally proximate social characteristics, such as occupation, wealth, or social engagement, some recent work of Elder and associates is also properly considered to belong in this cell (Crosnoe & Elder, 2002; Willson, Shuey, & Elder, 2007).

Cell C: Personological Explanations for Population Outcomes

Despite the collective character of the *explanandum* in row 2, demographers and other analysts of population outcomes often invoke personological explanations ranging from choice to ontogenetic change.

With regard to choice, consider population-level studies dealing with the transition to adulthood. Reflecting the idealization of increasing autonomy as a feature of advancing modernity, many such studies begin with structural explanations for behavior in the past but shift to personological explanations for behavior as we approach the present. Structural forces that constrained behaviors in the past are not hard to detect, but when we get closer to the present, the social structural mechanisms shaping human behavior are deemphasized in favor of choice-making. One example is provided by the work of John Modell (1989, 1995) on the transition to adulthood. In explaining cohort variations in such areas as schooling, premarital sex, marriage, and parenthood, Modell emphasizes the influence in earlier cohorts of social forces, such as "the market demand for labor" and "needs of the family economy." In more recent cohorts, however, increasing prosperity has meant that social structure has been losing its determinative force: "Young people . . . have increasingly taken control of the construction of the youthful life course" and "choose the timing of their own life course events and hence come increasingly to value the expression of personal choice in this as in other aspects of their lives" (Modell, 1989, pp. 326, 330). Other demographers have also frequently referred to choice, decision, or related terms like "preferences" and "options" in efforts to explain changes in marriage patterns and fertility (Cooksey & Rindfuss, 2001; Rindfuss, Choe, Bumpass, & Byun, 2004).

One irony of such interpretations is that, at least until recent decades, the presumed increase in personal freedom and choice was associated with greater conformity in behavior (see Dannefer, 1984, 1999a). For example, throughout the 20th-century United States and especially after World War II, a trend toward increased conformity among cohort members in transition to adulthood (Hogan, 1981) and in other life transitions was clearly evident. The interpretation typically offered for this finding has been, as in the previously given examples, increased prosperity in young adulthood, which provided increased degrees of freedom in choice and control; paradoxically, an increase in choice thus leads to an increase in conformity. We suggest that this can make sense only if one assumes that there is a strong set of impulses in human nature to differentiate from family of origin and marry soon after the period called adolescence. This is an example of the continued implicit reliance on the organismic model in sociological research.

An example of personological change driven explicitly by age-linked, ontogenetic characteristics for population outcomes is provided by the analysis of population cognitive aging by Alwin et al. (2008). They begin with an explicit assumption that

> *as a biological, neurological, social and cognitive process, cognitive aging can be defined as those time-dependent irreversible changes that lead to progressive loss of functional capacity for a point of maturity . . . these changes in the conditions of human frailty . . . are to some extent intrinsic within the organism rather than brought about by the outside environment. (p. 74)*

Cell D: Sociological Explanations for Population Outcomes

Row 2 concerns life course patterns studied at the collective level, which typically entails the study of population or cohort patterns. The use of sociological explanations for life course patterns of cohorts in later life is illustrated by studies of labor force exit (Henretta, 1992) and economic status (Crystal & Waehrer, 1996) and selective migration (Norman, Boyle, & Rees, 2005). Although such studies generally do not deny the influence of earlier life course experiences in determining later outcomes, they focus primarily on the significance of social factors encountered by cohorts as they move through later-life structures created by the state (e.g., Social Security) and the workplace (e.g., pension programs). These structures are seen not only as factors having an impact on the aggregate experience on cohorts in later life but also as forces that produce the internal stratification of cohorts (Crystal, 2006; Dannefer, 2003).

With the recent emphasis on structured inequality and cumulative dis/advantage processes as related to age, a growing number of cohort-level analyses have been interpreted in terms of sociological explanation, the right-hand cell of row 2.

For example, Crystal and Waehrer (1996) argue that income distributions characteristic of cohorts in later life are shaped "not only by the numerous vicissitudes of individual life events and choices, but also by policy choices implicitly in the design and regulation of retirement income systems" (p. S301). Using longitudinal data for several cohorts moving from middle age into later life, they show average income declines and increasing inequality within each cohort. Individuals within a cohort differentially encounter such later life course events as retirement, loss of spouse, illness, disability, and inheritance. The effects of these transitions on economic status, however, are mediated by larger structural forces related to the income system. Without attention to the stratification of the occupational structure and to policies regulating public and private pensions, health care, and taxes, one cannot understand cohort patterns of income distribution in later life.

A second illustrative example can be drawn from the work of Norman et al. (2005), who examined the relationship between area-level deprivation and health inequality over a 20-year period. Specifically, they compared changes in health status among migrants and nonmigrants to determine the net effect of living in an economically disadvantaged area. Although this study used a combination of individual- and area-level data, their purpose was to examine contextual effects on the observed health inequality in specific geographic regions.

Both of these studies suggest structural explanations for observed population patterns, but neither is able to examine in detail how particular social structures produce particular outcomes. Focusing on this limitation, Elder and O'Rand (1995) criticize cohort studies that "typically speculate about historical forces and fail to extend analysis to their actual investigation. At most we end with a plausible story that does not advance scientific understanding." This observation can be accepted as a challenge to identify and develop hypotheses to examine the role of social structural factors in producing observed cohort patterns of aging. Nothing is gained, however, if this critique is taken to justify a retreat to personological factors only or to avoid engaging the sociological imagination for a lack of data. Clear understanding of life course trajectories is not enhanced by ignoring how the extrusion of individuals through regulative and often age-graded structures shapes collective patterns of aging.

A critical conceptual distinction exists between sociological explanations of individual differences in a given outcome and population-level inequality.

The latter fits squarely in cell D because the observed patterns are population characteristics or processes that are influenced by social structure. Studies at the macrolevel, such as cross-national comparisons, belong in this cell, as do studies on a smaller population scale, such as neighborhoods, communities, and institutions. As we noted in our discussion of row 1 of the matrix, the difference between cell C, which has personological explanations, and cell D, which has sociological explanations, lies in the causal assumptions being made about postulated independent variables. Researchers must recognize population outcomes are influenced by social, political, or economic structure and can occur at the micro-, meso-, or macrolevel. Cell D has tremendous potential for understanding population life course processes but has heretofore been neglected in favor of individual-level measures and personological explanations.

Cells E and F: The Life Course as a Social Apparatus

Our conceptualization of the third row of life course *explananda* represents an expansion of its treatment in *Paths* as "a symbolic construct" because what is intended here is more than that. It concerns the life course as a socially constituted set of social practices, policies, and structures and a concomitant symbolic apparatus of age-related meanings, values, and norms. Thus, the phenomena in question here are different from the first two. In both of the first two, the *explanans* consist of actual individual people, whether treated as individuals or aggregated. This third category of phenomena is really *social structural, symbolic,* and *cultural* in nature. It refers to the life course (and age) as social phenomena—as a set of *social rules and practices* and as a *socially objectivated idea* that has plausibility in a given societal context as a set of publicly shared meanings and expectations for the course of human lives.

Accounts of the features of the life course as a symbolic construct are often cast in sociological terms, as indicated in cell F. Notwithstanding certain organismic and logical constraints on role sequences (e.g., puberty precedes biological parenting), the dramatic historical and cross-cultural diversity in the timing, sequencing, content, and orderliness of roles and activities dictates the importance of sociological approach here.

The power of social structure to organize the life course was a central theme of the classic essay by Leonard Cain (1964) that first articulated the connection between, as its title indicates, "Life Course and Social Structure." Perhaps the most familiar example of the life course as a social construction is the widely objectivated *institutionalized life course* of late modernity (Kohli, 1988, 2007). In welfare state economies and other modern states, age grading serves as a major organizer of what is defined as "normal" and "natural" human behavior, which is archetypically divided into the notorious "three boxes of life" (e.g., Riley & Riley, 1994).

The institutionalized life course includes an elaborate array of well-defined yet socially constructed markers the broad impact of which touches individuals whether or not they are able to conform to them. For example, the markers of transitioning to adulthood include economic and social independence from one's family of origin. Young severely disabled adults are often perceived as failing to reach adulthood because they are physically or mentally unable to maintain employment and/or achieve culturally important markers of independence

(Tisdall, 2001). The current debate over the possible deinstitutionalization of the life course in response to broader social forces simply underscores how intertwined the social constitution of the life course is, not with individual aging but rather with broadscale social forces.

The life course as a social apparatus also includes a symbolic approach that encompasses age norms, meanings, and values (e.g., Chudacoff, 1989; Dannefer & Shura, in press). This is well illustrated by the work of Riley and associates, which has included a focus on the meaning of age and the processes by which it changes. Especially relevant are their discussions of age norms and expectations deriving from societal age-grading (e.g., Riley, Kahn, & Foner, 1994). Their treatment provides a framework for analyzing age as a formal and informal criterion to encourage or impede entrance into and exit from roles, thereby regulating access to resources and opportunities.

Studies of specific organizations or subcultures that have documented the operation of age norms in local settings are also important contributions to this cell. For example, Burton (1990, 1996) has documented a quite distinct set of life course and age-related expectations in poor minority communities. Tragically, the truncated or abbreviated life course has been established as an expected feature of the life course of street gang members, whose lives are organized by a remarkably orderly progression of "career development" (e.g., from homeboy to original gangster) (Bing, 1992; Klein & Maxon, 2006). Work organizations also have their own cultural systems, of which age grading is often a part. Lawrence (1984, 1996) demonstrated the power of normative expectations about age appropriateness for certain career levels within a corporate setting.

From this perspective, age norms are explained in terms of the confluence of demographic change with social policies that have bureaucratized and increasingly institutionalized the life course in a matrix of formal and informal social regulation (cf. Kohli, 1988; Meyer, 1986). Over the past century, these societal developments produced a steady increase in the use of age as a formal role criterion for education, work, and retirement, creating the "three boxes of life" (Riley et al., 1994), and an unprecedented degree of life course transition and role conformity, especially for men (e.g., Glick, 1977; Hogan, 1981; Modell, Furstenburg, & Strong, 1978). Such a high degree of age-graded societal regulation (which tended to homogenize the major roles and transitions of tens of millions of people) produced a widely shared view of the life course and hence of age norms (Chudacoff, 1989). Historians have traced the forces underlying these changes back to earlier changes in the meaning and status of age, deriving from demographic changes in the age structure and technological change that shifted health expertise from the aged themselves to medicine (Achenbaum, 1979), and to still other technical and social changes that reshaped the age grading of work and school, creating new levels of age segregation and age awareness (Chudacoff, 1989). From this vantage point, then, the very concepts of age and life course are themselves historically contingent as culturally relevant and plausible constructs.

Although perhaps more commonly and plausibly cast in sociological terms, personological accounts of the source of the life course as symbolic construct are also available, and examples are located in cell E. One example of such an account is provided by the work of Riley and associates (Riley, 1978; Riley, & Riley, 1994). Her concept of *cohort norm formation* is an attempt to provide an action complement to the strong structural emphasis of the basic aging and society framework by explicating the role of individual behavior in creating population patterns.

Most personological accounts derive, at least implicitly, from the same kind of argument used by the historical demography in row 2. This cell contains work that views the culturally shared meaning of age—both age in general and being a particular age—as deriving from factors in the individual person. This is, of course, precisely the notion that is explicitly applied to old age when disengagement is said to be a realization of natural human tendencies. Despite its own age and its general disrepute, disengagement theory (Cumming & Henry, 1961) continues to resurface, as gerontological commentators regularly note. And in a context of a graying population, expanding health care potentials, and sharply rising health care costs, such theorizing is not irrelevant to economic arguments about aging. One recent reincarnation of disengagement can be found in Daniel Callahan's (1987) proposals that we think of a "full life" and an "expectable life course" of 70-odd years as a criterion of access to care. Such approaches provide a personologically based, organismic justification of contemporary age norms and of the biases they justify. This general point is relevant to current public debates on issues like withholding needed medical treatment from the very old and physician-assisted suicide. If the life course is seen as having an organismically determined end point within a certain age range, it is another argument for such practices and another form of social pressure to be visited on the aged individual in question.

Summary

In the mid-1970s, Glen Elder (1975) correctly referred to the life course as an "emerging field of inquiry" (p. 186). By the mid-1990s, the LCP had become the dominant perspective from which social scientists approached the study of aging, as reflected by the renaming of the American Sociological Association's section on aging as *Sociology of Aging and the Life Course* in 1997. Now, more than 10 years later, the LCP has been increasingly useful and widely applied in substantive domains of social science research. It nevertheless remains true, as Dannefer and Uhlenberg (1999) noted a decade ago, that the development of sociological theory to further our understanding of how social forces shape the life course is still in an early stage. From the perspective of social theory, the result is theoretical inadequacies in the formulation of life course issues, even though the term *life course* has a distinctly sociological heritage.

These theoretical inadequacies were the focus of the first section of this chapter. Discourse in the life course area has failed to acknowledge or utilize the basic insights concerning the unique role that social structure and interaction play in the constitution of individual lives and in the symbolic understanding of age and the life course. This tendency is evident even in the section name *Sociology of Aging and the Life Course* noted previously. Notably absent from both section titles is *age* (which identifies a structural dimension of social organization as opposed to the individual level)—an absence that invites a continuation of the tendency to obscure social structural aspects of the life course and to amplify the focus on individual aspects.

An adequate theory of the life course cannot ignore the unique features of the human organism (e.g., exterogestation, neoteny, and exceptional physical flexibility and resilience and cognitive capacities). These features of human physical anthropology mean that human development and aging require social interaction processes, and therefore the *explanation* of human development also requires an understanding of the integral and irreducible role of social interaction. Social interaction processes are almost always institutionalized to some degree in group practices, which thereby organize and structure social interaction, giving *social structure* an important and irreducible role in organizing life course patterns. Accordingly, we have proposed that attention to social interaction and social structure stand as first principles of life course analysis. Without them, human organisms do not become human beings, and there is no life course. However, the importance of social interaction and social structures is consequential to human development not only in the early years, but throughout the entire life course. As we illustrate in this chapter, social interaction and social structure operate as constitutive forces over the entire life course.

Given these principles, a theory of the life course cannot be based on the organismic model appropriate to other species, with its assumptions of a "natural" aging trajectory. Yet, as we have seen, common intellectual practices in the study of aging and the life course, such as the tendency to associate the importance of the social with change or the tendency to naturalize the institutionalized life course, continue to invite a reliance on unwarranted organismic assumptions.

The final section of the chapter expands the classification scheme set forth in *Paths*. Each of the three levels of phenomena (*explananda*)—individual, population, and structural-symbolic—stands as a legitimate and important focus for life course analysis. However, research in the first two categories has overemphasized key transition points and trajectories of individual life paths. Moreover, further attention should be paid to life course outcomes at the collective level as well as the social structuring and social construction of age.

Of the two classes of explanations (*explanans*), research on aging and the life course has relied primarily on personological factors, including inherent personality traits, individual choice, and early-life social context. As we note in the second section of the chapter, overreliance on these factors as well as ontogenetic aging as explanatory mechanisms has led to a neglect of sociological influences on the life course, both conceptually and methodologically. Too often, the explanatory force of social structural and temporally proximate social context is neglected, leaving us with the popular but naive perspective of individuals aging outside the influence of a social world. One need not contend that the social has the primary explanatory contribution to make to every imaginable life course outcome in order to appreciate the value of clarity with respect to the kinds of explanation that are being assumed and the kinds that are being excluded by the causal assumptions and/or data available to the life course researcher.

References

Achenbaum, W. A. (1979). *Old age in the new land: The American experience since 1790*. Baltimore: Johns Hopkins University Press.

Alwin, D. F., McCammon, R. J., Wray, L. A., & Rodgers, W. L. (2008). Population processes and cognitive aging. In S. M. Hofer & D. F. Alwin (Eds.), *Handbook of cognitive aging: Interdisciplinary perspectives* (pp. 69–89). Thousand Oaks, CA: Sage.

Alwin, D. F., & Wray, L. A. (2005). A life-span developmental perspective on social status and health. *Journal of Gerontology: Social Sciences, 60*(Special Issue 2), S7–S14.

Baars, J., Dannefer, D., Phillipson, C., & Walker, A. (2006). Introduction: Critical perspectives in social gerontology. In J. Baars, D. Dannefer, C. Phillipson, & A. Walker (Eds.), *Aging, globalization, and inequality: The new critical gerontology* (pp. 103–120). Amityville, NY: Baywood Publishing.

Baltes, P. B. (1979). Life-span developmental psychology: Some converging observations on history and theory. In P. B. Baltes & O. G. Brim, Jr. (Eds.), *Life-span development and behavior, Vol. 2.* New York: Academic Press.

Bass, S. A. (2007). The emergence of the golden age of social gerontology? *The Gerontologist, 47,* 408–412.

Belsky, J., Steinberg, L., & Draper, P. (1991). Childhood experience, interpersonal development, and reproductive strategy: An evolutionary theory of socialization. *Child Development, 62,* 647–670.

Bengtson, V. L., Horlacher, G., Putney, N. M., & Silverstein, M. (2008, August). *Growth and decline of religiosity across time and age.* Paper presented at the annual meeting of the American Sociological Association, Boston, MA.

Berger, P., & Luckmann, T. (1967). *The social construction of reality.* New York: Anchor Books.

Bing, L. (1992). *Do or die.* New York: HarperPerennial.

Birren, J. E. (1988). A contribution to the theory of the psychology of aging: As a counterpart of development. In J. E. Birren & V. L. Bengtson (Eds.), *Emergent theories of aging* (pp. 153–176). New York: Springer Publishing.

Buckley, W. (1967). *Social and modern systems theory.* Englewood Cliffs, NJ: Prentice Hall.

Burton, L. (1990). Teenage childbearing as an alternative life-course strategy in multigenerational black families. *Human Nature, 1,* 123–143.

Burton, L. (1996). Age norms, the timing of family role transitions, and intergenerational caregiving among aging African American women. *The Gerontologist, 36,* 199–208.

Cain, L. D. (1964). Life course and social structure. In R. E. L. Faris (Ed.), *Handbook of modern sociology* (pp. 272–309). Chicago: Rand McNally.

Callahan, D. (1987). *Setting limits: Medical goals in an aging society.* New York: Simon & Schuster.

Chudacoff, H. (1989). *How old are you? Age consciousness in American culture.* Princeton, NJ: Princeton University Press.

Clausen, J. A. (1993). *American lives: Looking back at the children of the Great Depression.* New York: Free Press.

Cooksey, E., & Rindfuss, R. R. (2001). Patterns of work and schooling in young adulthood. *Sociological Forum, 16,* 731–755.

Crosnoe, R., & Elder, G. H. Jr. (2002). Adolescent twins and emotional distress: The inter-related influence of non-shared environment and social structure. *Child Development, 73,* 1761–1774.

Crystal, S. (2006). Dynamics of late life inequality: Modeling the interplay of health disparities, economic resources, and public policies. In J. Baars, D. Dannefer, C. Phillipson, & A. Walker (Eds.), *Aging, globalization, and inequality: The new critical gerontology* (pp. 205–213). Amityville, NY: Baywood Publishing.

Crystal, S., & Shea, D. (2002). Prospects for retirement resources in an aging society. *Annual Review of Gerontology and Geriatrics, 22,* 271–281.

Crystal, S., & Waehrer, K. (1996). Later-life economic inequality in longitudinal perspective. *Journal of Gerontology: Social Sciences, 51,* S307–S318.

Cumming, E., & Henry, W. F. (1961). *Growing old.* New York: Basic Books.

Daatland, S. O., & Biggs, S. (2006). *Aging and diversity: Multiple pathways and cultural migrations.* Bristol: Policy Press.

Dannefer, D. (1984). Adult development and social theory: A paradigmatic reappraisal. *American Sociological Review, 49,* 100–116.

Dannefer, D. (1987). Accentuation, the Matthew effect, and the life course: Aging as intracohort differentiation. *Sociological Forum, 2,* 211–236.

Dannefer, D. (1999a). Freedom isn't free: Power, alienation and the consequences of action. In J. Brandstadter & R. M. Lerner (Eds.), *Action and self-development: Theory and research through the life span* (pp. 105–131). Thousand Oaks, CA: Sage.

Dannefer, D. (1999b). Neoteny, naturalization and other constituents of human development. In C. Ryff & V. W. Marshall (Eds.), *Self and society in aging processes* (pp. 67–93). New York: Springer Publishing.

Dannefer, D. (2002). Whose life course is it, anyway? In R. Settersten (Ed.), *Invitation to the life course* (pp. 259–268) Amityville, NY: Baywood Publishing.

Dannefer, D. (2003). Cumulative advantage/disadvantage and the life course: Cross-fertilizing age and social science theory. *Journal of Gerontology: Social Sciences, 58,* S327–S337.

Dannefer, D. (2008). The waters we swim: Everyday social processes, macro structural realities and human aging. In K. W. Schaie & R. P. Abeles (Eds.), *Social structure and aging.* New York: Springer Publishing.

Dannefer, D., & Shura, R. A. (in press). Experience, social structure and later life: Meaning and old age in an aging society. In P. Uhlenberg (Ed.), *Handbook of the demography of aging.* New York: Springer-Verlag.

Dannefer, D., & Uhlenberg, P. (1999). Paths of the life course: A typology. In V. L. Bengtson & K. W. Schaie (Eds.), *Handbook of theories of aging* (pp. 306–326). New York: Springer Publishing.

de Ribaupierre, A., Labouvie-Vief, G., Joye, D., Oris, M., Spini, D., & Widmer E. (Eds.). (in press). *Lifespan—Life course: Is it really the same? Linked lives and self-regulation.*

Dupre, M. E. (2007). Educational differences in age-related patterns of disease: Reconsidering the cumulative disadvantage and age-as-leveler hypotheses. *Journal of Health and Social Behavior, 25,* 1–15.

Elder, G. H., Jr. (1974). *Children of the Great Depression: Social change in life experience.* Chicago: University of Chicago Press.

Elder, G. H., Jr. (1975). Age differentiation and the life course. *Annual Review of Sociology, 1,* 165–190.

Elder, G. H., Jr. (1996). Human lives in changing societies: Life course and developmental insights. In R. B. Cairns, G. H. Elder Jr., & E. J. Costello (Eds.), *Developmental sciences* (pp. 31–62). New York: Cambridge University Press.

Elder, G. H., Jr. (1998). The life course and human development. In R. M. Lerner (Ed.), *Handbook of child psychology: Vol. 1. Theoretical models of human development* (pp. 939–991). New York: Wiley.

Elder, G. H., Jr. (2003). The life course in time and place. In W. R. Heinz & V. W. Marshall (Eds.), *Sequences, institutions and interrelations over the life course* (pp. 57–71). New York: Aldine de Gruyter.

Elder, G. H., Jr. (2006). Life course perspective. In G. Ritzer (Ed.), *The Blackwell encyclopedia of sociology* (4th ed., pp. 2634–2639). Malden, MA: Blackwell.

Elder, G. H., Jr., & O'Rand, A. M. (1995). Adult lives in a changing society. In K. S. Cook, G. A. Fine, & J. S. House (Eds.), *Sociological perspectives on social psychology* (pp. 452–475). Boston: Allyn & Bacon.

Ferraro, K. F., & Kelley-Moore, J. A. (2003). Cumulative disadvantage and health: Long-term consequences of obesity? *American Sociological Review, 68,* 707–729.

Ferraro, K. F., & Shippee, T. P. (in press). Aging and cumulative inequality: How does inequality get under the skin? *The Gerontologist, 49*(2).

George, L. (1993). Sociological perspective on life transitions. *Annual Review of Sociology, 19,* 353–373.

Glick, P. C. (1977). Updating the life cycle of the family. *Journal of Marriage and the Family, 39,* 5–13.

Gluckman, P., & Hanson, M. (Eds.). (2006). *Developmental origins of health and disease.* Cambridge: Cambridge University Press.

Gould, S. J. (1977). Human babies as embryos. In S. J. Gould (Ed.), *Ever since Darwin: Reflections on natural history* (pp. 70–78). New York: Norton.

Gubrium, J. (1993). *Speaking of life: Horizons of meaning for nursing home residents.* Chicago: Aldine.

Hagestad, G. O., & Dannefer, D. (2001). Concepts and theories of aging: Beyond microfication in social sciences approaches. In R. H. Binstock & L. K. George (Eds.), *Handbook of aging and social sciences* (5th ed., pp. 3–21). San Diego, CA: Academic Press.

Hareven, T. K. (1977). *Transitions: The family and the life course in historical perspective.* New York: Academic Press.

Heckhausen, J. (2006). *Developmental regulation in adulthood: Age-normative and sociostructural constraints as adaptive challenges.* New York: Cambridge University Press.

Henretta, J. (1992). Uniformity and diversity: Life course institutionalization and late life exit. *Sociological Quarterly, 33,* 265–279.

Hogan, D. (1981). *Transitions and social change: The early lives of American men.* New York: Academic Press.

Holstein, J., & Gubrium, J. (2000). *Constructing the life course.* Dix Hills, NY: General Hall.

Kelley-Moore, J. A., & Ferraro, K. F. (2004). The black/white disability gap: Persistent inequality in later life? *Journal of Gerontology: Social Sciences, 59,* S34–S43.

Klein, M. W., & Maxon, C. L. (2006). *Street gang patterns and policies.* New York: Oxford University Press.

Kohli, M. (1988). Social organization and subjective construction of the life course. In A. B. Sorensen, F. E. Weiner, & L. R. Sherrod (Eds.), *Human development and the life cycle* (pp. 271–292). Hillsdale, NJ: Lawrence Erlbaum Associates.

Kohli, M. (2007). The institutionalization of the life course: Looking back to look ahead. *Research in Human Development, 4,* 253–271.

Kohli, M., & Woodward, A. (2001). European societies: Inclusions/exclusions? In A. Woodward & M. Kohli (Eds.), *Inclusions and exclusions in European societies* (pp. 1–17). London: Routledge.

Lave, J., & Wenger, E. (1991). *Situated learning: Legitimate peripheral participation.*: Cambridge: Cambridge University Press.

Lawrence, B. (1984). Age grading: The implicit organizational timetable. *Journal of Occupational Behavior, 5,* 23–35.

Lawrence, B. S. (1996). Age norms: Why is it so hard to know one when you see one? *The Gerontologist, 36,* 209–220.

Lemert, E. (1975). Primary and secondary deviation. In S. H. Traub & C. B. Little (Eds.), *Theories of deviance* (pp. 167–179). Itasca, IL: F. E. Peacock.

Lerner, R. M. (1986). *Concepts and theories of human development* (2nd ed.). Reading, MA: Addison-Wesley.

Lucas, S. R. (1999). *Tracking inequality: Stratification, mobility in American high schools.* New York: Teachers College Press.

Maguire, E. A., Gadian, D. G., Johnsrude, I. S., Good, C. D., Ashburner, J., Frackowiak, R. S., et al. (2000). Navigation-related structural change in the hippocampi of taxi drivers. *Proceedings of the National Academy of Sciences of the United States of America, 97,* 4398–4403.

Marshall, V., & Clarke, A. (in press). Agency and social structure in aging and life course research. In D. Dannefer & C. R. Phillipson (Eds.), *International handbook of social gerontology.* London: Sage.

Matthews, S. (2002). *Sisters and brothers/Daughters and sons.* Bloomington, IN: Unlimited Publishing.

Meyer, J. (1986). The self and the life course: Institutionalization and its effects. In A. B. Sorenson, F. E. Weinert, & L. Sherrod (Eds.), *Human development and the life course* (pp. 199–216). Hillsdale, NJ: Lawrence Erlbaum Associates.

Modell, J. (1989). *Into one's own: From youth to adulthood in the United States.* Berkeley: University of California Press.

Modell, J. (1995). Did the good war make good workers? In K. P. O'Brien, & L. H. Parsons (Eds.), *The home-front war: World War II and American society* (pp. 139–156). Westport, CT: Greenwood.

Modell, J., Furstenberg, F. F., Jr., & Strong, D. (1978). The timing of marriage in the transition to adulthood: Continuity and change, 1860–1975. *American Journal of Sociology, 84,* 8120–8150.

Montagu, A. (1989). *Growing young* (2nd ed.). Granby, MA: Bergin & Garvey.

Morss, J. (1990). *The biologising of childhood.* Hillsdale, NJ: Lawrence Erlbaum Associates.

Morss, J. (1996). *Critical developments.* London: Routledge.

Norman, P., Boyle, P., & Rees, P. (2005). Selective migration, health and deprivation: A longitudinal analysis. *Social Science and Medicine, 60,* 2755–2771.

O'Rand, A. (1996). The precious and the precocious: Understanding cumulative disadvantage and cumulative advantage over the life course. *The Gerontologist, 36,* 230–238.

O'Rand, A., & Henretta, J. C. (1999). *Age and inequality: Diverse pathways through later life.* Boulder, CO: Westview Press.

Pallas, A. M., & Booher-Jennings, J. (2006, August). *Cumulative knowledge about cumulative advantage.* Paper presented at the annual meeting of the American Sociological Association, Montreal.

Pandey, S. C., Roy, A., Zhang, H., & Xu, T. (2004). Partial deletion of the CREB gene promotes alcohol-drinking behaviors. *Journal of Neuroscience, 24,* 5022–5030.

Parsons, T. J., Power, C., & Manor, O. (2001). Fetal and early life growth and body mass index from birth to early adulthood in 1951 British cohort: Longitudinal study. *British Medical Journal, 323,* 1331–1335.

Perry, B., & Svalavitz, M. (2006). *The boy who was raised as a dog: And other stories from a child psychiatrist's notebook: What traumatized children can teach us about loss, love, and healing.* New York: Basic Books.

Priestley, M. (Ed.). (2001). *Disability and the life course: Global perspectives.* New York: Cambridge University Press.

Riley, M. W. (1973). Aging and cohort succession: Interpretations and misinterpretations. *Public Opinion Quarterly, 37,* 35–49.

Riley, M. W. (1978). Aging, social change and the power of ideas. *Daedalus, 107,* 39–52.

Riley, M. W., Johnson, M. E., & Foner, A. (1972). *Aging and society: Vol. 3. A sociology of age stratification.* New York: Russell Sage Foundation.

Riley, M. W., Kahn, R., & Foner, A. (1994). *Age and structural lag: Society's failure to provide meaningful opportunities in work, family, and leisure.* New York: Wiley-Interscience.

Riley, M. W., & Riley, J. W. (1994). Age integration and the lives of older people. *The Gerontologist, 34,* 110–115.

Rindfuss, R. R., Choe, M. K., Bumpass, L. L., & Byun, Y. C. (2004). Intergenerational relations. In N. O. Tsuya & L. L. Bumpass (Eds.), *Marriage, work and family life in comparative perspective: Japan, South Korea and the United States* (pp. 54–75). Honolulu: University of Hawaii Press.

Rogoff, B. (2002). How can we study cultural aspects of human development? *Human Development, 45,* 209–210.

Rogoff, B. (2003). *The cultural nature of human development.* New York: Oxford University Press.

Rosel, N. (2003). Aging in place: Knowing where you are. *International Journal of Aging and Human Development, 57,* 77–90.

Rosenbaum, J. (1978). The structure of opportunity in school. *Social Forces, 57,* 236–256.

Rosenbaum, J. (1984). *Career mobility in a corporation hierarchy.* New York: Academic Press.

Rosenthal, R., & Jacobson, L. (1968). Pygmalion in the classroom. *Urban Review, 3,* 16–20.

Ross, C. E. (2000). Neighborhood disadvantage and adult depression. *Journal of Health and Social Behavior, 41,* 177–187.

Sampson, R. J., & Laub, J. H. (1993). *Crime in the making: Pathways and turning points through life.* Cambridge, MA: Harvard University Press.

Sampson, R. J., & Laub, J. H. (2005). A life course view of the development of crime. *The Annals of the American Academy of Political and Social Science, 602,* 12–45.

Schootman, M., Andresen, E., Wolinsky, F., Malmstrom, T. K., Miller, J. P., & Miller, D. K. (2006). Neighborhood conditions and risk of incident lower-body functional limitations among middle-aged African Americans. *American Journal of Epidemiology, 163,* 450–458.

Seifer, R., & Sameroff, A. J. (1987). Multiple determinants of risk and invulnerability. In E. J. Anthony & B. J. Cohler (Eds.), *The invulnerable child* (pp. 51–69). New York: Guilford.

Sorensen, A. B. (1986). Social structure and the mechanisms of life-course processes. In A. B. Sorensen, F. Weinert, & L. Sherrod (Eds.), *Human development: Multi-disciplinary perspectives* (pp. 177–197). Hillsdale, NJ: Lawrence Erlbaum Associates.

Symonds, M. E., & Gardner, D. S. (2006). The developmental environment and the development of obesity. In P. Gluckman & M. Hanson (Eds.), *Developmental origins of health and disease* (pp. 255–264). Cambridge: Cambridge University Press.

Tisdall, K. (2001). Failing to make the transition? Theorising the "transition to adulthood" for young disabled people. In M. Priestley (Ed.), *Disability and the life course: Global perspectives* (pp. 167–178). New York: Cambridge University Press.

Widmer, E., Burton-Jeangros, C., Bergman, M., & Dannefer, D. (Eds.). (in press). *Swiss Journal of Sociology.*

Willson, A. E., Shuey, K. M., & Elder, G. H., Jr. (2007). Cumulative advantage processes as mechanisms of inequality in life course health. *American Journal of Sociology, 112,* 1886–1924.

Wrosch, C., & Freund, A. M. (2001). Self-regulation of normative and non-normative developmental challenges. *Human Development, 44,* 264–283.

Yang, Y. (2008). Social inequalities in happiness in the United States, 1972 to 2004: An age-period-cohort analysis. *American Sociological Review, 73,* 204–226.

Yates, F. I. (1991). Aging as prolonged morphogenesis: A topobiological sorcerer's apprentice. In G. Kenyon, J. E. Birren, & F. F. Schroots (Eds.), *Metaphors of aging in science and the humanities* (pp. 199–218). New York: Springer Publishing.

Cumulative Inequality Theory for Research on Aging and the Life Course

22

Kenneth F. Ferraro
Tetyana Pylypiv Shippee
Markus H. Schafer

Robert Merton's (1968a, 1988) articulation of the Matthew effect in science is one of the key concepts that led to theoretical developments related to cumulative advantage and disadvantage.[1] The idea that early advantage can be leveraged for greater gain has since received conceptual development and empirical support in research on a variety of topics ranging from school-tracking systems to age heterogeneity. Merton's focus was how advantage accumulates, parallel

We appreciate the comments of Glen H. Elder, Jr., Stephani Hatch, Ann Howell, Shalon Irving, and Timothy Owens on an earlier version of this chapter. Address all correspondence to Kenneth F. Ferraro, Center on Aging and the Life Course, Purdue University, Young Hall, 302 Wood Street, West Lafayette, IN 47907-2108. E-mail: ferraro@purdue.edu; voice: 765-494-6388.

to what is considered a tournament-mobility model: early success provides opportunities for rapid career advancement. Advantage for some, however, often means disadvantage for others. Indeed, this is part of the metaphor of the Matthew effect: accumulating benefits for those already advantaged but accumulating loss for those who are disadvantaged early.

The concepts of cumulative advantage and disadvantage are useful for sociological inquiry, and our aim is to aid the development and application of these concepts for research on aging and the life course. We know that early life events and status rankings are important to later life, but a logical next step is to explicate how these early life experiences are translated into later outcomes. Do early events have effects that are inexorable in their impact? Can early disadvantage be overcome? Are there compensatory mechanisms that can counter the general principle that the "race is to the swift"? What role does human agency play in the process of cumulative disadvantage? These and many other questions merit attention if the concepts of cumulative advantage and disadvantage are to be transformed into a theory.

To enhance this transformation, we build on the contributions of others to develop a theory of *cumulative inequality*. Our approach to doing so is two-fold. First, useful theories have elements subject to falsification (Turner, 1982) and "sufficient formality" to differentiate closely related concepts (DiPrete & Eirich, 2006). Therefore, we explicate this theory in axiomatic form with propositions in order to make its elements empirically testable and subject to falsification. Second, although we draw from several sociological theorists and the literature on life course epidemiology, we give special attention to integrating life course theory into the study of cumulative inequality (Elder & Shanahan, 2006; Willson, Shuey, & Elder, 2007).

Cumulative Inequality Theory

Although our theoretical development draws heavily on the work of Dannefer (1987, 1988, 2003) and O'Rand (1996), we prefer to use a different name for this theoretical perspective: *cumulative inequality theory*. Our rationale for doing so is fivefold. First, the published record of CAD theory does not explicitly consider many elements that we deem essential to a theory for the study of cumulative inequality. One example that we articulate here is the intergenerational transmission of inequality. Thus, a slightly different phrase may help distinguish this articulation from the exemplary contributions of previous authors. Second, as is discussed, we think it is highly unlikely that cumulative advantage is the opposite of cumulative disadvantage. Whether the effect of disadvantage is parallel to that of advantage is an empirical question, but combining advantage and disadvantage in the name of the theory may be misleading. Third, cumulative inequality theory places the emphasis on system properties in generating inequality. Advantage and disadvantage are often seen as outcomes for given individuals, but the term *inequality* may help convey the importance of systemic properties in how individuals become stratified. Fourth, cumulative inequality theory gives explicit attention to *perceptions* of disadvantage rather than just the objective conditions of their situations, which has been the dominant approach in studies of accumulating disadvantage. Fifth, cumulative inequality is more concise than the phrase cumulative advantage/disadvantage.

We propose cumulative inequality as a middle-range theory—not derived from a single theory—but incorporating various theories in a synthetic way; it is, in Merton's (1968b) words, "consolidated into wider networks of theory" (p. 68). Cumulative inequality theory incorporates elements of macro- and microsociological content in an attempt to bridge both levels of analyses. Useful theories incorporate empirical generalizations and link hypotheses in a coherent framework. One of the ways to provide a coherent and useful framework is to develop axioms and propositions (Zetterberg, 1965).

To clarify what is meant by cumulative inequality (CI) theory, we offer five interrelated axioms—and propositions for each—that should facilitate both hypothesis testing and further development of the theory. We recognize that the axioms will be revised as empirical research accumulates and as others help illuminate theoretical linkages. The axioms are, nonetheless, a cogent way to articulate the essential elements of the theory and to direct future tests of it.

Social Systems Generate Inequality, Which Is Manifested Over the Life Course Through Demographic and Developmental Processes

Inequality is present in all societies, with some persons having more resources, opportunities, and influence than others. Although some viewpoints regard inequality as the result largely of personal action (human agency), we conceptualize the major antecedents of inequality as systematically structured. People make choices that influence inequality, but the choices available throughout the world are quite varied, signifying that human agency is "always constrained by the opportunities structured by social institutions and culture" (Elder, Johnson, & Crosnoe, 2003, p. 8). We will discuss human agency further, but we launch this axiom by recognizing the primacy of how inequality is systematically generated and, thereby, difficult to eliminate (Bourdieu, 1996).

Although many scholars recognize the existence of structural determinants of inequality, what CI theory adds is greater articulation of how these determinants are manifested through *demographic* and *developmental* processes. For this chapter, demographic processes refer to cohort-linked stimuli, events, and experiences. Developmental processes refer to age-linked stimuli, events, and experiences that can be observed in individuals. What may not be readily apparent, however, is that scores of scholars interpret these two sets of processes from a single indicator: age. Although gerontologists have long recognized that age is a crude indicator that is often confounded with period or cohort (the age–period–cohort [APC] confound), this fact often escapes the view of many studying how inequality accumulates over the life course.

As noted previously, inequality is systematically generated, and the cohort is a fundamental unit of social organization (Easterlin, 1987; Elder, 1974, 1998b). Not only do cohorts reflect the ages of persons who share a time of birth, but cohort membership marks population processes such as how large is the cohort into which a person is born and migration patterns. Cohorts also provide the context for development; they structure access to opportunity. Aging is highly dependent on social context, reflecting gene pools and social organization at that point in history.

Recognizing the demographic/developmental dialectic, CI theory holds that childhood conditions are important to adulthood. Based on research during the past decade, we now have compelling evidence that childhood conditions structure the life course. This is not just in terms of personality formation and stability but also in terms of achievement and well-being. Scholars have long seen the interconnectedness of life stages, but what has been most stimulating to this area of inquiry is whether early insults have long-term consequences. Are later-life outcomes dependent on childhood experiences? Does gestational health influence health in later life? The answers to these questions appear to be affirmative, but isolating the mechanisms for these long-term connections remains a matter of continuing inquiry (Barker, 2003; Holland et al., 2000; Irving & Ferraro, 2006).

Beyond childhood as a life stage, we assert that gerontologists would be wise to recognize that reproduction is a fulcrum for defining the life course trajectories and population aging. Missing from much of the discussion of cumulative disadvantage in gerontology is the pivotal role that reproduction plays in life course processes.

Puberty is widely accepted as a key biological step in the transition to adulthood, and reproduction is a marker for adulthood in many societies. But what follows reproduction? When we think of aging as a life stage of "growing older," we are probably referring to the *postreproductive* stage of life. There may be some arbitrariness to such demarcations of growing older, and the reproductive schedules of men and women are distinct. The point is that gerontologists would profit from greater attention to conceptualizing the reproductive period as a pivotal life phase (Waters, 2007), one that leads to nonlinearities in accumulation processes. In addition, CI theory privileges gender differences in the accumulation of inequality by noting the distinct processes for men and women that lead to inequality. Inequality exists *between* the sexes in part because of biology but *within* each sex because the accumulation processes are often distinct.

Biologists often refer to the postreproductive period as senescence. For instance, Spence (1989) describes senescence as "a term used to describe the group of deleterious effects that lead to a decrease in the efficient functioning of an organism with increasing age, and leads to an increased probability of death" (p. 8). This decrease in efficient functioning is most often attributed to an increase in molecular disorder (Hayflick, 1998). We think of defining the life course with more fluid boundaries but nonetheless feel that gerontologists should give greater attention to how the pre- and postreproductive stages of life sandwich the time during which individuals are able to reproduce.

As noted earlier, a major distinction between CAD and cumulative inequality theory is that the latter gives explicit attention to the intergenerational nature of inequality; family lineage is a major source of inequality (Pearlin, Schieman, Fazio, & Meersman, 2005; Wickrama, Conger, & Abraham, 2005). Despite the legacy of sociological research on the intergenerational transmission of inequality, we have not been able to identify systematic coverage of this topic in Dannefer's work on CAD. Angela O'Rand (2006), another major contributor to the development of the CAD theory, recently discussed "intergenerational flows of resources from older to younger members of the population" (p. 147), but we assert that the intergenerational nature of inequality is an *essential* element of how inequality is reproduced.

For instance, a growing body of research illuminates that many adult chronic diseases are the result of "longer-term consequences of the . . . complex accumulation and interaction, *across generations,* of early and later-life exposures" (Lynch & Smith, 2005, p. 2, emphasis added). Such statements challenge the notion of disadvantage starting and ending within one's lifetime, pointing instead to how inequality is passed across generations. We assert that family lineage is a major component of how social structures influence inequality over the life course.

Family lineage may influence the accumulation of inequality in many ways, but we identify four primary mechanisms: biological, social psychological, economic, and ecological. Biological processes are manifested via genetic and nutritional factors, social psychological via modeling and norms, economic via finances and wealth, and ecological via environmental and spatial arrangements. Any one of these mechanisms may be used to identify the influence of family lineage, but they frequently combine together.

Regardless of genetic background, ecology remains an important axis on which to advance the study of cumulative inequality. Ecological context is important as a mechanism for family lineage (e.g., shared environmental exposure), but this mechanism also unfolds over the life course. Moreover, status hierarchies are often correlated with spatial arrangements. For instance, poverty as a form of social disadvantage is often concentrated in geographic areas. Individuals of lower socioeconomic status tend to live in impoverished neighborhoods or rural areas that struggle to provide residents with social and economic resources, such as formal services or employment opportunities. Beyond the individual-level attribute of low income, there is the contextual effect of concentrated poverty that makes upward mobility more difficult to achieve. The bulk of the literature identifies hazards associated with segregation or poverty (Jackson, Anderson, Johnson, & Sorlie, 2000), but some forms of voluntary segregation may be associated with higher levels of social capital, which may be beneficial to physical and mental health (Lee & Ferraro, 2007). The point is that social systems generate inequality on multiple levels, and scientists are giving renewed attention to spatial effects in how inequalities develop.

Finally, multilevel models may have special utility for research on cumulative inequality. This should be straightforward with applying the contextual or clustered-observations model for analyzing how ecological forces shape inequality. A second application of multilevel models may be in dealing with the APC confound mentioned earlier. For time-specific social and behavioral phenomena, each factor may have important explanatory relevance, yet because of their linear dependency, each effect cannot be identified in standard applications of the general linear model. Yang and Land (2006) recently provided a solution for the APC confound by using a multilevel model approach, thereby allowing the analyst to examine explanatory factors at the level of age, period, and cohort and account for random variability at each level.

This is an important breakthrough for the study of cumulative inequality for at least two reasons. First, because social processes are inherently dynamic, inequalities take form over time. Time, as the APC challenge makes clear, however, occurs in multiple dimensions (biographical, historical, and generational time). A sound approach for studying age and inequality therefore must be very cautious in its a priori assumptions about differences between persons located within cohorts located within history and instead treat this multidimensionality as an empirical question. Second, the multilevel-model strategy makes statistically explicit the issue of heterogeneity by isolating the different levels of time and showing how much random variability exists at each level. A key assumption of cumulative inequality theory is that inequality is rooted in the structural components of social life, thus determining the extent of heterogeneity at age, period, and cohort levels.

Five propositions are developed from this axiom:

a. Childhood conditions are important to adulthood, especially when differences in experience or status emerge early in the life course.
b. Reproduction is a fulcrum for defining life course trajectories and population aging.
c. Influenced by genes and environment, family lineage is a key source of life course inequality, especially for the early stages of the life course.
d. Cohorts provide the context for development, structuring risks, and opportunities.
e. Given the confounding of age, period, and cohort, investigators should consider the inter- and intraindividual processes that lead to cumulative inequality and seek to explain variability on multiple levels and/or in multiple domains.

Table 22.1 summarizes each axiom and proposition and identifies relationships between CI theory and other theoretical perspectives. The table is intended not to be a comprehensive inventory but to identify key links in our development of CI theory. We cite mostly *theoretical* works that most closely link to our axioms and propositions, although the connections are less direct or nonexistent in some cases.

Disadvantage Increases Exposure to Risk, but Advantage Increases Exposure to Opportunity

The concepts of cumulative advantage and cumulative disadvantage have been used to explain the processes by which cohorts become differentiated and how the Matthew effect operates in shaping personal trajectories (Dannefer, 1988, 2003). Although Merton was focused on advantage, most applications of the concepts of cumulative advantage and disadvantage have focused on disadvantage or adversity (Hatch, 2005).

The underlying assumption for many scholars, however, has been that disadvantage and advantage accumulate inversely—the failure to accumulate advantage is presumed to be synonymous with the accumulation of disadvantage. Although this is possible, it may mask potential differences in the processes. Would we expect an *advantage* that is one standard deviation from the mean to have the same magnitude (absolute value) of an effect as a *disadvantage* one standard deviation from the mean? Most sociologists would likely attribute greater impact to *dis*advantages than to advantages. Thus, it may be useful to differentiate advantage from disadvantage, especially when testing differences in a quantitative variable. For instance, rather than treating income as continuous, Willson et al. (2007) found it useful to differentiate low income and high income

TABLE 22.1 Relationships Between Axioms and Propositions of Cumulative Inequality Theory and Other Theories or Perspectives

Axioms and propositions (abbreviated)	CAD (Dannefer, O'Rand)	Life course (Elder)	Other theories or perspective
1. *Social systems generate inequality—manifested over the life course via demographic and developmental processes.* a. Childhood conditions are important to adulthood, especially when differences in experience or status emerge early b. Reproduction is a fulcrum for defining life course trajectories and population aging c. Influenced by genes and environment, family lineage is critical to status differentiation early in the life course d. Cohorts provide the context for development, structuring risks and opportunities e. Consider inter- and intraindividual processes and use analytical techniques that explain variability on multiple levels or in multiple domains.	a. Health risks related to childhood disadvantage (O'Rand & Hamil-Luker, 2005) b. Family attributes affect health in later life; intergenerational flows of resources (O'Rand, 2003, 2006) c. Cohorts shape the reproduction of inequality (Dannefer, 2003; O'Rand, 1996) d. Inequality results from the interplay "between institutional arrangements and individual life trajectories" (O'Rand, 1996, p. 230).	a. Childhood conditions affect adult outcomes (Elder, 1998a; Elder & Johnson, 2003) b. Lives are interdependent (Elder & Johnson, 2003; Elder & Shanahan, 2006) c. Life course "embedded in and shaped by historical times and places" (Elder, 1998b, p. 3).	a. Childhood conditions are pivotal for life course development (Bronfenbrenner, 1979) b. The postreproductive period is characterized by less physiologic reserve (Waters, 2007) c. Inequality is transmitted across generations (Wickrama et al., 2005) d. Cohort flow is a vital process for age stratification (Riley et al. 1972) e. Multilevel models offer a rigorous way to account for the APC confound (Yang & Land, 2006).

(*continued*)

22.1 Relationships Between Axioms and Propositions of Cumulative Inequality Theory and Other Theories or Perspectives (*continued*)

Axioms and propositions (abbreviated)	CAD (Dannefer, O'Rand)	Life course (Elder)	Other theories or perspective
2. *Disadvantage increases exposure to risk, but advantage increases exposure to opportunity.* a. Consequences of advantage may not be the inverse of disadvantage b. Inequality may diffuse across life domains (e.g., health and wealth) c. Trajectories are affected by the onset, duration, and magnitude of exposures.	a. Disadvantage accumulates (Dannefer, 2003), leading to "other disadvantages" (O'Rand & Hamil-Luker, 2005, p. 117). Advantage arises via "cumulative process of differentiation" (Dannefer, 1988, p. 16) or a precocious work career (O'Rand, 1996).	a. Behavioral consequences can lead to "cumulating advantages and disadvantages" (Elder, 1998a, p. 7) b. Duration between transitions affects individual outcomes (Elder et al., 2003; Elder & Johnson, 2003).	a. Risks exist in chains (Kuh et al., 2003) b. Disadvantages lead to additional negative outcomes (George, 2003).
3. *Life course trajectories are shaped by accumulation of risk, available resources, and human agency.* a. Human agency and resource mobilization may modify trajectories b. Turning points in the life course may alter the anticipated consequences of a chain of risk c. The dialectic of human agency and social structure is essential to cumulative inequality	a. Modification of "cumulation processes" possible only within existing structural conditions (Dannefer, 1988, p. 16) b. Resource allocation shapes life course outcomes (Elman & O'Rand, 2004) c. Institutions, agency, and chance affect trajectories (O'Rand, 1996, 2003).	a. Resources and human agency affect trajectories (Elder & Shanahan, 2006; Hitlin & Elder, 2007) b. Study lives in motion (Elder, 1998a; Elder & Shanahan, 2006) c. Choice within structural constraints (Elder & Johnson, 2003) d. Resources affect rate of health change (Willson et al., 2007).	a. Social and biological resources can protect positive trajectories (Hatch, 2005) b. Personal agency affects stress management and social adjustment (Pearlin et al., 2005; Settersten, 1999; Thoits, 2006).

d. Unfavorable trajectories can be mitigated by the magnitude, onset, and duration of resources; resources can also accelerate favorable trajectories.			
4. *The perception of life trajectories influences subsequent trajectories.* a. Social comparisons shape trajectories b. Favorable life review linked to self-efficacy c. Perceived life course timing influences psychosomatic processes.		a. Perceptions of lived experience influence the life course (Elder & Shanahan, 2006).	a. Thomas theorem (Merton, 1995) b. Mastery shaped by status attainment, hardship, and coping (Pearlin et al., 2007).
5. *Cumulative inequality leads to premature mortality, perhaps giving the appearance of decreasing inequality in later life.* a. Cumulative inequality creates compositional change in a population b. Population truncation may give the appearance of decreasing inequality c. Test for selection effects d. Interpret results in light of event censoring and cohort inclusiveness.	a. Selective survival and sample attrition affect assessments of inequality in later life (O'Rand, 2003; O'Rand & Hamil-Luker, 2005) b. and d. Pseudovariable approach for predicted probabilities with incomplete data (O'Rand & Hamil-Luker, 2005).	a. Selective mortality complicates assessments of inequality (Willson et al., 2007) b. and d. Propensity scores to account for nonrandom selection (Willson et al., 2007).	a. Cohort flow is accompanied by cohort shrinkage (Riley et al., 1972) b. Magnitude of inequality affected by selective mortality (Noymer, 2001).

from a middling reference group, concluding that "long-term exposure to *advantage* produces more gradual rates of over-time health decline, while long-term exposure to *disadvantage* produces steeper rates of decline" (p. 1912, emphasis added). Viewed from an analytic perspective, there is value in testing for nonlinear relationships.

The distinction between advantage and disadvantage is also important because most people will simultaneously hold positions of advantage and disadvantage across life domains. A person may be economically advantaged but health disadvantaged nonetheless (or vice versa). Although disadvantages may cluster across a person's life, it is better to identify hierarchies within the multiple domains of the person's life rather than to presume omnibus disadvantage.

Although many scholars use the terms *disadvantage* and *risk* interchangeably, we draw a distinction here as well. We define *disadvantage* as an unfavorable position in a status hierarchy due to structural determinants and/or behavior that reflects the past and the present circumstances of one's life. By contrast, we refer to *risk* as the probability of a hazard or negative event occurring in the future. Once a risk eventuates in a negative outcome, it becomes a disadvantage; the pernicious cycle is that disadvantage heightens risk, which may lead to subsequent disadvantage. O'Rand and Hamil-Luker (2005) argue that "disadvantages lead to other disadvantages" (p. 117), and this is how many think of the phrase *cumulative disadvantage*. Although we agree with their statement, we believe that an important and logical next step is to identify the mechanisms by which disadvantage accumulates. We think it is useful to first conceive of disadvantage as increasing exposure to risks. This conceptualization provides room for resource mobilization and/or human agency to modify the process of how one disadvantage may lead to another (Settersten, 1999). Many trajectories have been reshaped by adequate resources and/or compensatory actions on the part of the person exposed to the risk (Thoits, 2006).

The mechanism specified herein is similar to a chain of risk as described in life course epidemiology. The concept of a *chain of risk* refers to "a sequence of linked exposures that raise disease risk because one bad experience or exposure tends to lead to another and then another" (Kuh, Ben-Shlomo, Lynch, Hallqvist, & Power, 2003, p. 779). Including risk in the conceptualization of how cumulative inequality operates also permits one to conveniently integrate findings regarding the onset and duration of exposures (Elder & Shanahan, 2006). When studying health, long-term exposure to risk is typically more important than short-term exposure, and this has been demonstrated in many studies such as exposure to low income (Willson et al., 2007) and obesity (Ferraro & Kelley-Moore, 2003; Schafer & Ferraro, 2007). The consequences of short-term risk exposure are more equivocal because onset can vary more than is the case for long-term risk exposure. Moreover, inequalities are shaped over the life course as a result of the magnitude, time of onset, and duration of exposures.

Disadvantages accumulate within specific life domains (e.g., health and wealth) but may also diffuse across domains. Negative health-related behaviors, for example, may raise the risk of disease, loss of income, and poor mental health. Given the tendency toward "stress proliferation—the propensity for stressors to multiply and 'spill over' into life domains beyond that in which the original stress occurred" (George, 2003, p. 170), it is likely that disadvantage in one domain may influence other areas in one's life (see also Pearlin et al., 2005).

Advantage, by contrast, refers to a favorable position in a status hierarchy. Although advantage may reduce risk exposure, there is another process that extends beyond risk reduction; advantage provides opportunities through distinct networks, resources, and prestige (i.e., Matthew effect). Opportunity refers to the probability of future achievement, and structural advantage provides greater opportunity. Seeding in tournaments is a simple illustration of this principle. Top-ranked competitors face the lowest-ranked opponents in the early rounds. Rankings do not guarantee success; they simply make it more likely.

One of the contributions from previous analyses of cumulative disadvantage is how it may alter the life course in enduring ways. Considerable variability exists in the consequences of disadvantage, which are usually negative (O'Rand, 2001) but can also be positive (e.g., health benefits of mild stress; Minois, 2000). Future research should identify how advantage and disadvantage shape opportunities and risks, which ultimately influence outcomes. Doing so requires attention to how life course trajectories are shaped and may be modified in an unanticipated way (i.e., two-tailed statistical tests). We should not underestimate the role of personal agency, especially for people who display resilience (Masten et al., 2004).

Three propositions may be articulated from this axiom:

a. The consequences of advantage may not be the inverse of the consequences of disadvantage.
b. Many individuals hold positions of both advantage and disadvantage across various life domains. Whereas inequality may diffuse across domains, it is useful to integrate additional life domains into studies of cumulative inequality (e.g., health and wealth).
c. Trajectories are shaped by the magnitude, time of onset, and duration of exposures. By magnitude, we refer to the degree to which an exposure deviates from a measure of central tendency (i.e., the severity or dose). (For exposure to physical activity, how do sedentary and athletic lifestyles compare to an average amount of activity?) By duration of exposure, we refer to the length of time that an individual experiences the condition (either risk or opportunity), and onset refers to when the exposure began.

As shown in Table 22.1, life course theorists and scholars in life course epidemiology have given priority to the concept of risk and opportunity exposure.

Life Course Trajectories Are Shaped by the Accumulation of Risk, Available Resources, and Human Agency

Trajectories do not develop in a vacuum; they are socially generated. We follow George's (2003) definition of trajectories as "long-term patterns of change and stability" (p. 162) that exist across a variety of outcomes. Thus, each person has many trajectories—examples include financial, functional, spiritual, and cognitive trajectories—and scientists seek to track change and stability within and between individuals on these outcomes. In physics, we think of a trajectory as the flight curve of a projectile. When an object remains in flight, we have the known trajectory (past) and a projection of the curve (future). Of course, outside forces may alter future movement. When major change occurs in a flight curve, we think of splines in the curve or inflection points to capture nonlinearities in the trajectory.

For example, one could argue that health is much more likely to change with transition points and nonlinearities; rarely does it proceed in a simple linear fashion, especially because illness onset often entails a social encounter. Thus, one way to conceptualize human trajectories is as a sequence of transitions (e.g., loss of functional capacity). This may also involve entry into and exit from different roles and "states" (Elder & Shanahan, 2006). Indeed, some transitions involve turning points that can redirect trajectories and contribute to life course discontinuities.

Rooted in social inequality, trajectories are strongly influenced by the accumulation of risk. As noted earlier, disadvantage increases exposure to risk, which, in turn, may lead to further disadvantage. Hence, the tenet *inequality accumulates*. Early disadvantage shapes the trajectory, most often bringing additional risks. As the risks accumulate, further disadvantage is likely to result unless measures are undertaken to offset the exposure to risks. A good start in life can have long-lasting effects for the individual and the cohort of which he or she is a member. This is not to say that the trajectory is fixed by early disadvantage, but that early disadvantage exposes one to additional risks—and early advantage provides additional opportunities (Easterlin, 1987).

A common approach to studying the enduring effects of resources is by testing an interaction term between age and the resource (e.g., Ross & Wu, 1996). This has been helpful for advancing research on cumulative inequality, but we think the research must move beyond this approach for at least two reasons. First, as described in axiom 5, such tests are highly dependent on sample composition and may be indicative of cohort rather than age (maturational) effects. Second, we assert that cumulative inequality is a more complex process than can be described with one interaction term, whether with cross-sectional or longitudinal data. We do not presume that the effect of early disadvantage is inexorable. Rather, a key question for the study of inequality is discovering which forces can alter the anticipated trajectory. (If not, what is the aim of public policy reform?) Although some may interpret cumulative disadvantage to require both the long-term effects of early disadvantage and heightened inequality in later life, we believe there are forces that can attenuate or counteract the consequences of early disadvantage, perhaps leading to reduced inequality. Chief among the modifying factors are available resources (Luthar, Cicchetti, & Becker, 2000; Merton, 1988; Schieman & Meersman, 2004).

Figure 22.1 is presented to illustrate how resource mobilization is critical to shaping trajectories—in this case how disability develops (Verbrugge & Jette, 1994). Although many studies of cumulative disadvantage focus on the long-term consequences of early disadvantage, we present five cases that begin at the same intercept but that diverge because of the onset and duration of resource mobilization. We contend that resource mobilization has the capacity to retard the disablement process, but rarely can it stop it during adulthood. In Figure 22.1, A represents the projected increase in disability without modification, B indicates late and short-lived resource mobilization, C indicates early and short-lived resource mobilization, D represents a trajectory affected by relatively late and sustained resource mobilization, and E represents early and sustained resource mobilization. These five trajectories were all disadvantaged

22.1

Illustration of disability pathways affected by the onset and duration of resource mobilization.

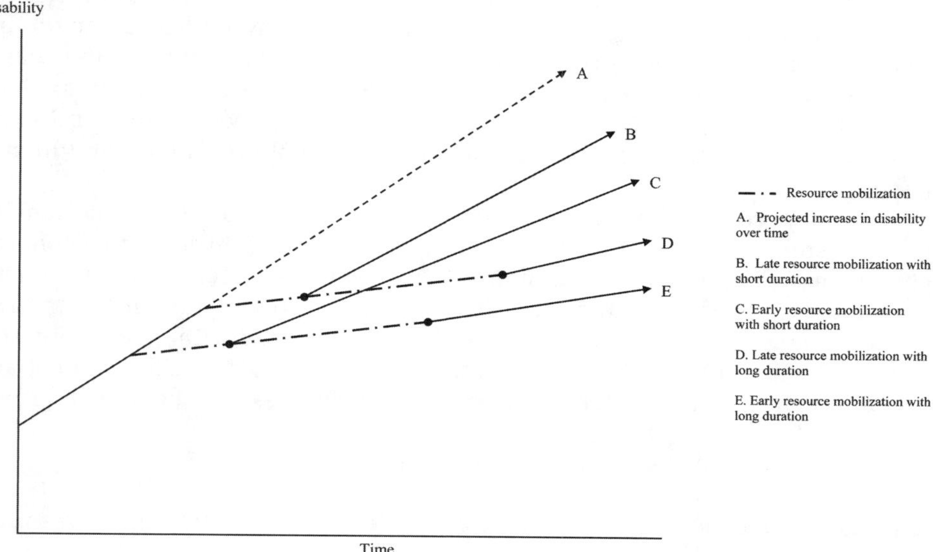

early, but their final observed levels of disability are affected by the timing of the resources—onset and duration. Moreover, in our illustration, the resource magnitude (or dose) was fixed. Parallel to axiom 2, however, we assert that unfavorable trajectories may be mitigated by the magnitude, onset, and duration of resources.

More generally, social, economic, and psychological resources can retard or accelerate trajectories. Individuals have a convoy of social relations over the life course, which may play a major role in shaping trajectories. Significant others help define situations and provide meaning for decisions over the life course. The information provided may not necessarily be correct or useful, but it helps define the situation, whether or not the person realizes it. Economic resources are recognized as the great compensator. As noted earlier, many tests of cumulative disadvantage theory have focused on the advantages experienced by persons with more education and higher incomes. Although financial resources are not the panacea for personal problems, they enable one to more easily resolve some disadvantages.

Psychological resources are also important in the development of trajectories, and there is a large literature on mind–body relations to underscore this assertion. If early disadvantage increases the likelihood of perceived failure, an individual may be less likely to envision overcoming the disadvantage. Conflict resolution, adaptation, and social participation are examples of important life course tasks, and psychological resources—both cognitive and emotional—are important for performing such tasks.

Structural influences are important for cumulative inequality theory (axiom 1), but axiom 3 counterbalances the structuralist view by considering the dialectic of structural forces and human agency. It is difficult to overstate the influence of structural forces, but neither should one neglect the influence of human agency (Hitlin & Elder, 2007). Some people face enormous disadvantage but emerge remarkably well by resource mobilization or by choosing wisely and/or expending extraordinary effort (Thoits, 2006). Such cases may be less common, but Black history in America provides exemplars to better understand the role of human agency against staggering odds (e.g., Rosa Parks). As stated in axiom 2, disadvantage increases exposure to risk, but axiom 3 is needed to identify trajectories as the product of risk accumulation, available resources, and human agency.

The importance of human agency in shaping trajectories is also manifest in the systematic study of resilience. For instance, living through the economic challenges of the Great Depression had a beneficial effect on mental health for middle-class women (Elder & Liker, 1982), and growing up during the Depression had a positive mental health effect on children with good adaptation (i.e., resilient) (Elder, 1974). Disadvantage is important, but social context and human agency may transform apparent disadvantages into beneficial effects (Thoits, 2006).

Four propositions are developed from this axiom:

a. Disadvantage accumulates, but trajectories may be altered by resource mobilization and/or human agency.
b. Turning points in the life course may alter the anticipated consequences of a chain of risk.
c. Human agency and social structure must be considered simultaneously in the development of the life course trajectories.
d. Unfavorable trajectories can be mitigated by the magnitude, onset, and duration of resources; resources can also accelerate favorable trajectories.

The Perception of Life Trajectories Influences Subsequent Trajectories

Although the word *trajectory* may not be used, most people are aware of the many changes they experience over the life course; it is their life story. Some persons may look at change in a shorter time frame, while others use more of a "wide-angle lens" for viewing their experiences. Indeed, lower socioeconomic status may be associated with a shorter-term horizon for conceptualizing change over one's life because of the financial exigencies of everyday living. Nevertheless, people have a sense that things are getting better, worse, or staying about the same. Cumulative inequality theory holds that perceptions of such change, whether positive or negative, are related to the subsequent shape of the trajectory (Carstensen, 2006).

In some ways, this may be viewed as an extension of proposition 3c (i.e., structure–agency dialectic), but it also incorporates elements of symbolic interactionism such as the Thomas theorem (Merton, 1995). People reflect on their lives, become aware of their place in hierarchies, and develop ways of thinking about their position in a social system. One's view of his or her status is *not* structurally determined. It can be understood only in light of the structure, but it is the perception of *relative* advantage or disadvantage that is most important. Actors seek meaning for their position, and the interconnectedness of human lives may predispose them to view their positions in ways that are parallel to their associates (Elder & Shanahan, 2006). Moreover, people seek out associates on the basis of their views, leading to homophily in reference groups.

The perception of upward socioeconomic mobility—real or imagined—may give a psychological lift to other perceptions of life course trajectories (Ennis, Hobfoll, & Schröder, 2000); see axiom 2b. The sense that one is doing better than one's parents, one's siblings, or one's own earlier experiences can be a source of confidence. If a person feels that his or her life is progressing at a good pace (e.g., ahead of one's cohort), this may be cause for attempting more ambitious activities or "coasting" after a gain has been reaped. Several studies show that perceptions of one's socioeconomic standing are better predictors of health than are objective measures of status (e.g., Sapolsky, 2004). In addition, perceptions of unmet need, regardless of actual need, have the power to elevate mortality risk (Blazer, Sachs-Ericsson, & Hybels, 2005).

School and family reunions are occasions that prompt evaluations of personal change, an opportunity to benchmark accomplishments. Pivot ages, such as 18, 21, 50, and 65, encourage one to consider life changes. The evaluations in the early years are more likely to be linked to occupational status achievement, while those in middle and later life are more likely geared to health issues or the status achievement of children. These evaluations are an important part of one's sense of achievement, and negative evaluations may initiate psychosomatic processes.

The sense of progress toward the "good life"—or the lack thereof—is consequential to well-being. A feeling of a lack of progress may stimulate one to work harder or, alternatively, to cut back on efforts to get ahead. In the latter case, believing that "the system" cannot be beat may lead to a type of fatalism, perhaps even a sense of resignation. In common vernacular, some people feel the wind in their face and slow down; others push harder into it. Social, economic, and psychological resources influence this disposition, but awareness of one's past trajectory is an important part of determining the shape of the future (Pearlin, Nguyen, Schieman, & Milkie, 2007).

There is a fairly substantial literature regarding how affective states influence health (e.g., Ryff, Singer, & Love, 2004; Steptoe, Wright, Kunz-Ebrecht, & Iliffe, 2006). Scores of studies show that dispositional optimism is correlated with health behaviors but that it has independent effects on health beyond simply avoiding behaviors such as smoking and excessive calorie consumption. Unfavorable life reviews, therefore, are likely to lead to more hopelessness and pessimism, which in turn have been shown to elevate mortality risk among older people (Stern, Dhanda, & Hazuda, 2001). We see both a direct effect of optimism on health as well as an indirect effect via selective participation in behaviors that can aid or compromise health.

Three propositions are derived from this axiom:

a. Personal review of the life course entails social comparisons about progress on trajectories.
b. A favorable review of a trajectory is associated with self-efficacy.
c. The sense of one's life course timing may influence psychosomatic processes.

As shown in Table 22.1, Elder and Shanahan (2006) contend that perceptions of lived experience are consequential over the life course. Dannefer and Uhlenberg (1999) acknowledge the symbolic interest of life course scholars but do not discuss how perceptions of life trajectories influence subsequent trajectories.

Cumulative Inequality May Lead to Premature Mortality; Therefore, Nonrandom Selection May Give the Appearance of Decreasing Inequality in Later Life

A basic premise of cumulative inequality theory is that inequality is consequential over the life course. Although it may be beneficial for some persons, especially those who are socially advantaged or possess a higher-than-average level of psychological resources (e.g., resiliency), cumulative inequality is likely to be deleterious for those who are structurally disadvantaged or exposed to many risks. If the risks accumulate to influence health, then accumulated disadvantage will result in premature mortality. Indeed, dozens of epidemiologic investigations show the importance of how social inequality is linked to mortality (Jackson et al., 2000). As Willson et al. (2007) recently concluded, "The process of cumulative inequality in health is shaped by the finite nature of the human life span and confronts forces of senescence and mortality over time" (p. 1892).

Although it may seem pedantic that social inequality is related to mortality risk, the consequences of this may not be fully appreciated. The difficulty exists in that the premature mortality associated with accumulated risks—selective survival—will result in *compositional change to a population.* Cohorts shrink in a nonrandom manner, leading some to refer to this process as leveling population heterogeneity. Moreover, it is possible that "cohort inversion" may occur: a cohort that was initially disadvantaged may appear better than before because mortality selection will remove persons with the most health problems from the population. Thus, mean scores may rise, giving the appearance of decreasing inequality (Noymer, 2001).

When characterizing an older adult population, it is tempting to refer to it as beset by disease, disability, and depression. Assuredly, these and other health-related outcomes are present, but the older adult population that survives may also be described as an elite—at least in comparison to those members of its cohort who died earlier. Perhaps more than any other distinguishing characteristic, the fact that advanced age represents survival speaks to the compositional change as cohorts age.

Both demographers and proponents of age stratification theory have long noted the importance of cohort shrinkage when interpreting the aging process (Riley, Johnson, & Foner, 1972). A recent article by Dupre (2007) uses multilevel models to effectively separate changes due to sample compositional from those due to the individual-level trajectory. His findings reveal that two hypotheses that have long been seen as competing—cumulative disadvantage and aging as leveler—are actually complementary. In studying the relationship between education and disease, Dupre found that compositional change led to a leveling of differences but that individual-level processes reflected cumulative disadvantage. This is a promising way to consider the importance of both compositional change and individual trajectories, reflecting the demographic and developmental processes involved in the accumulation of inequality (axiom 1).

It is also important to recognize more generally that special care needs to be given to interpreting the findings of cohort-centric studies designed to test cumulative inequality. Previous tests of cumulative disadvantage have been performed on samples of various ages; examples include 22 to 42 (Elman & O'Rand, 2004), 25 to 74 (Dupre, 2007), and 65 to 74 (Holland et al., 2000). The diversity in designs is good, but what if inconsistent findings on the same topic emerge from cohort-inclusive and cohort-centric studies? Although one may be drawn to the cohort-inclusive study for more compelling results, that study would have greater opportunity for nonrandom selection to be observed. If the investigators examined and tested for how the nonrandom mortality might shape the conclusions, the cohort-inclusive study may be preferred. If the investigators fail to account to selective mortality, however, there is probably a greater chance to be misled by the cohort-inclusive study. If nonrandom mortality is substantial, this may give the appearance of decreasing inequality.

Nonrandom mortality selection speaks more generally to the concept of event censoring. We assert that left and/or right censoring of events is critical to interpretations of cumulative inequality. For example, the Longitudinal Study on Aging II is a national sample of persons 70 years or older and contains exemplary information on functional limitations and disability. If one used this study to examine Black/White differences in disability, the higher mortality risk among Black people may make it more difficult to observe cumulative inequality because frail Black persons would likely be eliminated from the analysis. This may give the appearance of little or no racial difference in disability.

The issues of selection bias and event censoring are keener when one recognizes that surveys and experiments often add another layer of nonrandom selection. If experiments rely on volunteer subjects, the bias is often obvious. Even for surveys, however, the *ability to respond* is a favorable attribute. Persons in institutions and those physically or cognitively unable to respond to survey questions are often excluded. For longitudinal studies, the situation is even more complicated because continued availability and willingness to respond likely results in a positive bias in the sample subjects who provide the most data. Indeed, longitudinal research demonstrates how subjects with complete data often have less disease, disability, and depression at the study's start than those with incomplete data (Kelley-Moore & Ferraro, 2005).

All these processes converge to truncate a sample, and much of the truncation is probably due to social inequality. If inequality-induced truncation is operant, the distribution of inequality itself is bound to change over time. As such, it is likely that both population and sample truncation will result in the *appearance* of decreasing inequality in middle or later life. Investigators need to account for nonrandom selection in their generalizations regarding the effects of cumulative inequality on what may appear to be an increasingly select population and sample. With cohort shrinkage, investigators also need to test for statistical power to be certain that the lack of significant relationships is not due to insufficient power.

Four propositions are derived from this axiom:

a. Cumulative inequality will likely result in compositional change as a population ages; the greater the inequality, the more compositional change will transpire.

b. Population truncation and nonrandom selection in samples may give the appearance of decreasing inequality.
c. Studies of cumulative inequality should apply methods to test and, if need be, account for nonrandom selection.
d. The limitations of cohort-centric studies of cumulative inequality, especially if carried out within a narrow historic period, should be clearly identified. Scholars should attend to how event censoring may constrain conclusions.

As shown in Table 22.1, O'Rand (2003) and Willson et al. (2007) identify how selective survival and sample attrition may influence the assessment of inequality in later life.

Conclusion

Sociologists have long been interested in the pervasive and enduring effects of disadvantage such as poverty or child abuse. Research shows that such adversities may continue to affect individuals throughout the life course and that the disadvantage may compound over time. This is especially the case when the disadvantage is experienced early in life and/or when the available resources at the time of the original experience are not sufficient to compensate for the potential negative effects. In this context, we seek to better explain how inequality accumulates.

The five axioms and 19 propositions were presented to articulate a theory to explain core processes of how inequality accumulates over the life course. Cumulative disadvantage has proved to be an intriguing model of stratification processes, but we sought to provide greater formality to the model in order to develop a theoretical perspective with more elements subject to falsification.

We have drawn from cumulative disadvantage, life course, and other theoretical perspectives to synthesize a framework that provides new insights into the development of cumulative inequality. Part of our effort has been to seek points of integration between CAD and life course theory. Although the former is focused on population and cohort differentiation (Hagestad & Dannefer, 2001), we believe that much can be gained by the synthesis outlined herein. In doing so, cumulative inequality theory privileges the structural generation of inequality but counterbalances it with the structure–agency dialectic. Moreover, we do not view cumulative inequality as solely disparities in outcomes; rather, we view it as the process that leads to disparities in outcomes across the life course.

Note

1. Sociologists have shown keen interest in the concepts of cumulative advantage and disadvantage. This has been manifest in the study of earnings (Crystal & Shea, 1990), crime (Sampson & Laub, 1997), disease (Dupre, 2007), and health (Ross & Wu, 1996) as well as in DiPrete and Eirich's (2006) recent review of how cumulative advantage operates as a mechanism for inequality. Dale Dannefer (1987, 2003) has been one of the major architects of what he refers to as cumulative advantage/disadvantage theory (CAD) for understanding life course inequality and growing heterogeneity in later life. He defines CAD as the "systematic tendency for interindividual divergence in a given characteristic (e.g., money, status) with the passage of time" (Dannefer, 2003, p. 327). His focus has been on "a set of social dynamics that operate on a population, not individuals" (Douthit & Dannefer, 2007, p. 224).

References

Barker, D. J. (2003). *The best start in life.* London: Century.

Blazer, D. G., Sachs-Ericsson, N., & Hybels, C. F. (2005). Perceptions of unmet basic needs as a predictor of mortality among community-dwelling older adults. *American Journal of Public Health, 95,* 299–304.

Bourdieu, P. (1996). *The state nobility.* Stanford, CA: Stanford University Press.

Bronfenbrenner, U. (1979). *The ecology of human development: Experiments by nature and design.* Cambridge, MA: Harvard University Press.

Carstensen, L. L. (2006). The influence of a sense of time on human development. *Science, 312,* 1913–1915.

Crystal, S., & Shea, D. (1990). Cumulative advantage, cumulative disadvantage, and inequality among elderly people. *The Gerontologist, 30,* 437–443.

Dannefer, D. (1987). Aging as intracohort differentiation: Accentuation, the Matthew effect, and the life course. *Sociological Forum, 2,* 211–236.

Dannefer, D. (1988). Differential gerontology and the stratified life course: Conceptual and methodological issues. In G. L. Maddox & M. P. Lawton (Eds.), *Annual review of gerontology and geriatrics* (Vol. 8, pp. 3–36). New York: Springer Publishing.

Dannefer, D. (2003). Cumulative advantage/disadvantage and the life course: Cross-fertilizing age and the social science theory. *Journal of Gerontology: Social Sciences, 58,* S327–S337.

Dannefer, D., & Uhlenberg, P. (1999). Paths of the life course: A typology. In V. L. Bengtson & K. W. Schaie (Eds.), *Handbook of theories of aging* (pp. 306–327). New York: Springer Publishing.

DiPrete, T. A., & Eirich, G. M. (2006). Cumulative advantage as a mechanism for inequality: A review of theoretical and empirical developments. *Annual Review of Sociology, 32,* 271–297.

Douthit, K. Z., & Dannefer, D. (2007). Social forces, life course consequences: Cumulative disadvantage and "getting Alzheimer's." In J. M. Wilmoth & K. F. Ferraro (Eds.), *Gerontology: Perspectives and issues* (pp. 223–243). New York: Springer Publishing.

Dupre, M. E. (2007). Educational differences in age-related patterns of disease: Reconsidering the cumulative disadvantage and age-as-leveler hypotheses. *Journal of Health and Social Behavior, 48,* 1–15.

Easterlin, R. A. (1987). *Birth and fortune: The impact of numbers on personal welfare* (2nd ed.). Chicago: University of Chicago Press.

Elder, G. H., Jr. (1974). *Children of the great depression: Social change in life experience.* Chicago: University of Chicago Press.

Elder, G. H., Jr. (1998a). The life course and human development. In W. Damon & R. M. Lerner (Eds.), *Handbook of child psychiatry: Vol. 1. Theoretical models of human development* (5th ed., pp. 939–991). New York: Wiley.

Elder, G. H., Jr. (1998b). The life course as developmental theory. *Child Development, 69,* 1–12.

Elder, G. H., Jr., & Johnson, M. K. (2003). The life course and aging: Challenges, lessons, and new directions. In R. A. Settersten, Jr. (Ed.), *Invitation to the life course: Toward new understandings of later life* (pp. 49–81). Amityville, NY: Baywood Publishing.

Elder, G. H., Jr., Johnson, M. K., & Crosnoe, R. (2003). The emergence and development of life course theory. In J. T. Mortimer & M. J. Shanahan (Eds.), *Handbook of the life course* (pp. 3–19). New York: Kluwer Academic/Plenum Press.

Elder, G. H., Jr., & Liker, J. K. (1982). Hard times in women's lives: Historical influences across forty years. *American Journal of Sociology, 88,* 241–269.

Elder, G. H., Jr., & Shanahan, M. J. (2006). The life course and human development. In R. E. Lerner (Ed.), *Handbook of child psychology: Theoretical models of human development* (6th ed., pp. 665–715). New York: Wiley.

Elman, C., & O'Rand, A.M. (2004). The race is to the swift: Childhood adversity, adult education, and economic attainment. *American Journal of Sociology, 110,* 123–160.

Ennis, N. E., Hobfoll, S. E., & Schröder, K. E. E. (2000). Money doesn't talk, it swears: How economic stress and resistance resources impact inner-city women's depressive mood. *American Journal of Community Psychology, 28,* 149–173.

Ferraro, K. F., & Kelley-Moore, J. A. (2003). Cumulative disadvantage and health: Long term consequences of obesity? *American Sociological Review, 68,* 707–729.

George, L. K. (2003). What life-course perspectives offer the study of aging and health. In R. A. Settersten, Jr. (Ed.), *Invitation to the life course: Toward new understandings of later life* (pp. 161–188). Amityville, NY: Baywood Publishing.

Hagestad, G. O., & Dannefer, D. (2001). Concepts and theories of aging: Beyond microfication in social science approaches. In R. H. Binstock & L. K. George (Eds.), *Handbook of aging and the social sciences* (5th ed., pp. 3–21). San Diego, CA: Academic Press.

Hatch, S. L. (2005). Conceptualizing and identifying cumulative adversity and protective resources: Implications for understanding health inequalities. *Journal of Gerontology: Social Sciences, 60,* S130–S134.

Hayflick, L. (1998). How and why we age. *Experimental Gerontology, 33,* 639–653.

Hitlin, S., & Elder, G. H., Jr. (2007). Agency: An empirical model of an abstract concept. In R. MacMillan (Ed.), *Constructing adulthood: Agency and subjectivity in adolescence and adulthood, advances in life course research* (Vol. 11, pp. 36–67). New York: Elsevier.

Holland, P., Berney, L., Blane, D., Smith, G. D., Gunnell, D. J., & Montgomery, S. M. (2000). Life course accumulation of disadvantage: Childhood health and hazard exposure during adulthood. *Social Science and Medicine, 50,* 1285–1295.

Irving, S. M., & Ferraro, K. F. (2006). Reports of abusive experiences during childhood and adult health ratings: Personal control as a pathway? *Journal of Aging and Health, 18,* 458–485.

Jackson, S., Anderson, R., Johnson, N., & Sorlie, P. D. (2000). The relation of residential segregation to all-cause mortality: A study in black and white. *American Journal of Public Health, 90,* 615–617.

Kelley-Moore, J. A., & Ferraro, K. F. (2005). A 3-D model of health decline: Disease, disability, and depression among Black and White older adults. *Journal of Health and Social Behavior, 46,* 376–391.

Kuh, D., Ben-Shlomo Y., Lynch, J., Hallqvist, J., & Power, C. (2003). Life course epidemiology. *Journal of Epidemiology and Community Health, 57,* 778–783.

Lee, M.-A., & Ferraro, K. F. (2007). Neighborhood residential segregation and physical health among Hispanic Americans: Good, bad, or benign? *Journal of Health and Social Behavior, 48,* 131–148.

Luthar, S. S., Cicchetti, D., & Becker, B. (2000). The construct of resilience: A critical evaluation and guidelines for future work. *Child Development, 71,* 543–562.

Lynch, J., & Smith, G. D. (2005). A life course approach to chronic disease epidemiology. *Annual Review of Public Health, 26,* 1–35.

Masten, A. S., Burt, K. B., Roisman, G. I., Obradovic, J., Long, J. D., & Tellegen, A. (2004). Resources and resilience in the transition to adulthood: Continuity and change. *Development and Psychopathology, 16,* 1071–1094.

Merton, R. K. (1968a). The Matthew effect in science: The reward and communication systems of science are considered. *Science, 159,* 56–63.

Merton, R. K. (1968b). *Social theory and social structure.* New York: Free Press.

Merton, R. K. (1988). The Matthew effect in science, II: Cumulative advantage and the symbolism of intellectual property. *Isis, 79,* 606–623.

Merton, R. K. (1995). The Thomas theorem and the Matthew effect. *Social Forces, 74,* 379–424.

Minois, N. (2000). Longevity and aging: Beneficial effects of exposure to mild stress. *Biogerontology, 1,* 15–29.

Noymer, A. (2001). Mortality selection and sample selection: A comment on Beckett. *Journal of Health and Social Behavior, 42,* 326–327.

O'Rand, A. M. (1996). The precious and the precocious: Understanding cumulative disadvantage and cumulative advantage over the life course. *Gerontologist, 36,* 230–238.

O'Rand, A. M. (2001). Stratification and the life course: The forms of life-course capital and their interrelationships. In R. H. Binstock & L. K. George (Eds.), *Handbook of aging and the social sciences* (5th ed., pp. 197–217). San Diego, CA: Academic Press.

O'Rand, A. M. (2003). Cumulative advantage theory in life course research. In S. Crystal & D. F. Shea (Eds.), *Annual review of gerontology and geriatrics: Focus on economic outcomes in later life* (Vol. 22, pp. 14–30). New York: Springer Publishing.

O'Rand, A. M. (2006). Stratification and the life course: Life course capital, life course risks, and social inequality. In R. H. Binstock & L. K. George (Eds.), *Handbook of aging and the social sciences* (6th ed., pp. 145–162). Boston: Academic Press.

O'Rand, A. M., & Hamil-Luker, J. (2005). Processes of cumulative adversity: Childhood disadvantage and increased risk of heart attack across the life course. *Journal of Gerontology: Social Sciences, 60,* 117–124.

Pearlin, L. I., Nguyen, K., Schieman, S., & Milkie, M. (2007). The life course origins of mastery among older people. *Journal of Health and Social Behavior, 48,* 164–179.

Pearlin, L. I., Schieman, S., Fazio, E. M., & Meersman, S. C. (2005). Stress, health, and the life course: Some conceptual perspectives. *Journal of Health and Social Behavior, 46,* 205–219.

Riley, M. W., Johnson, M., & Foner A. (1972). *Aging and society: Vol. 3. A sociology of age stratification.* New York: Russell Sage Foundation.

Ross, C. E., & Wu, C.-L. (1996). Education, age, and the cumulative advantage in health. *Journal of Health and Social Behavior, 37,* 104–120.

Ryff, C. D., Singer, B. H., & Love, G. D. (2004). Positive health: Connecting well-being with biology. *Philosophical Transactions of the Royal Society of London, 359,* 1383–1394.

Sampson, R. J., & Laub, J. H. (1997). A life-course theory of cumulative disadvantage and the stability of delinquency. In T. P. Thornberry (Ed.), *Developmental theories of crime and delinquency* (pp. 133–161). New Brunswick, NJ: Transaction.

Sapolsky, R. M. (2004). Social status and health in humans and other animals. *Annual Review of Anthropology, 33,* 393–418.

Schafer, M. H., & Ferraro, K. F. (2007). Obesity and hospitalization over the adult life course: Does duration of exposure increase use? *Journal of Health and Social Behavior, 48,* 434–449.

Schieman, S., & Meersman, S. S. (2004). Neighborhood problems and health among older adults: Received and donated social support and the sense of mastery as effect modifiers. *Journal of Gerontology: Social Sciences, 59,* S89–S97.

Settersten, R. A. (1999). *Lives in time and place: The problems and promises of developmental science.* Amityville, NY: Baywood Publishing.

Spence, A. P. (1989). *Biology of human aging.* Englewood Cliffs, NJ: Prentice Hall.

Steptoe, A., Wright, C., Kunz-Ebrecht, S. R., & Iliffe, S. (2006). Dispositional optimism and health behaviour in community-dwelling older people: Associations with healthy ageing. *British Journal of Health Psychology, 11,* 71–84.

Stern, S. L., Dhanda, R., & Hazuda, H. P. (2001). Hopelessness predicts mortality in older Mexican and European Americans. *Psychosomatic Medicine, 63,* 344–351.

Thoits, P. A. (2006). Personal agency in the stress process. *Journal of Health and Social Behavior, 47,* 309–323.

Turner, J. H. (1982). *The structure of sociological theory.* Belmont, CA: Wadsworth.

Verbrugge, L. M., & Jette, A. M. (1994). The disablement process. *Social Science and Medicine, 38,* 1–14.

Waters, D. J. (2007). Cellular and organismal aspects of senescence and longevity. In J. M. Wilmoth & K. F. Ferraro (Eds.), *Gerontology: Perspectives and issues* (pp. 59–87). New York: Springer Publishing.

Wickrama, K. A. S., Conger, R. D., & Abraham, W. T. (2005). Early adversity and later health: The intergenerational transmission of adversity through mental disorder and physical illness. *Journal of Gerontology: Social Sciences, 60,* S125–S129.

Willson, A. E., Shuey, K. M., & Elder, G. H., Jr. (2007). Cumulative advantage processes as mechanisms of inequality in life course health. *American Journal of Sociology, 112,* 1886–1924.

Yang Y., & Land, K. C. (2006). A mixed models approach to the age-period-cohort analysis of repeated cross-section surveys, with an application to data on trends in verbal test scores. *Sociological Methodology, 36,* 75–98.

Zetterberg, H. L. (1965). *On theory and verification in sociology.* Stockholm: Almqvist & Wiksell.

Theorizing Lifestyle: Exploring Agency and Structure in the Life Course

23

Jon Hendricks
Laurie Russell Hatch

Importance of Lifestyle in Social Gerontology

The literature in social gerontology is replete with references to the effect of lifestyles on the experience of aging. In many of these works, lifestyle is used in a rather vague and generic fashion. Other approaches are more precise but vary widely in how the concept is defined, ranging from characteristic modes of being in the world to those quotidian routines of daily life that make up experience, undergird identity, and portend future possibilities. Ambiguities notwithstanding, lifestyles are far more portentous than might meet the eye and deserve thoughtful conceptualization and integration into the theoretical explication of life course experience.

Important contributions for such a project come from early social theorists as well as contemporary writers. The explication of lifestyles as explanatory frameworks in social science can be traced to the early 20th century, advancing industrialism, and the insights of Max Weber in particular. A Weberian approach to lifestyle conceives of an intrinsic connection between status groupings, styles of living, and life consequences (Weber, 1978). Weber relied on his conceptualizations of status groups and of lifestyles to draw a connection between denizens of particular social niches and normative experiences characteristic of that niche. Reaching beyond a focus on social class predicated on contributions to productivity, Weber identified status groups based on shared practices or styles of living, including both material and symbolic consumption, and other forms of conduct that connote collective social identities. He then relied on a canon of shared lifestyles to explicate social differentiation grounded in social location while leaving room for individual preference (Cockerham, Rutten, & Abel, 1997). Because of the communal and reciprocal nature of lifestyles, incumbents of a particular social setting develop elements of trust, normative expectations, sequencing, association, preference, and consensual worldviews (Weber, 1978). To draw on a concept from Durkheim, lifestyles promote within group cohesion, both reflecting and contributing to collective consciousness and to identifiable patterns of social differentiation. Lifestyles hence are seen as both cause and consequence of social differentiation, creating symbolic boundaries and communal conventions that connote membership groups (Katz-Gerro, 2006).

Among contemporary theorists, some writers have placed greater emphasis on structural groundings for lifestyle, whereas others have focused on individual choice. For example, Bourdieu (1990) stands out for his structural focus, emphasizing social capital and personal resources derived from a combination of structural locale and interpersonal relations. In contrast, Featherstone (1991) considers how lifestyle reflects personal tastes, self-expression, and personal identity, which also spawn behavioral choices and reaction patterns. This is not to say that contemporary theorists treat social structure and human agency as reverse sides of a coin; some writers, such as Giddens (1991), explicitly address the complex interconnections between structure and agency. In this regard, Giddens refers to the unity that both results in and derives from lifestyles and also to how shared lifestyles reproduce, unify, and channel individual choices.

From a sociological perspective, lifestyles encompass connections to collectivities of one or another type. By virtue of membership in definable social categories, actors find themselves with both shared preferences and characteristic modes of consumption regardless of whether these commonalities rise to the level of consciousness (Katz-Gerro, 2006). These issues are further explicated here.

In this chapter, we intend to take up the cudgel, outlining constitutive elements of lifestyles that must be considered when theorizing about their influence on life experiences, and how together these factors help shape the life course and ultimately old age. We begin by addressing how agency and structure have been conceptualized in the literature, including how these concepts have been linked to lifestyle via life choices and life chances. We then review some of the ways in which lifestyles have been conceived and utilized in social sciences explanations of aging, focusing especially on the health-related research traditions that have made up much of the aging and lifestyle literature to date. As will be evident in this chapter, the lion's share of attention in this literature has been on human agency; tensions and interplay between human agency and social structures often are unacknowledged or given short shrift.

We believe that lifestyles are helpful in elucidating the connection between human agency and social structures. In the final sections of the chapter, we outline dimensions of personal resources that undergird actors' perceptions of the choices and options that are available to them. These resources derive from actors' psychophysical capital; from their interpersonal relationships, family, and social capital broadly; as well as from actors' fiduciary resources, which encompass material as well as symbolic forms of exchange. We note how gender, ethnicity, and other socially important forms of diversity influence the resources available to and perceived by actors. Broadly, resources afforded or delimited by membership in recognized social categories are embedded within the public sphere and help to shape actors' life chances and pathways to and through old age—or, in other words, "lifestyle."

Lifestyle, Structure, and Agency

Issues of structure and agency are among those elusive concepts that have long riven social science, as far back to the 19th century at least. Interestingly, there is little consensus regarding what either structure or agency mean. Both are widely used and seemingly provide essential insights into experience. Let us consider each in turn.

Social structures are widely viewed as enduring institutional arrangements that give recognizable form to a group or society. As used in sociology, structure also refers to systems of beliefs, utile ideational processes and expectations that stem from collective experience and reinforce a sense of unity. It should be emphasized that structures do imply interrelationships, however, for they depend on their correlative position for their definition. For scholars working in a Durkheimian tradition, structures exert suzerainty over individual actors. Regardless of whether structure is taken to mean institutional provisions or relational arrangements, it does refer to collectivities standing independently of individuals yet internalized by individuals and shaping their worldviews. In a manner of speaking, structural circumstances can also be conceived of as resources providing a form of social capital available to actors as they make their way in the world.

The school of social theorizing known as structuralism emphasizes collective arrangements over personal volition in what is virtually a deterministic fashion (Sewell, 1992; Stones, 2006). Poststructuralism modifies that perspective considerably and highlights the internalization and reproduction of collective perspectives through the actions of actors. Giddens (1990), for example, conceived of the melding of structure and actors' actions in terms of what he called "structuration," meaning that there is no polarity between these phenomena but rather a reciprocal generativity. In phrasing that may sound slightly more familiar, Gordon and Longino (2000) alluded to personal regimes as "institutions writ small."

Agency, in turn, is generally believed to reside in the exercise of volition by individual actors or sometimes groups. That is not to say that individuals or groups act volitionally without being grounded in particular circumstances or by drawing from repertoires of plausible actions normatively sanctioned by their affinity groups. Agency or constructionist (and interactionist) theorizing tends to emphasize the production and reproduction of knowledge and interpretation, noting that actors do so with intentionality, practical consciousness, or habitus. Giddens's (1990, 1991) efforts to bridge the bifurcation of structure and agency are again helpful in this regard. Giddens notes that how actors interpret the world depends on where they stand in that world—that position permeates all aspects of an individual's life and is leavened into self-concepts and identity.

Some skeptics have referred to agency as a "red herring"—not really identifiable (Loyal & Barnes, 2000). There are of course a great many phenomena that are not readily identified, but that does not make them any less real. Obviously, part of the difficulty is that both agency and structure are abstractions that cannot be observed (King & Calasanti, in press). As Katz and Laliberte-Rudman (2005) point out, agency has been conceptualized in terms of subjectivity and reflexivity, empowerment, and personal choice, whereas structure has most often been used to refer to matters of constraint, domination, and macrolevel social reproduction.

As we alluded to at the beginning of this chapter, it would be a misperception to assume there is not a closer linkage between these phenomena and not necessarily a bifurcation at all. For example, Lockwood (1966) provides valuable insight when he points out that most actors visualize the societies to which they belong from the vantage point of their own milieus and their own experience. In so doing, he gave an explicit theoretical nod to the importance of agency and how identity and lifestyle provide the tie between structure and agency (Crompton, 1998; Katz & Laliberte-Rudman, 2005). In a manner of speaking, lifestyle may be thought of as a starting place of security, of surety, of direction, of anticipated futures.

Gubrium and Holstein (1995) resonate with Lockwood's line of reasoning as they point out that the accounts individuals create of themselves are shaped by their social locations and, we would add, the lifestyles that accrete as a result of those locations and the attendant resources configuring life chances (cf. Giddens, 1990; Katz & Laliberte-Rudman, 2005). In her prophetic assessment of issues of identity, Kauffman (1993) also speaks to the same point when she notes that shared meanings deriving from what Weber termed status groupings color how individuals see and interpret their worlds. Kauffman's contention—and that of Bourdieu—was that the ideational or cultural resources inherent in social categories are the source of lifestyles, habitus, and praxis that give rise to sense of self, social identity, and social reproduction.

Life Choices and Agency

The contention that actors are proactively agentic has been part of social science theorizing since the beginning, but there is a renewed interest in personal agency and its connection to perception, interaction, and objectivity running through early 21st-century social science. Weber himself recognized that individuals make choices, though in his opinion those choices are constrained by their membership alignments and shared lifestyles. Lewin's (1939) field theory and later Bronfenbrenner's (1979) work on the ecological context of human development follow in this same tradition but conceive of individual volition and action at the core of the ecological context and operating as a "perceiving unit" filtering environmental input in terms of an actor's priorities, mastery, and manipulation of his or her milieu. That is to say, "The self is the relational nexus to which all interaction and perception is perceived" (Hendricks, 1999, p. 189). It is as though there is an interpretive lens or practical consciousness operating, governed by the self-relevance of events and occurrences.

Hence, actors respond in accord with their intentional consciousness, selecting plausible courses based on their experiences and their anticipated futures as informed by their projects at hand. Interestingly, there is an importunate tendency to not attribute agency to older actors, even when allowing agency to their younger counterparts (King & Calasanti, in press). Whether this is because agency is more easily ascribed to those with whom one shares social proximity or for other reasons is difficult to say, but the reality is that older actors and especially impaired older actors are seldom discussed in terms of their personal agency (Barlett & O'Connor, 2007; Hazan, in press).

Putting the previous discussion in theoretical terms, as individuals prepare to act, they draw on their armamentarium, the aggregation of resources imparted to them by virtue of their "social addresses" within a given set of structural conditions. Although the terminology referring to social addresses dates to early in the 20th century, especially the work of Keeble, its current usage is grounded by Bronfenbrenner's (2001) effort to operationalize the pathway between sociological niches and their influence over individuals' worlds (Darling, 2007). Darling's (2007) point, in a nutshell, is that options for choices are embedded in experiences and by predispositions shaped by context, or social addresses.

Our contention in this chapter is that these shared groundings provide the stuff from which lifestyles and life experiences arise even as they are filtered by the intentional consciousness of the actors involved. As we have noted elsewhere (Hendricks & Hatch, 2006), individual actions and lifestyle choices do not play out in a vacuum but are the outcomes of ordered experience shared with others from comparable social addresses, tantamount to what have been termed "lifestyle enclaves" (Bellah, Madsen, Sullivan, Swidler, & Tipton, 1985). Lifestyles emerge from the relational bonds of associative status groups playing out in daily practices; they are interactive and relational, resulting in what might be termed a self-structure dialectic wherein each helps shape the other.

Life Chances and Structure

The concepts of life choices and life chances are often paired theoretically, the first referring to issues of agency and the second to opportunities and prospects circumscribed by structural conditions. A more nuanced view of the intersections between the two has been emerging in the literature. In speaking of social structures, a linkage is frequently made to social classes with their attendant resources, including distinctive lifestyles with all their ideational components making up social capital available to members as they encounter the world. The interaction of life's chances with life's choices can be said to be the mechanism by which the life course is given shape and old age is prefigured.

Attention to structural issues highlights situational factors that shape an actor's immediate realm of experience; structural conditions grounded in lifestyles and membership groups mitigate how life unfolds. In their explication of ensuing disparities that accrete for individuals from diverse social circumstances, Mirowsky and Ross (2003) coined the notion of "structural amplification" to convey the cascading consequence of social circumstances on individual actions. Cockerham et al. (1997) phrase a similar point (also in keeping with Weber's conceptualization) as "chance mitigates choice" (p. 224), that the structural circumstances in which individuals find themselves circumscribe the choices they can make. Or, to put it another way, it is difficult to break loose of one's social address, one's status groupings, if you will, despite individual initiative—initiatives are constructed within the strictures of the resources available.

In an effort to explicate the role of personal agency in the stress process, Thoits (2006) engages in a theorizing endeavor to identify the ways in which agentic purposeful acts may buffer what would otherwise be stressful events. Because coping resources are unequally distributed among various social statuses, greater attention to agency (and a subvariant that Thoits labels self-selection or self-construction of life's ebb and flow) may help unravel why comparable stressors have differential effects. As she notes, there are a number of theoretical and empirical gains to be achieved by paying greater attention to how agency modifies the experience of stress.

Beginning from the contention that stress is not equally distributed, Thoits (2006) sets out to examine whether psychological and social resources accompanying various status categories and social contexts make any difference in the resulting stress experienced by actors within those categories and contexts. She theorizes that positions within social structures provide variable social resources that, in turn, undergird those personal resources actors employ as they come to grips with life's eventualities. Actors are "socially placed, socially channeled, and socially shaped" (p. 318) in the exercise of personal agency.

Interestingly, controlling for life chances embodied in social class factors, which are virtually inseparable from lifestyle considerations to our way of thinking, means that most other factors relating to "healthy lifestyles" essentially disappear (Williams, 1995). In a salient analysis of long-term health conditions among 9,741 respondents to the Health and Retirement Survey, Hayward, Crimmins, Miles, and Yang (2000) found that socioeconomic circumstances and not risky health behaviors per se are responsible for race differences in mortality and morbidity across all health domains. Furthermore, prevalence rates are said to be traceable to long-term cumulative disadvantage or advantage within the fundamental social conditions of life.

In accounting for the diversity that appears to accompany the aging process, investigators have been slow to attend to the structural circumstances that anchor lifestyles and that are important sources of the variation that is now widely acknowledged to characterize older cohorts. We theorize that lifestyles and social resources deriving from social arrangements work in tandem to structure the life course, yielding cumulative advantages or disadvantages leading to one or another experience in older age (Dannefer, 2003; see also chapter 22 in this volume). In attempting to explain how personal histories affect future conditions, Bourdieu (1990), among others, speaks of the "active presence of past experiences" (p. 54). Bourdieu utilizes the concept of habitus to capture the generalized pattern of response shared by all who share a lifestyle. Blane (1999) makes much the same point in asserting that advantage or disadvantage experienced at any one point in the life course is likely to be preceded as well as followed by more of the same.

Cockerham et al. (1997) note Bourdieu's recognition that different situations may call forth different responses and assert that he was not being overly deterministic in explaining the origin of behavior. Rather, Bourdieu is cognizant that individuals' habituated dispositions for action are open systems that are fashioned by affinity groups. Nonetheless, the internalization of characteristic repertoires grounded in shared membership categories and their accompanying lifestyles is what prompts individuals to act in reasonably predictable ways. For Bourdieu (1990), lifestyles result from shared structural locations, from the resources derived from those locations, and from mutual practices or predispositions attributable to communal social addresses. He recognized that it is a symbiotic process; lifestyles are produced by collective conditions and reciprocally create collective worldviews that reinforce the originating structural conditions.

Our primary intention in this discussion has been to outline theoretical parameters for conceptualizing lifestyle and its constitutive elements. We next review how lifestyle has been utilized in social science explanations of aging. As will be evident in this review, prevailing approaches in the lifestyle literature can be distilled largely though not entirely to viewing lifestyle through the lens of individual choice and the initiation or maintenance of patterned individual-level behaviors. An individual-life focus, with an emphasis on agency and choice, is especially evident for psychological and health care frameworks. Attention to relational, collective, and social structural lifestyle influences and outcomes is growing, however, and draws largely on sociological frameworks.

Situating Lifestyle in Social Science Explanations of Health and Aging

Lifestyles as Individual Choice and Behavioral Practice

Lifestyle choices frequently are highlighted as responsible for many outcomes of interest to psychologists and health investigators. Despite a range of differences in the way the concept of lifestyle is used in these traditions, there is consensus that "lifestyle effects" show up in terms of social identities, personal habits, bodily regimes, and attitudes about health and well-being in their many guises as well as disease patterns (Cockerham, 2005). Individual traits, attributes, sensory processes, and innate predispositions are considered the scaffolding for personal choices, yielding lifestyle patterns.

Walters (1998) summarizes psychological conceptualizations of lifestyle in terms of what he calls the three "Cs," or cognition, conditions, and change. Briefly, the first "C," cognition, is conceived of as mental processing or patterned thinking. The second, conditions, is divided into intraindividual and external factors. Internal conditions include genetic endowments, intelligence, and personality traits that prepare an individual to perceive and process information and experience over the life course. Sensory acuities and physical capacities are fundamental to experience at every age; changes in either will redefine the nature of experience and thereby of lifestyles. A further intraindividual element within "conditions" revolves around motivation, whether innate or acquired, and influences attempts at mastery and control that are also seen as essential to the formulation of lifestyles. External conditions refer to surroundings and context, and conceptualization here takes up Lewin's (1939) contention that behavior plays out in the forum provided by circumstances and cannot be understood apart from those circumstances.

In social gerontology, Lawton (1985) and colleagues extended Lewin's attention to external circumstances via the concept of environmental press. By this, Lawton was referring to how physical circumstances interact with an actor's competencies to either facilitate adaptive responses or create a sense of enervation. In either instance, lifestyles may potentially be altered to match the extent to which environmental conditions impinge on feelings of mastery and competency to establish characteristic ways of being in the world.

The third "C" in Walters's framework refers to how change occurs as a consequence of these internal and external stipulations. Any stimulus that unsettles established patterns may also prompt changes in lifestyles—sometimes adaptive, sometimes maladaptive—the consequence being determined by the magnitude of the stimulus but also by personality factors, emotionality, temperaments, and motivational states (Hooker & McAdams, 2003). In terms of lifestyles, change may be conceived of as reflecting sense of control, efficacy, and adaptive capacity in the face of the complex of factors influencing individual behaviors and, thereby, how life unfolds (Moen & Chermack, 2005; Zarit, Pearlin, & Schaie, 2003). Then, too, changes in lifestyles are also conceived of as consequences of vulnerabilities in the face of declining capacities, displacing stimuli, inability to adapt, or motivational shifts (Hennen & Knudten, 2001).

A recurring theme in the health literature and within the medical model more generally is that personal beliefs, risky behaviors, and , indeed, volitional choices underlie many of the principal maladies affecting individuals—with personal responsibility seen as having primacy (Mechanic, 1978). It is commonly held that there is a direct correlation between risky behaviors and certain diseases, including some cancers, stroke, heart disease, hypertension, HIV/AIDS, and other morbidities, including obesity, alcoholism, drug use, smoking, and other outcomes, such as diet, dental hygiene, and exercise, among others (Cockerham et al., 1997). Ferraro (2006) reviewed the literature on unhealthy lifestyle practices and notes that all such behaviors are subject to change and that there is a strong link to what we label lifestyle factors associated with socioeconomic status and health status.

Cornaro's 16th-century *How to Live One Hundred Years and Avoid Disease* stands near the front of a long line of health promotion commentaries suggesting that individual regimes are responsible for long and healthy lives. Rowe and Kahn's (1998) research on successful aging stands as an exemplar of the contemporary end of the same line of experts advising lifestyle changes in order to improve prospects for healthy aging. The thrust of this scholarly tradition revolves around the twin suggestions that lifestyles are discretionary and, accordingly, that individuals are responsible for their own well-being. Generally health promotion campaigns, education, and risk management are the avenues for addressing personal lifestyle choices if behaviors are to be altered to improve well-being. One cannot come away from that literature feeling that there is much conceptualization about the impetus for the choices people make, only that they do make them. In fact, it is fair to say that the health promotion and intervention literature has most frequently focused on individual behavioral choices without looking at causative factors.

So, for example, the three-wave longitudinal investigation of 2,500 older people carried out by the SENECA project in nine European countries defines lifestyles strictly in terms of individual pathogenic behaviors, such as diet, smoking, using alcohol, being sedentary, and so on, as its definition of healthy and unhealthy lifestyles (Steen, 2003). A comparable perspective on individual behavior-linked definitions of lifestyles can be found throughout much of the health literature, especially in discussions of the compression of morbidity. In their prospective longitudinal study (1981–2006) of life expectancy among well-characterized male physicians, Yates, Djousse, Kurth, Buring, and Gaziano, (2008) conclude that modifiable healthy behaviors, such as not smoking, weight management, exercise, and comparable so-called lifestyle considerations, are associated with long life. According to literature cited in an editorial in the same issue of the *Archives of Internal Medicine,* these modifiable lifestyle factors predominate in determining longevity; approximately 35% of longevity can be attributed to genetic factors with the remainder due to nongenetic contributory factors gathered together under the label of malleable lifestyles (Hall, 2008).

Models for such "malleable lifestyles" have focused on issues such as locus of control and health beliefs as ancillary factors affecting individual decision making but without a great deal of theorizing about their basis. It is not an overstatement to say that in most of the dominant explanatory frameworks, health lifestyles are defined via an array of behavioral choices (smoking, diet, exercise, excessive alcohol consumption, and so on) without further reflection on what is reinforcing or dictating those choices (e.g., van Gool, Kempen, Penninx, Deeg, & van Eijk, 2007). Despite wide-ranging applications, some investigators maintain that such behavioral models are not particularly robust insofar as explaining health-related behaviors (Calnan, 1994; Campbell, 2000).

Broader Social Science/Sociological Approaches

Another branch of health investigators moves beyond the individualistic paradigm to couch both behavioral choices and health consequences in terms of collective patterns reflecting interpersonal ties, social networks, and options available within particular social environments (Abel, 1991; Cockerham et al., 1997; Cohen, 2004). These and other researchers cite mounting evidence that factors associated with social class and status groupings are associated with health practices and health outcomes though without necessarily exploring the mechanisms by which class or status link to personal behavior (Cockerham, 2005; Crawford, 1984; Williams, 1995). For example, in their investigation of the interaction of social status and diabetes, Wray, Alwin, McCammon, Manning, and Best (2006) identify risky behaviors (many of the same factors that are identified as "health lifestyles" in the health literature) that are linked with social status groupings and found that they were predictive of the incidence of diabetes among middle-aged and older adults. Blane (1999) offers a prophetic précis on how lifestyle factors influence health patterns over the life course, saying that "a person's biological status [is] a marker of their past social position and, through the structured nature of social processes, liable to selective accumulation of future advantage or disadvantage. . . . The social is, literally, embodied" (p. 64).

Sociologists most often speak of families, communities, status groups, or socioeconomic categories in conjunction with lifestyles. The social milieu is regarded as the source of ways of acting, feeling, thinking, and adapting to changes over the life course. It is fair to say that for a sociologist, lifestyles are conceived as being akin to careers in that they amount to durable arrangements that help structure experience over time (Pearlin, 1988).

The well-known Alameda, California, investigation of health statuses stands out for its finding that those individuals who were socially integrated had fewer health incidents 9 years later. Considerable evidence has been amassed to support the original findings of this study (e.g., Berkman & Glass, 2000; Cohen, 2004): aging individuals who are integrated into supportive networks find resources that mitigate negative outcomes. These networks also reinforce behavioral modifications, increasing the prospects of successful health-enhancing interventions. In their investigation of health and lifestyle among participants in health promotion programs in Italy, Lucchetti, Spazzafumo, and Cerasa (2001) create an array of individual behaviors (diet, smoking, exercise) but add to them family ties, friendships, and social participation. They identify positive attitudes, absence of regret, a sense of futurity, and extensive social interaction as more predictive of healthy lifestyles in their respondents and suggest that the array of social resources brought into play make a profound difference in receptivity to health promotion interventions.

In an exploration of health lifestyles in the American South, Snead and Cockerham (2002) appear to join those who stress an individualistic perspective when they speak of choices and practices operationalized as health lifestyle, defined by disadvantageous behaviors, such as smoking, poor dietary practices, inactivity, or excessive drinking. Yet they also emphasize that the linkage between social economic status and health behaviors can be attributed to lifestyle differences characterizing various social categories. That is to say, health lifestyles reflect individual choices from among options that are available to actors within their life situation (Cockerham, Abel, & Luschen, 1993). In other words, values of choice reflect values of membership groups.

In fact, the very premise of epidemiology is predicated on collective patterns deriving from some sort of overarching phenomenon (Lomas, 1998). Lomas identifies "caring communities," characterized by reciprocal trusting and supportive relationships, as keys to individual well-being. These relationships, the trust implicit in them, and the resources they provide are contingent on shared lifestyles, worldviews, and normative expectations—a "rich tapestry of trusted and valued social networks" that in all likelihood are predictive of positive health outcomes (see Campbell, 2000, p. 186). Health lifestyles hence can be conceptualized as derivatives of collectivities, from shared interactions stemming from the habitus that comes of communal lifestyles.

This discussion begs the question, What is the nexus between collectivities and individual behavior? Turner (1992) encapsulates the influence of mutual lifestyles in terms of the body becoming the site where cultural praxis is inscribed, meaning that collective perspectives play out in personal choices. And as Cockerham (2000) comments in his penetrating synopsis in the *Handbook of Medical Sociology*, lifestyles may be expressed via individual behavior, yet they must also be seen as a reflection of personal practices informed by group and socioeconomic membership categories with their accompanying socialization processes. These intersecting practices and processes can help social scientists explain what people do and why. In sum, lifestyles are the mechanisms through which broadly defined social categories show up in individual behaviors.

Theorizing Lifestyles: A Personal Resource Model

Theorizing Lifestyles

As reviewed in this synopsis, there are two parallel points of view regarding lifestyles that must be considered within the parameters of this discussion. A pervasive perspective in some quarters of the behavioral sciences has it that individuals make their own choices, of their own free will. For those who adopt such a point of view, lifestyle consequences are seen as resulting from personal choices. Yet another facet of the sociological tradition, in particular, is that although individuals may make their own choices, they do not do so entirely of their own free will. In the latter instance, an actor's actions are interpreted as corollaries of his or her membership groups.

Having said that, we herewith define lifestyles as "distinctive attributes or recognizable patterns of behaviors reflecting shared interests and life situations incorporating related values, attitudes and orientations that create characteristic identities" (Hendricks & Hatch, 2006, p. 303; Stebbins, 1997). Our definition is predicated on both collective forces nudging individuals toward certain courses and personal agency reflecting an actor's priorities and capabilities. In crafting this conceptualization, we leave room for both objective circumstances anchoring individuals and subjective reactions to those circumstances. Because of their synthetic quality, lifestyles may also be theorized as being the glue that holds many social science explanations of aging together.

Lifestyles forged from memberships, personal resources, and life-conduct choices create the patterns that social scientists label the life course. Whether explicitly recognized or not, lifestyle themes are what actors utilize in crafting their own narrative autobiographies. It is not an exaggeration to assert that lifestyle linkages are the bridge between macro- and microlevel phenomena that lie very near the center of social science. Each one reproduces the other, giving rise to "reference generators" that help keep the sociological puzzle integrated (Giddens, 1990; Sobel, 1981).

Having asserted that lifestyles are implicated in the experience of aging and the shape of the life course, it is necessary to spell out a few of the elements of such a claim—"to uncover the *why* and the *what* of occurrences and relationships" (Biggs, Hendricks, & Lowenstein, 2003, p. 1; Bengtson, Putney, & Johnson, 2005). Those who attend to theoretical developments in social gerontology agree that our explanations of human phenomena require a sound conceptual grounding if they are to have cumulative impact or to call out the interconnectedness and underlying processes. The purpose of what follows is to move in that direction, to spell out what we believe to be the constellation of factors contributing to lifestyles and to move beyond merely labeling lifestyles as important.

If social scientists are to theorize about lifestyles it is important to not disconnect context, capacity, experience, and meaning constructions (Hendricks & Hatch, 2006). Here we reiterate a claim we have made previously, namely, that lifestyles are constructed from the complex of resources available to actors and that these resources come from within multifaceted circumstances in which individuals find themselves. Some resources are grounded in status groupings or other social assemblages, some can be said to reside in individuals as achieved attributes, and some come from innate or inherent functional capacities. Of course, we also need to add that each of these likely evolves as part of the aging process. For purposes of this discussion, we describe these as iterations of social and human capital, and together they represent the range and types of resources actors utilize in establishing their lifestyles.

A Word About Social Capital as a Personal Resource

Before delineating more fully the personal resources that we believe help shape actors' choices, it is worthwhile to elucidate the concept of social capital. A great deal of the current conceptualization about the social resources people use to make their way in the world stems from the work of Bourdieu, Coleman, Putnam, and, closer to gerontology, Lin. In his explication of four overlapping forms of capital, Bourdieu (1991) was explicit in stating that singularly and in combination each is a resource available to individuals as they negotiate passage through life. Earlier we mentioned his term *habitus,* or coordinated and interdependent patterns of thought, deriving from shared language and socially meaningful relations. These stand as virtually impartible predicates to an actor's perceptual schema and also underlie the reproduction of social relations, or their institutionalization, if you will, that give rise to discernible lifestyles and to interpersonal relationships.

To introduce the concept a bit more fully, social capital may be thought of as comprising of those resources that come with memberships and shared experiences within groups ranging from the family on through to informal and formal associations and socioeconomic status. Sociologists have been theorizing about its role in shaping experience since the inception of the discipline. It is our contention that social capital, the social resources that derive from membership in socially meaningful categories and interpersonal associations, is a constitutive element of lifestyle as well as social identity and is instrumental in shaping all experience. Bourdieu (1991) is the progenitor of contemporary usage, and he grounds social capital within the ambit of institutionalized relationships and their appurtenances. He stresses that social capital also paves the way toward access to other resources and to the development of human capital (see also Coleman, 1988). Despite substantial complexity in operationalizing the concept of social capital, it does provide a valuable heuristic perspective on the roles played by a variety of resources that are no less critical than financial resources in channeling life experience.

Although he takes a somewhat divergent tact on social capital, Coleman (1988) observes that it is embedded in social structures, organizations, and relations and thereby facilitates actors' actions within the context of that structure.

Coleman was speaking specifically of how social resources shape the cognitive and social development of young people, pointing to a causal relationship between access to social resources and early educational success—noting in the process that social relations are the stuff of social capital and the vehicle by which information, norms, expectations, or trust are shared and learned. Putnam (1996) puts a slightly finer point on social capital as a feature of social life, networks, and so on that paves the way toward cooperative action and shared goals. Because of the mutuality and shared associational life within social categories, transaction costs are minimized; hence, the concept of social capital helps explain interpersonal attractions and associations (Schuller, Baron, & Field, 2000; Szreter, 2000).

To further conceptualize social capital, it might help to illustrate by means of analogy. Social capital can be thought of as one of those invisible forces that affect our lives. Although there are technical reasons why slipstreaming among racers or birds flying in a "V" formation helps facilitate the progress of one another, suffice it to say their close relationship optimizes expenditures of energy. In the case of human beings, comparable closeness brings about learning, sharing, and supporting. Following House and Kahn (1985), we would assert that social capital includes types of informational, emotional, and instrumental resources that individuals can tap into to help facilitate certain forms of action or to buffer vagaries encountered along the way. Not only is social capital a resource available to individuals, but it bespeaks of a close, even infrangible connection that entails relatively moderate if any opportunity costs.

Much of the seemingly ubiquitous social network analyses widely reported in the literature of social gerontology could be construed as speaking to the empirical foundations of social capital. For example, Ensel and Lin (2000) utilized a number of quite sophisticated measures to examine the relationship between psychological stress and physical distress in diverse age-groups. One of their hypotheses referred to the role of social resources, operationalized through a close set (alpha = .71) of social support items revolving around ties with and perceptions of relationships with friends, companions, or confidants. Their results suggest that social resources mediate the effects of stressors on distress among respondents in three age-groups but with some interesting differences in the temporality of stressors most likely to be ameliorated by social resources. In search of similar empirical support, Nilsson, Rana, and Kabir (2006) undertook a small-scale cross-sectional analysis of quality of life among elderly people in rural Bangladesh. They operationalized social capital as the extent of an individual's informal interpersonal ties with family and friends, whether the person claimed membership in various community-level organizations and associations, and whether the person had voted recently (as a measure of social engagement). Not unlike Ensel and Lin, they found that respondents with higher social capital scores also reported better quality of life and sense of well-being.

Personal Resources

We would contend that three dimensions of personal resources are available as actors make their way in the world. Each is also constitutive of lifestyles, and each underpins an actor's perception of choices and options available to him or her. First, among the resources relevant to an actor's course of action is a social-familial dimension deriving from what we just noted about social capital. The social-familial dimension of resources revolves around interpersonal relationships, family, and extrafamilial supportive networks or contacts. These relationships are one form of social capital providing anchorage as well as resources utilized by individuals as they experience life. Of course, not all relationships are positive, but all positive relationships do contain affirmational promise as well as emotional and instrumental assistance. We touch on entitlements as another aspect of social capital later in this chapter.

Second, physiological-psychological resources are among the types of human capital individuals carry with them. O'Rand (2001) speaks of these same resources as a form of psychophysical capital. When fully functional, these resources facilitate engagement with the world, and when diminished, for whatever reason, they necessitate adaptation. Changes in health status or biological functioning, whether through environmental assaults, poor behavioral choices, or genetic programming, have palatable effects disrupting ability to maintain homeostasis. We regard physiological-psychological resources as a form of human capital used to negotiate the life course and evolving over the course of life. Singularly and in combination, they affect actors' ability to engage the environment around them and the matrix of meaning they construct as a consequence.

Third, options and choices reflect the means one has available for bargaining. Fiduciary capability is no less valuable than social and human capital and is one of those instrumental resources individuals call on to exercise control, to trade, and to negotiate. Mostly fiduciary resources can be equated to monetary resources, but other token currencies couched in one or another social context are also included, as they, too, are relevant to exchange. In addition to enabling an individual to bargain his or her way in the world, fiduciary resources carry symbolic relevance, connoting social status and circles of confidence by virtue of their shared recognition.

None of these resources is absolute or even ordinal in nature. Much of their value reflects the context in which they play out. Accordingly, both physical and social environments must be factored into the constitution of lifestyles. As we pointed out previously, modes of being in the world are grounded by capacities and capabilities for dealing with the environmental conditions. Lawton (1985) had physical circumstances in mind when he initially spoke of environmental press, but we would add that social environments are also germane to the creation of lifestyles. There are also a variety of exogenous factors that affect how lifestyles are constructed and their effects are cumulative over time.

Other Factors Relevant to a Theory of Lifestyles

Gender and Ethnicity

Thus far, we have spoken of lifestyles, capital, and the array of resources individuals employ as though there were no intervening or mitigating factors as far as how they play out. There is considerable research evidence suggesting that such issues as gender, ethnicity, sexuality, and other forms of diversity do in fact affect lifestyles and the resources available to make one's way in the world (Dannefer, 2003; Hatch, 2000; see also chapter 22 in this volume). For example,

Hakim (2000) is among those who maintain that lifestyle choices for women and for men involve distinct dynamics, unique to their circumstances but influenced by societal impositions and even by generational shifts that subvert the stability of the life course. Burt (1998) provided a major service to those who would theorize about social capital when he noted the presence of what he terms a "gender puzzle" within institutionalized relationships. By that he meant that what might be a resource for one gender is not necessarily a resource or form of capital for the other. For those who are considered "one of us," social capital is readily available; for those falling outside that category, membership and participation may not carry the same benefits. The point relevant to a theory of lifestyles is the inherent relativity of resources and that they cannot be taken as unconditional.

Gender-based norms also enter into the determination of lifestyles. In an analysis of psychological distress experienced by women and men and the resulting health lifestyles in three areas of the former Soviet Union, Cockerham, Hinote, and Abbott (2006) found that women verbalize far more distress yet fewer women than men drink (while both genders smoke) as a coping mechanism. Because of normative expectations, women were not as drawn to alcohol, traditionally putting the welfare of their families ahead of personal coping needs. Habitual dietary excesses were a coping mechanism for both men and women, however, as food was an acceptable means of finding comfort for both genders. As they looked over the health lifestyles of men and women in a culture undergoing rapid social change, Cockerham and colleagues conclude that psychological distress influences health lifestyle practices in virtually all instances but that it plays out differently for women and men based on acceptable norms for dealing with difficulties.

Role of the Public Sphere in Lifestyles

State institutions, ideologies, and public policies provide key macrolevel dimensions for theorizing about lifestyles. From legislation establishing parenting provisions to education policies, mandated occupational policies, and labor force participation to health care and retirement entitlements, the state is central to how life unfolds. Public provisions are part of the social capital that influences life chances and shape the pathway to and through old age. As we noted previously, the provision of leisure activities, from national parks to "senior citizen" engagements, is widely regarded as among the rights of citizenship in most Western nations at least. Although the state exists on a macrolevel and is seemingly far removed from individual lifestyles, the opposite is true: it is intimately involved.

In a conceptually innovative look at health lifestyles in Russia following the breakup of the Soviet Union, Cockerham, Snead, and DeWaal (2002) utilized the concept of lifestyles to examine whether macrolevel political ideologies of reigning governments might affect individuals' health behaviors. Taking a cue from the unprecedented rise in mortality after the fall of the Soviet Union, Cockerham and colleagues brought their conceptually sophisticated notions of lifestyles to the task of examining whether an adverse psychosocial environment promotes feelings of apathy, alienation, or diminished personal responsibility affecting health locus of control and whether these declines constrain individuals' practice of positive health lifestyles. Utilizing a regression model for five health variables reported by more than 8,000 respondents, they conclude that the collectivist ideology of the Soviet Union, characterized as a "*Homo Soveticus*" personality, fostered a kind of passivity that did not lead to positive health choices and that after the breakup those who preferred a return to Soviet principles practiced less personal responsibility for their own health. Although they call for further analysis prior to concluding that macrolevel ideologies play a pivotal role in health practices, they do assert that in countries where the habitus of lifestyles emphasizes individual choices, healthy lifestyles are more prevalent.

Lifestyle as an Integrative Framework in Explaining Aging

We have argued that lifestyle provides an integrative linkage between micro- and macrolevel considerations of constitutive elements of the life course. The connection between individual action and membership in recognized social categories represents a central—though not the sole—linkage elucidated by lifestyle. As integrated practices, lifestyles manifested by individuals reflect personal choices, to be sure, but they also express normative considerations of membership groups.

There are a couple of significant illustrations of the notion of lifestyles that help to underscore its relevance for understanding the experience of life and of aging. Despite the effects (direct) of socioeconomic status on health being widely documented, the mechanisms by which socioeconomic status plays out are not well understood. In a follow-up to the Hayward et al. (2000) investigation mentioned previously, Crimmins, Hayward, and Seeman (2007) felt that a closer examination of those mechanisms was in order. What is the portent of differing socioeconomic categories, and what are the pathways by which socioeconomic status comes to make a difference? The answer likely lies in the fact that membership in diverse socioeconomic statuses carries with it the prospect of very different life experiences from childhood to old age; such things as leisure, proximate circumstances, health care, attitudes about health care, and so on play out in patterned fashion. As Crimmins and colleagues aver, socioeconomic status is more than income or educational attainment; it implies long-term differences in resources, the structure of opportunities, access to knowledge, and the accumulation of experience reflecting individual and social capital. As they say, higher social statuses not only are associated with fewer risky health behaviors but also confer more psychological resources (e.g., mastery and control) with which to deal with adversity. One of the most striking admonitions offered in their discussion is the call for better conceptualization of why socioeconomic status matters, and they call for greater theorizing as well as better operationalization.

In an exploration of the role played by social and personal resources associated with differential socioeconomic status groupings, de Leon and Glass (2004) make two points pertinent to this discussion. First, they point out that personal and social resources, accruing to individuals as a consequence of their linkages and interactions with others, what we referred to as social capital, modulate all manner of assaults and adversities, thus helping to optimize adaptation to the aging process. Second, they point out that these resources are, in turn, a product of sociocultural environments and what they describe as the ecology of social structures and personal resources.

Conclusion

Weber's seminal contributions notwithstanding, it was not until late in the 20th century that social scientists started to explicate issues of lifestyle. Despite widespread assertions that socioeconomic status, structural locale, and social networks make a difference in well-being and the experience of aging, the mechanisms by which these and other factors actually affect experience have not been well explicated. Only recently have investigators begun to examine those mechanisms and suggest that lifestyles may provide the connection. As Higgs and Gilleard (2006) aver, well-being in later life is increasingly seen as an outgrowth of lifestyles and identity rather than as merely a consequence of residual incomes and previous occupations.

The array of personal and social resources available to actors is a crucial component of the construction of their lifestyles. In the personal resource model outlined in this chapter, resources are described as making up three distinct dimensions that work in combination to shape lifestyles. In addition to those resources, the context in which they play out and a range of other exogenous factors enter into the equation.

Our goal has been to highlight the importance of lifestyle theorizing as an explanatory template in assaying the experience of old age. Here and in an earlier publication (Hendricks & Hatch, 2006) we join Crompton (1998), Giddens (1991), Bourdieu (1991), and Cockerham (2000), among others, in contending that lifestyles provide an integrative theoretical framework for making sense of many aspects of experience, including the diversity that is widely acknowledged to characterize older cohorts. We are of a mind to say that lifestyles are the active linkage between structural locale, socioeconomic status, and any number of outcomes across the life course. By addressing lifestyle issues, the focus is shifted from actors as individuals to actors as members of broader social categories whose actions and identities are shaped by virtue of their membership in those categories. There is still "an urgent need to understand and explain . . . issues at a theoretical level . . . as they relate to the core problems of sociological theory concerning the relationship between structure and agency" (Williams, 1995, p. 581), and it is our contention that lifestyles may do exactly that.

References

Abel, T. (1991). Measuring health lifestyles in comparative analysis: Theoretical issues and empirical findings. *Social Science and Medicine, 32,* 899–908.

Barlett, R., & O'Connor, D. (2007). From personhood to citizenship: Broadening the lens for dementia practice and research. *Journal of Aging Studies, 21,* 107–118.

Bellah, R., Madsen, R., Sullivan, W., Swidler, A., & Tipton, S. (1985). *Habits of the heart: Individualism and commitment in American life.* Berkeley: University of California Press.

Bengtson, V. L., Putney, N. M., & Johnson, M. L. (2005). The problem of theory in gerontology today. In M. L. Johnson (Ed.), *The Cambridge handbook of age and ageing* (pp. 3–20). Cambridge: Cambridge University Press.

Berkman, L., & Glass, T. (2000). Social integration, social networks, social support, and health. In L. Berkman & I. Kawachi (Eds.), *Social epidemiology* (pp. 137–173). New York: Oxford University Press.

Biggs, S., Hendricks, J., & Lowenstein, A. (2003). The need for theory in gerontology. In S. Biggs, A. Lowenstein, & J. Hendricks (Eds.), *The need for theory: Critical approaches to social gerontology* (pp. 1–12). Amityville, NY: Baywood Publishing.

Blane, D. (1999). The life course, the social gradient, and health. In M. Marmot & R. G. Wilkinson (Eds.), *Social determinants of health* (pp. 64–81). Oxford: Oxford University Press.

Bourdieu, P. (1990). *The logic of practice.* Cambridge: Polity Press.

Bourdieu, P. (1991). *Language and symbolic power.* Cambridge: Polity Press.

Bronfenbrenner, U. (1979). *The ecology of human development.* Cambridge, MA: Harvard University Press.

Bronfenbrenner, U. (2001) *Making human beings human: Bioecological perspectives on human development.* Thousand Oaks, CA: Sage.

Burt, R. S. (1998). The gender of social capital. *Rationality and Society, 10,* 5–46.

Calnan, M. (1994). "Lifestyle" and its social meaning. *Advances in Medical Sociology, 4,* 69–87.

Campbell, C. (2000). Social capital and health: Contextualizing health promotion within local community networks. In S. Baron, J. Field, & T. Schuller (Eds.), *Social capital: Critical perspectives* (pp. 182–196). Oxford: Oxford University Press.

Cockerham, W. A. (2000). The sociology of health behavior and health lifestyles. In C. Bird, P. Conrad, & A. Fremont (Eds.), *Handbook of medical sociology* (5th ed., pp. 159–172). Upper Saddle River, NJ: Prentice Hall.

Cockerham, W. A. (2005). Health lifestyle theory and the convergence of agency and structure. *Journal of Health and Social Behavior, 46,* 51–67.

Cockerham, W. A., Abel, T., & Luschen, G. (1993). Max Weber, formal rationality, and health lifestyles. *Sociological Quarterly, 34,* 413–425.

Cockerham, W. A., Hinote, B. P., & Abbott, P. (2006). Psychological distress, gender, and health lifestyles in Belarus, Kazakhstan, Russia, and Ukraine. *Social Science & Medicine, 63,* 2381–2394.

Cockerham, W. A., Rutten, A., & Abel, T. (1997). Conceptualizing contemporary health lifestyles: Moving beyond Weber. *Sociological Quarterly, 38,* 321–342.

Cockerham, W. A., Snead, M. C., & DeWaal, D. F. (2002). Health lifestyles in Russia and the socialist heritage. *Journal of Health and Social Behavior, 43,* 42–55.

Cohen, S. (2004). Social relationships and health. *American Psychologist, 59,* 676–684.

Coleman, J. (1988). Social capital in the creation of human capital. *American Journal of Sociology, 94*(Suppl.), 95–120.

Crawford, R. (1984). A cultural account of health: Control, release and the social body. In J. McKinley (Ed.), *Issues in political economy of health care* (pp. 60–103). New York: Tavistock.

Crimmins, E. M., Hayward, M. D., & Seeman, T. (2007). Race/ethnicity, socioeconomic status, and health. In N. Anderson, P. Bulatao, & B. Cohen (Eds.), *Critical perspectives on racial and ethnic difference in health in later life* (pp. 310–252). Washington, DC: National Archives Press.

Crompton, R. (1998). *Class and stratification: An introduction to current debates.* Cambridge: Polity Press.

Dannefer, D. (2003). Cumulative advantage/disadvantage and the life course: Cross fertilizing age and social science theory. *Journal of Gerontology: Social Sciences, 58,* S327–S337.

Darling, N. (2007). Ecological systems theory: The person in the center of the circles. *Research in Human Development, 4,* 203–217.

de Leon, C. F. M., & Glass, T. (2004). The role of social and personal resources in ethnic disparities in late-life health. In N. Anderson, P. Bulatao, & B. Cohen (Eds.), *Critical perspectives on racial and ethnic difference in health in later life* (pp. 353–404). Washington, DC: National Archives Press.

Ensel, W., & Lin, N. (2000). Age, the stress process, and physical distress: The role of distal stressors. *Journal of Aging and Health, 12,* 139–168.

Featherstone, M. (1991). *Consumer culture and post-modernism.* Thousand Oaks, CA: Sage.

Ferraro, K. (2006). Health and aging. In R. Binstock & L. George (Eds.), *Handbook of aging and the social sciences* (6th ed., pp. 238–256). San Diego, CA: Academic Press.

Giddens, A. (1990). Comments of the theory of structuration. *Journal for the Theory of Social Behaviour, 20,* 75–80.

Giddens, A. (1991). *Modernity and self-identity.* Stanford, CA: Stanford University Press.

Gordon, C., & Longino, C. (2000). Age structure and social structure. *Contemporary Sociology, 29,* 699–703.

Gubrium, J. F., & Holstein, J. A. (1995). Individual agency, the ordinary, and postmodern life. *Sociological Quarterly, 36,* 555–570.

Hakim, C. (2000). *Work–lifestyle choices in the twenty-first century: Preference theory.* Oxford: Oxford University Press.

Hall, W. J. (2008). Centenarians: Metaphor becomes reality. *Archives of Internal Medicine, 168,* 262–283.

Hatch, L. R. (2000). *Beyond gender differences: Adaptation to aging in life course perspective.* Amityville, NY: Baywood Publishing.

Hayward, M., Crimmins, E. M., Miles, T., & Yang, Y. (2000). The significance of socioeconomic status in explaining the racial gap in chronic health conditions. *American Sociological Review, 65,* 910–930.

Hazan, H. (in press). Essential others: Anthropology and the return of the old savage. *International Journal of Sociology and Social Policy, 29.*

Hendricks, J. (1999). Practical consciousness, social class, and self-concept: A view from sociology. In C. Ryff & V. Marshall (Eds.), *The self and society in aging processes* (pp. 187–222). New York: Springer Publishing.

Hendricks, J., & Hatch, L. R. (2006). Lifestyle and aging. In R. Binstock & L. K. George (Eds.), *Handbook of aging and the social sciences* (5th ed., pp. 301–319). San Diego, CA: Academic Press.

Hennen, J., & Knudten, R. (2001). A lifestyle analysis of the elderly: Perceptions of risk, fear, and vulnerability. *Illness, Crisis and Loss, 9,* 190–208.

Higgs, P., & Gilleard, C. (2006). Departing the margins: Social class and later life in a second modernity. *Journal of Sociology, 42,* 219–241.

Hooker, K., & McAdams, D. (2003). Personality and adult development: Looking beyond the OCEAN. *Journal of Gerontology: Social Sciences, 58,* P296–P304.

House, J., & Kahn, R. (1985). Measures and concepts of social support. In S. Cohen & S. Sume (Eds.), *Social support and health* (pp. 83–108). New York: Academic Press.

Katz, S., & Laliberte-Rudman, D. (2005). Exemplars of retirement: Identity and agency between lifestyle and social movement. In S. Katz (Ed.), *Cultural aging: Life course, lifestyle, and senior worlds.* Peterborough, ON: Broadview Press.

Katz-Gerro, T. (2006). Lifestyle. In G. Ritzer (Ed.), *Blackwell encyclopedia of sociology* (pp. 2644–2646). London: Wiley-Blackwell.

Kauffman, S. (1993, Spring/Summer). Reflections on "The ageless self." *Generations,* 13–16.

King, N., & Calasanti, T. (in press). Ageing agents; social gerontologists empowerment of old people. *International Journal of Sociology and Social Policy, 29.*

Lawton, M. P. (1985). The elderly in context: Perspectives from environmental psychology and gerontology. *Environment and Behavior, 17,* 501–519.

Lewin, K. (1939). Field theory and experiment in social psychology: Concepts and methods. *American journal of Sociology, 44,* 868–897.

Lockwood, D. (1966). Sources of variation in working class images of society. *Sociological Review, 14,* 244–267.

Lomas, J. (1998). Social capital and health: Implications for public health and epidemiology. *Social Science & Medicine, 47,* 1181–1188.

Loyal, S., & Barnes, B. (2000). "Agency" as a red herring in social theory. *Philosophy of the Social Sciences, 31,* 507–524.

Lucchetti, M., Spazzafumo, L., & Cerasa, F. (2001). Italian people aged 50–75 years enrolled in a health promotion program: Health and lifestyle. *Educational Gerontology, 27,* 439–453.

Mechanic, D. (1978). *Medical sociology.* New York: Free Press.

Mirowsky, J., & Ross, C. (2003). *Education, social status, and health.* New York: Aldine de Gruyter.

Moen, P., & Chermack, H. (2005). Gender disparities in health: Strategic selection, careers, and cycles of control. *Journal of Gerontology: Social Sciences, 60* (Special Issue 2), 99–108.

Nilsson, J., Rana, A. K., & Kabir, Z. N. (2006). Social capital and quality of life in old age: Results from a cross-sectional study in rural Bangladesh. *Journal of Health and Aging, 18,* 419–434.

O'Rand, A. (2001). Stratification and the life course: The forms of life-course capital and their interrelationships. In R. Binstock & L. K. George (Eds.), *Handbook of aging and the social sciences* (5th ed., pp. 197–213). San Diego, CA: Academic Press.

Pearlin, L. (1988). Social structuring and social values: The regulation of structural effects. In H. O'Gorman (Ed.), *Surveying social life* (pp. 252–264). Middletown, CT: Wesleyan University Press.

Putnam, R. D. (1996, March). Who killed civic America? *Prospect,* 66–72.

Rowe, J., & Kahn, R. (1998). *Successful aging.* New York: Random House.

Schuller, T., Baron, S., & Field, J. (2000). Social capital: A review and critique. In S. Baron, J. Field, & T. Schuller (Eds.), *Social capital: Critical perspectives* (pp. 1–38). Oxford: Oxford University Press.

Sewell, W. (1992). A theory of structure: Duality, agency and transformation. *American Journal of Sociology, 98,* 1–29.

Snead, M. C., & Cockerham, W. C. (2002). Health lifestyles and social class in the deep south. *Social Inequalities, Health and Health Care Delivery, 20,* 107–122.

Sobel, M. (1981). *Lifestyle and social structure: concepts, definitions, analyses.* New York: Academic Press.

Stebbins, R. (1997). Lifestyle as a generic concept in ethnographic research. *Quality and Quantity, 31,* 347–360.

Steen, B. (2003). A "healthy" lifestyle in old age and its relation to health and disease. *Age and Ageing, 32,* 365–366.

Stones, R. (2006). Structure and agency. In G. Ritzer (Ed.), *Blackwell encyclopedia of sociology* (pp. 4861–4864). London: Wiley-Blackwell.

Szreter, S. (2000). Social capital, the economy, and education in historical perspective. In S. Baron, J. Field, & T. Schuller (Eds.), *Social capital: Critical perspectives* (pp. 56–77). Oxford: Oxford University Press.

Thoits, P. A. (2006). Personal agency in the stress process. *Journal of Health and Social Behavior, 47,* 309–323.

Turner, B. (1992). *Regulating bodies.* London: Routledge.

van Gool, C., Kempen, G., Penninx, B., Deeg, D., & van Eijk, J. (2007). Chronic disease and lifestyle transitions: Results from the longitudinal aging study Amsterdam. *Journal of Aging and Health, 19,* 416–438.

Walters, G. D. (1998). Three existential contributions to a theory of lifestyles. *Journal of Humanistic Psychology, 38,* 25–40.

Weber, M. (1978). *Economy and society* (G. F. Roth & C. Wittich, Ed. & Trans.). Berkeley: University of California Press. (Original work published 1922)

Williams, S. J. (1995). Theorising class, health, and lifestyles: Can Bourdieu help us? *Sociology of Health & Illness, 17,* 577–604.

Wray, L., Alwin, D., McCammon, R., Manning, T., & Best, L. (2006). Social status, risky health behaviors, and diabetes in middle-aged and older adults. *Journal of Gerontology: Social Sciences, 61,* S290–S298.

Yates, L. B., Djousse, L., Kurth, T., Buring, J. E., & Gaziano, J. M. (2008). Exceptional longevity in men: Modifiable factors associated with survival and function to age 90 years. *Archives of Internal Medicine, 168,* 284–290.

Zarit, S., Pearlin, L., & Schaie, K. W. (Eds.). (2003). *Personal control in social and life course contexts.* New York: Springer Publishing.

24 The New Terrain of Old Age: Hallmarks, Freedoms, and Risks

Richard A. Settersten Jr.
Molly E. Trauten

Great shake-ups seem to be afoot in every period of life, so much so that the whole of human experience feels in flux. In this chapter, we turn attention to the changing terrain of *old age*. First, we explore some of its new or emerging hallmarks along with some of its shifting sands and mines that create both new risks and opportunities for old people. Then we consider some of the specific markers that now punctuate the process of becoming and being old; we contemplate the meanings of age (and of *agelessness*) along with a range of alternative markers that define movement into and through life's final decades. Finally, we reflect on some of the social skills and psychological capacities that may be especially helpful—and even necessary—for navigating this new terrain.

Each of these fronts is ripe for theoretical advances and empirical investigation. The issues we raise along the way pose many significant challenges to existing theories of aging and to the task of generating new theories. They offer precious opportunities to rethink theories of aging—what can be kept, what must be recast, what must be discarded, and what might be created anew to do better by the complexities of aging and old people in a complicated world.

New and Emerging Hallmarks of Old Age

Altered Terms of Life, Illness, and Death

In the past century, significant reductions in mortality, morbidity, and fertility—the very factors that have created aging societies—have also transformed human experience. These demographic changes have permitted shake-ups in the organization of the entire life course and in the nature of educational, work, family, and leisure experiences (for illustrations, see Settersten, 2007c). The same demographic changes have also created a longer, healthier landscape for old age, making it possible for individuals to become and be "old" in brand-new ways. Old age extends multiple decades, but it comprises of early and late phases that are often extremely different from one another.

Ultimately, these changes have made a long and healthy life more certain, and death more predictable, than ever before. Individuals can now count on surviving close to eight decades, if not longer, with much of this time lived jointly with loved ones. Individuals can also expect major encounters with chronic illness to be confined to old age, often followed quickly by death (the so-called compression of morbidity; see Fries, 2005). Such changes, which are relatively recent historical phenomena, are absolutely remarkable but are by no means universal, as populations in some parts of the world face starkly different realities.

Theories of aging would benefit from and even be revolutionized by renewed attention to the "demographic imperative"—of what it means to live in a society populated by many old people and, in particular, by many old women given their longer life expectancy; of how the demographic parameters that produce aging societies have not only altered old age but have also created reverberations in every life period before it; and of how social institutions and policies, which guide or govern every sphere of life, may lag behind the times and need to be rearchitected to reflect contemporary demographic conditions.

The Individualization of Old Age

Age-based norms are painstakingly documented for children in terms of height, weight, intelligence, and social and emotional development; extensive batteries of valid and reliable tests are available to measure these statuses. The same is clearly not true of adult life, for which variability is now a central hallmark. Beginning in the middle part of the 20th century, adults moved lockstep through a set of well-timed and well-ordered role transitions related to education, work and retirement, and family. At the time, research emphasized the developmental tasks and social expectations that distinctly marked movement through life's stages—including old age. Recent decades have witnessed the crumbling of traditional timetables for such transitions in terms of both when and in what order they occur. There has been proliferation of a wide range of timetables, and even the elimination of timetables altogether.

Relative to the first half of adulthood, however, one can argue that the terrain of old age has never been well defined. Yet all around us, we can point to examples of individual behavior and ambitions in old age that *defy* age-based expectations. But what *are* those expectations exactly? It seems easier to recognize the things that shatter our assumptions than to recognize the things that fit and be fully aware of the assumptions we take for granted—whether in our everyday lives or in theories and research on aging. So what is it that we assume individuals are to be doing or striving for in old age? How are these decades to be filled? Is it that there are no scripts for old age, few scripts, or new scripts that are in the process of being developed?

Age, as we elaborate on later, has become a poor predictor of self-concepts, of achievements or failures, of the anticipations of things yet to come, and of capacities to cope with change. The task of theorizing about old age becomes more difficult when these decades are understood to be highly variable and unstable, leaving little regularity to describe or explain.

Existing theories of aging and the life course have little to say about what people of a particular age or life period share—for example, what is it that "old people," as a group or as individuals, have in common across the multiple decades that compose "old age"? Existing theories have little to say about what makes one life period different from another—for example, how is "old age" distinct from "middle age"? And existing theories have little to say about when one period of life begins and another ends—for example, when does "old age" start, and what marks movement between the "young-old," old-old," and "oldest-old" periods or between the "third" and "fourth" ages, terms so often referenced in the aging literature? Together, these constitute pressing questions for theoretical and empirical advances related to aging and the life course.

Perhaps nowhere is the degree of variability among people in an age-group greater than it is among old people, as individuals' life experiences over at least six decades of adulthood culminate in what seem like personalized constellations of experiences that are as unique as one's fingerprints. The highly individualized routes taken through old age presumably only exacerbate the variability we would already expect to find among old people. Yet some things about late life, such as normative declines in physical and cognitive health, may be postponed but not escaped. In this sense, becoming and being old can also come with a set of common experiences that are often deemphasized and to which we later turn.

New Freedoms and Risks in Old Age

The new landscape of adulthood brings flexibilities for people of every age, including those who are old, to live their lives in ways that are congruent with their personal interests and wishes. But these new freedoms also bring new risks. This seems particularly true of old age. For old people, the future seems open but also fragile, unpredictable, dwindling, and compressed. Choices now seem greater, but these choices may also seem heavier and come with unknown consequences. Any fallouts must also be negotiated and absorbed by individuals and their families rather than by governments, markets, or other entities (at least in the context of American policy). The trend toward individualization means that old people are increasingly left to their own devices to determine the directions that the ends of their lives will take. Old people are largely on their own with only the safety nets they can create with the resources they have, whether through personal and family resources or through social skills and psychological capacities, to be discussed shortly.

The experimental nature of "do-it-yourself" biographies, to use Beck's (2000) provocative phrase, in later life may make them vulnerable to breakdown. When old people choose or find themselves on pathways that are not widely shared with others or reinforced by institutions or policies, they may lose important sources of informal and formal support. In old age, these losses may come at a high price, particularly for those individuals and groups already at risk, because there may be less time to recover and fewer personal and social resources to marshal in compensatory ways. Moreover, policies meant to help old people may end up hurting them if they are based on outdated models of life that do not reflect contemporary experiences and opportunities. These points highlight the need to redefine and broaden thinking about the groups of people who are at risk as they move through life—and, in the case of old age, arrive with long histories of risk that greatly influence the freedoms or constraints that individuals feel during life's final decades.

In the absence of clear scripts for life, including old age, one must ask what happens over time to the mental health of individuals when there is no shared framework within which to assess themselves and others. How can people make plans, set goals, and take action, knowing all the while that their lives will be continually altered in ways that cannot be predicted and can be only partially controlled? What are the implications for how societies might function when age-based norms vanish? These are central challenges for theorizing aging and the life course in postindustrial societies.

No matter how such variability arises, it should become the friend rather than the enemy of theorists of aging. Variability is not something that should be wished away for simplicity's sake; it should instead be actively seized to produce fresh and innovative theories of aging that do right by the complexity of our subject matter.

The Big "Ifs": Old Age as a Highly Contingent Period

Uncertainty has been part of life in every historical period, but there can be no doubt that the nature and even level of uncertainty today is quite different than just half and full centuries ago (for hypotheses, see Settersten, 2007b). The ability to plan a life of one's own and project possibilities long into the future rests on having a relatively certain future to begin with. The decreases in mortality, morbidity, and fertility noted earlier now make it more possible to plan. The mere fact that individuals can count on long and largely healthy lives is an enormous luxury—and, in the larger historical picture, a fairly recent phenomenon. Many of the key concerns of contemporary times—in every domain of life and sector of society—could not have emerged even half a century ago (or at least not in the same way) precisely because basic conditions of life and of death were so different.

Yet the precondition of a long and largely healthy life is not a universal phenomenon, even today. In many parts of the world, life simply *cannot* be counted on—whether in nations experiencing political and economic upheaval, war, and violence or in developing countries characterized by very poor health conditions, high rates of poverty, and high rates of mortality, even among the young.

Despite these important exceptions, one can still argue that old people today face lives with far *greater* predictability and choice than ever before—afforded partly through longer life and better health and partly through their better aggregate standing on financial and other indicators of well-being relative to prior cohorts.

Being able to count on an old age, however, is not the same as being able to predict *how* those years will be experienced or *whether* the balance of experiences will be positive. Indeed, we argue that one of the primary ways in which old age today is distinct from younger life periods is that *the later years have a highly contingent quality*. The fact that old age is longer and highly variable seems to have made its contingent quality more salient. Old age is embodied with so much possibility—yet its potentials, if they are to be realized, depend on some big "ifs" that cannot be predicted or controlled.

These big "ifs" especially relate to life, health, and resources: *if* I am (or my partner is) still alive, *if* I am (or we are) healthy, *if* I (or we) can manage financially, *if* I (or we) can live independently, *if* my (or our) children are able or willing to help, and so on. As these contingencies come undone, so too do the futures that have been counted on or taken for granted. For individuals and their families, the ways in which these big "ifs" play out are themselves conditioned by dimensions such as social class, family resources and ties, cohort, and gender. These same forces are at work in creating shifting sands and mines in the larger social terrain of old age—to which we now turn.

Shifting Sands and Mines of Old Age

The Great Divide: Social Class

In the future, social class will almost certainly become the most powerful factor in determining aging and life course experiences and in creating "cleavages" within societies (see also Furstenberg, 2003; Kohli, 2007). Disparities related to social class are growing on indicators of all kinds; inequalities generated by social class will likely trump inequalities that stem from gender, race, and ethnicity and will wield additional power *through* these other statuses. Individuals with adequate resources early in life often accumulate resources over time, while those with few or no resources stay the course at best (see also Dannefer, 2003; chapter 22 in this volume). This results in significant disparities in financial, social, and other resources by old age. The chasm between those who do and those who do not have resources leaves people in positions and with experiences that are worlds apart. This chasm is likely to persist—and even grow—in the future.

Social class must therefore be a central focal point for theories of aging in all substantive areas. Social class is at present remarkably absent in scholarship and policy-making on aging. Yet most aspects of aging and old age are—or can be expected to be—shaped by social class: life expectancy, physical and psychological health, family structure and relationships, social integration and engagement, personal resources, and so forth. Given this, theories of aging must be sensitive to how these different worlds of old age are related to and even produced by social class and how patterns of aging are products of earlier inequalities.

It is also important to consider intersections between social class and other social dimensions. Consider the revolutionary racial-ethnic population changes already under way and on the horizon, particularly those related to immigration dynamics. Such transformations are radically altering the face of aging in the United States and bringing challenges that must be understood and prepared for. These are not pure changes in racial-ethnic composition; they are also about social class. Race, ethnicity, and immigration status are tightly coupled with social class in America, so much so that it is difficult to address one without the other.

Understanding the growing diversity of the population is therefore not just about understanding *difference*; it is about understanding differences that generate and are generated by *inequality*. Both difference and inequality must be incorporated into theories of aging. In fact, the issues we posed earlier about the need to revisit the "demographic imperative" (which concerns the implications of the shifting *age* structure of the population) should also be posed for the shifting *racial-ethnic* composition of the population: What does it mean to grow old in an increasingly diverse and unequal society and to grow old as a member of one of these groups? How is diversity altering the terrain of old age and creating reverberations in periods of life before it? How might the social institutions and policies that serve old people be rearchitected in light of it? These questions demand exploration and will require (and also lead to) new theories to guide them.

Similarly, the generational equity debate that surfaced a few decades ago and attempted to pit children and old people against one another in a struggle for public resources seems dead for the moment. It is possible that real tensions between age-groups could manifest themselves in bigger and stronger ways in the decades ahead as the visibility and demands of the aged population increase. It seems more likely, however, that subgroups of people *within* the aged population will have greater competing needs—especially by social class and wealth, and by health status. Old people in good standing on these fronts seem faced with a wide array of choices. But the most vulnerable of old people will not only have fewer choices; they will also have fewer capacities and resources on which to draw as they make those choices, further exacerbating their existing vulnerabilities. These chasms seem likely to fracture any political power that older people, as a group, might have over younger groups.

These and other cleavages will make aging and the life course even greater sources of political regulation and conflict and of public controversy and struggle (see also Kohli, 2007). Theories of aging, in turn, must reflect and inform these explicitly *political* aspects. Welfare states are an important part of this equation, as they, along with families, powerfully determine how old age is experienced by providing different packages of resources that create stronger or weaker scaffolding for old people as they move through life's final decades (see also chapters 29 and 32 in this volume).

Families as Risk Absorbers—and Risk Creators

As the period of old age has become more protracted, individualized, and open to new vulnerabilities and risks, the family is often the primary institution called on to absorb the costs of these risks. The abilities of families to manage this long and complex period varies extensively by the resources they possess or those they can access through formal and informal ties. Experiences in old age therefore seem very different depending on personal and family resources and connections—and so, again, social class rears its head. Old people in relatively privileged families may have the luxury to use their later years for purposes of exploration—to return to school, to switch careers or work as desired, to volunteer, to pursue activities aimed at personal growth and development, and the like (see also chapter 23 in this volume). Such patterns are actively chosen and permitted by personal resources and health status. In contrast, for old people in less privileged families these possibilities seem more tenuous and out of reach, as they may be required to work beyond retirement age, as life must be managed with limited means or poor health, and as family members struggle to stay afloat and cannot readily provide or buy support. These two different profiles of life experiences in old age result from very different educational, work, and family trajectories that, again, seem tied to early family resources and personal options.

While family relationships can offer help and protection in old age, as in the rest of life, it is equally important to remember that family relationships can also create risks—for both men and women alike. Many assumptions in social policies about the presence and nature of family relationships are inherited from the past and no longer warranted (for illustrations, see Settersten, 2007a). This is especially true in light of dramatic changes in marriage, divorce and remarriage rates, as well as other aspects of family life—patterns that seem likely to diversify further in the future (see Bianchi, Robinson, & Milkie, 2006). These changes have brought new complexities, disruptions, and ambiguities to relationships, leaving them potentially more fragile than before in old age and every period of life (for illustrations, see Settersten, 2007c). At the same time, longer lives and better health have made possible more durable, active, and intense social relationships; a wider and more varied mix of family, family-like, and nonfamily ties; and the ability to inhabit family and other roles in novel ways (for illustrations, see Putney & Bengtson, 2003; Riley & Riley, 1996; Settersten, 2007c).

The Future Is Already Here: Revolutions in Cohort Composition and Experiences

Future cohorts will enter and navigate old age with different characteristics, experiences, resources, expectations, and needs than those of the past. But the future of aging is already here. It can be partly understood by getting more intimately acquainted with cohorts who are *not yet old*. Understanding the middle aged is particularly important, for they are next in the queue. For example, doom-and-gloom public discourse surrounding the baby boom generation has focused on how its size has strained the social institutions through which it has moved during early and middle adulthood. There is little doubt these challenges will continue as members of the baby boom move through old age. But it is important to remember that the physical, psychological, and social statuses of the boomers are extremely favorable relative to cohorts past—or at least the early cohorts of boomers. In fact, one could argue that in the future there may not be another group of people who enter old age as *uniformly* well positioned as these early boomers. (The cohorts that make up the tail end of the baby boomers do not seem as advantaged as the earlier members of the generation.) Important theoretical advances will be found by probing the implications of their better positions for all aspects of aging as well as by probing their assumptions about and perspectives on old age, which will yield insights into the new and emerging models of old age for which they are striving (see also Moen, 2003, on the notion of "midcourse").

Yet we should also become intimately acquainted with cohorts currently in early adulthood. These cohorts are experiencing a significantly prolonged transition to adulthood, with delays accompanying many specific transitions—leaving home, finishing school, starting work, being married or partnered, and having children (e.g., Settersten, Furstenberg, & Rumbaut, 2005). Relative to other cohorts, younger generations are in some ways better off and in some ways worse off—but their worldviews are clearly different from previous cohorts and the routes they are taking toward adult roles and responsibilities are more circuitous. Their lives will not match the linear models of the life course that underlie many contemporary educational, work, and family policies; these mismatches will likely play out in ways never before seen, whether in early adulthood, midlife, or old age. As these young adults grow older, they, like the boomers, will further challenge much of what we now take for granted in theories, research, and public policies of aging. The lives of each of these cohorts have been subject to very different historical circumstances than the cohorts on whom scientific knowledge of aging has thus far been based.

All of these shifts—from the baby boomers to current young adults and so on—serve as reminders that lives and times seem always to be in flux and that change is the rule rather than the exception. As change occurs, we cannot treat "new" conditions as if they have somehow become permanent, which we so often do. Such conditions will eventually be displaced by new ones. In addition, even change we deem to be positive is certain to challenge our work as scientists—and our existence as human beings. It is easy to say that change has occurred. It is much harder to specify what precisely has changed, which parts matter more for which kinds of functioning and which kinds of people, and the mechanisms through which the effects of social change can be traced. Theories of aging must address dynamic phenomena—in individual lives, in families, and in societies—ideally cutting across these levels to understand how change on one level affects and is affected by change on other levels. Yet the constant presence of change, coupled with the fact that it often feels so remote and hard to assess, is what makes its incorporation into theories of aging so difficult.

Breakups in the Gendered Life Course

Trends in women's educational attainment, employment, and earnings suggest that women's lives are converging with men's despite the fact that on some dimensions, such as economic standing, their aggregate status remains lower.

To date, women's family relationships have been more active and positive and have offered greater protection for women than for men (chapter 28 in this volume). Yet there may be long-term negative legacies for women's relationships, marked by divorce and remarriage and by commitments to education and employment, the consequences of which remain unknown. Regardless, recent cohorts of women will have hopes for and experiences in old age that are sure to differ from past cohorts of women. It is important to explicate how the changing choices and circumstances of women earlier in life will flavor and even determine the choices and circumstances they face later in life. It is also interesting to wonder whether women's lifelong commitments to diverse and multiple roles might also make it easier for women to adjust to change and manage hardships when they are old.

Men's family relationships are especially important to watch, particularly the connections between men and children. Surprisingly, a range of social indicators reveal that men are, as a group—and contrary to public perception—becoming *less* intensely involved with and committed to children (e.g., Eggebeen, 2002). Divorce is particularly important to understand because it often leads to a loss or restriction of fathers' ties to children.

One begins to wonder, then, what these trends will mean for men's future experiences in old age. The picture is bleak if men's social relationships in late life become even more tenuous than they are today. At the same time, it is possible that subgroups of men who clearly *are* making bigger investments in children will therefore have relationships that become protective in later life. There is also evidence that cohorts of young men currently entering adulthood have more fluid attitudes about masculinity and manhood, which may improve the look and feel of old age for men in the future (see also Cohler & Smith, 2006).

Old age may also offer novel powers and possibilities for men's relationships. Aged men seem to lose interest in or care less about the judgments of other men, and it is the acceptance of other men, not women, that most prominently shapes definitions of masculinity and manhood (Turner, 2006). In being secure in one's own masculinity and liberated from the approval of others, old age may provide men with greater freedom and time to explore relationships and express themselves in new ways.

It is important to note that trends in educational and occupational attainment, earnings, and family formation often differ dramatically for particular subgroups of men and women—especially by social class and by race or ethnicity. Theorists must remain mindful of how the differential attainments and experiences of these subgroups earlier in life will leave individuals in different financial, social, and psychological standings in old age (see also chapter 22 in this volume).

Markers of Becoming and Being Old

Age and Agelessness

When does old age begin, and what markers signify entry into and calibrate movement through it? Traditional markers of entry into old age—at least in many Western nations—have been tied largely to chronological age and eligibility for old-age programs and entitlements and to retirement from work (e.g., Leisering, 2003). These markers, embedded in laws and policies, are important forces in how old age is socially constructed and personally experienced (Hendricks, 2004). Historically, the age of eligibility for Social Security and pensions in the United States—age 65—was long synonymous with "old age." There is a need to examine, in contemporary times, the ages that Americans now associate with "old," to know whether public definitions have changed as eligibility criteria for age-based entitlements have been raised, as retirement patterns have become variable, as old age has grown longer and generally healthier, and as age itself has lost its relevance as an index of individuals' maturity, roles and statuses, and needs. Nonetheless, the encoding and reifying of age in social policy determines the content of particular life periods and affects how individuals think about themselves and others as they occupy those periods.

Interestingly, research on "age identity" and "subjective age identity" (e.g., Barrett, 2003, 2005; Kaufman & Elder, 2002, 2003) has consistently revealed discrepancies between how old individuals actually are and how old they report feeling, looking, and acting. Taken together, this research suggests aggregate trends for people to begin reporting younger subjective ages than chronological ages in the second half of life. There is great resistance to labeling oneself as "old," even among people who would be classified as old on the basis of ages that far exceed criteria for old-age policies and programs. "Old" is a label that seems far easier to apply to others than to oneself. Adopting and fostering a "youthful" identity can serve as a mechanism of self-enhancement, especially for individuals in youth-oriented cultures like the United States (Barrett, 2003). But at what point does the maintenance of a youthful identity, as a self-enhancement mechanism, become limited in its effectiveness—and even leave individuals unable to experience old age for all that it is, good and bad? Still unclear are the points or conditions under which individuals ultimately evaluate themselves or others in ways that are consistent with or even surpass their chronological ages. Many factors surely affect how "old" or "young" individuals feel relative to others or to themselves at earlier times and in what specific ways they feel older or younger. Much remains to be learned about these processes and the meanings of age in different contexts.

Gerontologists and aging advocacy organizations have been prophets of agelessness, going to great lengths to promote positive images of old people and old age and to combat negative stereotypes—so much so that even the use of term "old" has become taboo. This sentiment is further reflected in the social world, in which media, the "antiaging" industry, and cultural norms emphasize the ability or need to defy aging. Ironically, these messages end up restricting rather than expanding the models of aging for public consumption because they communicate that *defying* aging is the primary way to *go about* aging. In this sense, the preoccupation with being age*less* itself becomes a marker of old age, for agelessness is something that seems largely sought by and marketed to people who *are* old, rather than young.

Amidst all this agelessness, one must ask whether aging professionals—including theorists and researchers—do old people a tremendous disservice in the process. Too strong an emphasis on the powers and potentials of aging threaten to obscure from our lenses the real underbellies of aging and old age—not only the normative physical and cognitive declines experienced by many people but, more important, the individuals and groups whose conditions deviate from these norms. The dark sides of aging need to be acknowledged if they are to be understood and handled effectively.

Beyond Age: Alternative Markers

Somewhat ironically, age *itself* has lost some of its relevance as a straightforward marker of *old* age. So what is it, then, that signals to individuals that they are becoming or are old? Little is known about the specific markers on which individuals rely, how they judge and apply these markers to themselves and others, and what these markers mean to different kinds of people in diverse life circumstances. Investigating these issues will guide theories of aging in important new directions. To promote discussion, let us offer some good candidates to be explored, many of which can be extracted from existing literature:

- Increasing prospects of failing health or chronic health conditions
- Declining physical and cognitive statuses and the onset of multiple conditions
- The growing salience of health concerns in individuals' self-definitions
- A growing fear of losing control over one's life, driven by the declining body
- A dwindling time horizon and the need to come to terms with one's mortality
- An increased search for meaning in life
- A growing concern for younger generations and acts of generativity
- The death of parents, spouses, and friends
- Moving up the family "ladder" and especially assuming the top position once parents have died
- Becoming a grandparent or great-grandparent
- Seeing one's children reach middle age or one's grandchildren reach adulthood
- Shrinking social networks
- Being perceived or treated by others in ageist ways
- Retiring, whether chosen or forced
- Drawing on Social Security or Medicare
- Moving to a long-term care or retirement community

This list is by no means exhaustive, but it does contain what we imagine to be among the most poignant subjective markers of aging and old age. Of course, the experiences and interpretations of these markers will be conditioned by the characteristics and circumstances of individuals or vary across social class, gender, racial-ethnic, and other groups. Whether such experiences are welcomed or avoided, or positively or negatively evaluated, will also to a great extent be found in the eye of the beholder.

It is important to note that these markers make up a *process* that is likely to be understood and experienced gradually. Some of these markers may be more significant—in their perceptibility or in how they matter for one's self—than others, depending on their qualities (e.g., whether they are anticipated, controllable, typical, desirable, or acute). Some markers may also be understood and experienced in interconnected and bundled ways rather than singly.

One can imagine that achieving an identity as "old," like that of an "adult" earlier in the life course (Settersten, in press), happens slowly and is punctuated with notable "old age" moments that signal to individuals and those around them that they are changing. One can also imagine that old age is often reached without much fanfare or, for that matter, much recognition by oneself or others. This process may even be met with some resistance or denial, such that signals may be dismissed or explained away—until they become more rhythmic or dense and must ultimately be confronted by and incorporated into the identities of individuals and the views of others around them.

While we have described these alternative markers as extending "beyond age," it would be naive to suggest that they are not age related. These markers may not occur lockstep at predictable, fixed ages, but they are experiences that many old people share despite their differences. Indeed, many seem like essential parts of what it means to be human. If these experiences are acknowledged as such, they may carry the potential to unify and connect groups of people who might otherwise have—or think themselves to have—little in common.

What to Pack: Necessary Skills and Capacities for Navigating Old Age

In light of the changing contours of old age, it is important to understand the social skills and psychological capacities that may be particularly helpful to individuals as they make their way. Given the highly individualized and contingent nature of old age, individual characteristics and resources have become increasingly important in determining experiences than heretofore. These skills and capacities may serve as alternative or additional forms of "capital" in negotiating old age, especially in compensating for its uncertainties and for the often weak scaffolding provided by some families and welfare states. To stimulate discussion, we offer a few skills and capacities that would seem to have widespread applicability in many contexts and populations. These include the following:

- ***Interdependence***—reflected in wide and strong webs of relationships with others. These relationships include networks of loosely connected acquaintances who might provide access to valuable opportunities and resources and potential protections (what Granovetter [1983] called "the strength of weak ties"). Still, more superficial connections like these are not likely the stuff from which major personal responsibilities, obligations, or sacrifices are borne. A small number of meaningful relationships seem especially critical to ensuring strong protections for old people when it is (inevitably) required. Unlike *dependence,* fears about which are particularly strong in the United States, the notion advanced here with respect to *interdependence* is not about completely relying on others for one's own welfare but rather about both making and maintaining positive, healthy, mutual, and reciprocal relationships that contribute to the well-being of both parties (see also chapter 14 in this volume).
- ***Fluid self-definitions***—as adaptation during old age, like earlier life periods, may be facilitated by being open and committed to experimenting

with a range of selves. Old age would seem to offer important opportunities for individuals to reclaim selves they once left behind or to try on selves they have longed to explore. Of course, this can be done to a greater or lesser extent depending on one's health and resources. But the new terrain of old age may make it advantageous and even necessary for individuals to *actively strive* for fluid and dynamic self-definitions in an effort to maximize their opportunities during a risk-laden portion of life.

- ***The ability to plan for and set realistic goals***—but goals characterized by *flexibility* and *openness* to new and unexpected experiences.
- ***The capacity for intimacy and close social relationships***—in an effort to form and maintain healthy, supportive relationships and strengthen interdependence with others.
- ***The capacity for intergroup relationships***—in being able to understand and relate to one's own "group" as a single group within a diverse society and, more important, in being open to and having relationships with members of other groups.
- ***Reflective capacity and "developmental regulation"***—in possessing self-awareness and the ability to take into account the feelings and behaviors of others before acting and in being able to exercise self-control and restrain one's impulses in accordance with social norms.
- ***Self-efficacy***—in being able to manage disappointment and be persistent when confronted with setbacks, foreclosed opportunities, or failures.

Many of these skills and capacities seem interrelated, with higher or lower levels of one promoting higher or lower levels of the others. Yet as a bundle, they would seem to foster adaptation and resilience in the face of uncertainty, risk, shifting opportunities, and unexpected or difficult experiences. There are, of course, existing and even large bodies of literature on each of these skills and capacities, but little of it has explored interconnections among these skills and capacities or their joint relevance or influence in old age. There are also many other skills and capacities that can and should be considered in theories and research on aging. The particular characteristics mentioned here, however, seem especially important for the most vulnerable of elders who have few other social resources at their disposal with which to protect themselves. Yet elders from more privileged backgrounds probably possess higher levels of these capacities and skills, as most of these things are associated with higher educational, work, and financial statuses. As a result, these additional types of "capital" may further protect those who already have access to other kinds of resources. One could also argue that these skills and capacities have been equally important for navigating old age in the past and are equally desirable in earlier periods of life. These remain important open empirical questions for future scholarship.

Conclusion

This chapter begins with an exploration of the new terrain of *old age*. We have tried to delineate some of its emerging hallmarks as well as some of its shifting sands and mines—all of which create new constellations of risk *and* opportunity for old people, their families, and societies. We have reflected on some of the things that may now mark movement into and through old age as well as some of the social skills and psychological capacities that may be helpful in navigating these decades. On each of these fronts, we have pointed to issues that bring significant challenges to existing theories of aging and to the generation of new theories. As these issues are addressed or further explored, they are sure to prompt theoretical and empirical advances in gerontology. Indeed, many of the ideas we have put forward are tentative and in need of comprehensive and systematic investigation.

So many of the issues we have raised also seem to be occurring in or have reverberations for other periods of life. In some ways, the whole of human life seems in flux, and some of the hallmarks, risks, and opportunities of old age may also be shared with earlier periods of adult life—especially the protracted and variable transition to adulthood (for comparison, see Settersten, 2007b).

The task of explicating the changing terrain of old age, then, becomes inextricably linked to explicating the changing terrain of the entire life course. Aging and the life course cannot be separated. Indeed, greater attention to the life course in recent years has revolutionized gerontology because it has demanded that aging be understood as a lifelong process and old age as a product of the past. But in emphasizing the variability that results from these long histories, such a perspective has also caused us to lose sight of what it is that old people have in common *precisely because* they are old and *despite* their differences. Theories of aging must now grapple more seriously with these tensions between commonness and difference.

Similarly, theories must also address how aging and old age today are similar to and different from earlier historical periods. There seems to be a tendency to assume that little about aging and old age today was true just a few decades ago. In writing this chapter, we have ourselves been guilty of making this assumption. Might it be possible that there *are* some aspects of aging and old age that are enduring and timeless?

Finally, old age is the sole period of life in which only those individuals who inhabit it can truly know it. Old age is something *toward which* most people are moving, not *from which* they are leaving or have already left, as is the case with childhood, adolescence, and early adult life. Most people who create expectations, conduct research, make policies, and engage in practice related to old people and old age *are not themselves old.* This seems true of most gerontologists, including the contributors to this *Handbook of Theories of Aging*, which is a centerpiece in the field. We are outsiders to the very people and phenomena we hope to understand. We can only assume what it is like to be old, though we have all had direct experiences with old people in our families and our society. These assumptions and experiences affect what we do (or do not do) with and for old people. This predicament creates challenges for theory and research. It also suggests that our knowledge base might itself have a questionable quality, especially if it is not firmly anchored in the voices and perspectives of old people who can, with great depth and texture, tell us firsthand what it is actually like.

References

Barrett, A. E. (2003). Socioeconomic status and age identity: The role of dimensions of health in the subjective construction of age. *Journal of Gerontology: Social Sciences, 58B,* S101–S109.

Barrett, A. E. (2005). Gendered experiences in midlife: Implications for age identity. *Journal of Aging Studies, 19,* 163–183.

Beck, U. (2000). Living your own life in a runaway world: Individualization, globalization, and politics. In W. Hutton & A. Giddens (Eds.), *Global capitalism* (pp. 164–174). New York: New Press.

Bianchi, S. M., Robinson, J. P., & Milkie, M. A. (2006). *Changing rhythms of American family life.* New York: Russell Sage Foundation.

Cohler, B. J., & Smith, G. D. (2006). The dilemma of masculinity and culture. In V. H. Bedford & B. F. Turner (Eds.), *Men in relationships: A new look from a life course perspective* (pp. 3–26). New York: Springer Publishing.

Dannefer, D. (2003). Cumulative advantage/disadvantage and the life course: Cross-fertilizing age and social science theory. *Journal of Gerontology: Social Sciences, 58B,* S327–S337.

Eggebeen, D. J. (2002). The changing course of fatherhood: Men's experiences with children in demographic perspective. *Journal of Family Issues, 23,* 486–506.

Fries, J. F. (2005). The compression of morbidity. *Milbank Quarterly, 83,* 801–823. (Original work published 1983)

Furstenberg, F. F., Jr. (2003). Reflections on the future of the life course. In J. T. Mortimer & M. J. Shanahan (Eds.), *Handbook of the life course* (pp. 661–670). New York: Kluwer Academic/Plenum Press.

Granovetter, M. (1983). The strength of weak ties: A network theory revisited. *Sociological Theory, 1,* 201–233.

Hendricks, J. (2004). Public policies and old age identity. *Journal of Aging Studies, 18,* 245–260.

Kaufman, G., & Elder, G. H., Jr. (2002). Revisiting age identity: A research note. *Journal of Aging Studies, 16,* 169–176.

Kaufman, G., & Elder, G. H., Jr. (2003). Grandparenting and age identity. *Journal of Aging Studies, 17,* 269–282.

Kohli, M. (2007). The institutionalization of the life course: Looking back to look ahead. *Research in Human Development, 4,* 253–271.

Leisering, L. (2003). Government and the life course. In J. T. Mortimer & M. J. Shanahan (Eds.), *Handbook of the life course* (pp. 205–225). New York: Kluwer Academic/Plenum Press.

Moen, P. (2003). Reconfiguring careers and community service for a new life stage. *Contemporary Gerontology, 9*(3), 87–94.

Putney, N. M., & Bengtson, V. L. (2003). Intergenerational relations in changing times. In J. T. Mortimer & M. J. Shanahan (Eds.), *Handbook of the life course* (pp. 149—163). New York: Kluwer Academic/Plenum Press.

Riley, M. W., & Riley, J. W., Jr. (1996). Generational relations: A future perspective. In T. K. Hareven (Ed.), *Aging and generational relations over the life course* (pp. 526–532). New York: Walter de Gruyter.

Settersten, R. A., Jr. (2007a). The new landscape of adult life: Road maps, signposts, and speed lines. *Research in Human Development, 4,* 239–252.

Settersten, R. A., Jr. (2007b). Passages to adulthood: Linking demographic change and human development. *European Journal of Population, 23,* 251–272.

Settersten, R. A., Jr. (2007c). Social relationships in the new demographic regime: Potentials and risks, reconsidered. *Advances in Life Course Research, 12,* 3–28.

Settersten, R. A., Jr. (in press). Becoming adult: Meanings and markers for young Americans. In M. Waters, P. J. Carr, M. Kefalas, & J. Holdaway (Eds.), *Coming of age in America.* Berkeley: University of California Press.

Settersten, R. A., Jr., Furstenberg, F. F., Jr., & Rumbaut, R. (Eds.). (2005). *On the frontier of adulthood: Theory, research, and public policy.* Chicago: University of Chicago Press.

Turner, B. F. (2006). In the company of men: Collective independence and self-construal in masculinity. In V. H. Bedford & B. F. Turner (Eds.), *Men in relationships: A new look from a life course perspective* (pp. 167–196). New York: Springer Publishing.

Theorizing Feminist Gerontology, Sexuality, and Beyond: An Intersectional Approach

25

Toni Calasanti

Despite growth in the study of old men and masculinities (e.g., Calasanti, 2004; Calasanti & King, 2005, 2007; Davidson, Daly, & Arber, 2003; Russell, 2004), feminist gerontology continues to be seen as a specialized approach within gerontology overall, unable to contribute to knowledge about aging in general. In this chapter, I contend that feminist gerontology is inclusive in that it theorizes *gender relations* and thus the experiences of both women and men. Further, I argue that a focus on intersecting inequalities is critical to understanding those experiences of aging and that feminist gerontology is uniquely able to offer scholars a lens through which to view these intersections. To demonstrate these points, I briefly outline the emergence of feminist gerontology and discuss intersections of gender with other systems of inequality, including age.

I am indebted to Neal King for his thoughtful comments and editing of earlier drafts of this chapter.

Next, I challenge feminist gerontologists to take seriously inequalities based on sexuality, to which scholars often allude but rarely discuss in depth. I end with a discussion of whether the potential of feminist approaches to aging would be enhanced by dropping the use of the "f" word and adopting a different moniker.

Feminist Gerontology: A Brief Overview

Spurred by the 1970s women's movement, in the 1980s, some scholars of aging began to question the lack of explicit attention paid to aging women. For instance, women were routinely excluded from retirement research (Gratton & Haug, 1983). The presumed split between private and public spheres fostered a belief that paid labor was central only to men's identities and that, especially for married women, "retirement is usually irrelevant" (Bixby & Irelan, 1969, p. 144).

Initial calls to address women's omission from aging research often led simply to adding women to samples and placing them into models and theories derived from men's experiences. Conceptually, gender remained an individual attribute within such models, and, as Gibson (1996) notes, scholars tended to discuss gender differences in old age in ways that treat men as the implicit standard against which women are assessed. As a result, scholars noted differences between men's and women's labor force participation histories and women's subsequent lower retirement benefits but failed to ask why women's work histories were more intermittent, why Social Security rewards stable participation, why dependent-spouse benefits amount to only half of the retired-worker benefit, or whether women and men garner similar workplace returns for similar human capital attributes.

Feminist gerontology emerged in the 1990s, partly in response to this failure to theorize the relations of inequality that underlie gender differences. It examined women's experiences from their own standpoints, but it has allowed scholars to reformulate methods and derive theories that incorporate men's experiences as well. Its critical approach to gender inequality has led some feminist gerontologists to theorize the larger system of intersecting *relations* of inequality, a project shared with other groups of scholars, driven by overlapping social movements (e.g., labor, civil rights, gay/lesbian, and Gray Panthers).

In its theories of such systems of inequality, feminist gerontology recognizes that both women and men have gender and that their experiences are structured by *gender relations:* dynamic, constructed, institutionalized processes by which people orient their behaviors to ideals of manhood and womanhood, influencing life chances as they do so. Gender is not a biological given but is what people collectively agree that natural sex attributes mean. Societies organize on the basis of gender such that what people take to be masculine and feminine influences and reflects gendered divisions of labor, the performance of which people evaluate and reward in a differential fashion. Thus, the gender identities that emerge in social interaction also serve to privilege men—give them unearned advantages—while they usually disadvantage women, even as people resist and reformulate seemingly "natural" gender differences and meanings.

Gender relations are embedded in patterns of behavior such that they are generally invisible, taken for granted, and unquestioned, as they reflect the way that social institutions, such as paid work or family, normally operate. The systematic nature of gender relations means that even though individuals enact them, gender relations are not dependent on any one person's actions or intentions. Because men's privileges are intimately tied to women's disadvantages, the situation of one group cannot be understood without at least implicit reference to the position of the other.

For instance, beginning with women's experiences of retirement has revealed the ways in which men's and women's experiences of this transition are related. To be sure, women's responsibility for domestic labor shapes their retirement by lowering their potential income; it also means that when they leave the labor force, they relinquish only their paid labor and maintain their unpaid work. In this sense, the meaning of "freedom" in retirement for women includes continued labor, even though they may be happy with this time in their lives. The contribution of feminist theory was to move beyond simply noting women's deviations from the model of retirement built for male breadwinners and to theorize the ways in which collective efforts to see that women lived up to ideals of gendered labor shaped their work lives.

Divisions of domestic and paid labor also influence men's lives—both their greater retirement income potential and their relative freedom. That is, husbands' abilities to enjoy successful careers and financial security in old age or the choice of what work (if any) to perform in retirement rest on the domestic labor of their wives (Calasanti & Slevin, 2001).

Theories of such gender relations explain what might otherwise appear anomalous, such as the ways in which subordinate status can result in strengths while privilege can be harmful. For instance, women's immersion in the work of daily life, including kin keeping, provide them resources in later life that men may not enjoy at that stage. Not only do such networks offer social support in old age; for those with fewer material resources, such networks may also ensure a decent quality of life. Because men are not responsible for domestic life, they often access social networks through their wives. Thus, some men can be highly dependent on their wives for social and material resources, and men who are not married often have smaller networks (Barker, Morrow, & Mitteness 1998; Davidson et al., 2003).

Intersecting Inequalities

For many gerontologists with ties to liberatory social movements that demand attention to inequality, the picture of retirement painted here would be inadequate without a sense of its place in a larger system of *intersecting inequalities*. Recent feminist gerontologists have argued that just as gender shapes aging, so too do other hierarchies influence both gender and aging (e.g., Calasanti, 2004; Calasanti & Slevin, 2001; Connidis, 2001; McMullin, 2000). Thus, while feminist gerontologists may focus on gender at points in their analyses, they recognize that old men and women do not exist apart from their racial and ethnic, sexual, and class-based locations. For instance, if we look only at gender, we see a much higher incidence of poverty among old women. But when we look at intersections with race, we find that Blacks—men and women—have higher poverty rates than do White women (Social Security Administration, 2006). No doubt, this results in part from White women's ability to align themselves with those with greater privilege (i.e., White men). Similarly, Black women who live alone have a much higher incidence of poverty than their male or White counterparts despite longer labor force histories (Administration on Aging, 2007). Recognition of the importance of such intersections is increasingly common in feminist gerontology and has extended to the study of privilege as an ongoing accomplishment—something, for instance, that men must continually struggle to achieve.

Multiple masculinities, based on intersecting inequalities, shape men's behaviors but usually operate in orbit around a hegemonic set of ideals characteristic of any society's ruling elites (Connell, 1995). This process of struggling to achieve or maintain masculinity (hegemonic or an alternative form) influences the old-age experiences of men in many ways, some of which are debilitating. Men's attempts to achieve dominant ideals of masculinity may lead them to take physical risks that women do not take. Such actions may differ by class based on cost and accessibility, such that car racing is the activity of choice for poorer or working-class men, while skydiving fits the bill for men of higher class (Courtenay, 2000). Further, exclusion from legitimate avenues for economic success based on race, class, and sexuality can result in the construction of alternative masculinities that both repudiate accepted ideals and threaten health. The resultant street culture can include such behaviors as excessive drinking and drug use, demonstrations of physical prowess and risk taking, and dangerous sexual behavior (Anderson, 1999). These practices are just some of those that can influence men's health in later life, in similar and different ways, by social location.

By way of theorizing intersecting inequalities, such feminist theorists as Young (1990) have given us criteria by which we can assess systems of privilege and oppression. Based on these criteria, we might define a group as oppressed to the extent that they experience economic marginalization, powerlessness and a lack of authority and status, and stigmatization. Those who are privileged use their greater resources to control those who are disadvantaged and justify these inequalities through ideologies that deem them to be "natural" and thus beyond dispute or based on social necessity or the will of a higher power (Calasanti & Slevin, 2006; King, 2006). Recently, feminist gerontologists have used these criteria to theorize old age itself as a social location, part of a system of age relations that intersects with other forms of inequality.

Age Relations

Similar to gender relations, the term *age relations* encompasses the ways in which age serves a social *organizing principle* such that different age-groups gain *identities and power* in relation to one another. That societies are organized on the basis of age is widely accepted, as is the notion that individuals and groups gain identities as they strive to live up to age-specific ideals of behavior (Hendricks, 2003). Relatively unexplored by most social gerontologists, however, is whether and how such age-based organization matters for life chances (McMullin, 2000). Analytically, this implies that old age does not simply exacerbate existing inequalities but is instead embedded in age-based power relations such that being old, in and of itself, confers a loss of power for all those designated as "old" regardless of their possible advantages on other social hierarchies. A detailed exposition of inequalities in relation to the criteria for a system of privilege and oppression is beyond the scope of this chapter (but see, e.g., Calasanti, 2003; King, 2006); here I only briefly address these.

Economic marginalization is apparent in the multiple studies that show that older people experience labor market discrimination in relation to hiring, earnings, and job stability (Bytheway, 1995; Encel, 1999). Such ageism intersects with gender to further reduce unemployed older women's job opportunities (McMullin & Berger, 2006). And beyond the workplace, the vast majority of old people must depend on Social Security for financial solvency. In 2006, Social Security provided at least half of all income for two-thirds (65%) of eligible beneficiaries and a full 90% or more income for more than one-third (34%) (Social Security Administration, 2007). Even with Social Security, more than a third (35%) of Blacks are poor or near poor; 30% of Hispanics are similarly situated, as are 29% of unmarried women (Social Security Administration, 2006). Yet during times of fiscal austerity, politicians tend to protect younger groups at the expense of expenditures for older people, often using inadequate or faulty demographic projections to make such decisions (Wilson, 2000).

In their daily lives, old people experience powerlessness in their loss of authority and their ability to exert control over their bodies and personal decisions. For example, doctors withhold information, services, and treatment from old patients more often than with younger clients (Robb, Chen, & Haley, 2002). They take the complaints of old people less seriously, often simply ascribing reported symptoms to "old age" (Quadagno, 1999). At the same time, the increasing biomedicalization of aging means that some old people lose their ability to make decisions about medical care and their bodies because doctors simply turn to drug use rather than other curative treatments (Estes & Binney, 1991; Wilson, 2000).

Finally, the stigma and cultural devaluation that accrue to old age are evidenced by the number of people trying to avoid the physical markers of aging through such strategies as spending time at gyms and the use of surgical and nonsurgical cosmetic techniques and products, a wide range of dietary supplements, and drugs to produce erectile penises. Further, the equation of old age with disease and decline legitimates limiting the rights and authority of old people. Ideologies of old people's physical frailty and their economic dependence on paid workers both reflect inequalities and reinforce their differential treatment (King, 2006). Such ideologies are internalized by old people themselves so that they avoid identifying themselves as old (Minichiello, Browne, & Kendig, 2000) and thus are unlikely to band together to counter these views and promote their interests. In this manner, old people become depicted as "others" who are not fully deserving of citizenship rights (Wilson, 2000).

While feminist gerontologists have begun to make inroads into the topic of age relations, one form of inequality often added to the list of important systems of oppression and privilege but still untheorized is that based on sexuality. In order to demonstrate the ways in which feminist theory mixes with scholarship inaugurated within other overlapping social movements and thus contributes to a larger study of inequality, I discuss the intersections of relations of age, gender, and sexuality.

Sexuality

Sexuality fits the criteria for privilege and oppression outlined previously: inequalities in terms of wealth, authority and status that are justified by ideologies that posit such inequalities as natural and beyond dispute. Nonheteroseuxals are both stigmatized and subject to various methods of control, including violence (Rubin, 1984; Stein, 2008), and they lose in terms of status, income, and wealth (Badgett, 2001; Heaphy, 2007). This situation is exacerbated by the fact that, at the federal level alone, "1,138 statutory provisions [use] marital status [as] a factor in determining or receiving federal benefits, rights, and privileges" (Hereck, 2006, p. 614), including Social Security and other entitlement programs, access to affordable housing, employee benefits, death benefits, and tax breaks. The obvious financial benefits that advantage married couples relative to those who are single are exacerbated by similar state provisions (Hereck, 2006). And contemporary arguments against allowing nonheterosexuals to marry are based in ideologies that maintain that that which is not heterosexual is unnatural (in terms of nature or god) or goes against the social good (maintenance of family). In these ways, sexuality constitutes a relationship of privilege and oppression.

To begin, *heteronormativity* (norms, beliefs, and practices that naturalize heterosexuality) is a key organizing principle of society (Stein, 2008). That is, the assumption of heterosexuality as natural lies at the heart of social organization, shaping the experiences of people of all sexual preferences: not only are nonheterosexual persons disadvantaged by a range of social practices based on the notion that women and men naturally desire to mate with members of the other group, but avowed heterosexuals both are "policed" (Stein, 2008) and receive unearned advantages as result. To the extent that such advantages are often unseen, a focus on people who are oppressed on the basis of sexual orientation reveals not only the sources and depth of their disadvantage but also the invisible advantages that heterosexuals enjoy daily.

Although we live in a society in which the reality of sexuality is taken for granted, it has not always been the case that people have taken any particular activity to connote "sex" or any particular orientation (Rupp, 2001). The construction of certain behaviors as sex is social, and as is the case with gender, race, ethnicity, and old age, societies construct heterosexual and nonheterosexual people differently, with those differences both reflecting and perpetuating inequality. Sexuality is thus more than identity (Heaphy, Yip, & Thompson, 2004); it is basic to social organization and "an important focus of power and resistance" (Heaphy, 2007, p. 194).

Social relations of sexuality developed in relation to changing modern forms of labor. First, the concept *sexuality* gained its meaning over the course of the 19th century's industrializing process, as moral reformers concerned with disciplining labor and consumption invent labels for reckless, instinctual, unproductive activity and posed those newly coined sexualities (e.g., masturbation, prostitution, and homosexuality) as threats to social order (Bristow, 1997; Greenberg, 1988; Laqueur 1990, 1992, 2003). As a social organizing principle, sexuality was thus distinct from gender relations in which men barred women from professional and citizen status (Rubin, 1984; Ward, 2008).

Only at the end of the 19th century did sexual identity emerge as a salient issue, with the coining of such terms as "heterosexual" and "homosexual."[1] Those terms became relevant as middle-class parents and medical professionals concerned themselves with the development of boys into laborers and especially into professionals whose work would require discipline. The terms also came into more popular use as urban, homosexual communities appropriated them to identify themselves as political agents and thus rally in their own defenses against state persecution (D'Emilio, 1983; Greenberg, 1988; Sedgwick, 1992).

Rubin (1984) argues that in contemporary society, notions about what counts as appropriate sexuality not only extract harsh legal and economic penalties on those who do not conform but also effectively control all people's behaviors. Further, sexuality intersects with other forms of oppression such that those who are marginalized by other systems of inequality tend to feel the brunt of such control. For instance, sexual violence has been used to control and exploit African American women (Collins, 2004); the myth of Black men as rapists justified lynching as a form of sexual violence and social control (Davis, 1981). More recently, research has explored the role of whiteness (including White masculine archetypes, such as frat boys, surfers, and jocks) and class in constructing "believable" heterosexual masculinity (Ward, 2008).

Sexuality relates to labor in a second manner that also affects its intersection with other relations of oppression. Ideals of sexuality include opposite-sex couples engaged in marital, reproductive activity and exclude those who do not conform to this ideal from occupational and family-based privileges. *Compulsory heterosexuality* refers to the set of institutionalized pressures on women to form sexual relationships with men, ranging from social exclusion to eugenics to rape (McLaren, 1999; Rich, 1986). All women are subject to these pressures such that single, unmarried women are suspect and treated as deviant, though in the contemporary context, censure for singlehood varies by class (e.g., middle-class women may be expected to complete higher education first) and race (e.g., the lack of marriageable men increases the likelihood that Black women will be single).

Drawing on decades of feminist scholarship, especially the demonstration of the centrality of unpaid labor to social life, Acker (2006, 2008) outlines a feminist political economy. By taking women's unpaid labor into account, she reconceptualizes the economy as based on *provisioning:* providing what is socially recognized as needed for individual and community survival. Such economic activity, which involves production, social reproduction, and distribution, need not involve monetary exchange and thus includes many unpaid activities—done in the contemporary United States mainly by women under the pressure of compulsory heterosexuality. Acker argues that provisioning takes a particular form within capitalism, which was created predominantly by White men. Production and power are centered in corporations, far from households and families, and the "norms of heterosexuality are deeply embedded in this gendered organization of 'public' production and household activity" (Acker, 2008, p. 106).

From this standpoint, reproductive labor appears as central to political economy, and the exploitation of women's labor appears to rest on compulsory heterosexuality. Heteronormativity thus helps to shape a social order in which women are to provide unpaid, reproductive labor that benefits men and bolsters their status in the public realm. Further, Connell (1987) argues that heterosexuality is key to hegemonic masculinity, as women's exploitation is institutionalized in marriage; thus, homosexual masculinity is a key form of subordinated masculinity.

What a political economic analysis reveals is a system of sexual oppression—appropriation and control of labor—that is analytically distinct from but shaped by intersections with race, class, and gender. For instance, the sexualities that come under the greatest scrutiny as dysfunctional tend to include those that seem either undisciplined or unproductive—the latter including that of people past retirement age. Old people find themselves stigmatized either as overly passive and retiring if they abstain or as disgusting if they seek intercourse (Calasanti & King, 2005; Katz & Marshall, 2003). In addition, all women are pressured to provide unpaid labor, the greatest benefit of which goes to those with the most advantaged positions—that is, White, well-to-do men who can both support dependents financially and amass greater wealth as a result. The implications of these intersections have important consequences for later life, some of which are outlined next.

Gender, Sexuality, and Aging

The negligible attention paid to sexuality and aging in mainstream gerontological literature is no doubt attributable in part to the assumption that analysis of sexuality applies to a small group. What feminist gerontology argues instead is that sexual oppression and privilege influences all old people and thus should play an important role in aging theory, research, and practice. In this section, I briefly discuss some of the ways in which scholarship that takes sexuality seriously would proceed. I focus on intersections with gender and age relations for reasons of space, but other intersections must be considered as well.

The scant research on old sexuality focuses on identity (e.g., Fullmer, Shenk, & Eastland, 1999; Rosenfeld, 2003). Although some research maintains that nonheterosexual identity shapes aging in positive ways, usually because of presumed skills gained in relation to managing their nonheterosexual identity, other research suggests that nonheterosexual persons can be lonely and isolated (Friend, 1991; Heaphy, 2007). To be sure, issues of identity shape the aging experiences of nonheterosexuals in significant ways that heterosexuals do not have to consider. For instance, expected and actual discrimination makes caregivers for gay and lesbian elders reluctant to request services, especially medical or in-home services, even if they can afford these, for fear of biased treatment (Brotman et al., 2007; Cantor, Brennan, & Shippy, 2004). Variation in publicly acknowledged partner status can present caregivers additional limits on general mental health (Fredriksen, 1999) and on the effectiveness of their advocacy for the care receiver (Brotman et al., 2007). Similarly, the fact that health care providers often overlook questions of sexuality for all clients and are often uncomfortable with these topics adds to the discomfort older gays and lesbians feel in relation to the long-term care system, a system that has already been intolerant of gays and lesbians (Brotman, Ryan, & Cormier, 2003). Examples of "survival strategies" in such contexts include a woman who changed her last name to her partner's so that providers would think they were sisters (Brotman et al., 2003).

However, this focus on sexual identity as "the key determining factor of later life experience" is both problematic and should be augmented with investigation of how other inequalities shape old lives (Heaphy, 2007). While some of this variation may be due to cohort differences in terms of the historical period in which persons came to identify themselves as gay or lesbian (Rosenfeld, 2003), the consequences of nonheterosexuality for aging go far beyond identity. For instance, Heaphy (2007) argues that the dominant discourses concerning differences between men and women, particularly in relation to heterosexual love and family, shape their actions within the economic sphere and make women economically dependent on men—which in turn has important ramifications for men's and women's financial positions in later life.

The impact of sexuality can be seen both over the life course and in relation to policies derived for old age. A brief overview of financial security in later life provides examples. The workplace discrimination faced by nonheterosexuals affects hiring, job safety, and mobility, resulting in lower wages (Badgett, 2001), and includes workplace policies that deny health coverage to such persons as partners and nonbiological children of partners and so on. People justify such discrimination both in terms of the association of homosexuality with the range of undisciplined sexualities and in terms of the deviation of homosexuality from ideals of reproductive heterosexuality. Stigmatized as disorderly and unproductive, lesbians, gay men, and other sexual minorities remain targets of labor policies that reduce their life chances. That discrimination has cumulative effects and places many lesbian and gay seniors at financial and health risk in later life, particularly as this status intersects with gender, class, and racial/ethnic inequalities. Thus, Heaphy (2007) finds that lesbians are disadvantaged in the labor market because of their gender, especially those who had been married and had been engaged in care work. Thus, even if it is the case that being nonheterosexual encourages greater economic independence for lesbians (in relation to heterosexual women), thereby enhancing their financial position in later life, they are still subject to gender-based discrimination.

Consider also the heteronormativity embedded in federal policies for old people, such as Social Security and Medicare. This disadvantages many old people, across a range of social locations. It excludes from benefits nonheterosexuals while subjugating women and men of color who are likely to earn lower wages in their racialized occupational niches and thus collect lower benefits in old age. Those who cannot legally marry cannot collect benefits on the basis of their partners' work histories. Women remain dependent on their heterosexual bargains: not only is the dependent spouse's benefit only 50% of the retired worker amount (more than 90% of those who collect as dependent spouses are women), but Social Security is calculated in such a way (assuming the economic dependence of a spouse) that some dual-earner couples receive less in Social Security benefits than if they had had the same income but that income was brought home by one traditional breadwinner. Social Security thus serves as an example of compulsory heterosexuality; the legislation not only assumes but reinforces heterosexual women's dependence on men while penalizing those who do not follow these sexual dictates. Nonheterosexual people are also constrained from reaping the health benefits—financial and in terms of social support—that accrue to marriage (de Vries, 2007).

Incorporation of sexuality challenges us to rethink aging theories and research in all realms. In relation to informal caregiving, a focus on gender alone might reveal the ways in which men and women draw on gender repertoires as they perform their care work. Such repertoires consist of the skills and resources that people develop over their life course that affirm their gender identities. Caregiving experiences (and sources of stress) differ for men and women to the extent that their skills allow them to perform care work as they believe they should, according to their senses of selves as men and women. For instance, men tend toward more managerial styles, performing care work in a more task-oriented fashion, while women approach it with more empathy (Calasanti, 2006; Rose & Bruce, 1995). Thus, caregiving husbands report relatively little distress because they find enjoyment in the sense of task accomplishment and are better able to compartmentalize the loss of marital reciprocity, whereas women, for whom caregiving is generally not new, grieve for the lost emotional relationships (Rose & Bruce, 1995). The belief that women are more natural caregivers appears to create higher standards against which many of the women hold their care work, resulting in greater stress when problems arise. By contrast, men convey that they would work hard at giving care, but because such work is not a part of their self-concept as men, difficulties did not detract from their identities as husbands and men (Calasanti, 2006). Other research also suggests that caregiving husbands will discuss instrumental and not affective matters (Russell, 2004), a tendency that also fits with masculine identity.

Such research has taken for granted the way in which *heterosexuality* shapes gender repertoires by assuming a marital relationship with different roles for husbands and wives. Among present cohorts of older men and women, for example, wives were to perform the bulk of the domestic labor and child care and thus developed self-identities as nurturing, whereas most husbands worked at occupations that emphasized problem solving and control and thus developed self-identities rooted in task accomplishment (Calasanti, 2006). Gay men and lesbians are socialized in the same culture; they learn the same gender roles. But same-sex couples cannot fall back on notions of "husbands" or "wives" as they engage in their intimate relationships and must negotiate who will perform what domestic labor. Thus, research finds that gay and lesbian couples tend to be relatively egalitarian (Heaphy, 2007). Gender matters, but it does so differently in nonheterosexual contexts. Gay men may develop both the workplace skills and the identities noted previously, while they also learn aspects of domestic labor that husbands are relatively likely to forgo because they cannot assign responsibility for it to wives. How such gender repertoires influence care work is unknown.

Similarly, research shows that husbands typically rely on wives for emotional support; Russell (2004) suggests that this means caregiving husbands may experience greater isolation than do caregiving wives. Given that gay men do not have wives, how does their being men shape their experiences of isolation? The links between gender and sexuality are complex, so no obvious answers pertain. Gendered assumptions for both heterosexuals and nonheterosexuals are resistant to change as they are "internalized, reconfirmed and shored up through institutionalized social practices, relations and discourses" (Heaphy, 2007, p. 201) across the life course. Thus, research on heterosexual couples in retirement finds that, despite women's increased labor force participation and some changes in gendered behaviors, women mostly retain responsibility for domestic labor, even when husbands opt to "help out" (Calasanti & Slevin, 2001).

The intersections of gender with ageism can take many forms, shaped by heterosexual and nonheterosexual contexts. Research on the antiaging industry finds that among those assumed to be heterosexual, aging women are valued only to the extent that they continue to be attractive to men; such appeal is based not so much on being active and healthy as on looking youthful. Once this diminishes, women who are deemed to be old shift from being sexually exploited to being sexual *castoffs*. In light of ideals of sexual *productivity* that shape the larger relations of compulsory heterosexuality, old women's assertion and desire appears in popular culture as a joke if at all. By contrast, White, well-to-do men can stave off ageism to the extent that they are able to compete with younger men in performance—they must be "sexually functional" (Katz & Marshall, 2003) and able to compete at work and not allow themselves to become in any way "feminine" through hormonal changes that are thought to sap their prowess and masculinity (Calasanti & King, 2005, 2007).

The status of old gay sexuality as doubly unproductive affects women and men. Older lesbians often say that youth is less important in their culture than for heterosexual women (Heaphy, 2007) because they are not as subject to the "male gaze." However, in addition to the caution that internalized gendered values and assumptions are often resistant to change, research shows a similar resistance to changing ageist values and assumptions among those who are old (Hurd Clarke, 1999; Minichiello et al., 2000). Thus, Slevin (2006) finds that older lesbians' experiences and practices often contradict their claims that their community is more accepting of older women; they engage in distancing tactics from those who might be deemed "old," worry about losing weight, and approve of cosmetic surgery for looking younger. At the same time, gay men are more likely to feel that "the visible signs of ageing had marked them as undesirable in gay culture" (Heaphy et al., 2004, p. 898), and some older gay men indicate a preference for younger partners (Heaphy, 2007).

Many older gays and lesbians speak of ageism, noting that "beauty, and youthfulness are values that reign supreme within most gay and lesbian communities" (Brotman et al., 2003, p. 198). Perhaps as a result of this—and despite the fact that nonheterosexual communities can provide important sources of support over the life course—a significant minority of both gay men and lesbians report feeling isolated from such community supports (Brotman et al., 2007; Heaphy, 2007). Those who had been very couple focused but whose relationships ended (for whatever reason) find it hard to become a part of a community. Age was a critical reason, particularly for gay men who allude to the emphasis on youth and physical appearance within gay male culture (Heaphy et al., 2004). Although participants in one study felt that such exclusion was less true among lesbians, still, one-third of lesbians surveyed (compared to one-half of men) felt unwelcome in nonheterosexual places as they aged. Along these lines, Heaphy (2007) notes gender differences in the extent to which nonheterosexual communities provide gays and lesbians resources for dealing with aging. Both gay men and lesbians talk of their "self-made communities" and support networks, but while lesbians point to the ways they participate in mutual care and talk about their communities in positive ways, gay men are more likely to say that they would like to receive care from their communities and said that they felt excluded from their communities in some ways.

In part, this ageism is manifest in the lack of attention that gay and lesbian communities pay to issues faced by their older members, particularly in contrast to the amount of time and energy that is spent "articulating and responding to the needs of its younger members" (Brotman et al., 2003, p. 198). Such older members feel that this is directly attributable to the ageism within both gay and lesbian communities. Some gay men and lesbians have remarked on their increasing invisibility in both heterosexual and nonheterosexual communities. That is, despite the possibility that being open about their lives could put them at risk, many nonheterosexuals were very engaged in their local community, and many developed protective strategies. However, they have found that getting older reduced their risks of being identified as nonheterosexual (Heaphy et al., 2004); they realized that they become more invisible sexually—but also in every way—as they age. Because they are old, they are seen as asexual; they thus become nonthreatening to heterosexuals while becoming more invisible within their communities.

Thus do the relations of sexuality and age, imbricated as they are with modern systems of labor and social control, intersect in the lives of old people. This framework, drawn from the feminist study of gender inequality as well as the scholarship inspired by other social movements of the 20th century, provides critical explanations of old people's experiences unavailable from most life course and more traditional gerontological perspectives.

Discussion: Where Do We Go From Here?

My goal in this chapter has been to show that, with its emphasis on intersecting power relations, feminist gerontology provides a framework for exploring the intersections of a range of inequalities and their effects on women and men. When one begins with an understanding of the inextricable links between privilege and disadvantage, it becomes apparent that, in fact, gender—and hence feminist gerontology—relates to all old people. Further, just as consideration of the intersections of power relations have led scholars of gender to recognize multiple masculinities and femininities (Connell, 1995), so too does the intersection of age relations with other social locations reveal multiple "old ages"—discourses and practices that vary by gender, race, ethnicity class, and sexual preference.

Theories of inequality in old age include political economy and feminist theories; these can be and often are fruitfully joined (e.g., Estes & Associates, 2001; McMullin, 2000). But this conjunction appears to be one sided. That is, while feminist gerontologists often utilize the macrolevel contributions of political economy in understanding various old-age experiences, most political economists do not employ feminist gerontology to complicate their own work. While they may *acknowledge* gender, race, ethnicity, and sexuality (among other hierarchies) as important, they also tend to treat those as epiphenomena without fundamental theoretical import. The difference lies in how theorists treat relationships among forms of inequality. The intersectional view is apparent in the ways in which feminists such as Acker (2008) makes clear that our theorizing should "focus on the relational and reinforcing processes of mutual and emergent reproduction of gender, class, race, and sexuality" (p. 197) (and, I would add, age). Thus, she discusses class as "gendered and racialized"; class does not stand on its own.

An additional explanation for the relative disuse of this theoretical tradition may lie in the use of the term *feminism* to describe this approach, a label that may allow many scholars to assume that it deals only with women. I have maintained my tie to "feminist gerontology" to honor its roots, to insist on respect for the perspective and for those who are disadvantaged as well as advantaged, and in resistance to those who would co-opt or blunt the critique of feminists by acting as if we live in a "postfeminist" society. At the same time, as feminist approaches more broadly and feminist gerontology in particular continue to evolve, it may be that the term does not adequately convey the import of the perspective. *Feminist* connotes gender, but as the discussion here makes clear, even when gender relations are the focus, they also constitute but one form of inequality. And to the extent that this is the case, feminist theorizing has learned from and incorporated theories (and social movements) related to other forms of inequality as well. A name that reflects these aspects of feminist gerontology and the central emphasis on power relations may be needed.

Note

1. Prior to the modern era, what we now define as sexual activity between persons of the same sex was typically neither seen as sexual nor marked as "same sex." Rupp (2001) argues that status differences, such as those based on age, were more salient. Thus, age was critical in determining the character of sex acts in ancient Athens; adult male citizens of Athens penetrated younger men (as well as other social inferiors), an activity that was thought to be as educative as much as sexual. Similarly, 17th-century Japanese men were expected to desire sexual relationships with boys as well as women; in some cultures in New Guinea, moving into male adulthood is marked by formal rituals in which boys ingest older men's semen (Rupp, 2001).

References

Acker, J. (2006). *Class questions: Feminist answers.* Lanham, MD: Rowman & Littlefield.

Acker, J. (2008). Feminist theory's unfinished business: Comment on Andersen. *Gender & Society, 22,* 120–125.

Administration on Aging. (2007). *Profile of older Americans: 2007.* Washington, DC: U.S. Department of Health and Human Services.

Anderson, E. (1999). *Code of the street: Decency, violence, and the moral life of the inner city.* New York: Norton.

Badgett, M. V. L. (2001). *Money, myths, and change: The economic lives of lesbians and gay men.* Chicago: University of Chicago Press.

Barker, J. C., Morrow, J., & Mitteness, L. S. (1998). Gender, informal social support networks, and elderly urban African Americans. *Journal of Aging Studies, 12,* 199–222.

Bixby, L. E., & Irelan, L. M. (1969). The Social Security Administration program of retirement research. *The Gerontologist, 19,* 143–147.

Bristow, J. (1997). *Sexuality.* London: Routledge.

Brotman, S., Ryan, B., Collins, S., Chamberland, L., Cormier, R., Julien, D., et al. (2007). Coming out to care: Caregivers of gay and lesbian seniors in Canada. *The Gerontologist, 47,* 490–503.

Brotman, S., Ryan, B., & Cormier, R. (2003). The health and social service needs of gay and lesbian elders and their families in Canada. *The Gerontologist, 43,* 192–202.

Bytheway, B. (1995). *Ageism.* Buckingham: Open University Press.

Calasanti, T. M. (2003). Theorizing age relations. In S. Biggs, A. Lowenstein, & J. Hendricks (Eds.), *The need for theory: Critical approaches to social gerontology for the 21st century* (pp. 199–218). Amityville, NY: Baywood Publishing.

Calasanti, T. M. (2004). Feminist gerontology and old men. *Journal of Gerontology: Social Sciences, 59,* S305–S314.

Calasanti, T. (2006). Gender and old age: Lessons from spousal caregivers. In T. Calasanti & K. Slevin (Eds.), *Age matters: Re-aligning feminist thinking* (pp. 269–294). New York: Routledge.

Calasanti, T., & King, N. (2005). Firming the floppy penis: Age, class, and gender relations in the lives of old men. *Men and Masculinities, 8,* 3–23.

Calasanti, T., & King, N. (2007). "Beware of the estrogen assault": Ideals of old manhood in anti-aging advertisements. *Journal of Aging Studies, 21,* 357–368.

Calasanti, T. M., & Slevin, K. F. (2001). *Gender, social inequalities, and aging.* Walnut Creek, CA: AltaMira Press.

Calasanti, T. M., & Slevin, K. F. (Eds.). (2006). *Age matters: Re-aligning feminist thinking.* New York: Routledge.

Cantor, M. H., Brennan, M., & Shippy, R. A. (2004). *Caregiving among older lesbian, gay, bisexual and transgender New Yorkers.* New York: National Gay and Lesbian Task Force Policy Institute.

Collins, P. H. (2004). *Black sexual politics: African Americans, gender, and the new racism.* New York: Routledge.

Connell, R. W. (1987). *Gender and power.* Cambridge: Polity Press.

Connell, R. W. (1995). *Masculinities.* Berkeley: University of California Press.

Connidis, I. (2001). *Family ties and aging.* Thousand Oaks, CA: Sage.

Courtenay, W. H. (2000). Constructions of masculinity and their influence on men's well-being: A theory of gender and health. *Social Science and Medicine, 50,* 1385–1402.

Davidson, K., Daly, T., & Arber, S. (2003). Exploring the social worlds of older men. In S. Arber, K. Davidson, & J. Ginn (Eds.), *Gender and ageing: Changing roles and relationships* (pp. 168–185). Philadelphia: Open University Press.

Davis, A. (1981). *Women, race, and class.* New York: Random House.

D'Emilio, J. (1983). Capitalism and gay identity. In A. B. Snitow, C. Stansell, & S. Thompson (Eds.), *Powers of desire: The politics of sexuality* (pp. 100–113). New York: Monthly Review Press.

de Vries, B. (2007). LGBT couples in later life: A study in diversity. *Generations, 31,* 18–23.

Encel, S. (1999). Age discrimination in employment in Australia. *Ageing International, 25,* 69–84.

Estes, C. L., & Associates. (2001). *Social policy & aging: A critical perspective.* Thousand Oaks, CA: Sage.

Estes, C. L., & Binney, E. A. (1991). The biomedicalization of aging: Dangers and dilemmas. In M. Minkler & C. L. Estes (Eds.), *Critical perspectives on aging: The political and moral economy of growing old* (pp. 117–134). Amityville, NY: Baywood Publishing.

Fredriksen, K. (1999). Family caregiving responsibilities among lesbians and gay men. *Social Work, 44,* 142–155.

Friend, R. A. (1991). Older lesbian and gay people: A theory of successful aging. *Journal of Homosexuality, 20,* 99–118.

Fullmer, E. M., Shenk, D., & Eastland, L. J. (1999). Negating identity: A feminist analysis of the social invisibility of older lesbians. *Journal of Women & Aging, 11,* 131–148.

Gibson, D. (1996). Broken down by age and gender: "The problem of old women" redefined. *Gender & Society, 10,* 433–48.

Gratton, B., & Haug, M. R. (1983). Decision and adaptation: Research on female retirement. *Research on Aging, 5,* 59–76.

Greenberg, D. F. (1988). *The construction of homosexuality.* Chicago: University of Chicago Press.

Heaphy, B. (2007). Sexualities, gender and ageing: Resources and social change. *Current Sociology, 55,* 193–210.

Heaphy, B., Yip, A. K. T., & Thompson, D. (2004). Ageing in a non-heterosexual context. *Ageing & Society, 24,* 881–902.

Hendricks, J. (2003). Structure and identity—Mind the gap: Toward a personal resource model of successful aging. In S. Biggs, A. Lowenstein, & J. Hendricks (Eds.), *The need for theory: Critical approaches to social gerontology* (pp. 63–87). Amityville, NY: Baywood Publishing.

Hereck, G. M. (2006). Legal recognition of same-sex relationships in the United States. *American Psychologist, 61,* 607–621.

Hurd Clarke, L. (1999). "We're not old!": Older women's negotiation of aging and oldness. *Journal of Aging Studies, 13,* 419–439.

Katz, S., & Marshall, B. (2003). New sex for old: Lifestyle, consumerism, and the ethics of aging well. *Journal of Aging Studies 17,* 3–16.

King, N. (2006). The lengthening list of oppressions: Age relations and the feminist study of inequality. In T. Calasanti & K. Slevin (Eds.), *Age matters* (pp. 47–74). New York: Routledge.

Laqueur, T. W. (1990). *Making sex: Body and gender from the Greeks to Freud.* Cambridge, MA: Harvard University Press.

Laqueur, T. W. (1992). Sexual desire and the market economy during the industrial revolution. In D. C. Stanton (Ed.), *Discourses of sexuality: From Aristotle to AIDS* (pp. 185–215). Ann Arbor: University of Michigan Press.

Laqueur, T. W. (2003). *Solitary sex: A cultural history of masturbation.* New York: Zone Books.

McLaren, A. (1999). *Twentieth-century sexuality: A history.* Oxford: Blackwell.

McMullin, J. A. (2000). Diversity and the state of sociological aging theory. *The Gerontologist, 40,* 517–530.

McMullin, J. A., & Berger, E. D. (2006). Gendered ageism/age(ed) sexism: The case of unemployed older workers. In T. Calasanti & K. Slevin (Eds.), *Age matters* (pp. 201–223). New York: Routledge.

Minichiello, V., Browne, J., & Kendig, H. (2000). Perceptions and consequences of ageism: Views of older people. *Ageing & Society, 20,* 253–278.

Quadagno, J. (1999). *Aging and the life course.* Boston: McGraw-Hill.

Rich, A. C. (1986). Compulsory heterosexuality and lesbian existence. In *Blood, bread, and poetry: Selected prose, 1979–1985* (1st ed., pp. 23–75). New York: Norton.

Robb, C., Chen, H., & Haley, W. (2002). Ageism in mental health care: A critical review. *Journal of Clinical Geropsychology, 8,* 1–12.

Rose, H., & Bruce, E. (1995). Mutual care but differential esteem: Caring between older couples. In S. Arber & J. Ginn (Eds.), *Connecting gender & ageing* (pp. 114–128). Buckingham: Open University Press.

Rosenfeld, D. (2003). *The changing of the guard: Lesbian and gay elders, identity and social change.* Philadelphia: Temple University Press.

Rubin, G. S. (1984). Thinking sex: Notes for a radical theory of the politics of sexuality. In C. Vance (Ed.), *Pleasure and danger: Exploring female sexuality* (pp. 267–319). Boston: Routledge.

Rupp, L. J. (2001). Toward a global history of same-sex sexuality. *Journal of the History of Sexuality, 10,* 287–302.

Russell, R. (2004). Social networks among elderly men caregivers. *Journal of Men's Studies, 13,* 121–142.

Sedgwick, E. K. (1992). *Between men: English literature and male homosocial desire.* New York: Columbia University Press.

Slevin, K. F. (2006). The embodied experiences of old lesbians. In T. Calasanti & K. Slevin (Eds.), *Age matters* (pp. 247–268). New York: Routledge.

Social Security Administration. (2006). *Income of the aged chartbook, 2004.* Washington, DC: Office of Research, Evaluation, and Statistics.

Social Security Administration. (2007). *Fast facts and figures on Social Security, 2007.* Washington, DC: Office of Research, Evaluation, and Statistics.

Stein, A. (2008). Feminism's sexual problem: Comment on Andersen. *Gender & Society, 22,* 115–119.

Ward, J. (2008). Dude-sex: White masculinities and "authentic" heterosexuality among dudes who have sex with dudes. *Sexualities, 11,* 415–435.

Wilson, G. (2000). *Understanding old age.* Thousand Oaks, CA: Sage.

Young, I. M. (1990). *Justice and the politics of difference.* Princeton, NJ: Princeton University Press.

26 Theorizing Across Cultures

Peggye Dilworth-Anderson
Monique D. Cohen

The ever-growing and diverse older population in the United States requires that researchers and theorists understand diversity beyond racial categories and changes in the numbers of group members. At the numerical level, the older adult population is increasing at a faster rate than any other subgroup in America. In 2002, the older population numbered 35.6 million; this was an increase of 3.3 million, or 10.2%, since 1992 (U.S. Census Bureau [hereafter Census], 2002). Among the aging population, the percentage of older adults who are members of minority groups will grow between 2000 and 2050 at an even faster rate than the White majority. Minority populations are projected to represent 26.4% of the aging population (65 years or older) in 2030, up from 17.2% in 2002 (Census, 2000). Between 2000 and 2030, the White population 65 years and older is projected to increase by 77% compared with 223% for older minorities, including

Hispanics (342%); African Americans (164%); American Indians, Eskimos, and Aleuts (207%); and Asians and Pacific Islanders (302%) (Census, 2000).

When considering diversity in later life beyond numbers and static categories, it is important to consider cultural differences between groups as a major way of understanding what the numbers actually mean. In this discussion, we refer to Goodenough's (1999) definition of culture as a set of shared symbols, beliefs, and customs that shape individual and group behavior. Goodenough (1999) suggested that culture provides guidelines for speaking, doing, interpreting, and evaluating one's actions and reactions in life. In addition, his concept of cultural frame provides further insight into how individual characteristics and experiences, such as gender and age, can influence cultural beliefs and values (Goodenough, 1981). He suggested that cultural frames allow us to understand how an individual's culture is developed through the incorporation of the totality of one's experiences, interactions, and thoughts with the norms and expectations one perceives as being held by other group members. Therefore, because of differences in individual cultural frames, people can simultaneously be cultural group members and hold cultural beliefs that are not shared by some members of the group (Goodenough, 1981).

Theorizing across cultures in later life is indeed a large intellectual and conceptual endeavor. The process of theorizing across cultural groups, however, is not viewed here as a new process for every group that we study. Instead, we propose that once a culturally competent theorizing process or approach is in place, theorizing across cultural groups becomes more likely. With this in mind, this chapter provides several streams of discussion on ways that researchers and theorists can approach theorizing across and about diverse older cultural groups. Our first discussion provides insight into what we describe as some fundamentals for understanding theorizing across cultures that address cultural values and beliefs. The second discussion focuses on what we call the firewall of cultural theorizing. The third section addresses how theory and methods inform each other. We end the chapter with some discussion on retooling and theorizing across cultures.

Some Fundamentals: Cultural Metaphors and Values

Metaphors can provide insight into why and how cultural groups behave and interact in certain ways (DeJong, 2004). Different cultural groups use distinct metaphors to express their experiences, which often have historical connections that are passed from one generation to the next within a culture. In the African American culture, for example, the circle has represented both the confinement of bondage and a sense of belonging within their cultural community. The circle has also been seen as protective and nurturing and may have helped to create closeness and intimacy to bind family relationships among some immigrants (Greenfield, 1984). The fence, another metaphor of some cultural groups, sets limits about who comes in and who is kept out.

We believe that cultural values of a group can give more concrete meaning to the metaphors when theorizing across cultures in later life. Cultural values can inform theorizing across cultural groups because they provide an understanding of "being" for a people. Values are defined in this discussion as internal criteria for evaluation (Hechter, 1993). More specifically, values can be defined as "principles, or criteria, for selecting what is good (or better or best) among objects, actions, ways of life, and social and political institutions and structures. Values operate at the level of individuals, institutions, and entire societies" (Hechter, 1993, p. 155). They are standards that guide individual actions, even though they may change over time because of individual, group, historical, and societal factors. They give more than insight; they provide some explanation and understanding of a persons or group's life. Values also provide direction for behavior and give parameters for acceptable and unacceptable behavior within groups. They also tell us what to expect of ourselves and what to expect of others within our primary groups, such as families. Similar to metaphors, values provide an understanding of how individuals experience themselves and others. Dilworth-Anderson, Burton, and Klein (2005) stated that the metaphors we live by are created by the values we hold, based in part on the experiences that shape our lives. Thus, metaphors provide images and meanings, and values provide the vehicle through which they become real in everyday life.

Of course, theorists themselves also bring their own values, assumptions, and history to the theorizing process that impact their approaches to understanding diverse cultural groups. An examination of one's own background and experiences, which will include values, may be a necessary prerequisite for the study of culturally diverse groups. Such examination may lead to understanding the limitations of existing theoretical paradigms and traditions, which shape how groups are approached at many levels. The importance of values in the study of culturally diverse groups challenges researchers to move beyond perspectives and theories that are laden with researcher's values but have been presented as though they were scientific truths. Ideas, conceptual views, and theoretical perspectives are invented by humans, who are products of their experiences and, more relevantly, their values and assumptions. It is important to acknowledge that even a researcher's predisposition for asking certain questions and propensity for conducting research in a certain method is influenced by the researcher's values. Moreover, whether acknowledged or not, values guide most of what a person thinks and does. Therefore, awareness of our own values is viewed here as an important part of theorizing.

The Firewall of Cultural Theorizing

A firewall of cultural theorizing provides insight into and knowledge about the boundaries of our theories regarding diverse cultures. These boundaries should serve to encompass the cultural values relevant to the group while keeping out the influence of our own values. Cultural metaphors and values can inform creating these boundaries, and they can help researchers formulate and pose important culturally relevant questions. Can the people we are theorizing about recognize that we are interpreting them and their lives? In other words, are we theorizing within the boundaries of the lived experiences of diverse cultural groups? How do we recognize when we have moved *too far* from the cultural reality of any group, and, equally important, do we know the cultural reality of the group? When we ask these types of questions about a group, particularly about their cultural metaphors and values and their historical and sociopolitical realties, we are helping to create a "firewall" of culturally competent boundaries of our theoretical thinking. Further, the firewall of theorizing should always emphasize the importance and significance of another people's culture in order to develop competent boundaries of our theoretical thinking. Equally important in creating this firewall is how we can maintain it and make it effective. We propose that culturally competent and relevant theories and methods are needed to help maintain an effective theoretical firewall.

The Informing Links Between Methods and Theories

When Methods Inform Theorizing

We believe that no one method is best or most appropriate for informing theorizing about diverse cultures. Multimethod approaches (e.g., quantitative and qualitative interviews, observations, and focus groups) have been identified as helpful in theorizing about diverse cultures. For example, ethnographic interviews and information from focus groups can inform developing theoretical concepts, and the methods can inform interpreting findings. More important, we believe, as noted earlier, that the critical issues are those that relate to informing us how these methods will yield better theorizing about diverse cultures. The use of grounded theory, coupled with survey research, for example, is very useful in helping to create and expand theoretical thinking. Therefore, we propose that, in collaboration with survey research, grounded theorizing, a method that generates culturally relevant concepts, be used. Grounded theory, which was first introduced by Glaser and Strauss (1967) in the early 1960s, has been specifically used in the analysis of qualitative data, allowing researchers to systematically identify and extract concepts and relationships among variables from the data (Strauss, 1987). Grounded theory takes an emic understanding of the world whereby categories of information drawn from respondents themselves help make implicit belief systems explicit. It involves using an inductive process to collect, analyze, and interpret information gathered from cases (Glaser & Strauss, 1967; Strauss & Corbin, 1998). Any concepts derived through using this approach are thought to be culturally relevant because they emerge from the cultural agendas and meanings that respondents assign to the phenomena being studied. The grounded theory approach may be a particularly viable method for developing culturally relevant ways of thinking and theoretical perspectives for studying diverse cultures. Further, using the grounded theory approach, one could identify traditional themes and concepts that emerge and new or different ones that are culture specific. When culturally relevant, these methods should also allow for defining and giving meaning to certain concepts from a cultural frame of reference.

A grounded theory approach also works well with certain theoretical perspectives and methods. For example, perspectives on the social construction of reality (Berger, 1967; Berger & Luckmann, 1966) can be used to interpret findings from qualitative studies, which fits well with using a grounded theory approach to gathering and interpreting information. These perspectives suggest that the very fabric of social order is determined by the meanings assigned by its members as well as the interpretations that they make in legitimizing what they have created.

The use of the community-based participatory research (CBPR) approach is another methodological approach that informs conducting research as well as creating and expanding theoretical thinking about culturally diverse older populations. This is a collaborative approach to research that equitably involves all partners in the research process and recognizes the unique strengths that each brings. One of the major components of this approach is the involvement of both the researchers and the communities they study in helping to frame the research topic. Community members (in this instance culturally diverse communities) can also contribute their expertise and share responsibility and ownership of the research project. The CBPR approach promotes colearning, involves a cyclical and iterative process, disseminates findings to all partners, and involves a long-term commitment by all partners (Israel, Schulz, Parker, & Becker, 1998). Because there is, at best, an emerging body of information to inform theorizing across cultures, CBPR can help establish a frame of reference from which to think about and better understand different cultures. This approach will facilitate using different and diverse means to help in reframing and developing new conceptual frameworks to be used in the study of diverse cultures.

The examples of the methods and approaches available to researchers to inform theorizing have both theoretical and substantive value. Grounded theory allows for developing new themes or concepts and conceptual frameworks. These methods also offer multilevel explanations of research problems and questions. Researchers using participatory methods have found community input invaluable in the design and adaptation of research instruments to make the tools user friendly, applicable, and culturally appropriate (Andrews, Bentley, Crawford, Pretlow, & Tingen, 2007).

When Theorizing Informs Methods

Existing conceptual and theoretical ideas can inform and provide guidance to designing research studies in diverse cultures in later life. For example, the sociocultural perspective and a constructivist approach provide conceptual guidance for understanding how to include diverse populations in research. A sociocultural perspective suggests that human beings are not limited to their biological inheritance, as other species are, but are born into an environment that is shaped by the activities of previous generations and that higher-order functions develop out of social interaction. This perspective notes that meaningful experiences are interpreted within the human sphere of one's own culture and that individuals cannot be understood apart from their embeddedness in social and symbolic systems in their culture (Vygotsky, 1986). Similarly, a constructivist approach suggests that the human experience emphasizes meaningful action by developing the self in complex and unfolding relationships, which take place within a cultural and social context (Kukla, 2000). Thus, people exist and grow in living webs of relationships that define and give meaning to their experiences.

The conceptual guidance from the sociocultural perspective and constructivist approach directs us to the important role that cultural and social worlds play in recruiting participants for our research. To recruit diverse cultural groups into research, it is important to have knowledge about their worlds, or contexts, and also have an understanding of the beliefs, values, and attitudes common within their cultural groups. Moreover, knowledge about cultural norms and values and attitudes among diverse cultures can be used to help select and train interviewers, develop questionnaires, select and develop measures, conduct pilot studies, and interpret findings. It also allows for developing sensitivity to situations and circumstances that could influence the interviewing process.

Theorizing about older diverse cultures through the life course perspective can also inform the methods that are used to study them. This perspective incorporates the views and information from sociology and psychology, economics, anthropology, history, and elsewhere. It looks at the distinctive series of roles and experiences through which the individual passes as he or she ages from birth to death and inquires into the impact of various changes on these patterns (Bengtson & Allen, 1993). Further, by focusing on the actual experiences of individuals from birth to death, the life course approach provides an understanding of the range and diversity of one's life and that of the group. Fry (2003), points out that lives are also understood through society and culture. Even the concept of time is subject to this influence whereby the past is often measured against the transitions of others. In short, the life course perspective emphasizes the transactional influence between economic, political, social, and cultural developments and individuals' reactions to them.

Because older adults have a history, this history encourages the use of the life course perspective as a useful methodological tool in the future. The life course perspective puts individuals and groups at center stage through their interconnected lives and by serving as mediators between developing individuals and societies (Hagestad, 2003; Hagestad & Call, 2007). Through using a life course perspective, our methods go beyond using cross-sectional data. Instead, this theoretical approach requires that a longitudinal methodology be used. To methodologically capture the complexity of what this perspective emphasizes, longitudinal data must be collected to provide good foundational information for theorizing across cultural groups in later life. For example, when researching and theorizing about family development in Native American families, it is important to know the cultural values of the people. Cultural values of the Native American population are centered on a collectivist framework (Swisher & Pavel, 1994). The value of the community permeates through the population at all age levels. Generally, Native American traditional values consist of the importance placed on community contribution, sharing, cooperation, being, noninterference, community and extended family, harmony with nature, a time orientation toward living in the present, preference for explanation of natural phenomena according to the spiritual, and a deep respect for elders (Garrett, 1999). In addition to these, there are other values, such as a holistic approach to health, collectivism, caution, and the cultural value of modesty. This type of information needs to be used in developing better and more inclusive conceptual models, for example, to address health disparities across the life cycle.

We believe that moving the theoretical discourse on theorizing across cultures requires linking much of the discussion provided thus far. When such linking occurs, we have the tools for theorizing across cultures. Therefore, existing methods and theories will inform each other and new ideas emerge from the process about cultural groups. Selecting methods and theories to inform further theorizing will require using multimethods and theories that allow capturing the experiences and lives of cultural groups. Therefore, research questions need to be framed in the context of other social constructs (i.e., age, gender, sexual orientation, disability, social class, language barriers, and religious and spiritual orientations) that require examining the multiple concerns of various cultural groups (Dilworth-Anderson & Boswell, 2006). By merely controlling for race of individuals, as is often done in research, or even by stratifying by age, the richness of social and cultural contexts may be lost (Dilworth-Anderson, Williams, & Gibson, 2002). Although we believe that these types of studies have been the necessary foundation for current theorizing, by incorporating cultural issues we move the discourse even further. This discourse would go beyond racial and ethnic differences. Instead, it would address the culture of a group by examining within- and between-group variations that allow for understanding both cultural complexity and heterogeneity.

Example: Linking Theory and Methods

The following study provides a unique opportunity both to use theorizing to inform methods and to use methods to inform theorizing. The title of study is "Perceiving and Giving Meaning to Dementia in Diverse Groups," the aims of which are the following: (a) to identify and describe cultural values and beliefs that influence how families perceive and give meaning to dementia, (b) to examine the influence of culture and other social factors (e.g., socioeconomic status, geographic location, and so on) on the level and type of help caregivers seek when caring for an older relative with dementia, and (c) to examine the influence of culture and other social factors on physical functioning, general health, and depression of caregivers.

Using Theorizing to Inform Methods

Since the purpose of the study was to understand the influence of culture and other social factors across diverse caregiving populations, we decided to use a sociocultural perspective and a constructivist approach to inform the study methodology. As we have already discussed, both of these theoretical ideas emphasize the importance of environment, particularly the complexities of relationships and social interaction, on the beliefs, values, attitudes, and behaviors of individuals. We used these theories to shape the conceptual framework for our study and to guide our strategy for recruitment, data collection, data analysis, and interpretation of results. To do this, we designed each aspect of the study keeping in mind that the beliefs, values, attitudes, and behaviors of each individual caregiver were rooted in a sociocultural context that included factors external to the individual.

For example, recognizing the importance of relationships and the family context in the caregiving experience, we recruited families into the study as opposed to individual caregivers. It is important and necessary to consider the family as a caregiving unit because each individual caregiver does not exist in a vacuum. Instead, each caregiver is influenced by and dependent on other caregivers in the family. The sample for the study consisted of 10 African American, 10 White, and 10 Native American families caring for an older relative with dementia. To accurately reflect the relationship dynamics of each family, we conducted 2- to 3-hour family focus groups instead of individual interviews. Each family unit included a primary caregiver who requested the participation of up to five additional family members who also shared some of the caregiving responsibilities. We allowed the families to decide on the number of family members they wanted to participate in the focus groups to allow for cultural variations in caregiving structures. With respect to recruitment, many of the caregivers were recruited in environments that reflected their social and cultural worlds, such as churches and community events. Often, community recruiters who shared their social and cultural context recruited the caregivers.

The sociocultural perspective and constructive approach also heavily influenced our data collection procedures. We designed a semistructured interview protocol that allowed us to explore how caregivers, both as individuals and as a family, constructed perceptions about and gave meaning to their loved one's dementia. We also probed caregivers about the level and type of help they sought as a family and the processes through which they collectively made help-seeking decisions. The questions allowed us to develop a profile of both their cultural-historical background (e.g., values and meanings assigned to dementia symptoms) and their sociopolitical conditions (e.g., perceived access to health care services).

To get a more comprehensive view of how culture and other social factors influenced caregivers, we supplemented the focus groups with quantitative data. Specifically, the caregivers completed demographic questionnaires that assessed the sociodemographic characteristics, caregiving responsibilities, and health status of each caregiver. In addition, we collected information from the primary caregiver about the perceived health and functioning of the care recipient as well as the care recipient's medical records. This information enabled us to gather a profile of each individual family member as well as the collective family unit so that we could better understand how the social profile of caregivers helped shape their perceptions, meanings, and experiences.

Consistent with the sociocultural perspective and constructivist approach we used, throughout the data collection process, we were sensitive to the cultural diversity of our sample and the resulting need to develop materials and methods that were appropriate for each group. For example, we consulted focus group specialists and community members to ensure that the focus group protocol was culturally sensitive, relevant, and appropriate. During this process, we identified portions of the interview guide that, for some families, could be interpreted differently than we intended or that could be construed as insensitive. Consequently, we modified the document slightly to replace those portions with culturally relevant words and phrases. At the suggestion of a community liaison, to respect the deep-rooted spirituality of some of the Native American caregivers, we changed the focus group protocol to begin each session with a word of prayer from a Native American community leader who was present during all the interviews. Furthermore, although one moderator conducted all the focus groups, the note taker always shared the same race as the family being interviewed.

Using Methods to Inform Theorizing

Just as theorizing can inform methods, methods can in turn inform theorizing, and this project provided an opportunity for both processes to be enacted. Since we collected qualitative data (i.e., focus group interviews) about a topic with a limited amount of previous research (i.e., cultural influences on perceptions of dementia and on caregiving), we decided to use a grounded theory approach to shape our strategy for analyzing and interpreting the data. Grounded theory is frequently used to analyze and interpret qualitative data because it allows researchers to systematically uncover concepts, themes, and relationships between variables (Strauss, 1987). Grounded theory enabled us to approach data analysis and interpretation without expectations and assumptions about what we thought the data should show. Instead, we were able to allow the data to show us what was important. Thus, we were able to identify culturally relevant concepts, themes, values, and processes that were assigned by the caregivers themselves. It is important to note that, throughout this process, we continued to work within the sociocultural and constructivist framework, noting that culture and family dynamics heavily influenced the caregivers' responses to questions and interaction throughout the focus groups.

We analyzed the data using a software package designed to facilitate analysis of qualitative data. First, we independently read a sample of four focus group transcripts to get a general understanding of the themes present in data. We used open coding to identify a provisional list of codes congruent with the key ideas initially extracted from the data. We convened as a team to refine the list of codes and used it to systematically code all the transcripts in the study. This was an iterative process that involved continual additions, amendments, and deletions to the original code list to better reflect the data. Second, we employed axial coding to identify concepts that emerged in the data. Third, we used selective coding to group the concepts into larger categories that would help us generate theory. Finally, we used the categories to identify how culture influenced the perceptions and meanings caregivers attributed to dementia as well as their caregiving experience, including their help-seeking behaviors and resulting health status.

As an example, one theme that emerged during data analysis was the caregivers' dilemma of coping with "negative" emotions, such as anger and resentment, which they perceived as being undesirable. Understanding the effect of culture on caregivers' coping skills and emotion management was not an original aim of the study. However, because we used a grounded theory approach to analyze the data, we were able to identify that this theme, which was implicit across interviews, was important, and we were able to extract it from the data to make it explicit. For instance, during the open coding process, we developed codes to identify instances in which caregivers dismissed dementia symptoms as unimportant or not problematic or would distance themselves emotionally from the care recipient when they were overwhelmed with emotion. During axial coding, we decided to combine these and similar codes and discovered a new concept in which caregivers developed a coping style that caused them to occasionally disengage themselves from the care recipient. We identified this disengagement as a domain of coping and also identified four other coping domains—humor, reliance on faith, preempting (i.e., avoiding) conflict with the care recipient, and seeking support. During selective coding, we compared the use of coping domains across groups and found that there were cultural differences with respect to the frequency with which each group used each coping domain. We also noticed that caregivers often used multiple domains depending on the situation to which they were coping. For example, caregivers often used humor in concert with disengagement. We used this information to develop coping categories that we called coping styles. For instance, caregivers who simultaneously used both humor and disengagement were described as having a coping style we coined "managed distress."

In summary, this process of using theorizing to inform methods and using methods to inform theorizing has allowed our research team to begin developing culturally relevant coping concepts, provided foundational information for developing a coping measure that will be tested in a larger culturally diverse sample, and provided data to inform developing a larger, more comprehensive study on stress and coping within a cultural context among caregivers in diverse groups.

Retooling and Theorizing Across Cultures

We call this section "retooling" because when the linking process between methods and theories discussed previously is working, we propose that new ways of thinking will emerge to help create a new and different mind-set about how to study and theorize about diverse cultures in later life. Although a multidisciplinary approach is being encouraged to help create this different mind-set, our own values and beliefs, discipline-bound truths, and "learned" expertise may serve as barriers. Nevertheless, we propose that several processes are needed to move beyond these barriers. As noted earlier, it is important to know and recognize the role of our values and those of the groups we study and theorize about in shaping our thinking and work. Moving to a new mind-set may include using different frameworks, conceptual models, and theories to capture the richness of cultural diversity in aging. It may also require applying old methods differently and, equally important, using different methods and cross-disciplinary methods as well as mixed methodologies. Additionally, this retooling may require additional training of investigators (Curry & Jackson, 2003; Levkoff & Sanchez, 2003). Ultimately, retooling begs to ask different and relevant questions and to use different methods and approaches that can capture the realities and lived experiences of diverse groups.

Conclusion and Discussion

Social sciences, as well as other sciences, have made progress in first acknowledging and addressing the value of diversity in research and theory. This progress is now moving to another level that looks beyond racial and ethnic categories and toward acknowledging that diversity in the 21st century should move to the level of inclusion. Diversity speaks to differences, while inclusion allows for acknowledging the complexity of differences and accepting them as a way to explain how we should theorize about and study diverse groups in later life. Acknowledging this complexity allows us to view diversity in later life beyond numbers and static categories.

Theorizing about diverse cultures will require an involved intellectual and conceptual process in which the values of both the cultural groups and the researchers must be considered. We believe that an examination of one's own background and experiences, which includes values, may be a necessary prerequisite for this theorizing process since our values, assumptions, and history impacts our approach to understanding diverse groups. Further, researchers need to be aware of the boundaries of our theories regarding diverse cultures. In other words, they should ask questions and assess the cultural relevance of theories instead of assuming that they are universally appropriate scientific truths. One way of doing this is by constructing a symbolic firewall of cultural theorizing that includes the values relevant to the group while excluding the values imposed by the researcher. Once a culturally competent theorizing process or approach has been developed, it does not have to be reinvented for every group.

Theorizing across cultures will further require that both methods and some existing theories inform theorizing about diverse cultures now and in the future. Existing conceptual and theoretical ideas can inform and provide guidance to designing new ways to theorize about and study diverse cultures in later life. Finally, to achieve most of what we have discussed in this chapter, we believe that some retooling may be required to help create a new and different mind-set about how to study and theorize about diverse cultures in later life.

References

Andrews, J. O., Bentley, G., Crawford, S., Pretlow, L., & Tingen, M. S. (2007). Using community-based participatory research to develop culturally sensitive smoking cessation intervention with public housing neighborhoods. *Ethnicity and Disease, 17,* 331–337.

Bengtson, V. L., & Allen, K. R. (1993). The life course perspective applied to families over time. In P. G. Boss, W. J. Doherty, R. LaRossa, W. R. Schumm, & S. K. Steinmetz (Eds.), *Sourcebook of family theories and methods: A contextual approach* (pp. 469–504). New York: Springer Publishing.

Berger, P. L., & Luckmann, T. (1966). *The social construction of reality: A treatise in the sociology of knowledge.* Garden City, NY: Doubleday.

Berger, S. M. (1967). Social structure and mediated learning. *Journal of Personality and Social Psychology, 7,* 104–108.

Curry, L., & Jackson, J. (2003). The science of including older ethnic and racial group participants in health-related research. *The Gerontologist, 43,* 15–17.

DeJong, M. (2004). Metaphor and the mentoring process. *Child & Youth Care Forum, 33,* 3–17.

Dilworth-Anderson, P., & Boswell, G. (2006). Cultural diversity and aging: Ethnicity, minorities and subcultures. In G. Ritzer (Ed.), *The Blackwell encyclopedia of sociology.* Oxford: Blackwell.

Dilworth-Anderson, P., Burton, L. M., & Klein, D. M. (2005). Contemporary and emerging theories in studying families. In V. Bengtson, A. Acock, K. Allen, P. Dilworth-Anderson, & D. Klein (Eds.), *Sourcebook of family theory and research* (pp. 35–58). Thousand Oaks, CA: Sage.

Dilworth-Anderson, P., Williams, I. C., & Gibson, B. E. (2002). Issues of race, ethnicity, and culture in caregiving research: A 20-year review (1980–2000). *The Gerontologist, 42,* 237–272.

Fry, C. L. (2003). The life course as a cultural construct. In R. A. Settersten (Ed.), *An invitation to the life course: Toward new understandings of later life* (pp. 269–294). Amityville, NY: Baywood Publishing.

Garrett, M. T. (1999). Understanding the "medicine" of Native American traditional values: An integrative review. *Counseling and Values, 43,* 84–98.

Glaser, B. G., & Strauss, A. (1967). *The discovery of grounded theory: Strategies for qualitative research.* Chicago: Aldine de Gruyter.

Goodenough, W. H. (1981). *Culture, language, and society.* Menlo Park, CA: Benjamin/Cummings.

Goodenough, W. H. (1999). Outline of a framework for a theory of cultural evolution. *Cross-Cultural Research, 33,* 84–107.

Greenfield, P. M. (1984). A theory of the teacher in the learning activities of everyday life. In J. Lave & B. Rogoff (Eds.), *Everyday cognition: Its development in social context* (pp. 117–138). Cambridge, MA: Harvard University Press.

Hagestad, G. O. (2003). Interdependent lives and relationships in changing times: A life course view of families and aging. In R. A. Settersten Jr. (Ed.), *Invitation to life course: Toward new understandings in later life* (pp. 135–159). Amityville, NY: Baywood Publishing.

Hagestad, G. O., & Call, V. A. (2007). Pathways to childlessness. *Journal of Family Issues, 28,* 1338–1361.

Hechter, M. (1993). Values research in the social and behavioral sciences. In M. Hechter, L. Nadel, & R. E. Michod (Eds.), *The origin of values* (pp. 1–28). Hawthorne, NY: Aldine de Gruyter.

Israel, B., Schulz, A., Parker, E., & Becker, A. (1998). A review of community-based research: Approaches to improve public health. *Annual Review of Public Health, 19,* 173–202.

Kukla, A. (2000). *Social constructivism and philosophy of science.* New York: Routledge.

Levkoff, S., & Sanchez, H. (2003). Lessons learned about minority recruitment and retention from the Centers on Minority Aging and Health Promotion. *The Gerontologist, 43,* 18–26.

Strauss, A. (1987). *Qualitative analysis for social scientists.* New York: Cambridge University Press.

Strauss, A., & Corbin. M. (1998). *Basics of qualitative research: Grounded theory procedures and techniques* (2nd ed.). Thousand Oaks, CA: Sage.

Swisher, K. G., & Pavel, D. M. (1994). American Indian learning styles survey: An assessment of teacher knowledge. *Journal of Educational Issues of Language Minority Students, 13,* 59–77.

U.S. Census Bureau. (2000). *National population projections: Total population by age, sex, race, and Hispanic origin.* Retrieved May 15, 2008, from http://www.census.gov/population/www/projections/natsum-T3.html

U.S. Census Bureau. (2002). *The 65 and over population: 2000.* Retrieved July 8, 2005, from http://www.census.gov/prod/2001pubs/c2kbr01-10.pdf

Vygotsky, L. (1986). *Thought and language.* Cambridge, MA: MIT Press.

27 Out of the Armchair and Off the Veranda: Anthropological Theories and the Experiences of Aging

Christine L. Fry

By the early 20th century and certainly by the mid-20th, the social sciences had abandoned attempts to arrive at grand theories of social life. Following the critique of Merton (1957), the pursuit of theories of the middle range is much more desirable because of the ability to better operationalize and evaluate these theories. Grand theory was viewed with increased skepticism because of armchair speculation and often the just-so stories involved. The emphasis on middle-range theory, combined with increased specialization within and across the social sciences and the technological ability to manage and analyze data, has narrowed the scope of the questions investigated. The net effect is a much finer grained but fragmentary understanding of parts of social life. In gerontology, this has resulted in the frequent lament about a data-rich but theory-poor discipline and to complaints about microfication (Bass, 2006;

Hagestad & Dannefer, 2001). Anthropological contributions to gerontology for the most part have avoided most of these pitfalls for a number of reasons.

First, grand theory in anthropology has always been data rich. For instance, Edward Tylor (1889) had 350 cultures in his paper arguing the evolutionary laws for the development of family structures. Lewis Henry Morgan (1877) actually sent out questionnaires to missionaries and colonial administrators to substantiate his systems of affinity and consanguinity. Likewise, Sir James Frazier's *The Golden Bough* (1922) is loaded with examples. The reason we no longer subscribe to these theories is they were a rather sterile effort with a society-specific agenda of justifying the latter phases of European mercantilism. The universal history involved was an overly simple story of progress from a lower state to that of the European civilization of the 19th century.

Second, as anthropology was created, a distinctive theory of measurement evolved. This is the invention of fieldwork and the methodology of participant observation. Early anthropologists had to rely on travelogues and the reports of missionaries and colonial administrators. Fieldwork began with the work of Spencer and Gillin (1899) in the outback of Australia and the Torres Strait Expedition of 1898 to the north of Australia. Immediately, it became obvious that primary data collection over a considerable length of time vastly improved not only the depth of knowledge but also the quality of that knowledge. It was not until 1918, when Bronislaw Malinowski stepped onto that isolated beach in the Trobriand Islands, that anthropology got out of the armchair and off the veranda. At the heart of this new method is that by sharing the culture and its setting with informants through long-term residence, the ethnographer learns about life in that context through a wide variety of specific data collection strategies. The resulting ethnography is a representation of social and cultural life heavily informed by the native's point of view. Ethnographies more often than not present a comprehensive or holistic view of how things work and are understood in the context under investigation. The resulting data can be used to evaluate the theory that guided the research or can be used in cross-cultural comparisons. Perhaps the most famous statement on participant observation is Malinowski's own in the first chapter of *Argonauts of the Western Pacific* (1922).

Third, because anthropology is concerned with humans at all times and all places, comparison across time and cultures is rather central to the discipline. This has some obvious advantages for anthropological theory. The immersion in data collection in an alien world forces the observer to see the world through native eyes. Consequently, the researcher's own cultural assumptions are drawn into question and sometimes turned on their head. A single culture study with no comparison runs the risk of missing culture altogether (Fry, 2006). Why should we see culture when it is common sense? Unfortunately, theories driven by common sense often result in obvious and not very interesting generalizations. By taking the stance of "we the alien," we use the diversity in other cultures as a mirror not only to better understand our own but also to construct theories that are counterintuitive.

Theories have to be about something in order to make generalizations. Anthropology has contributed to gerontological theory in a number of ways by maintaining a holistic and big-picture perspective. In this chapter, I focus on four issues:

1. Theories of cultural transformation through time and across cultures
2. Theories of culture and the life course
3. Theories about the problem of old age
4. Anthropological and gerontological theories of age

Theories of Cultural Transformations and Aging

One of the initial questions about older people concerned cultural change and how it affected their circumstances. Leo Simmons was among the first to document the experiences of aging in simpler societies. Although *The Role of the Aged in Primitive Society* (Simmons, 1945) is not a theory of change, it did dispel the myth of "paradise lost" by indicating that the killing of frail older people was not rare. The first explicit and systematic theory of change and older people was that of Donald Cowgill and Lowell Holmes. In *Aging and Modernization* (1972), they linked urbanization, education, health technology, and economic factors as contributing to the marginalization of older adults. Theories of change come and go. Modernization has been replaced by globalization. A problematic aspect of many theories of change is that they are teleological. In linking past features to a projected future, an ideological societal agenda lies at the heart of the theory. Like the universal history of humankind of Tylor (1889) and Morgan (1877), it is progress, positive or negative. Modernization was the faith of the post–World War II era with the hope that the entire world would end up as the United States. Globalization is alarmed about increased inequality and poverty as "free" markets engulf the globe. One strategy to get away from teleological arguments and change has been to reduce the scope of the research by focusing on specific circumstances in a case study. Another strategy has been to adapt evolutionary theory to social phenomena.

The theory of Darwinian natural selection informs most of biology, and in anthropology it is strong in biological anthropology, historical linguistics, and the parts of sociocultural anthropology concerned with ecology. As early as the 1960s, major efforts were made to develop this perspective as appropriate for culture (Sahlins & Service, 1960). It is not surprising that selection works quite well with cultural phenomena. Both Darwin and Wallace acknowledged the influence of Thomas Malthus on their theory. In fact, there are strong parallels between natural selection and the "invisible hand" of Adam Smith. However, for selection to work with cultural phenomena, we have to slightly alter how we view culture. It cannot be a "complex whole" or the "superorganic" or a thing. Instead, we have to view culture as a pooled set of knowledge and values.

The way in which societies change or maintain a relatively stable course is through the decisions that are made about daily activities or likely futures. Knowledge informs these decisions, and values enable actors to sift through alternatives for what they think are the right options. Selection occurs, and the diversity of pooled knowledge shifts. Some ideas are thought to be wrong; they may be argued against or their proponents eliminated, and the information may eventually be forgotten. Other ideas appear to work and are used. New ideas can be borrowed or invented in flashes of insight. The resulting decisions and actions can have impacts for individuals or a larger community. In a stratified society, some individuals are more powerful, and with their influence and position in an attention structure they constitute a significant selective mechanism. They impose their understandings and values on their subordinates.

By embracing this view of culture as a pooled knowledge about a design for living, we are inviting additional questions other than the consequence of change for older people. For instance, to what extent does the knowledge of older people dominate the cultural pool? Do younger people seek their elder's wisdom and counsel? In cultures without writing (Goody, 1987), knowledge is retrieved differently than in those with writing. The experience of older people is sometimes essential in dealing with circumstances that look like novelty to a novice. They have simply been around long enough to have encountered the situation before. Some have argued that it is old people who are the creators of a culture (Amoss, 1981). For instance, Nisa, a !Kung woman in the Kalahari Desert, frequently commented to her biographer (Shostak, 1981) that at the time she knew nothing. In the absence of teachers and schools, it was the old people who gave her knowledge.

Another line of questions deals with the knowledge about old age and how it is used. What constitutes a "good old age"? Not surprisingly, considerable agreement exists across cultures but is spelled out in quite different ways in each context. Underlying positive aging are issues related to health, material security, social life and family, and concerns related to personhood (Fry et al., 1997). What support should be given to older people, and when should it be terminated? Comparative research has demonstrated that when an older person is classified as "decrepit," the behavior of others can change dramatically (Glascock, 1997). A frail elder may be provisioned, but in more than 50% of the societies in the sample, they were scorned, and even decisions were made about them that hastened their death. This was in the same societies where intact older people were cared for, respected, and loved.

If we take a long view of change, we return to the progressive nature of what has been identified as "general evolution." This is concerned with the diversification of human cultures, mostly in the past 10,000 years. This bigger picture sees an unfolding of intensification of production, creation of wealth, concentration of power, social stratification, and population growth. What happens to old age in all this? For the most part, greater wealth has brought greater security but not always. Older people are disadvantaged in economies where it is impossible to accumulate wealth. Both the pressure to produce mostly by foraging and the premium on mobility create major problems for the old. With sedentism and domestication, the old often find themselves as family elders and managers of the family enterprise, making decisions that affect not only themselves but their children as well. Stratification usually results in lifelong trajectories. If one's family is disadvantaged or one is disadvantaged when young, old age will also be disadvantaged. In spite of increased wealth, it is not distributed equally, for poverty is the companion of stratification. The last part of our evolutionary story is the appearance of capitalism during the closing of the 18th century in Europe. It is here that "the problem" of old age begins.

Theories About the Experiences of the Life Course

Initially, gerontology coalesced around old age. The basic questions were the following: Why did it happen and What could we do about the associated problems, especially of health and poverty? However, it became quite apparent that theoretically the exclusive focus on old age was problematic. First, as a life stage, being old has no sharp and explicit boundaries. Individuals become old through a combination of health issues, withdrawal from the labor force, entitlements, self-identification, or none of these. The ages at which these happen are so variable that it is difficult to chronologically pinpoint when a person becomes old. In addition, with chronological age as well as heterogeneity in other characteristics, researchers began to classify old age into the "young-old," the "old-old," and the "oldest-old" with equally vague boundaries. Second, the exclusive focus on old age was theoretically ill advised. Aging is so gradual as to be almost imperceptible, and as a life stage, what happens in earlier life stages shapes the experiences in later stages. Consequently, gerontological theory encompassed the life course. As a researchable unit, the life course proved to be theoretically rewarding but has its challenges (Settersten, 1999). Most notably is the vastness and diversity of lives in any society. But as we probe deeper into the underlying questions, we find order in what could be a labyrinth. The questions I focus on in this chapter are (a) How does a society define time and age? and (b) How does a society use that knowledge?

Cultural Conceptions of Time and Age

Lives are experienced through a combination of memories of a past and the anticipation of a future. Cultural knowledge is used to interpret the "lost worlds" of the past and to integrate memories with a present. As the future is negotiated and created, knowledge and experience are temporally incorporated with the past and present. Time and knowledge of time is central to the life course. Culturally, there are two ways to conceptualize time. The first is relative time, and the second is absolute time. Things, events, are ordered in time. In relative time, something happens either before or after something else. A person is either younger or older than someone else. We may never know how much older or how long ago something happened or for how long we must wait for it to happen simply because time is not measured. We can know only temporal order or sequence. The second conception of time does involve some kind of measurement. Measurement is the imposition of culture on natural regularities that, for the most part, are not regular. For instance, the day is 24 hours long only 3 days out of the year. The solar year is not 365 days plus 6 hours long. Twenty-four time zones are not a built-in feature of the rotation of the earth. With measurement, however, time becomes absolute. Temporal order is reckoned in some form of metric units. It is possible to tell exactly when something happened and the temporal distance between events. Indeed, we can measure the age of about anything given enough technology.

Lives are experienced mostly through the inexactitude of relative time. Individuals pass through the routines of daily life without necessarily needing to know how long it takes. In fact, we might ask, Why do people need the cultural knowledge to measure time? Calendars and clocks are major cultural inventions involving a lot of work and even centuries to create. The most convincing reason for temporal measurement is the need to control nature by anticipating a future and developing a strategy to deal with it. Clock time and calendar time are associated with the need to plan, coordinate activities and people, and make predictions about the future. The measurement of time most simply involves dividing a cycle into equal units. For clocks, the daily rotation of the earth is divided into 24 60-minute hours. For calendars, the yearly orbiting of the earth around the sun is divided into named and numbered days. From the invention of calendars comes the idea of age. Most calendars also number years anchored in some event in the distant past. The Christian calendar (Gregorian) is rooted in time before and after the birth of Christ. Other calendars are linked to different culturally significant events. With a sufficiently long count of years and anchoring events that are divorced from local politics, calendars take on the appearance of being independent of culture. They are not. Similarly, the construction of chronological age is based on a calendar by the logical operation of subtracting the year of birth from the present year to determine the number of years lived. For most people in the 21st century all around the globe, it would be odd not to know their age, the year, the month, and the day of birth. In fact, this cultural knowledge of a time line is used in items to medically determine whether a person is demented.

Culture and Age Structuring

Theories of the sociocultural aspects of life courses have developed notions of age norms (Neugarten, Moore, & Lowie, 1965), age stratification (Riley, Johnson, & Foner, 1972), and age cohorts. Encompassing all these ideas is a concept of age structuring. How a society organizes the interdependency between people of the same and different ages is the structuring of the life course as individuals pass through that society from birth to death. This involves not only the allocation of privileges, power, access to goods and services, and social support but also what it takes to achieve a good life along a meaningful temporal trajectory. Age structuring involves the way a society uses age to manage its members. Controlling people as they pass through their lives is accomplished through varying degrees of formality. Informal arrangements involve fairly complete knowledge of a context and employ such sanctions as negative gossip or the supernatural to shape behavior. Formal arrangements, on the other hand, are often based on explicit criteria and less knowledge of context and in shaping behavior and choices using legal sanctions.

In trying to classify the diversity of life courses across cultures, a productive way is to consider both the formality of the age structure and the conceptualization of time. In Table 27.1, four types of life course are outlined. I consider these types primarily through the formality in age structuring as (a) age-ambiguous life courses, (b) age-aware life courses, (c) age-explicit life courses, and (d) age-forced contexts.

27.1 Classification of Life Courses Based on Measurement of Age and the Requirement That Age Be Known by an Individual or Not

	Relative age, nonchronological measurement	Absolute age, chronological measurement
Informal knowledge of age (noncompulsory)	Age-ambiguous life courses: In these cultures, lives are understood in terms of maturational differences. Others are seen as senior or junior to a specific ego. Because these lives are defined largely through kinship, this type of life course has been called a generational life course.	Age-aware life courses: These cultures have calendars that enable the calculation of chronological age, but it is often not used to organize social life. Only a few will know their ages since the date of birth has to be recorded.
Formal knowledge of age (compulsory)	Age-forced contexts: A colonizing society imports ideas of chronological age and requires age estimates of local populations.	Age-explicit life courses: Age is explicitly used to organize life stages and to regulate access to markets, especially the labor market. This has been called a staged life course.

Age-Ambiguous Life Courses

In small-scaled societies, as recently as the 20th century, life courses were experienced in relative time. No one knew their age, nor was it important to know their age. For instance, Lorna Marshall (1976) notes for the !Kung, a foraging society in the Kalahari Desert of South Africa, that

> *they have no calendar, and they do not count years. They can only vaguely place events in time by saying that they were children or young men or old men when the event occurred. Often they point to someone and say, "I was the age of that person." They reckon the recent past by the seasons; they may remember two or three dry or rainy seasons back and can place the birth of a child, for instance, within that range, but after that they lose track. Placing events in measured time is not significant to them. (p. 53)*

Maturational differences, on the other hand, are important and are structured into social life and productive activities. Since these societies are small scaled, birth orders and genealogy make it rather straightforward to figure out who is senior and who is junior to a specific ego. A few of these societies, such as the Herero of southern Africa, have named years. Individual Herero do know the name of the year of their birth, but it takes an anthropologist to translate this into chronological age. The daily routine and the yearly cycle are undoubtedly experienced much as they would be with clocks and calendars. The main difference is that in these smaller-scaled societies, people look for clues in nature or the moon to anticipate seasonal changes. There is no need to know exactly the interval between full moons or how much older or younger one is than another person.

Life courses based on relative time can be classified as "generational life courses." This is very tempting because the age gap between parents and children and birth orders between siblings are convenient markers of relative age. However, we must be cautious in making generations a proxy for time (Kertzer, 1982). Although reproduction takes place in time, the resulting cohorts confuse temporal measurement even in relative terms. With large families and a long interval of reproduction (20 years or more), the boundaries of a generation become confused. A mother may have a child after her oldest child has begun her reproductive career. Depending on perspective, a grandchild may be older than a child, or an aunt may be younger than her niece. These life courses are better described as "age ambiguous."

Age does not appear to be a central feature to organize people. Instead, it is maturity, skills, ability, and a host of personal qualities, including kinship, that are important. Maturity, of course, implies physical growth as well as social adulthood as evidenced in marriage, parenthood, and operating a household. Relative age operates adequately under these circumstances. There is no reason to be able to answer the question, "How old are you?"

A notable exception to this is a phenomenon known as "age classes." Here males are stratified by some criteria that look a lot like age. The male population is grouped into explicit sets or classes. As the set grows older, its entire membership moves into the next-older set, pushing that set into more senior ranks. Societies that are organized in this manner have posed a fairly esoteric problem in social anthropology. Ethnographically, we find age classes in Africa, especially East Africa, and in Australia, lowland South America, and Native North America on the Great Plains. From the perspective of gerontology, these societies could serve as small-scaled models of age stratification and cohort flow. Unfortunately, age classes have very little to do with age other than age as maturity. Although the specifics are quite variable (Bernardi, 1985), the class is based on generations. To make the boundaries clear, rites of passage initiate young boys and mark the transitions across classes. Rules governing class membership get very elaborate in attempting to keep maturity and place in the system relatively compatible (Stewart, 1977). A minimal rule ensures that a father and a son cannot belong to the same class. Yet we know ethnographically that sometimes men who are physically too young are forced into the most senior rank and out of the action. Likewise, boys who are far too immature are forced into adult roles. In addition, some men do not participate and suffer lower status. Reasons for this type of organization are multifunctional, ranging from incorporating young males into the world of adult men as juniors; mobilizing younger males for raiding, defense, and even army regiments; positioning power with older males; and reducing intergenerational conflict.

Age-Aware Life Courses

Most societies do have some form of a calendar to arrange activities and ceremonial life in a yearly round. Lunar cycles work quite well and are the basis of the Jewish and Islamic calendars. Because these cycles are not synchronized with the solar year, periodic adjustments must be made. Calendars are important and do all sorts of things within a culture. They predict when it is the best time to plant agricultural products. They distinguish between the sacred days and those that are profane. They define the days of work and marketing and those days created as a holiday. Astrologically, they can tell humans when things are predicted to be good and the days to be avoided. They also help in figuring out the answer to the question, "How old are you?"

Calendars are not new. They appear 18,000 years ago in the Magdalenian of France in the form of calendar sticks (Marshack, 1991). But the more formalized calendars with numbered years, named months, and named and numbered days were not invented until the appearance of politically centralized societies and especially archaic states. The Christian calendar, based on the older Julian calendar, saw the Gregorian reform of 1582 to better approximate the solar year. By the 16th century in Europe, we begin to see the day, month, and year of birth recorded in church records.

If these calendars help individuals to figure out their age, is it important to do so? If a state does not require knowledge of age, then it is not important to know age. The individuals who know their age are most likely literate and lead fairly public lives. Even where individuals are required to know their age, if records of their birth are destroyed (e.g., courthouse fires), they most usually only approximate their age. Thus some but not most of the population have knowledge of their age.

Age-Explicit Life Courses

In societies where calendars record the years and states require knowledge of and evidence of birth years, the vast majority of a population lives an age-explicit life course. We find these societies in the 19th century of Europe and North America and by the 20th century in the nations of the globalized world. Historically, the roots to age explicitness appear in the Enlightenment of Europe. The French Revolution brought with it a concern for rational measurement and vital statistics. In Europe of the late 18th century, a new organization of society was also being negotiated. Feudalism was being replaced by nation-states. Liberty and freedom were prevalent ideological themes. Yet human beings could not really be "free" since they had to be integrated into a social order. The new social order involved different forms of integration. Individuals were no longer nested into a feudal hierarchy around a chain of authority, protection, and obligation based on nobility and kings. The archaic economy of tribute evolved into capitalism, largely integrated through accommodating legal systems enforcing contracts, financial institutions, and markets. As Durkheim (1964) noted, integration involved an organic solidarity involving a division of labor based on heterogeneity and interdependency. Society became increasingly bureaucratized into what Max Weber (Scaff, 1989) would call "an iron cage." Social relationships became less face-to-face and less personal. Universal criteria came to dominate decision making about citizens. In short, a new form of citizenship was created.

Age as a universal criterion is central to citizenship. We see this clearly in the U.S. federal census across the 19th century with an increased refinement and concern with chronological age. In the first federal census of 1790, there were two age categories for males (above and below 16) and none for females. By 1840, for the first 20 years, age was in 5-year intervals and 10-year intervals past 20. The census of 1850 was the first modern census with every person individuated along with their ages. This reached its apex in 1900, when not only age but also the year and month of birth were elicited. The refinement in age categories is because the state and other institutions are using age to regulate and manage people. In the census, age is a proxy for all sorts of things, ranging from able-bodied workers and men who can serve in the military. Demographically, we use age to estimate possible futures of fertility, mortality, and dependency. Date and place of birth became mandatory on state-issued documents such as passports, driver's licenses, and Social Security cards.

Age and the age grading of the life course is a product of the rationalization of production (Kohli, 1986). Yet culturally, it goes far deeper than rationalization and the requirement that one know his or her age and can prove it. Age is entangled in the duties and privileges of citizenship. Historically, the life course differentiated into two life stages: childhood/adolescence and adulthood. Childhood as a period of life is comparatively new (Aires, 1962). Child labor laws defined the lower age for labor force participation. Children became defined as dependent on parents and as being culturally incompetent. Educational institutions arrange children into narrow age grades to make them into citizens by teaching them basic skills in math and literacy and to impart knowledge of the state and nation in history and social studies curricula. Laws explicitly prevent adolescents from enjoying the privileges of adulthood by setting age norms on such activities as voting, driving, working, marriage, and consumption of alcohol and tobacco. The duties for subadult citizens are to prepare for adulthood by acquiring the knowledge and skills that make one a useful adult citizen. Parents invest in children because, with lower fertility, there are fewer of them and because, with reduced infant mortality, they are likely to survive into adulthood. Adulthood became the longest life stage with all the freedoms and privileges of maturity. The main duties of adult citizens are to be law-abiding workers and to pay their taxes. Adults are also expected to provide for families and to see children through their preparation into adulthood. Old age did not figure into this life course until late in the 19th century and into the 20th with state-managed entitlements such as old-age pensions or Social Security to ameliorate old-age poverty. As citizens, older adults are expected to withdraw from the labor force and to still consume and pay their taxes.

Age-explicit societies have in effect boxed in adulthood between adolescence and old age defined largely through the legal structure of those societies. Gerontology has incorporated this structure into the three boxes (Best, 1980), or the tripartite life course. This model does capture the structure of the life course as defined by contemporary nation-states. However, is that the way people who live this life course experience it? In Project AGE, we asked people in seven different communities around the world how they viewed the life course. Using a card sort technique, we asked individuals to sort social persona identified by culturally relevant criteria into life stages (Keith et al., 1994). Two interesting results for this discussion were discovered. First, those individuals from age-ambiguous contexts had difficulty sorting persona into life stages. This was in the Kalahari Desert of southern Africa among the !Kung and the Herero and in western Ireland, which was economically depressed. The institutions requiring knowledge of age were minimally present. On the other hand, individuals in age-explicit contexts, in the United States, eastern Ireland, and Hong Kong, had far less difficulty arranging persona by age.

Second, if age-explicit contexts organize the life course into the three major stages, then we would expect the informants in these societies to do likewise. To the contrary, we discovered an average of five life stages with as many as 10 in these sites. It is only by probing deeper into an interpretation and exploration of meaning that we see the impact of this life course on the way people understand what is either ahead of them or behind them. In age-explicit contexts, it is a combination of getting established and assuming or releasing responsibility. At the start of adulthood, people are just getting started and trying to get themselves established. Being established means taking on responsibilities for jobs and families along with other things. Once children mature, one becomes free of some responsibilities, and finally one retires from the responsibility of jobs into a world of leisure. In this life course, it is rough in the beginning, as all sorts of decisions have to be made that will shape future fortunes. The image is that it gets better as one gets older with increased seniority and associated benefits on the job. This may be a view from the mid- to late 20th century, when the majority of workers worked for one corporation for most of their lives. This positive view may well be challenged by job commitments that are now lasting less than 2 years.

Age-Forced Contexts

Colonizing societies bring with them temporal measurement, which is imposed on indigenous populations for whom numbered years and birthdays are irrelevant. Nevertheless, census takers and other agents are compelled to determine age. Often, the ages are estimates only. One Navajo woman reported that "there was no calendar in the Hogan where she was born and that when the government came, her mother reported the month of her birth by its Navajo name". Correctly or not, March was entered in the record; the woman herself subsequently chose a date in the middle—March 15—and said regarding the year of her birth, "I might be older, too" (Griffin, 1989, p. 91). Likewise, anthropologists bring with them a chronocentrism when living among and observing the lives of people for whom age is ambiguous. Methods for determining age are often included in ethnographies. Even though chronological age is irrelevant to the people observed, it is used to describe life courses primarily because of the centrality of age to the intended audience who will read the ethnography. The agents of age-explicit societies force their understanding of age onto the members of age-ambiguous societies.

Culture, the Life Course, and Meaning

A very fertile avenue to understanding the experiences of aging is the diversity of cultural contexts, life courses, and age structuring. It is culture that gives meaning to time and age as well as providing actors with the knowledge of how to use their time and manipulate their age. With that knowledge, humans develop strategies to deal with everyday life and to make longer-range plans. Decisions are made to deal with the economic and political framework within which lives are lived. But culture is more than economics and politics. Humans acquire values with which they aspire to the good life and try to avoid the negatives. With nearly a half century of research on the well-being of older people, the main axis for a good old age or any age at all consists of health, material security, social issues, and ideas of personhood. How these are understood are culturally specific but can be seen as variants on a central theme. Culture and knowledge are noted for diversity. Life takes place in diverse locations locally and globally. By and large, most people live in localized communities. It is here that they organize their worlds. They make decisions about whom to work for and with whom to cooperate. They play political and economic games. They create families. Other institutions are created and participated in, such as religious organizations or voluntary associations. Because culture as a phenomenon is ideational, it has no sharp boundaries. Localized communities are shaped by national and global forces that vary over time. As individuals mature and age, they shape and are shaped by these contexts. Over one's life, an individual may pass through several communities or be linked to several contexts, including even international linkages. Meaning is found, and opportunities are seized or lost. Cultural contexts are natural arenas in which to evaluate theories about the experiences of aging.

Theories About the Problem of Aging

Across time and cultures, for most of humanity's existence, old age has not been a society-wide problem. Old age has had its problems for the 100,000 years that humans have been able to sustain long lives physically and culturally. Any issues arising in older individuals were addressed by their kin, sometimes positively, sometimes negatively. Historically, old age as a social problem is well understood (Haber, 1993). Disability, old-age poverty, and the prospects of the almshouse, the state mental hospital, or the county home became reality for a significant number of older men and women. Old age, like childhood, is a culturally constructed stage of life and one that is problematic (Katz, 1996). By combining poverty, disability, and dependency ratios with apoplectic demography, increased longevity is viewed as a national problem. Increasing cohorts of older people are feared as having the potential to bankrupt nations faster than military conflicts. Why did old age begin to be a social problem in the 19th century of Europe and North America?

Theoretically, we turn to economic anthropology. The industrial revolution brought the invention of capitalism. This new economic order transformed the political and economic organization of the societies it expanded into. In archaic economies based on a domestic mode of production or even on tribute, no individual was divorced from a producing unit. Families or other organizations such as guilds gave their members a safety net for when they reduced their productivity or could no longer work. Capitalism intensified production by separating production from domestic control. The majority of work takes place in factories or commercial establishments where it can be supervised and regulated for efficiency. Capitalism also introduced labor as a commodity to be sold for wages. Commodification of labor is positive as long as one works. One can meet consumption needs and plan ahead. However, when one can no longer work, the consequences are rather obvious and negative. The structure of this economy creates old-age poverty, especially for those who worked in low-paying jobs all their working lives.

The problem of old age is more than poverty, although that is a large part of it. In his capitalistic utopia, *The Wealth of Nations,* Adam Smith (1776) envisions an economy that works through markets fine-tuned by an "invisible hand." A free market has little interference in state regulation other than the necessary infrastructure of finance, law, and transportation. As capitalism expanded, a number of industrial complexes emerged, including the best-known military industrial complex. Corporate entities within a complex and across complexes are integrated through a series of power domains (Adams, 1988) and markets. Corporations, in either producing goods or providing services, recruit workers from yet another market, the labor market. The entire economic structure of these capitalistic societies is integrated through a division of labor based on interdependency and heterogeneity. This is the familiar "organic solidarity" identified by Durkheim (1964) a long time ago. It is the organization of the labor market that is problematic for older adults.

Like archaic economies that created wealth through tribute, capitalism also uses inequality to make wealth. The labor market is segmented into jobs requiring specific skills and responsibility and rewarding workers with high pay as compared to unskilled and menial work. Laborers entering this market bring with them the advantages or disadvantages of age, gender, race, class, and ethnicity. The labor market should not be a free or unregulated market. Commodities, goods, and services do not need pensions and do not need health care. Human beings, laborers, do. Nation-states in Europe and in North America have responded to problematic issues in old age by taxing wages to fund the part of the redistributive economy that is responsible for programs such as Social Security or Medicare in the United States. However, as corporations have expanded offshore and into global markets in search of cheap labor, it is apparent that old age has been left out (Walker, 2005). In many underdeveloped nations, the redistributive economy is not large and is committed to repayment of debt to the World Bank or to funding programs targeted toward children. With over half the world's workers earning less than U.S.$2 per day, there is little wealth to tax and nothing to defer for retirement on the part of the workers. David Ricardo's famous theory of "the iron law of wages" has never been actualized, but we could be seeing some of the effects. Even in the heartland of capitalism, wages have stagnated, and debt has steadily risen since the 1970s. With inadequate pensions and health care plans, many of the baby boomers in the United States plan to work longer to maintain economic security (Mermim, Johnson, & Murphy, 2007).

If poverty abatement and access to affordable health care for older people is a goal in the 21st century around the globe, theoretically we have two strategies. The first is to strengthen the redistributive part of the economy and the programs that provide economic security and that underwrite health services. The second is to make adjustments in the labor market and how it is regulated.

Anthropology and Gerontological Theories of Age

Gerontology has had its share of theories, some of which approach the status of a grand theory attempting to explain the essence of our phenomenon. For instance, in the 1960s, disengagement theory (Cumming & Henry, 1961) explained the engagements of adulthood and the ultimate mutual disengagement of society and old people. This was abandoned partly on ideological grounds but also because it was an oversimplification. Disengagement has returned, however, in modified form for the oldest-old (Johnson, 1987). Gerontologists continue the search for a comprehensive theory. Handbooks are produced with the state-of-the-art findings from each discipline and specialized area comprising gerontology. As we ride our gerontological carousels reaching for the golden ring, we find ourselves disappointed. Our questions become more specialized with the resulting picture more fragmented.

Perhaps a rewarding activity is to step back onto the veranda and settle into the armchair. There are good reasons to return to the armchair. Grand theory and its advantages are encouraged. In speculation we also find creativity. Gerontology is a complicated field of inquiry encompassing multiple types of phenomena and many distinctive disciplines. Anthropology is even more complicated in attempting to deal with the origin and diversity of humans (biologically, socially, and culturally) for more than 10 million years all over the globe. Conventional wisdom simply divided anthropology into the four subfields of biological anthropology, archaeology, sociocultural anthropology, and anthropological linguistics. This division, however, invites specialization and fragmentation. A moment of insight for me occurred when, as a then beginning and somewhat overwhelmed graduate student, I talked with my major professor, Edward Spicer. The topic was the organization of my growing library. He said, "Statics and dynamics." After glancing at the books in his office, I said, "Of course." In a very simple but deep-structure way, the anthropological pieces of the puzzle fell together. The four fields became issues of change and stability.

What would a grand theory of gerontology look like? The mission of gerontology is very different from that of anthropology. Human aging involves journeys through time as individuals are born, mature, grow old, and ultimately die. Our simple, deep-structure, theoretical thread has to be time. Unfortunately, time is elusive, and we have difficulties in understanding what it is. On the other hand, we can measure time with great exactitude and tell the age of about anything from humans to little chunks of ancient carbon. Even physics, with the most developed theories about time, offers gerontology little useful advice and encouragement. Time is also meaningless and sterile, but if we are to study aging, we must deal with time (Baars & Visser, 2007). Since time never caused anything, it cannot be a variable. Yet aging is a temporal phenomenon. It is not time but what happens in time that are our variables. Since a lot of things happen in time to a lot of different phenomena, analytically it is necessary to think of dimensions or levels. These are not surprising and have been discussed a number of times by a number of authors. In wrestling with time simultaneity of temporal measurements, Schaie (1965) identified the age–period–cohort confounds. Neugarten and Datan (1973) introduced the distinctions between life time, social time, and historical time, again occurring simultaneously in human lives. The most obvious dimensions follow a hierarchy of phenomena and the associated disciplines. These are the physical, the chemical, the biological, the psychological, the social, and the cultural along with humanitarian interests. The potential for integration is quite clear and is evident in the way we have organized our professional gerontological organizations, such as the Gerontological Society of America. The real potential is in linkages across dimensions. This is more difficult given disciplinary agendas, the nature of funding, and the organization of research. However, it is not difficult to see linkages between the behavioral, social, and cultural. Humans use their brains to learn and store knowledge to negotiate their social worlds, make decisions, and organize their lives as they grow older.

Time tips the emphasis toward change. Aging is a journey that can last a century. Aging is not a race to death. It is slow and gradual. Thus, theories should incorporate the variables that prevent systems from rapid collapse. Organization is far more interesting than disintegration. Folk wisdom tells us that aging is a breakdown on all fronts when it is not. Humans are biologically programmed to remain intact for a very long time, and medically, socially, and culturally, we extend it even further.

Finally, our theories should be relevant to the mission of gerontology. An academic community incorporating scientific and humanitarian perspective in addressing issues of aging is only a part of gerontology. A large part of our enterprise is directed to power and politics. Since the invention of gerontology, gerontologists have been unified by their interests in the welfare of older people. In a very real sense, the mission of our discipline is to put old age back into the societies that have evolved in the past three centuries and that are evolving around the globe and the economies of which are organized by capitalism. Theoretically, change occurs when powerful people use the pooled knowledge in their attention structure, combined with their values, to make decisions. The net effect of change is to reduce the variation in knowledge and values. To include old age in capitalism, the knowledge we create and the theories we construct must become a part of that pooled knowledge. Obvious targets are politicians and the political process, but not all powerful people are politicians, and political and economic theory is probably not relevant to their influence. Thus, a broad based set of theories loosely linked in a temporal framework could increase gerontological knowledge in our cultural pool.

Perhaps we should ask the "So what?" question. Do we really need an integrated, comprehensive, grand theory that would explain everything there is to know about aging? Or, better, do we already have adequate theories for what gerontology is trying to accomplish? In a perfect world, a grand theory would also be ideal. At minimum, it would provide a paradigm with which to put the pieces of the jigsaw puzzle together and see the larger picture. Unfortunately, the world is not perfect. In an interdisciplinary enterprise such as gerontology, we work within the division of labor of the contributing disciplines. It is here that we link theory and research with issues of social policy and practical problems of aging. Handbooks—and especially the three editions of this handbook on theories of aging—encourage us to ponder our scientific foundations and to keep reaching for that golden ring.

References

Adams, R. N. (1988). *The eighth day: Social evolution as the self-organization of energy.* Austin: University of Texas Press.

Aires, P. (1962). *Centuries of childhood: A social history of family life.* New York: Vintage Books.

Amoss, P. (1981). Cultural centrality and prestige for the elderly: The Coast Salish case. In C. L. Fry (Ed.), *Dimensions, aging, culture and health* (pp. 47–64). Brooklyn, NY: J. F. Bergin.

Baars, J., & Visser, H. (Eds.). (2007). *Aging and time: Multidisciplinary perspectives.* Amityville, NY: Baywood Publishing.

Bass, S. (2006). Gerontological theory: The search for the Holy Grail. *The Gerontologist, 46,* 139–144.

Bernardi, B. (1985). *Age class systems.* London: Cambridge University Press.

Best, F. (1980). *Flexible life scheduling.* New York: Praeger.

Cowgill, D. O., & Holmes, L. D. (Eds.). (1972). *Aging and modernization.* New York: Appleton-Century-Crofts.

Cumming, E., & Henry, W. E. (1961). *Growing old, the process of disengagement.* New York: Basic Books.

Durkheim, É. (1964). *The division of labor in society.* New York: Free Press. (Original work published 1893)

Frazier, J. (1922). *The golden bough: A study in magic and religion.* London: Macmillan.

Fry, C. L. (2006). Whatever happened to culture? In D. J. Sheets, D. B. Bradley, & J. Hendricks (Eds.), *Enduring questions in gerontology* (pp. 159–176). New York: Springer Publishing.

Fry, C. L., Dickerson-Putman, J., Draper, P., Ikels, C., Keith, J., Glascock, P., et al. (1997). Culture and the meaning of a good old age. In J. Sokolovsky (Ed.), *The cultural context of aging: Worldwide perspectives* (pp. 99–124). Westport, CT: Bergin & Garvey.

Glascock, A. P. (1997). When is killing acceptable: The moral dilemma surrounding assisted suicide in America and other societies. In J. Sokolovsky (Ed.), *The cultural context of aging: Worldwide perspectives* (pp. 56–70). Westport: CT: Bergin & Garvey.

Goody, J. (1987). *The interface between the written and the oral.* New York: Cambridge University Press.

Griffin, J. (1989). *Life is harder here: The case of the urban Navajo woman.* Hurst, TX: Southwestern American Indian Society.

Haber, C. (1993). Over the hill to the poorhouse: Rhetoric and reality in the institutional history of the aged. In K. W. Schaie & W. A. Achenbaum (Eds.), *Societal impact on aging: Historical perspectives* (pp. 90–113). New York: Springer Publishing.

Hagestad, G. O., & Dannefer, D. (2001). Concepts and theories of aging: Beyond microfication in social science approaches. In R. H. Binstock & L. K. George (Eds.), *Handbook of aging and the social sciences* (5th ed., pp. 3–21). San Diego, CA: Academic Press.

Johnson, C. (1987). *Life beyond 85 years: The aura of survivorship.* New York: Springer Publishing.

Katz, S. (1996). *Disciplining old age: The formation of gerontological knowledge.* Charlottesville: University Press of Virginia.

Keith, J., Fry, C. L., Glascock, A. P., Ikels, C., Dickerson-Putman, J., Harpending, H. C., et al. (1994). *The aging experience: Diversity and commonality across cultures.* Thousand Oaks, CA: Sage.

Kertzer, D. I. (1982). Generation and age in cross-cultural perspective. In M. W. Riley, R. P. Ables, & M. S. Teltelbaum (Eds.), *Aging from birth to death: Sociotemporal perspectives* (pp. 27–50). Boulder, CO: Westview Press.

Kohli, M. (1986). The world we forgot: A historical review of the life course. In V. W. Marshall (Ed.), *Later life: The social psychology of aging* (pp. 271–303). Beverly Hills, CA: Sage.

Malinowski, B. (1922). *Argonauts of the western Pacific: An account of native enterprise and adventure in the archipelagos of Melanesian New Guinea.* London: Routledge.

Marshack, A. (1991). *The roots of civilization: The cognitive beginnings of man's first art, symbol and notation.* Mount Kisco, NY: Moyer Bell.

Marshall, L. (1976). *The !Kung of Nyae Nyae.* Cambridge, MA: Harvard University Press.

Mermin, G. B. T., Johnson, R. W., & Murphy, D. P. (2007). Why do boomers plan to work longer? *Journal of Gerontology: Social Sciences, 62,* S286–S295.

Merton, R. K. (1957). *Social theory and social structure.* Glencoe, IL: Free Press.

Morgan, L. H. (1877). *Ancient society.* New York: World Publishing.

Neugarten, B. L., Moore, J. W., & Lowie, J. (1965). Age norms, age constraints, and adult socialization. *American Journal of Sociology, 70,* 710–717.
Neugarten, B. N., & Datan, N. (1973). Sociological perspectives on the life cycle. In P. B. Baltes & K. W. Schaie (Eds.), *Life-span developmental psychology: Personality and socialization* (pp. 53–71). New York: Academic Press.
Riley, M. W., Johnson, M., & Foner, A. (1972). *Aging and society: Vol. 3. A sociology of age stratification.* New York: Russell Sage Foundation.
Sahlins, M. D., & Service, E. R. (Eds.). (1960). *Evolution and culture.* Ann Arbor: University of Michigan Press.
Scaff, L. A. (1989). *Fleeing the iron cage: Culture, politics, and modernity in the thought of Max Weber.* Berkeley: University of California Press.
Schaie, K. W. (1965). A general model for the study of developmental problems. *Psychological Bulletin, 64,* 92–107.
Settersten, R. A. (1999). *Lives in time and place: The problems and promises of developmental science.* Amityville, NY: Baywood Publishing.
Shostak, M. (1981). *Nisa: The life and words of a !Kung woman.* Cambridge, MA: Harvard University Press.
Simmons, L. W. (1945). *The role of the aged in primitive society.* New Haven, CT: Yale University Press.
Smith, A. (1776). *An inquiry into the nature and causes of the wealth of nations.* London: Strahan & Cadell.
Spencer, W. B., & Gillen, F. J. (1899). *The native tribes of central Australia.* London: Macmillan.
Stewart, F. H. (1977). *Fundamentals of age group systems.* New York: Academic Press.
Tylor, E. B. (1889). On a method of investigating the development of institutions. *Journal of the Royal Anthropological Institute of Britain and Ireland, 18,* 245–256, 261–269.
Walker, A. (2005). Towards an international political economy of ageing. *Aging & Society, 25,* 815–839.

Theorizing About Families and Aging From a Feminist Perspective

28

Katherine R. Allen
Alexis J. Walker

In this chapter, we define theory from a feminist perspective and apply it to the substantive area of families and aging. Like family studies and aging studies, feminist theorizing is inherently interdisciplinary. Feminist theorizing has activist origins as well. In order to appreciate the value that feminist theory brings to the study of families and aging, we situate our consideration of feminist theorizing about families and aging into a historical context. We document the history of feminist theorizing in the academy from its origins in two divergent locations: feminist activism, evident in the women's movement for social change (Freedman, 2002), and postpositivist theorizing, still dominant in most theory-building efforts today (Bengtson, Acock, Allen, Dilworth-Anderson, & Klein, 2005). Then we describe the development and uniqueness of feminist contributions, apply feminist theory to families and aging, and raise feminist questions for new research on older women's family lives.

We tell this story because feminist theorizing has brought impassioned scholarship into the academic study of families and aging and made social change an explicit goal of inquiry and practice (Allen, 2000; Thompson & Walker, 1995; Walker, 2000). We concur with the feminist view that knowledge is power and exists not just for its own sake but also to make changes in the ruling relations of society (Smith, 1999). The power of a feminist approach is to expose the fault lines between the local particularities of people's everyday/everynight activities with the abstracted, objectified, extralocal forms of social organizations that exert control over social life (Smith, 1999).

We cannot improve women's lives, old people's lives, students' lives, and our own lives if we neither know our history nor take a position on where we have been and where we wish to go. Those for whom the particular subjugated histories matter at the most private and political levels must take the responsibility for writing those histories for themselves, lest others (re)write their histories for them (Kolondy, 1998). Losing the narratives and history of our collective past contributes to the continued subordination of women, old people, and racial-ethnic minorities (e.g., Collins, 2000; Heilbrun, 1988; hooks, 1989; Ray, 2006). The ability of feminism and other liberation movements to be "history-in-process with a future—depends on our ability to reproduce ourselves in subsequent generations and to pass on what we have learned so that the wheel does not need to be reinvented by every generation" (Friedman, 1995, pp. 28–29).

Defining Theory

Feminist Theory Is Grounded in Women's Lived Experience

We define theory from a feminist perspective, where theoretical explanation and subjective practice are entwined. Feminist inquiry avoids the traditional theory/practice split (Smith, 1999). Theory is not viewed as some objective reality independent of the knower's subjective perception and experience. In this way, theory is itself a practice (Smith, 1999). Writing about what we observe, or "writing the social," is the process of "finding out how to make active, present, and observable the theoretical, conceptual, ideological, and other forms of thought" (Smith, 1999, p. 7). Feminists develop a critical eye for seeing well and at the same time recognizing that knowers are "embodied" or situated in specific contexts, thus rendering multiple interpretations. There is no one perfect perspective that all observers can agree on. Feminists critique the mainstream view that "general" knowledge is neutral and obtainable through the scientific discovery process (Code, 2006).

By deconstructing the gender-neutral posture of androcentric science, so-called real science is exposed as harmful to women. The language and tools used to obtain knowledge that satisfies the androcentric mandate objectifies women as unknown, unknowing, and unknowable (Code, 2006). Knowledge production procedures thus reinforce the status quo, and scientists themselves are complicit in re-creating the social order. Feminist inquiry, instead, begins from a different starting point: women's standpoint (Smith, 1987). Given that women's experiences have been ignored, distorted, and misrepresented, feminists pay attention to women's lived experiences and take subjectivity, oppression, and empowerment into account (Acker, Barry, & Esseveld, 1983).

Women's lived experience provides a radically new location for theorizing because feminists have unmasked the partiality of the universal male subject. That is, the accepted standard of knowledge has been an androcentric subject in which White, Western, educated, propertied, heterosexual masculinity has been idealized (Code, 2006). Women's exclusion from what counts as knowledge has profound consequences. Feminist methods of theory and practice use the situation at hand—women's subjective experience—to write women back into existence (Collins, 2000; Fonow & Cook, 1991; Smith, 1987).

Feminist Standpoints and Families

Feminist methods of theorizing and practice are necessary for uncovering new knowledge because only certain kinds of women—those who are derivative of idealized males—have been "seen" and thus represented in our theories of families. The women who have been written into social science theory conform to the stereotypes of the Standard North American Family, consisting of a breadwinner father, his stay-at-home wife, and their dependent biological children (Smith, 1993). Feminists critique these portrayals of women as objectified and inaccurate. Women are not seen as embodied individuals negotiating their way through their life experiences (Sprague, 2005). Variations on this normative theme are positioned in binary form as deviant (e.g., married mother versus single parent and parent versus childless) or are ignored altogether in the traditional family studies literature (e.g., gay and lesbian parents).

This portrait of the family, in particular, omits old people because they do not fit within the confines of the early stages of marriage and parenthood that correspond to the family life cycle (Bengtson, 2001; Connidis, 2001; Walker, Allen, & Connidis, 2005). Older adults, especially those who are childless and unmarried, are absent from family theories as well (Allen, 1989; Wenger, Scott, & Patterson, 2000). Theorizing about the family life of old people and about old people in families means that to account for why things are the way they are, we must learn to see deeply, beyond taken-for-granted assumptions. This process begins with and takes seriously people's own perspectives on how their lives unfold (Allen & Walker, 2006). Thus, a feminist perspective on families and aging attends to how women's lives have been ignored or distorted in family studies and exposes how the lives of old people are made invisible in related disciplines as well. Considering this distortion of knowledge and the desire to change course on behalf of women, old people, and families, we next consider how the investigations of gender, families, and aging intersect.

Interdisciplinarity: Families, Aging, and Women's Studies

Family studies (Cheal, 1991; Sprey, 1990), gerontology (Bengtson, Acock, et al., 2005), and feminism (Reinharz, 1992; Spender, 1983) are inherently interdisciplinary. In each of these disciplines, multiple points of view are needed to examine the dynamic complexity of the phenomena involved. Interdisciplinary perspectives are not additive but dialectic and dialogic (Gergen, 1999). Interdisciplinarity is not about taking a theme and gathering two or three sciences around it. Rather, interdisciplinarity selects a substantive issue, in this case, older women's family lives, and creates something new.

The transformative nature of interdisciplinary experience triples when all three issues are placed in the center of vision: families, aging, and gender; that is, interdisciplinarity as practiced from a feminist perspective is transformative (Floyd-Thomas, Gillman, & Allen, 2002). Whether in gerontology or family studies, complex inquiry about structure, process, and agency in real life cannot be experienced at arm's length (Allen, 2000; Bengtson, Putney, & Johnson, 2005; Mills, 1959). A feminist perspective makes this method of inquiry critically self-conscious and accountable (Stanley, 1990).

Historical Perspective on Feminist Theorizing About Families and Aging

Family studies and aging studies share a common academic history in that positivism is the epistemological paradigm accounting for most of the theory-building efforts in these fields (Bengtson, Putney, et al., 2005). A positivist epistemology is consistent with the scientific method by emphasizing an objective reality that can be known independent from the knower. Feminist theory and the process of theorizing on and behalf of aging families depart from positivist theory by questioning the dominant ideology and critiquing oppressive narratives and practices (Allen & Walker, 2006).

A feminist perspective is critical of the positivist approaches to science that flourished in the mid-20th century, beginning with the way gender was constructed (Code, 2006; DiPalma & Ferguson, 2006). The male vantage point and masculinity were the taken-for-granted superior subjects, and the female vantage point and femininity were the presumed inferior other (Harding, 1986). In circumstances where gender differences were emphasized (alpha bias), women were clearly the losers, but in situations where gender differences were denied (beta bias), women's inferior status was rendered invisible (Hare-Mustin & Marecek, 1990). Both alpha bias and beta bias impeded steps for change, constructing the problem only as *between* differences and not in terms of intersections *among* differences.

Jessie Bernard (1972) initiated the feminist revolution in family studies by demonstrating that gender neutrality in families is a myth. In her critical analysis of social inequality in heterosexual marriage, she studied how gender differences are played out in social relations. Bernard argued that marriage was not a unitary experience but rather was comprised of "his" and "hers." She demonstrated that men's experience of marriage was more positive and that women's experience was more ambivalent.

Subsequently, prevailing assumptions that families were centers of love and support, that motherhood was women's calling, and that men were the breadwinners and women the caregivers—these and many more assumptions were called into question by feminist theory and research (Thorne, 1982). Women's development as full persons was sacrificed by the demands of motherhood, and motherhood was not an experience or status that all women naturally desired (Rich, 1986). Working-class women and nearly all women of color were both breadwinners and caregivers (Dill, 1988; Glenn, 1987). Separate spheres existed only for middle-class White women and then only for a very short time during the demographic anomaly of the postwar 1950s (Coontz, 1992).

Normative approaches to the idealized modern nuclear family could not explain the diversity of women's lives over the life course, nor could they explain the diversity in structures that characterized families since the last half of the 20th century.

Not only were women in real life paying attention to the disjuncture between their lived experience and the ideology of being a good wife and mother (Freidan, 1963), but by the 1970s, women who studied families over the life course, too, experienced the disjuncture between mainstream theories used to explain social relations and the realities of their own and other women's lives. Insightful observations about family sociology as wives' sociology, because women were the source of most data (Safilios-Rothschild 1969), began a new way of thinking about "sex roles" in family studies and related disciplines (Fox & Murry, 2000; Osmond & Thorne, 1993).

The awakening of women to their second-class status and of feminist academics to the limitations of the disciplines show how contemporary feminist approaches are grounded in the second wave of the women's liberation movement (Freedman, 2002). This movement, gaining full steam in the 1970s, forced academic feminists to look at the way their disciplines were studying women's lives and to call into question what counted as knowledge (Bowles & Klein, 1983; Walker & Thompson, 1984). Only a perspective critical of the status quo could show the tension in women's lives between reality and ideology. The critical perspective—holding in tension what is normative and viewing it through multiple lenses of lived experiences—is what makes feminist theory different from mainstream social science theory about families and aging. A feminist perspective applied to family studies is a description of what is treated as different, a reaction to being silenced and made invisible, and a desire to enact change (Walker & Thompson, 1984).

Today, there are a multitude of feminisms and many versions of feminist theory. Differences in feminist theorizing range from viewing gender as a key organizing principle to seeing that gender cannot be disentangled from all the etceteras that intersect with gender (e.g., race, class, sexual orientation, and age) (DiPalma & Ferguson, 2006). Yet contemporary feminist thought shares the common assumption, despite nuances in language and perspective, that the various power/privilege asymmetries of gender, race, class, sexual orientation, and the like are major and intersecting (not competing) influences on people's everyday lives (Code, 2006; Freedman, 2002). Intersectionality has become the key concept in feminist theorizing (Collins, 2000, 2005). For each person, social stratifications combine in unique ways to constrain individual lives and also operate to focus group oppression and privilege.

Social stratifications also create unique opportunities for agency. Numerous individual and collective resistance efforts have led to alterations in oppressive social structures (for a discussion of work on the productive and reproductive labor of poor racial-ethnic women in urban neighborhoods, see Naples, 1992). In recognizing the tension between constraining structures and opportunities for agency, feminists champion the need for political theorizing that leads to social change (Andersen, 2005). Ultimately, this practical goal to change society by and on behalf of women is at the core of feminist theorizing (Smith, 1987).

Feminist Epistemologies

As noted previously, feminist theorizing of today has multiple origins. Two of the most pronounced are its activist roots in the women's liberation movement and in other civil rights movements of the second half of the 20th century (Freedman, 2002) and in the critical discourse about academic disciplines that occurred in the 1960s and 1970s. This discourse challenged positivism and its problematic assumptions of objectivity, which posited that scientists are apart from the social world they study (Smith, 1987). It criticized the framing devices characteristic of social science, such as logical dichotomies (e.g., nature/nurture, micro/macro, and work versus family), which perpetuate systems of domination, as well as a focus on the individual without attention to the interpersonal, sociocultural, and historical context (Sprague, 2005). A feminist perspective gives permission to stand outside the accepted modes of inquiry and to ask new and often subversive questions about the status quo.

Feminist theory was also influenced by social constructionist and other postmodern approaches that self-consciously questioned the connections between authority and power (Sprague, 2005). In social constructionism, feminists pay attention to the fact that knowledge is produced in a particular social context. We scrutinize and deconstruct ideas, theories, and methods for "complex and even contradictory meanings" (Sprague, 2005, p. 38). We attend to the relational context of research, including the connections between researchers and subjects, researchers and each other, and researchers and others in the social world. Feminist theorists differ, however, in the degree to which they depart from objectivity.

Harding (1986) proposed a taxonomy of feminist epistemologies that can be understood in terms of how far each departs from traditional empiricism. All three feminist epistemologies reject the ideals of universal conceptions of man, knowledge, reason, and morality, but there are some distinctions as we discuss here. Furthermore, in the past two decades since Harding first proposed the taxonomy, feminist thinking has evolved, and distinctions among categories are no longer plausible. Indeed, nearly all feminist thinking can be characterized as some version of postmodern thinking, with intersections of empiricism and standpoint integrated as well.

Feminist Empiricism

As with a traditional empiricist perspective, feminist empiricism states that knowledge requires an evidentiary basis. Feminist empiricism differs from the traditional viewpoint, however, by acknowledging that knowledge is shaped by its creators. Classical empiricists require that "evidence must come from ideal observation conditions where knowers figure as self-reliant, neutral information processors whose access to 'the evidence' is assured by their simply encountering it" (Code, 2006, p. 153). Knowledge is embodied and cannot be separated from the knower or from its construction. The goal of feminist science, then, is to produce knowledge that is both rigorous and informed by feminist values (nonsexist, nonracist, and the like). Feminist empiricism is still a politicized form of inquiry but one that generates strong objectivity. Objectivity, as practiced by feminist empiricism, is not inherent in the neutral observation procedure but becomes a social achievement.

Feminist Standpoint Theory

Feminist standpoint theorists go beyond the individualism of feminist empiricism and focus on the power structures that infuse knowledge production in the social-material world (Code, 2006). This position critiques patriarchy as responsible for disproportionately privileging men through a hierarchical sex/gender system. A feminist standpoint can be achieved through the difficult process of consciousness raising and political action, where women come to understand the myth of gender neutrality and to expose the structures underlying the system of domination and subordination. Clearly, a more powerful tool—a radical standpoint—than empiricism is needed to challenge the structural factors that shape women's practices and consciousness in the everyday world (Smith, 1987).

Feminist Postmodernism

Feminist postmodern epistemologies take an even more radical step away from the realist notion of objectivity. At the same time, feminist postmodernists have trouble with the standpoint idea of women's subjectivity and are deconstructive about the very notion of gender as a category in and of itself. Feminist postmodern theories say that gender does not stand alone but intersects with other salient relations of power. Knowledge is contested, incomplete, and partial. Gender itself becomes impossible because "no useful generalization about it can be made, and thus the term becomes difficult to use at all" (DiPalma & Ferguson, 2006, p. 134). Feminist postmodernists are also contentious about the value of subjective experience. By criticizing the instability and opacity of subjectivity, postmodernism makes it difficult to take women's lives and commitments seriously (Code, 2006). The very feminist project of empowerment and social change is called into question.

New Possibilities for Theorizing

As interdisciplinary scholars in family studies and gerontology, we are accustomed to combining and integrating theories and investigating the situation at hand. As feminist scholars, we stress the importance of subjective perspectives and situated knowledge. Thus, we posit that an interdisciplinary approach can be comfortable with difference and contradiction and that we can combine theories, even those with divergent epistemological origins. Just as all feminist epistemologies are critical of the neutral standpoint of "general knowledge," that is, knowledge posited as existing apart from the knower (Code, 2006), so, too, are the theories we integrate in order to understand women's family lives over the life course.

Thus, we approach the process of theorizing—explanation and understanding—from life course, feminist, and social constructionist points of view (Walker et al., 2005). To integrate theories that have some divergent epistemological principles (e.g., life course is grounded in an empirical worldview), the knower must be comfortable with ambivalence. Theoretical pluralism is dialectical and dialogic: contradictions, paradoxes, and tension are the tools one uses to search for ways to answer questions. Doing all three means asking questions at different levels and asking different kinds of questions simultaneously.

Feminists examine the opportunities and constraints linked to gender and age as well as other major social locations at three levels: the individual, the interactional, and the institutional (Ferree, 1990; Risman, 2004). At the individual level, we look at the development of old, gendered selves. At the interactional level, we attend to diverse cultural expectations for old relative to young people and women relative to men even when they are in identical structural positions. At the institutional level, we find age- and gender-specific rules for how resources and material goods are to be distributed (Risman, 2004). We find examples in the feminist family gerontology literature, a literature that goes back and forth between theory and data for a richer understanding of women's lives.

Combining insights from critical theory and symbolic interaction, Connidis and McMullin (2002) reconceptualized the construct of sociological ambivalence, theorizing it as rooted in sets of structured social relations. They highlighted the role of social structure in creating differences between groups in power, privilege, and opportunity on the basis of age, gender, class, race, and so on. These differences are evident in conflicting norms embedded in institutional resources and requirements such as roles. The contradictions inherent in socially structured conditions become evident in social interactions, creating mixed feelings or ambivalence in individual thoughts, feelings, and motivations. Ambivalence thus becomes a property of all social relations, which must be negotiated and renegotiated over time.

Willson, Shuey, and Elder (2006) pursued an ambivalence framework in their study of the relationships between adult children and their aging parents and parents-in-law. Their research highlighted social relations as structured by gender and by kinship. Because gender structures family life and paid work, it is a power structure that influences the differential distribution of resources and privileges within families, leading women to have fewer resources than men. Having fewer resources means they are less able to resist normative obligations. Caregiving is expected of women, and they are expected to enjoy it as well as the opportunity to experience closeness with the family members for whom they are caring. For these reasons, women were expected to and did experience greater ambivalence than men in their relations with other women, with in-laws, and with family members in poor health. Further, daughters who provided aid to family members also experienced more ambivalence than those who did not provide assistance. Their research contributed to feminist theorizing about family ties as embedded in sets of structured social relations that create power differences with consequences for individual lives.

Similarly, Sarkisian, Gerena, and Gerstel (2007) addressed the intersections of gender, ethnicity, and class in their study of extended family integration among Euro-Americans and Mexican Americans. The authors challenged two dominant theories of ethnicity and kin ties, one positing superintegration and the other positing disintegration. The superintegration perspective argues that Latino/a families—especially Mexican American families—are more likely than Euro-American families to live near relatives, to maintain contact, and to provide more and more types of help to family members. The disintegration perspective argues the opposite: that Latino/a families are less likely than Euro-American families to provide help and support to their kin. They argued that the inability to resolve this debate was rooted in part by decisions to include women and men together in data analysis. Doing so ignored the intersectionality of ethnicity, gender, and class as well. The authors studied women and men separately and found evidence that gender and class were more important than culture in kin support. Their data showed that family integration is a multidimensional construct—that Mexican Americans demonstrated greater proximity and more coresidence than Euro-Americans but lower rates of financial aid. They also found that Euro-American women were less likely than Mexican American women to help with child care and household work. The findings highlighted the importance of an intersectional perspective of gender, class, and ethnicity in family integration.

Finally, Schmeeckle (2007) studied gender dynamics among adult children in stepfamilies who acquired stepparents during their childhoods. Whereas most research focuses on children with stepfathers, she included stepmothers as well. Unlike other studies of stepfamilies, she highlighted gender and not only family structure as key. Her findings pointed to traditional gender practices in parenting (by mothers and fathers) and in stepparenting (by stepmothers and stepfathers). Like biological mothers, stepmothers, too, functioned as kin keepers, helping adult children to renegotiate relationships with their biological fathers from whom they had become distant. Her findings highlight the master status of mother for women, even for stepmothers.

Feminist Questions for Women, Families, and Aging

To conclude, we end with some important feminist questions about what we want to know in order to understand, explain, validate, and change older women's family lives. Unlike mainstream disciplines, feminist theorists challenge the "prominent individual syndrome" (Spender, 1983, p. 366), with its image of a lone scholar spending "his" life on the development of a singular theory. Feminist theorizing is a collective endeavor that is inextricably linked to praxis (Smith, 1987).

Theorizing about gender, generation, and age has the potential to redress fundamental questions about the experiences of older women and men in families because it acknowledges the explicit connections between social structures and lived experiences over the life course (Walker, 1999). Theorizing from a feminist approach allows us to get more comfortable with the challenges of uncertainty as knowers. We are not omnipotent, independent of the frame in which knowledge is constructed. Our research reports cannot be sanitized or stripped of their humanity. Yet we still claim an allegiance to accountability standards of trustworthiness, empowerment, and change. Our goal is to open our eyes, to see deeply, to see well, and to not be afraid to challenge and to be challenged.

One of the most difficult challenges scholars face in trying to incorporate multiple social locations into our consideration of intersectionality is the lengthening list of oppressions (King, 2006). The temptation is to ignore difference and intersectionality altogether, but a feminist perspective challenges us to try, even when efforts are clumsy and need revision. For example, we are interested in how adult siblings experience inequality. To examine this issue, we integrate feminist, life course, and social constructionist perspectives in order to examine multiple viewpoints from siblings in the same families. We presume not a "family" perspective but rather many perspectives that are like a moving target. By considering multiple perspectives, structures, questions, and so on together, we can discover a new view of the experience of inequality—as perceived and observed—among older adults.

We also acknowledge the pioneering efforts of scholars who brought intersectionality to the feminist project in families and aging. Colleen Johnson stands out as a researcher for whom such definitions may not apply but whose work is a precursor to the kind of scholarship we champion in this chapter. Her interdisciplinary research has been highly influential for feminist thinking about families and aging. Johnson, an anthropologist by training, investigated intergenerational issues in all her studies, and her research on divorced families (Johnson, 1988) demonstrated the demise of the modern nuclear family. In subsequent work, feminist family scholars applied her ideas to investigate postmodern arrangements in families (Allen, Blieszner, Roberto, Farnsworth, & Wilcox, 1999), thus bridging disciplines and creating something new. We acknowledge as well the old women whose everyday lives help to motivate our desire for social change. Our generation of researchers builds on women's lives and feminist scholarship—telling the history, moving into new territory, ceding the knowledge to others, and enabling it to grow.

References

Acker, J., Barry, K., & Esseveld, J. (1983). Objectivity and truth: Problems in doing feminist research. *Women's Studies International Forum, 6,* 423–435.

Allen, K. R. (1989). *Single women/family ties: Life histories of older women*. Newbury Park, CA: Sage.

Allen, K. R. (2000). A conscious and inclusive family studies. *Journal of Marriage and the Family, 62,* 4–17.

Allen, K. R., Blieszner, R., Roberto, K. A., Farnsworth, E. B., & Wilcox, K. L. (1999). Older adults and their children: Family patterns of structural diversity. *Family Relations, 48,* 151–157.

Allen, K. R., & Walker, A. J. (2006). Aging and gender in families: A very grand opening. In T. M. Calasanti & K. F. Slevin (Eds.), *Age matters: Re-aligning feminist thinking* (pp. 155–174). New York: Routledge.

Andersen, M. L. (2005). Thinking about women: A quarter century's view. *Gender & Society, 19,* 437–455.

Bengtson, V. L. (2001). Beyond the nuclear family: The increasing importance of multigenerational bonds. *Journal of Marriage and Family, 63,* 1–16.

Bengtson, V. L., Acock, A. C., Allen, K. R., Dilworth-Anderson, P., & Klein, D. M. (2005). Theory and theorizing in family research: Puzzle building and puzzle solving. In V. Bengtson, A. Acock, K. Allen, P. Dilworth-Anderson, & D. Klein (Eds.), *Sourcebook of family theory & research* (pp. 3–33). Thousand Oaks, CA: Sage.

Bengtson, V. L., Putney, N. M., & Johnson, M. L. (2005). The problem of theory in gerontology today. In M. L. Johnson (Ed.), *The Cambridge handbook of age and ageing* (pp. 3–20). Cambridge: Cambridge University Press.

Bernard, J. (1972). *The future of marriage.* New York: Bantam.

Bowles, G., & Klein, D. (Eds.). (1983). *Theories of women's studies.* London: Routledge.

Cheal, D. (1991). *Family and the state of theory.* Toronto: University of Toronto Press.

Code, L. (2006). Women knowing/knowing women: Critical–creative interventions in the politics of knowledge. In K. Davis, M. Evans, & J. Lorber (Eds.), *Handbook of gender and women's studies* (pp. 146–166). London: Sage.

Collins, P. H. (2000). *Black feminist thought: Knowledge, consciousness, and the politics of empowerment* (2nd ed.). New York: Routledge.

Collins, P. H. (2005). *Black sexual politics: African Americans, gender, and the new racism.* New York: Routledge

Connidis, I. A. (2001). *Family ties and aging.* Thousand Oaks, CA: Sage.

Connidis, I. A., & McMullin, J. A. (2002). Sociological ambivalence and family ties: A critical perspective. *Journal of Marriage and Family, 64,* 558–567.

Coontz, S. (1992). *The way we never were: American families and the nostalgia trap.* New York: Basic Books.

Dill, B. T. (1988). Our mothers' grief: Racial ethnic women and the maintenance of families. *Journal of Family History, 13,* 415–431.

DiPalma, C., & Ferguson, K. E. (2006). Clearing ground and making connections: Modernism, postmodernism, feminism. In K. Davis, M. Evans, & J. Lorber (Eds.), *Handbook of gender and women's studies* (pp. 127–145). London: Sage.

Ferree, M. M. (1990). Beyond separate spheres: Feminism and family research. *Journal of Marriage and the Family, 52,* 866–884.

Floyd-Thomas, S. M., Gillman, L., & Allen, K. R. (2002). Interdisciplinarity as self and subject: Metaphor and transformation. *Issues in Integrative Studies, 20,* 1–26.

Fonow, M. M., & Cook, J. A. (1991). Back to the future: A look at the second wave of feminist epistemology and methodology. In J. Cook & M. Fonow (Eds.), *Beyond methodology: Feminist scholarship as lived research* (pp. 1–15). Bloomington: Indiana University Press.

Fox, G. L., & Murry, V. M. (2000). Gender and families: Feminist perspectives and family research. *Journal of Marriage and the Family, 62,* 1160–1172.

Freedman, E. B. (2002). *No turning back: The history of feminism and the future of women.* New York: Ballantine.

Freidan, B. (1963). *The feminine mystique.* New York: Dell.

Friedman, S. S. (1995). Making history: Reflections on feminism, narrative, and desire. In D. Elam & R. Wiegman (Eds.), *Feminism beside itself* (pp. 11–53). New York: Routledge.

Gergen, K. J. (1999). *An invitation to social construction.* London: Sage.

Glenn, E. N. (1987). Gender and the family. In B. B. Hess & M. M. Ferree (Eds.), *Analyzing gender* (pp. 348–380). Newbury Park, CA: Sage.

Harding, S. (1986). *The science question in feminism.* Ithaca, NY: Cornell University Press.

Hare-Mustin, R. T., & Marecek. J. (Eds.). (1990). *Making a difference: Psychology and the construction of gender.* New Haven, CT: Yale University Press.

Heilbrun, C. G. (1988). *Writing a woman's life.* New York: Ballantine.

hooks, b. (1989). *Talking back: Thinking feminist, thinking black.* Boston: South End Press.

Johnson, C. L. (1988). *Ex familia: Grandparents, parents, and children adjust to divorce.* New Brunswick, NJ: Rutgers University Press.

King, N. (2006). The lengthening list of oppressions: Age relations and the feminist study of inequality. In T. M. Calasanti & K. F. Slevin (Eds.), *Age matters: Re-aligning feminist thinking* (pp. 47–74). New York: Routledge.

Kolondy, A. (1998). *Failing the future: A dean looks at higher education in the twenty-first century.* Durham, NC: Duke University Press.

Mills, C. W. (1959). *The sociological imagination.* London: Oxford University Press.

Naples, N. A. (1992). Activist mothering: Cross-generational continuity in the community work of women from low-income urban neighborhoods. *Gender & Society, 6,* 441–463.

Osmond, M. W., & Thorne, B. (1993). Feminist theories: The social construction of gender in families and society. In P. G. Boss, W. J. Doherty, R. LaRossa, W. R. Schumm, & S. K. Steinmetz (Eds.), *Sourcebook of family theories and methods: A contextual approach* (pp. 591–623). New York: Plenum Press.

Ray, R. E. (2006). The personal as political: The legacy of Betty Friedan. In T. M. Calasanti & K. F. Slevin (Eds.), *Age matters: Re-aligning feminist thinking* (pp. 21–45). New York: Routledge.

Reinharz, S. (1992). *Feminist methods in social research.* New York: Oxford University Press.

Rich, A. (1986). *Of woman born* (10th anniv. ed.). New York: Norton.

Risman, B. J. (2004). Gender as a social structure: Theory wrestling with activism. *Gender & Society, 18,* 429–450.

Safilios-Rothschild, C. (1969). Family sociology or wives' family sociology? A cross-cultural examination of decision-making. *Journal of Marriage and the Family, 31,* 290–301.

Sarkisian, N., Gerena, M., & Gerstel, N. (2007). Extended family integration among Euro and Mexican Americans: Ethnicity, gender, and class. *Journal of Marriage and Family, 69,* 40–54.

Schmeeckle, M. (2007). Gender dynamics in stepfamilies: Adult stepchildren's views. *Journal of Marriage and Family, 69,* 174–189.

Smith, D. E. (1987). *The everyday world as problematic: A feminist sociology.* Boston: Northeastern University Press.

Smith, D. E. (1993). The Standard North American Family: SNAF as an ideological code. *Journal of Family Issues, 14,* 50–65.

Smith, D. E. (1999). *Writing the social: Critique, theory, and investigations.* Toronto: University of Toronto Press.

Spender, D. (1983). Modern feminist theorists: Reinventing rebellion. In D. Spender (Ed.), *Feminist theorists: Three centuries of key women thinkers* (pp. 366–380). New York: Pantheon.

Sprague, J. (2005). *Feminist methodologies for critical researchers: Bridging differences.* Walnut Creek, CA: AltaMira Press.

Sprey, J. (1990). Theoretical practice in family studies. In J. Sprey (Ed.), *Fashioning family theory: New approaches* (pp. 9–33). Newbury Park, CA: Sage.

Stanley, L. (Ed.). (1990). *Feminist praxis: Research, theory and epistemology in feminist sociology.* London: Routledge.

Thompson, L., & Walker, A. J. (1995). The place of feminism in family studies. *Journal of Marriage and the Family, 57,* 847–865.

Thorne, B. (1982). Feminist rethinking of the family: An overview. In B. Thorne & M. Yalom (Eds.), *Rethinking the family: Some feminist questions* (pp. 1–24). New York: Longman.

Walker, A. J. (1999). Gender and family relationships. In M. B. Sussman, S. K. Steinmetz, & G. W. Peterson (Eds.), *Handbook of marriage and the family* (2nd ed., pp. 439–474). New York: Plenum Press.

Walker, A. J. (2000). Refracted knowledge: Viewing families through the prism of social science. *Journal of Marriage and the Family, 62,* 595–608.

Walker, A. J., Allen, K. R., & Connidis, I. A. (2005). Theorizing and studying sibling ties in adulthood. In V. L. Bengtson, A. C. Acock, K. R. Allen, P. Dilworth-Anderson, & D. M. Klein (Eds.), *Sourcebook of family theory & research* (pp. 167–190). Thousand Oaks, CA: Sage.

Walker, A. J., & Thompson, L. (1984). Feminism and family studies. *Journal of Family Issues, 5,* 545–570.

Wenger, G. C., Scott, A., & Patterson, N. (2000). How important is parenthood? Childlessness and support in old age in England. *Ageing & Society, 20,* 161–182.

Willson, A. E., Shuey, K. M., & Elder, G. H., Jr. (2006). Ambivalence in the relationship of adult children to aging parents and in-laws. *Journal of Marriage and Family, 65,* 1055–1072.

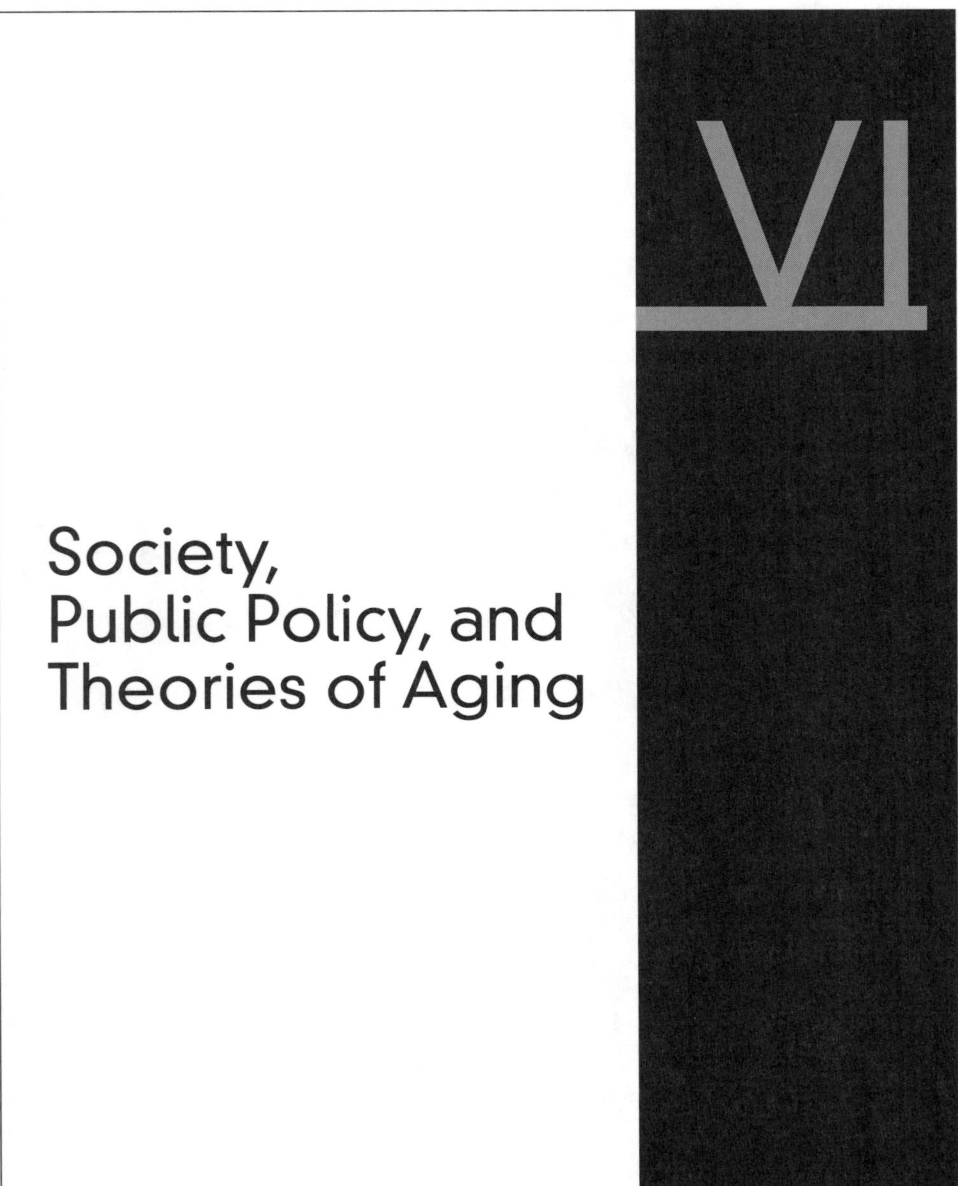

VI

Society, Public Policy, and Theories of Aging

From Industrialization to Institutionalism: Theoretical Accounts of Aging Policy Development in the United States

29

Robert B. Hudson

There can be little doubt that older people have today assumed a special place in the American social policy and political landscape. They constitute a large and growing population, they are increasingly well organized, and they are the recipients of public benefits that are the envy of every other social policy constituency in the nation.

It is the purpose of this chapter to review and assess different theoretical approaches that may help account—in all or in part—for these fairly recent and remarkable developments. While there is some variety in how welfare state analysts have organized and distinguished between these approaches (Myles & Quadagno, 2002; Pampel & Williamson, 1992; Skocpol, 1991), each has identified a fairly common set of alternatives. The organization here centers on seven separate (though potentially reinforcing) possibilities. These, in turn, can be clustered into two economic, three society-centered, and two state-centered approaches.

The two economic theories—the logic of industrialization and neo-Marxist—represent contrasting functionalist representations of how emerging industrial economies conditioned welfare state development. Both approaches are centered on the unrelenting economic forces of the industrial age, the former emphasizing the massive increase in economic resources and consequent social dislocations and the latter focusing on the inevitable consequences of wealth being concentrated in fewer and fewer hands. The aged, understood as an increasingly notable demographic presence, play an important role in each of these understandings.

The society-centered approaches bring into play the values, behaviors, and actions of individuals and groups that inform and structure the demands made of government tied to individual and social well-being. The first of these, based on cultural norms, is usually discussed under the rubric of national values. This lens has often been focused on American social policy developments because of the country's "exceptionalist" political culture. However, as this culture allegedly impedes broad-based welfare state developments as seen in Europe, the aged emerge as a rather unique beneficiary group, being indulged where others are denied. A second society-centered approach finds working-class mobilization central to welfare state developments; workers come to influence or even organize political parties, using their strength of numbers to press for benefits that they are unable to gain from owners in the money-dominated economic realm. The aged are found to gain (or lose) relative advantage depending on the success of these forays by labor into politics.

The third society-centered approach looks to the participation of individual and organized interests manifested as groups or as constituencies rather than as classes. Groups organize around various "identities" individuals may have, and in modern society these may be more particularistic than class goals. In a nation such as the United States, where working-class cohesion was never firmly established, multiple demands organized along these lines emerge. By the 1980s, the aged in the United States could be very easily identified as one such interest.

The third theoretical clustering is "state centered," directing attention to the autonomy and cohesion of public and quasi-public institutions. These institutional elements include formal constitutional conditions, such as federalism and governmental structure; quasi-public entities, such as political parties; and, importantly, the product of those structures, that is, *public* policy. It is worth distinguishing between two variants of state-centered theory, one focused on the state itself and the second on the policy outcomes. How the state is structured and, in particular, how much autonomy its incumbents—both political and administrative—enjoy is critical to the first of these. The second understands the policies generated by the state to have critical effects in shaping and constraining subsequent political activity. Put differently, policy is understood here as an independent rather than as a dependent variable in explaining welfare state developments. A rich literature focusing on age-related policy has in recent years come to serve virtually as the leading exhibit in pushing this perspective to the theoretical fore.

The following pages review these seven theoretical understandings. Each discussion frames the particular approach, places it in both the American and comparative contexts, and finally finds the place of the aged in these understandings. As will be seen, there exists a rich literature on the first two of these three elements; the principal value added of this presentation finds itself in the aging-related material, the old—until quite recently—having been often treated more in passing than as central players in social policy development.

The Logic of Industrialization

The birth of the modern welfare state in Western nations occurs in the wake of the process of industrialization and urbanization in the 19th century. Analysts vary on how dominant was the role of industrialization alone, but none questions its essential contribution. It is also the case that the aged—through both their emerging plight and their growing numbers—provide a key link between the forces of industrialization and early welfare state development.

At the most basic level, industrialization made possible the accumulation of resources not possible in preindustrial society. Industrial organization and technological advances grew symbiotically and make investment, not only consumption, possible. By so doing, surpluses could accumulate, allowing for social welfare expenditures among other uses. It is over the use of these surpluses that capitalist and anticapitalist ideologues have struggled since the dawning of industrialization. These twin processes of industrialization and urbanization disrupt traditional economic, social, familial, and geographic relationships. The status that older people enjoyed in agricultural economies, where farmers have considerable control over their own employment and where "landed property is power" (Gratton, 1986), wanes with the onset of industrialization. Over time, workers become disabled or exhausted, and owners demand ever-higher levels of productivity, especially during the "the industrial efficiency" movements of the late 19th and early 20th centuries. For their part, families find the economic utility of children lessens in urban settings, abetted by small and squalid living arrangements. "At this point, all of the things that happen to old people become much more tragic" (Wilensky & Lebeaux, 1958, p. 77). In this "resources plus needs" formulation, the old come to hold a relatively unique, if very unfortunate, place. Their family supports have been undermined (fewer children, higher divorce, and disabled kin), and their economic value has been diminished (physically weak and technologically backward).

It is here that the state steps in, performing something of a regulatory function by instituting programs to provide for those necessarily (and appropriately) forced from the productive economy. The proximate factors that might make this so—sympathy, assuring work for the young, and responding to pressures from adult children—are not specified by this approach; however, cross-national analyses covering welfare state expansion from inception through the 1970s find the aged to be a strong correlate if not an established engine of public social expenditure growth. In Wilensky's (1975) words, "As economic level climbs, the percentage of aged climbs, which shapes spending directly; with economic growth the percentage of aged goes up, which makes for an early start and swift spread of social security programs" (p. 27).

At one level, what Myles and Quadagno (2002) refer to as the weaker version, this approach is hard to fault: it would be hard to account for welfare state growth absent the effects of economic growth and population aging. Importantly, these forces are at work today as well as they were yesterday. Numerous analysts have posited economic growth as the absolutely essential (if not sole) factor (Cameron, 1978) behind the explosion in post–World War II social welfare expenditures. Indeed, the potentially dominant role of economic growth (today associated more with technology than industrialization)—played down in the 1980s and 1990s by those emphasizing political factors in accounting for welfare state expansion—has received renewed attention in explaining assaults on the welfare state since the mid-1970s. That is, if economic growth fuels expansion, why would economic stagnation not contribute to program contraction? Yet, while welfare state cutbacks have been observed in numerous national settings over the period (Huber, Stephens, & Ray, 1999), there remains disagreement about whether the economics and politics of austerity are the mirror image of the economics and politics of expansion (Pierson, 1994).

A stronger version of the economic development approach is more contested. Cross-nationally, there is great variation between levels of economic growth on the one hand and the growth and size of welfare states on the other, a divergence that strongly suggests that forces other than the narrowly economic must be at work. Perhaps most notable is the United States, where industrial growth was early and fierce yet where social welfare spending has long lagged behind (Skocpol, 1991). A critique of this approach holds that it does not account for the proximate activities that generate change. For example, it does not take a terribly advanced understanding of human behavior to intuit that it is relatively easy to raise public revenue when gross domestic product (GDP) is expanding, but countries have done so at far different rates nonetheless.

These larger debates about welfare state growth aside, the place of the aged in the industrialism approach is notable. In historical context, population aging appears as a driver of pension and (later) health care spending, and today analysts on both sides of "the coming crisis in age-related spending" debate employ a GDP/aging expenditure ratio to make their points—based on very different assumptions (Gist, in press; Teles, 2007). There is some irony in this concern being driven by population aging (i.e., the aging of the baby boomers) in that the causal arrows are again up for grabs: whereas population aging presumably helped drive welfare state development 100 years ago, it is also the case today that the enormity of welfare state expenditures has centrally contributed to the imposing presence represented by this generation of seniors. If this is at least partially the case, the role of industrialization and economic growth must be augmented by other theoretical considerations that will be encountered in this chapter.

Neo-Marxist Theory

A second deterministic approach borrows from and modifies Marxist arguments about the logic of capitalism and the relentless imperative toward concentration of wealth into fewer and fewer hands. More than the original, contemporary Marxist theory finds in the welfare state an expanded, if limited, role for the state itself. Beyond being a handmaiden to capitalism in abetting capital accumulation (infrastructure, education, and security), the state takes on the burden of caring for those who cannot meet the demands of labor imposed by organized capital. At the very time the state is doing capitalists' bidding by preparing workers with skills to assume new occupations, the state also plays a legitimating role by enacting programs to prevent widespread suffering for those who cannot measure up. As Piven and Cloward (1971) put it, "Without work, people cannot conform to familial and communal roles; and if the dislocation is widespread, the legitimacy of the social order itself may come to be questioned" (p. 7).

In this understanding, the welfare state leads vulnerable populations to believe that the overall system can be reasonably supportive of them even if they have been cast out of the labor market. In something of an updated version of the original Marxian false-consciousness formulation, the populace sees in these interventions beneficence rather than control. This is accomplished through a pervasive yet subtle power mechanism whereby one party succeeds in "influencing, shaping, or determining [a second party's] very wants" (Lukes, 1974, p. 34). In so doing, the welfare state performs what Edelman (1964) terms a quiescent function.

Prior to the rise of a "critical gerontology" literature in the 1990s, the aged had not been centrally featured in these discussions, although they had been implicitly addressed in many (Gough, 1979; O'Conner, 1973). In borrowing from neo-Marxist literature, critical gerontology "differs from other gerontological perspectives by viewing the situation of the aged as the product of social structural forces rather than natural or inevitable individual and psychological processes" (Estes, 1991, p. 21). Thus, income maintenance policy for the old should be understood not merely as offsetting physical declines in late life but rather as a means to remove older workers from the industrial labor force (Graebner, 1974) in the name of promoting economic efficiency. Modern health care interventions for the old are less about addressing their indisputable needs than about siphoning public monies into the largely private hospital, nursing home, and mental health industries (Estes & Binney, 1991). The success of these efforts can be partially understood as the result of overt power of dominant private sector actors, but a more adequate explanation is found again in the false-consciousness idea, here applied to the old, wherein "people accept as legitimate the conditions that lead to their own exploitation" (Hendricks & Leedham, 1991, p. 55).

The most interesting case for testing neo-Marxist and critical gerontology tenets on older people in the United States is found in the Townsend movement of the 1930s. As elders suffered perhaps more than any other population, Francis Townsend proposed that each of them receive $200 per month on the condition that they spend it immediately (in order to stimulate the economy) and agree not to work (in order to free up jobs for younger workers). The movement caught fire and, at its height during the Depression, there were hundreds of Townsend chapters with tens of thousands of adherents. How much pressure it generated on the Roosevelt administration as it designed its Social Security legislation is a matter of scholarly debate (Amenta, 2006; Orloff, 1988), but Roosevelt's Committee on Economic Security was keenly aware of its presence (Witte, 1963). The neo-Marxist interpretation holds that

Old-Age Insurance is best understood as a means of appeasing older people and, in so doing, defanging the Townsend movement. In lieu of the Townsend Plan, "What the old folks got instead—if it did not entirely placate them, it placated their public supporters—was the Social Security legislation." Ultimately, this "meager concession spelled the demise of the movement" (Piven & Cloward, 1971, p. 101).

Critical gerontology's placating hypothesis is one of several that can tie the Townsend movement and the Social Security Act to one another. Not to be lost in this theoretical discussion, however, is that the most notable social movement that comes out of the Depression is by and about old people. Nowhere else have older people ever been organized to such a degree. Moreover, this was no radical movement; it was carried on by "solid folk" (Piven & Cloward, 1971) and was overtly intended to restore, not to overthrow, the prevailing system. While the logic of the neo-Marxist approach can hold—Social Security did hasten the movement's demise—the need to calm conservative old people rather than radical workers says a good deal about the American political culture, to which attention turns next.

Political Culture and Values

An "exceptionalist" and reinforcing set of national values served as the predominant theme in post–World War II writings about the unique place the United States appeared to occupy in comparative welfare state development (Orloff, 1988). Americans' historical attachments to individualism, self-reliance, voluntarism, free markets, and a Protestant-based moralism were seen as instrumental both in understanding the etiology of poverty and ill health and in limiting the role government should play in their amelioration (Rimlinger, 1971). Poverty and ill health were attributed largely to individual failings and immoral behavior, a diagnosis that left little room or justification for government involvement (Rosenberg, 1962). In early New England, the "old and the disabled were proper objects of relief, but not the able-bodied poor, who received harsher treatment" (Quadagno, 1988, p. 25). During this period, Americans warmed to Herbert Spencer's juxtaposing Charles Darwin and Protestantism, "a philosophy of liberation from the trammels of government" (Fleming, 1963, p. 127).

This value set poses a direct challenge to the logic of industrialization approach since the country underwent massive economic dislocations in the almost complete absence of public intervention on behalf of those dislocated. While other countries were instituting unemployment, health care, and pension policies, social policy efforts in the United States were limited largely to the regulatory and "good government" initiatives of the Progressives. And even these followed the more substantive European developments by more than a decade. Theda Skocpol's work highlighting early Civil War pensions and state-level mothers' pensions has served as a partial correction to these earlier understandings of how delayed American developments were and, as such, adds a cautionary note about the national values argument. Nonetheless, these benefits' being confined to veterans, women, and children was in sharp contrast to the European experience where the needs, grievances, and demands of the working class were the essential ingredient.

Differences in national value structures also inform conceptual understandings of different welfare regimes. Under one formulation, the exceptionalism of the United States takes on particular salience. In a series of lectures delivered at Oxford in 1949, British sociologist T. H. Marshall (1964) delineated three types of citizenship—civil, political, and social—that have marked the evolution of modern societies and contrasted their pattern of development cross-nationally. Civil citizenship encompassed a basic set of rights necessary to freedom in the modern world: the right to liberty, the right to property, and the right to the evenhanded administration of justice. A second set of rights were political ones, the right to vote, to organize, and to hold office. The third stage was social rights, referring to economic security and the right to enjoy a reasonable level of well-being understood not only in terms of absolute well-being but also in terms of relationship to one's fellow citizens.

Writing at a time when the postwar Labour government was building the British welfare state, Marshall guardedly forecast that the historical victories involving civil and political citizenships would be joined by the social. Not only was it happening in Britain, but it had already happened to a significant degree in the Continental and Scandinavian nations; indeed, in Germany, social citizenship had preceded the civil and political, leading to a highly paternalistic state and one, tragically, open to demagoguery given the relative absence of vital free and participatory spheres.

As for the United States, it clearly and famously succeeded at the civil and political stages, both sets of rights being firmly established before anywhere else, including Britain. The Bill of Rights, early White manhood suffrage, and expansions of organizing rights set the United States apart for many years, although with the very notable omission of women and African Americans (Fraser & Gordon, 1992). Yet the third stage has never developed as fully as elsewhere. The "right" to health care, to decent housing, to employment, and to a decent standard of living has never been codified here in a manner to seriously approach most other nations. There may be more than one way to account for this relative failing, but an entrenched set of deeply rooted exceptional values is certainly high on the list.

Value salience can also help account for rationales associated with American social policy interventions when they did ultimately occur. Franklin Roosevelt and his advisers were nearly obsessed with the work disincentives that might be associated with New Deal initiatives. Writing of that and subsequent periods, longtime Social Security Commissioner Robert Ball (2000) repeatedly emphasized how important the idea of work was to all discussions:

> *Private pensions, group insurance, and social insurance all belong, along with wages and salaries, to the group of work-connected payments, and it is this work connection, the fact that it is earned, which gives social insurance its basic character. (p. 43)*

Indeed, the controversy that sprung up about extending Old-Age Insurance to cover survivors in 1939 centered on the absence of any work history among those individuals.

The values perspective can also help account for what many observers see as major gaps in American social policy. Most notable is the absence of any kind of family allowance policy acknowledging the costs and contributions of child rearing in the modern world. American policy toward young families, especially low-income young families, has been marked by exclusionary (Ryan, 1971), residual (Wilensky & Lebeaux, 1958), and behaviorist (Marmor, Mashaw, & Harvey, 1990) policies, most recently associated with welfare reform and the Temporary Assistance to Needy Families program. Lawrence Mead's (1998) writings on the need for a "new paternalism" to guide the unworthy poor ("Individuals need self-restraint. . . . Those who would be free must first be bound" [p. 109]) rival the writings of William Graham Sumner a century earlier ("The ill-endowed are also made radically unfree by yielding up their claim to fend for themselves" [quoted in Fleming, 1963, p. 129]).

Focusing finally here on the aged, the national values perspective has much to offer theoretically. Indeed, both sympathy for the aged and antipathy for much of the remaining population is a very suggestive framework. "Firsts" for the aged in the United States include Civil War pensions for northern veterans in 1862, old-age assistance and old-age insurance in 1935, Disability Insurance in 1956 (initially only for those over age 50), Medicare in 1965 (for the old alone until 1972), and Supplemental Security Income (SSI) in 1972 (for the poor old, blind, and disabled). Because the old were assumed to be poor and frail, they alone could pass the American values litmus test around work and self-sufficiency. This also made the aged a favored group among social policy reformers who wished to institute benefits that would ultimately extend beyond the aged to other population groups.

Working-Class Mobilization

This approach to understanding welfare state development has the organized presence of industrial workers at center stage. Not to be confused with neo-Marxist theories, analysts here see workers as having "agency" and as actively challenging the presumed imperatives of monopoly capital. Because the presence of workers and their economic and political organizations—unions and parties—are readily measured, assessing the utility of the working-class-struggle approach is more straightforward than addressing the imperatives and values addressed previously.

In this model, "politics matters" in that industrial workers use their numbers and organizations to impact the political system. If the strike is the workers' economic weapon, the vote is the workers' political one. And because in free market economies workers will always outnumber owners, the political realm is a fertile one, especially when parties organize to mobilize and channel worker concerns. The organizational element is critical; the extension of political democracy absent effective organization is not sufficient to generate needed pressures on the existing system. Early on in the European experience, expansion of the franchise largely through the efforts of left-wing parties (and by conservative parties trying to co-opt workers) created political opportunities propitious for welfare state development.

There is a well-established empirical literature supporting the positive relationship between left-wing legislative presence and welfare state growth (Cameron, 1978; Esping-Andersen, 1985). The logic of the theory is, obviously enough, that social democratic parties will prevail, form governments, and enact expansive programs. That, of course, happened, but one also finds that the approach can be operative even when rightist parties are in power. This occurred most famously in the case of Bismarck's creation of the German welfare state in the 1880s. Antecedent to this but related would be Conservative Prime Minister Benjamin Disraeli extending the franchise to workers in 1860s Britain; in both cases, a co-optation hypothesis—paternalistic privilege of the right indulges the emerging working class in order to forestall the further organization of the left.

Not surprisingly, very little is said of the American experience in these discussions. As has been well documented, in comparative perspective the United States failed to generate permanent, sizable, or cohesive left-wing political (or economic) movements. On the economic side, there were periodic appearances (e.g., the Industrial Workers of the World and the Knights of Labor), but these were mercurial and fleeting. When mainstream labor did organize, it was the more skilled craft unions that first emerged, ultimately to form the American Federation of Labor (AFL). Far from an orthodox leftist union leader, the AFL's founder, Samuel Gompers, opposed federal unemployment insurance well into the early years of the Depression. In the political domain, an American Socialist Party emerged around the turn of the century—Eugene Debs won nearly 7% of the vote in the 1912 election—but the Democratic Party has served as the closest approximation of a leftist party in the United States for more than a century.

A vast literature exists on why "socialism failed in America" (Greenstone, 1969; Lipset & Marks, 2001). Most obviously at work are the exceptionalist values discussed earlier. Geography and the frontier have long been argued to have played a role in dispersing the disgruntled and defusing tensions. Much has been laid to race and ethnic animosities, whereby "blood being thicker than class" vitiates attempts to bring workers of different backgrounds together. And, of course, employers vehemently opposed organizing efforts on behalf of workers and attacked workers and their leaders who attempted organization. As a result of these various factors, it is widely agreed that the United States failed to generate a viable and cohesive political movement based on the working class.

There are interesting ramifications of this failure for the emerging older population. On the one hand, an effective working-class movement would appear to benefit the aged, if only because current workers would become old, and pension benefits were almost always included as one of a package of worker demands. Indeed, pensions can be seen as a way for workers to press for (future) benefits in a manner that was less threatening to employers than were demands for improvements in current wages and working conditions. As Myles (1984) argues, pensions are a form of deferred wage, and because most jobs were onerous but necessary, the promise of future leisure time through the pension mechanism was appealing. That American workers pressed for and received some private pension (and, later, public) coverage is consistent with the working-class-struggle approach. In fact, invoking Marshall's terminology, Myles sees these pensions as "a citizen's wage." Because public pensions have come to constitute a comparatively enormous portion of American welfare state expenditures and because pension and health benefits were the lion's share of fringe benefits negotiated for by workers, the aged in the United States can be seen as both conceptually and economically advantaged through leftist (or at least progressive) efforts at benefit expansion. The passage of Medicare in the 1960s serves as further evidence of this advantage. Its passage has been partially attributed to organized labor trying to push union-funded retiree health care costs—another form of deferred income—off onto the public sector so that those energies and resources could be channeled into efforts on behalf of current workers (Quadagno, 2005).

On the other hand, as Pampel and Williamson (1992) observe, the workings of this theory could be seen as inimical to the concerns of the aged. To the extent that the theory postulates and behaviors might follow, organized labor's political action efforts might work to exclude other groups. In addition to the aged, these might include women and populations of color, who might or might not be workers. Certainly, the segregationist impulses of mainstream American labor would serve to substantiate such a concern.

As for current workers, there is no reason to believe that pensions would be the number one bargaining item unless circumstances forced other more immediate concerns of workers off of the table. Unemployment and workers' compensation benefits certainly might be seen as more central. Moreover, as Pampel and Williamson (1992) note, intergenerational tensions might emerge for unions (and, conceivably, the Democratic Party) in a situation where there was a call for imposition of higher dues or taxes in order to support pension benefits for current retirees. Despite these theoretical possibilities, the dangers of such a split are reduced in the American case by, once again, the limited impact of purely working-class political movements. The recent erosion of union membership, to say nothing of an influx of hard-to-unionize low-wage immigrant workers, makes this potential working-class "threat" to the old a marginal possibility at best.

Democratic and Group Participation

Perhaps the most commonly presented construct of "how a (social policy) bill becomes a law" in the United States centers on how interests are articulated, aggregated, and realized. In the classic democratic participation model, citizens express their views through voting, letter writing, campaigning, and contributing; interest groups are organized around clusters of citizen concerns and carried by them to political parties and directly into the halls of government; and political parties join separate demands into coherent platforms as a means of structuring political debate (Easton, 1957).

Associated very much with pluralist theories of the political system (Polsby, 1963), this model has both empirical and normative dimensions. Mainstream political science saw these pluralistic impulses as marking how American government worked from World War II through the 1960s, but it was widely held that the pluralists often conflated depictions of how the system worked with how they preferred it to work. Subscribing very much to an "order paradigm" (Horton, 1966), the pluralists saw individual and group competition taking place within a larger world of shared values and common assumptions. Voter, group, and party competition functioned not unlike the workings of the free economic market, with myriad demands being muted and compromises being forged. In all this, the government served as something of a referee, ratifying the winners and losers and lending formal recognition to the balance of political powers at any given point in time. A growing tide of criticism (Lowi, 1967; Parenti, 1970) and events of the 1960s and 1970s led to the model's fall from grace. Nonetheless, the pluralists' desire to document and defend democratically stable political systems in light of the widespread failure of democratic governments earlier in the century was more than understandable.

There can be no question that the basic ingredients of the model were (and are) very much in evidence in the United States. Long seen as a nation of joiners, the United States has more interest groups, many of them highly particularistic, than found elsewhere. Whereas political parties in other nations do, in fact, perform critical aggregating functions around candidate selection and policy formulation, in the United States it is said to be "K Street"—home to hundreds of special interests, many of them generously funded—where disproportionate influence on these key functions is effectively exercised. The logical basis for this reality derives in part from what the United States does not possess; lacking strong working-class structures or consciousness and marked by a highly fragmented constitutional structure, the policy process in the United States itself becomes balkanized. Put differently, of the two so-called demand theories presented here, the unit of analysis in the pluralistic model is groups; in the social democratic model, it is classes.

If the democratic participation model worked as advertised, it would represent a highly reasoned if comparatively underorganized political system. Over time, however, observers found many elements to fault with both its workings and its outcomes. As most famously argued by Lowi (1967), referring to the model as "interest group liberalism," the group process does not yield bargaining and negotiated outcomes. Many unfiltered demands indulging numerous program constituencies sail through a fragmented committee structure in Congress and through a maze of subcabinet agencies in the executive branch. Beyond the excessive "noise" created by such a system, there are also negative distributional consequences, with "have" groups being better able to organize, generate resources, and press their demands, creating, in Lowi's words, "a system of privilege." Yet other theorists see no checks at work offsetting the relentless series of demands that those in search of governmental largesse make, resulting potentially in "an overload of democracy" (Buchanan & Tullock, 1962; Niskanen, 1971) and impeding governance itself.

The aged present a fascinating case study of the potential validity of the interest group model and its limitations, both empirical and normative. They are a large and growing population, they are very active politically, they are extremely well organized, they have particularistic policy concerns, and roughly one-third of the federal budget is devoted to their interests. As they say, that is a very potent political cocktail. However, it need be kept in mind that correlation is not causation, and, as we will see subsequently, exactly how the cocktail is mixed may make all the difference.

It is first important to note that the aged's organized presence in Washington is reinforced by its imposing electoral standing. Not just a large population, seniors now have higher participation rates than any other age-group (U.S. Bureau of the Census, 2004). In off-year and primary elections, that disproportionate presence is even more pronounced. Yet it is equally important to observe that older people vote much like younger ones in general elections (Binstock, 2000), suggesting that their particularistic interests do not necessarily determine their voting decisions. Of course, since no candidate campaigns on an antiaging platform, this "nonevent" becomes a potent illustration of how elders exercise a "second face of power" (Bachrach & Baratz, 1962), namely, keeping unwanted alternatives off the political agenda altogether. There is little evidence that voting patterns of older people directly shape aging-related policy results, but a fair summation of older voters' place in the policy process may simply be that "they are there, and they are aware."

Seniors' interest group presence in Washington is formidable, and it is here that the potential exercise of "the first face of power" is in full view. Organizations ranging from AARP (with 34 million members) to the National Academy of Elder Care Attorneys and the American Society of Consulting Pharmacists are among 54 organizations that constitute the Leadership Council of Aging Organizations (an organization of aging organizations). A few of the members, such as AARP, are mass-membership organizations, but the majority represent professionals and other providers with interests in Washington serving older Americans.

While these organizations' significant presence is beyond dispute, their exact role in securing the enormous benefits today's elders enjoy is a matter of some controversy. Certainly, there has been much commentary in both popular (Peterson, 1999; Samuelson, 2005) and scholarly circles (Pratt, 1976; Price, 1997), pointing—usually with alarm—at the influence the organized aged have in Washington. AARP has been portrayed as the capital's most powerful group, and its support of President Bush's Medicare Part D prescription drug program is widely believed to have been critical to its passage (Iglehart, 2004).

In many other legislative episodes, however, it has been difficult to isolate a determinative role that the groups have played. Since the groups themselves have only been organized quite recently—AARP and the National Council of Senior Citizens were the first, both dating back only to the late 1950s—they played no role in the formative years of aging policy. And accounts of particular legislative episodes report mixed results as well. In each of the following cases, the organized aged and their allies were engaged, but evidence of their role in determining ultimate policy outcomes is more mixed: Social Security (Campbell, 2003; Derthick, 1979a), Medicare (Marmor, 1970), SSI (Burke & Burke, 1974), the repeal of the Medicare Catastrophic Coverage Act (Himelfarb, 1995), and private pension benefit protection (Madland, 2007).

These cautionary comments do not ignore the reality that the aged and their organized representatives have assumed a major place in American political life. It is no longer possible, as it was 50 years ago, for politicians to ignore older people as they went around their business. The question of concern here, however, is how different theoretical approaches understand and account for what has now become that imposing presence. In the democratic and group participation model, the literal presence of the aged is less mediated than in any of the competing approaches. Nonetheless, imposing as seniors' political presence may now be does not necessarily account for aging-based welfare state development, appealing as that direct linkage may appear.

The Role of the State: Structure

Having reviewed two functionalist theories and three society-centered ones, we turn our attention to the role of the state in aging-related welfare state developments. In a literal sense, it is, of course, the state that formally enacts and funds policies of all sorts. Yet in the approaches reviewed thus far, the role of the state is remarkably marginal. Industrialization theory sees it as responding in some quasi-automatic and unspecified way to an emerging combination of technological innovation and human suffering, neo-Marxists see it as abetting organized capital in a wholly subordinated manner, the working-class approach sees the state as the prize that one or the other of two class-based interests will control, and the pluralism inherent in the democratic organized interest model finds state actions as largely a ratification of the balance of organized group influence within the polity.

The 1980s saw the reemergence of the state as a central analytical ingredient in accounting for welfare state developments. The center of attention in political science's very early years—Woodrow Wilson wrote famously about it while at Princeton (Robertson, 1993)—was that the role of the state lost standing to the alternative approaches discussed previously, especially in the post–World War II years. Two scholars in particular are associated with this reemergence of interest in the state. Theodore Lowi (1964) suggested that what the state does critically affects the subsequent political process, not simply the reverse, as suggested by social democratic and democratic process approaches. At the 1981 American Political Science Association, Lowi and his cochair, Sydney Tarrow, argued, "We do not reject the perspective that focuses on the political process, or on political behavior—even when it is *mass* behavior—but we argue that processes and behavior can best be studied within the context of institutions" (quoted in Robertson, 1993, p. 20).

Theda Skocpol and colleagues have produced a significant literature over the past 20 years under the rubric of "bringing the state back in," the essential argument being, "States conceived as organizations claiming control over territories and people may formulate and pursue goals that are not simply reflective of the demands or interests of social groups, classes, or society" (Skocpol, 1985, p. 9).

The essence of the argument is that state structures play an independent role in shaping political activity and political outcomes. These structures include all significant elements of the state—formal constitutional structures and quasi-public institutions, such as political parties. Robertson (1993) sees measures of both *political capacity* and *political coherence* as being critical in state-centered analysis. Three key measures of capacity are the boundaries of legitimate governmental intervention, fiscal capacity, and expertise of legislators and administrators. Coherence involves two dimensions: the extent to which authority within a level of government is unified or fragmented and the autonomy possessed by different levels of government.

If not once again exceptional, the American experience is at least notable if we briefly examine it against these five items. In comparative perspective, the boundaries of legitimate governmental action in the social policy realm are noticeably narrow. The exceptionalism of the national values perspective weighs in heavily here, as does the Marshall formulation noting how far social citizenship trails behind the civic and political in the United States. A famous passage from Thomas Paine captures Americans' historical disdain for the state: "the more perfect civilization is, the less occasion it has for government, because the more does it regulate its own affairs and govern itself."

Fiscal capacity of the national government was historically weak, one of many examples being that the budget of the U.S. State Department was drawn exclusively from consular fees until just before World War I. While slowing the gap modestly, the United States continues to spend considerably less on social welfare functions than do other advanced nations (see Table 29.1).

The United States also trails other nations in critical aspects of administrative expertise. For myriad reasons, the civil service in the United States has never enjoyed the autonomy and prestige of its counterparts in other nations. In France, for example, a majority of senior civil servants and a significant number of senior politicians are graduates of L'Ecole National d'Administration, the training academy of France's political elites. The traditions about the administrative sphere of government differ sharply on either side of the Atlantic. In Europe, the autonomy of the state is long established and taken as an institutional reality across a range of critical social activities (Nettl, 1968). This is in direct contrast to the experience in the United States, where "the civil administration of the early twentieth-century American state was quite weak, given the lack of an established state bureaucracy and the dispersion of authority inherent in U.S. federalism and the division of powers" (Orloff, 1988, p. 59).

The lack of cohesiveness of America's political structures is known, if not fully appreciated, by generations of students. Cohesion was intentionally attenuated from the beginning: a federal restructure with divided areas of sovereignty, separated branches of government, checks and balances, a bicameral legislature (with the Senate embodying overt state-level representation), and

29.1 Gross Public Social Expenditure as a Percentage of Gross Domestic Product, 2003

Australia	17.9
Belgium	26.5
Canada	17.3
Denmark	27.6
France	28.7
Germany	27.3
Norway	25.1
Sweden	31.3
United Kingdom	20.6
United States	16.2

Source: Organization for Economic Cooperation and Development, Social Expenditure Database for 2003.

staggered elections within and between the legislative and executive branches. Samuel Huntington (1966) argues that American governmental institutions are more incoherent than even the textbook version of checks and balances would suggest. In short, "sovereignty was divided, power was separated, and functions were combined in many different institutions" (p. 392). In Huntington's analysis, it is America's consensual society that makes this institutional chaos possible: "In America, the ease of modernization within society precluded the modernization of the political system. The United States thus combines the world's most modern society with the world's most antique politics" (p. 406).

Why this state of institutional events would impede social policy development is not hard to deduce. In the bastardized words of a popular advertisement, "You expect less of the American government, and you get it." Limited capacity and coherence—especially when intended—does not bode well for the reformers' agenda. That, in the 19th century, all levels of American government were marked as well by high levels of patronage and cronyism adds fuel to the fire. In short, in the eyes of the theory's proponents, weak political institutions can go a long way toward explaining America's peculiar social policy posture.

In addition, for purposes here, it also can be used to account for how the aged have fared in these United States. The most interesting application comes in Theda Skocpol's widely heralded rethinking of when America's version of the welfare state actually began. As indicated, for decades scholars have pointed to the New Deal period as when the United States entered the welfare policy game, occasionally with the grudging acknowledgment that the Progressives at the turn of the century made tentative moves in that direction. Yet in her work highlighting the importance of Civil War pensions and so-called mothers' pensions, Skocpol (1992) argues that, however selectively, the United States preceded what famously occurred elsewhere. By the late 19th century, these payments were roughly equal to any expenditure category in the federal budget, and in 1910, about 28% of men over aged 65—more than half a million—were receiving these benefits.

More interesting than their size, however, is their theoretical relevance: these pensions were awarded in great numbers to farmers and townspeople not central to industrialization, and they were not demanded by industrial workers or principally extended to them (Skocpol, 1992). Instead, pension expenditures expanded greatly until the end of the century, caught up in a uniquely American political process whereby they moved from "relatively straightforward compensation for wartime disabilities into fuel for patronage politics" (p. 120). Of course, coterminous with the growth of these politics was the aging of the veterans themselves; the combination of the "distributive politics" (Lowi, 1964) associated with politicians' ability to dispense benefits quite freely and beneficent attitudes toward the old proved a powerful policy combination. In Skocpol's (1992) words, the Civil War pension "evolved from a generous partially utilized program of compensation for combat injuries and deaths into an even more generous system of disability and old-age benefits which were taken up by 90 percent of the union veterans surviving in 1910" (pp. 109–110). In short, political incoherence and limited fiscal capacity did not impede the ability of elected representatives to inaugurate social welfare benefits for the old.

A second and last application of this perspective to old-age policy in the United States centers on the role of government civil servants in the welfare state enterprise.

That such individuals were central to European developments has been well established (Beer, 1966; Heclo, 1974). In perhaps the first of the state-centered monographs, *Modern Social Politics in Britain and Sweden,* Heclo (1974) reviews and downplays the roles of industrialization, elections, political parties, and interest groups: "At no time did organizations of the aged or pensioners themselves play any prominent part" (p. 156). Rather, he concludes that "the bureaucracies of Britain and Sweden loom predominant in the policies studied" (p. 301).

Despite the capacity and coherence shortcomings in the United States (or perhaps because of them), there are important instances of policy elites making a critical difference in social policy developments. And many of these involved the aged. Most notable in this regard is Franklin Roosevelt's Committee on Economic Security, which fashioned the original Social Security Act. As Ikenberry and Skocpol (1987) bluntly conclude, "The policy process through which Social Security was planned and drafted in the mid-1930s was strikingly closed" (p. 405). Martha Derthick has famously chronicled how closed was Social Security policymaking from the beginning through the mid-1970s. Two commissioners, Arthur Altmeyer and Robert Ball, held the job for two-thirds of the period and longer if one realizes Ball's influence in the years both preceding and following his officially holding the job. As to their relationship to the elected officials with whom they interacted, *Derthick* (1979a) concluded,

> *Program specialists in executive bureaus are one of the principal sources of supply for politicians who are looking for ideas for things to do. In the case of social security, for several decades they were almost the only source of supply. (p. 210)*

Policy elites inside government were critical to later successes, again disproportionately involving the aged. Wilbur Cohen, Oscar Ewing, and two key congressional figures—Senator Patrick McNamara of Michigan and Representative Aime Forand of Rhode Island—centrally fashioned Medicare strategy from the mid-1950s until its enactment in 1965 (Marmor, 1970). John Veneman, undersecretary of the Department of Health, Education, and Welfare, was the central actor in the phoenix-like transformation of President Nixon's failed Family Assistance Plan for Aid to Families with Dependent Children into the SSI program, providing a modest guaranteed income for the poor old, blind, and disabled in 1973 (Burke & Burke, 1974).

In the American case, the working of policy elites was far less institutionalized than in the European case. But these key actors, working in an admittedly semi-incoherent political system, seized critical moments and were able to strike when the policy moment was hot. And in these efforts, they often seized on the plight of the aged and the sympathy they engendered in the American context. In this manner, the aged served as something of an "ideological loss leader" for these reformers, eager not only to help the aged but also to use them in hopefully advancing policy agendas to other groups as well (Hudson, 1978).

The Role of the State: Policy

In various ways, each of the perspectives mentioned previously addresses factors and actors who may be seen as responsible for the timing and shape of welfare state policies. This last perspective reverses the causal arrows by asking, instead, to what degree the policies shape subsequent political activity. Here, policy becomes an independent variable affecting politics and, in turn, future policy. This hypothesis derives directly from the state-centered perspective in that policies, being formal product of states, both contribute to and derive from state autonomy and capacity.

Schattschneider (1935) was the first to identify and examine the phenomenon of how "policy causes politics" in his early discussion of tariff policy. Later investigations of "policy types" (Lowi, 1964; Wilson, 1973) demonstrated how the scope and distributive consequences of various enactments shaped subsequent activity. More recently, Schneider and Ingram (1993) added yet another key dimension, inquiring how the power and political construction of particular "target populations" can create arenas generating very different political processes. In particular, different policies can draw individuals into the political system, alienate them from it, or leave them indifferent. Policies are a powerful mechanism in attaching citizens to the political world; they can see what government can do for them or what it may do to them. Because levels of political participation have been declining and Americans' civic engagement has been called into question (Putnam, 1995), the role of public policy in fostering citizen involvement has normative as well as empirical ramifications.

Contemporary scholars have shown the impact that governmental policy can have. Skocpol's treatment of Civil War pensions reveals how patronage politics developed out of what was initially a reasonably constricted set of benefits but where the policy created political opportunities. Suzanne Mettler (2007) has shown how enactment of the GI Bill following World War II both contributed to broad-based economic gains and "also prompted higher levels of subsequent involvement in civic and political activities" (p. 196). Given the extraordinary growth in social welfare expenditures after 1960, the argument can be made more broadly: government spending on behalf of individual citizens created widespread interest in and commitment to the broader civic enterprise. During this period, the New Deal programs grew dramatically (after very little growth in their early years), and the Great Society programs of the Kennedy/Johnson years were enacted as well. By the mid-1970s, as Mettler notes, one sees "the expansion of the American welfare state, the growth of the middle class and the reduction of economic inequality, and high levels of positive attitudes and civic involvement among citizens" (p. 196).

Within this policy → politics template, the place of older people has a stunning presence. In part it is because the programs—Social Security, Medicare, a large part of Medicaid, and numerous lesser ones—dominate the federal domestic spending landscape. But the connection and timing between the growth in policies and the subsequent actions of older citizens and their interest groups is yet more remarkable. Looking at the role of aging-related interest groups, a simple chronology hints at this possibility as one notes that notable policy enactments and expansions appear to have preceded rather than followed interest group developments. Thus, AARP had virtually no policy presence until the 1970s, and, even then, one of its first political positions was to oppose as inflationary a 1972 Democratic proposal to raise Social Security benefits by 20% (Pratt, 1976). Somewhat later, Walker (1983) determined that more than one-half of the 43 aging-related interest groups in his study came into being after 1965, the breakthrough year that saw the enactment of Medicare, Medicaid, and the Older Americans Act. In Walker's words,

> *In all of these cases, the formation of new groups was one of the* consequences *of major new legislation, not one of the* causes *of its passage. A pressure model of the policymaking process in which an essentially passive legislature responds to petitions from groups of citizens who have spontaneously organized because of common social or economic concerns must yield to a model in which influences for change come as much from inside the government as from beyond its institutional boundaries. (p. 403)*

Actions subsequent to passage of the Older Americans Act—a program funding an array of social and in-home services to people aged 60 and above—provide a concrete example of this process at work. The state agencies charged with administering the program formalized their trade association, the National Association of State Units on Aging, in the years after 1965; the substate agencies, brought into existence through amendments in 1972, created their trade association, the National Association of Area Agencies on Aging, in the wake of that authorization (Hudson, 1994). Groups of nutrition, transportation, and legal service providers were also formed subsequent to these amendments.

Yet more compelling evidence of the policy generating politics chain is seen in the creation of seniors themselves as a self-identified political constituency. In her pathbreaking book *How Policies Make Citizens: Senior Political Activism and the American Welfare State,* Andrea Campbell (2003) documents how the growing presence of older Americans in the political process owes much of its existence to the expansion of Social Security. In carefully crafted research juxtaposing public opinion and voting data with Social Security program expansion, Campbell shows how levels of political consciousness, participation, and salience followed in the wake of Social Security's growth. Seniors are the only group for which electoral participation in presidential elections over the past 40 years has actually increased, while the participation rates of voters aged 18 to 24, 25 to 44, and 45 to 64 have each declined. In relative terms, a higher proportion of seniors now vote than does any other age-group; in 1964, they exceeded only the youngest group. In addition, Campbell shows that participation rates of seniors in other forms of political activity—letter writing, campaigning, and contributing—have also increased in both relative and absolute terms.

In assessing these findings, Campbell (2003) concludes that Social Security, in dramatically improving the economic well-being of older people, created both time and interest—what Pierson (2007) calls material and cognitive incentives—for seniors to involve themselves in political matters more heavily than had ever been the case:

> *Senior mass membership groups did not create Social Security policy. Rather, the policy helped create the groups. Social Security's effects on individuals—the increases in income, free time due to retirement, and political interest—enhance the likelihood of group membership. Social Security created a constituency for interest group entrepreneurs to organize, just as it defined a group for political parties to mobilize. (p. 77)*

While the causal role of policy is the principal contribution of this analysis, the secondary effects of policy's role is equally important. Thus, at "time 1," public policy may have been critical in the creation and institutionalization of the organized aging, but at "time 2," the groups become critical in efforts to expand or—more recently—to defend the policies against outside encroachment. Put differently, the Walker/Campbell argument does not dismiss the role of interest groups; rather, it helps explain both their origins and the dynamic—that is, benefit protection—that keeps formal members or informal adherents tuned in to their messages. In short, while AARP may be the biggest lobby in Washington, it would not be where it is if (a) Social Security had not helped galvanize the elderly and (b) Social Security and other programs were not there as a policy fulcrum around which AARP could rally the membership.

Conclusion

In these pages, I have reviewed seven approaches that may help account for the prominent place of the aged in America's truncated welfare state. That the aged have fared better than other groups in the United States is beyond dispute, although it is worth noting that in European welfare states, where working-age and younger populations have been much more generously provided for than in the United States, the European aged are still relatively better off than those in the United States. Smeeding (2006), using standardized poverty rate data from the Luxembourg Income Study, finds the United States with the highest rate of poverty of 11 rich nations and the second-highest rate of poverty among the elderly (after Ireland) of those nations. See Table 29.2.

It is neither necessary nor possible to find any one of these approaches accounting for the entirety of aging-related policy events. Some may be more

29.2 Relative Poverty Rates: Percentage Below 50% Median Adjusted Income, Overall and for Elders

Nation	Overall (rank)	Elders (rank)
United States	17.0 (1)	28.4 (2)
Ireland	16.5 (2)	48.3 (1)
Italy	12.7 (3)	14.4 (6)
United Kingdom	12.4 (4)	23.9 (3)
Canada	11.4 (5)	6.5 (10)
Germany	8.3 (6)	12.2 (7)
Belgium	8.0 (7)	17.2 (5)
Austria	7.7 (8)	17.4 (4)
Netherlands	7.3 (9)	2.0 (11)
Sweden	6.5 (10)	8.3 (9)
Finland	5.4 (11)	10.3 (8)
Overall average	10.3	17.0

attuned to particular time periods of particular episodes, but even then, no single perspective can be expected to explain the totality of events.

That said, some theoretical speculations are in order to conclude this voyage through American old-age policy. First, it seems fair to conclude that the aged have been transformed from being a group defined overwhelming by need into a fully institutionalized population quite capable of articulating its own interests. The elites and reformers that have historically made the policy case on behalf of older people have no contemporary equals. The likes of Arther Altmeyer, Robert Ball, Arthur Flemming, and Claude Pepper are nowhere to be found around aging policy today (Browdie, 2004). But more important, the landscape has changed; aging policy has become institutionalized and routinized.

Second, in Schattschneider's (1960) famous words, "the scope of conflict has expanded." As Derthick (1979b) was among the first to observe in a late 1970s article, "How Easy Votes on Social Security Came to an End," the closed decision-making circle she described in *Policymaking for Social Security* has ceased to exist. Whether generationally or ideologically motivated (Hudson, 1999; Williamson & Watts-Roy, in press), organized resistance has brought to an end Social Security's long existence in splendid isolation. Indeed, these twin factors—the new institutional presence of the aged (in both politics and policy) and the ideological and fiscal pressures bearing down on this presence—have created something of a perfect political storm.

Third and last, if this loggerhead is be broken as the baby boomers enter old age, it may be the result of a reassessment of what old age is and who, in fact, the old are. People aged 65 and older enjoy an aggregate level of well-being that is stunning in comparison to the situation 50 years ago; for example, poverty levels are down by a factor of four, and health insurance coverage has risen from less than half to virtually the entire older population. Having celebrated those developments in the face of looming fiscal pressures, the question then emerges whether benefits should be cut either through increasing age of eligibility or through some other mechanism. To further raise the age of eligibility for full Social Security benefits would, in policy terms if not beyond, have old age begin at, say, age 75. Doing so would certainly save enormous sums and would probably arguably improve program's target efficiency. Yet to do so might well have the ethically charged consequence of "re-residualizing the aged," literally re-creating them as the singularly vulnerable group of a century ago.

Despite aging populations, globalization, and other contemporary pressures, it is not at all clear that the welfare state in general or America's "old age welfare state" will be retrenched. It is clear, however, that the aged's new policy and political presence will represent an impressive counterweight against those who would pare away existing benefits.

References

Amenta, E. (2006). *When movements matter: The Townsend Plan and the rise of Social Security.* Princeton, NJ: Princeton University Press.

Bachrach, P., & Baratz, M. (1962). The two faces of power. *American Political Science Review, 56,* 947–952.

Ball, R. (2000). *Insuring the essentials: Bob Ball on social security.* New York: Century Foundation Press.

Beer, S. H. (1966). *British politics in the collectivist age.* New York: Alfred A. Knopf.

Binstock, R. H. (2000). Older people and voting participation: Past and future. *The Gerontologist, 40,* 18–31.

Browdie, R. (Ed.). (2004). Advocacy and aging. *Generations, 28*(1), 5–7.

Buchanan, J., & Tullock, G. (1962). *The calculus of consent: Logical foundations of constitutional democracy.* Ann Arbor: University of Michigan Press.

Burke, V., & Burke, V. (1974). *Nixon's good deed.* New York: Columbia University Press.

Cameron, D. R. (1978). The expansion of the public economy: A comparative analysis. *American Political Science Review, 72,* 1243–1261.

Campbell, A. L. (2003). *How policies make citizens: Senior political activism and the American welfare state.* Princeton, NJ: Princeton University Press.

Derthick, M. (1979a). *Policymaking for Social Security.* Washington, DC: Brookings Institution.

Derthick, M. (1979b). How easy votes on Social Security came to an end. *Public Interest, 54,* 94–105.

Easton, D. (1957). An approach to the analysis of political systems. *World Politics, 9,* 383–400.

Edelman, M. (1964). *The symbolic uses of politics.* Urbana: University of Illinois Press.

Esping-Andersen, G. (1985). *Politics against markets: The social democratic road to power.* Princeton, NJ: Princeton University Press.

Estes, C. (1991). The new political economy of aging: An introduction and critique. In M. Minkler & C. Estes (Eds.), *Critical perspectives on aging* (pp. 19–36). Amityville, NY: Baywood Publishing.

Estes, C., & Binney, E. A. (1991). The biomedicalization of aging: Dangers and dilemmas. In M. Minkler & C. Estes (Eds.), *Critical perspectives on aging* (pp. 117–134). Amityville, NY: Baywood Publishing.

Fleming, D. (1963). Social Darwinism. In A. Schlesinger (Ed.), *Paths of American thought* (pp. 123–146). New York: Houghton Mifflin.

Fraser, N., & Gordon, L. (1992). Contract versus charity: Why is there no social citizenship in the United States? *Socialist Review, 22,* 45–67.

Gist, J. (in press). Population aging, entitlement growth, and the aging. In R. B. Hudson (Ed.), *Boomer bust? Economic and political issues of the graying society.* Westport, CT: Praeger.

Gough, I. (1979). *The political economy of the welfare state.* London: Macmillan.

Graebner, W. (1974). *A history of retirement.* New Haven, CT: Yale University Press.

Gratton, B. (1986). The new history of the aged: A critique. In D. Van Tassel & P. Stearns (Eds.), *Old age in a bureaucratic society* (pp. 217–221). Westport, CT: Greenwood.

Greenstone, J. D. (1969). *Labor in American politics.* New York: Vintage Books.

Heclo, H. (1974). *Modern social politics in Britain and Sweden.* New Haven, CT: Yale University Press.

Hendricks, J., & Leedham, C. (1991). Dependency or empowerment: Toward a moral and political economy of aging. In M. Minkler & C. Estes (Eds.), *Critical perspectives on aging* (pp. 51–66). Amityville, NY: Baywood Publishing.

Himelfarb, R. (1995). *Catastrophic politics: The rise and fall of the Medicare Catastrophic Coverage Act.* University Park: Pennsylvania State University Press.

Horton, J. (1966). Order and conflict theories of social problems as competing ideologies. *American Journal of Sociology, 71,* 701–713.

Huber, E., Stephens, J., & Ray, D. (1999). The welfare state in hard times. In H. Kitschelt, P. Lange, G. Marks, & J. Stephens (Eds.), *Continuity and change in contemporary capitalism* (pp. 164–193). Cambridge: Cambridge University Press.

Hudson, R. B. (1978). The graying of the federal budget and its consequences for old-age policy. *The Gerontologist, 18,* 428–440.

Hudson, R. B. (1994). The Older Americans Act and the defederalization of community-based care. In P. Kim (Ed.), *Services to the aged: Public policies and programs* (pp. 41–76). New York: Garland.

Hudson, R. B. (1999). Conflict in today's aging politics: New population encounters old ideology. *Social Service Review, 73,* 358–379.

Huntington, S. (1966). Political modernization: America vs. Europe. *World Politics, 18,* 378–414.

Iglehart, J. (2004). The new Medicare prescription drug benefit: A pure power play. *New England Journal of Medicine, 350,* 826–833.

Ikenberry, G. J., & Skocpol, T. (1987). Expanding social benefits: The role of Social Security. *Political Science Quarterly, 102*(3), 389–416.

Lipset, S. M., & Marks, G. (2001). *It didn't happen here: Why socialism failed in the United States.* New York: Norton.

Lowi, T. J. (1964). American business, public policy, case-studies, and political theory. *World Politics, 16,* 677–715.

Lowi, T. J. (1967). The public philosophy: Interest group liberalism. *American Political Science Review, 61,* 5–24.

Lukes, S. (1974). *Power: A radical view.* London: Macmillan.

Madland, D. (2007). The politics of pension cuts. In T. Ghilarducci & C. E. Weller (Eds.), *Employee pensions: Policies, problems, and possibilities* (pp. 187–214). Champaign, IL: Labor and Employment Relations Association.

Marmor, T. (1970). *The politics of Medicare*. Chicago: Aldine.

Marmor, T., Mashaw, J., & Harvey, P. (1990). *America's misunderstood welfare state.* New York: Basic Books.

Marshall, T. H. (1964). *Class, citizenship and social development.* Garden City, NY: Doubleday.

Mead, L. (1998). Telling the poor what to do. *The Public Interest,* no. 132, 97–112.

Mettler, S. (2007). The transformed welfare state and the redistribution of voice. In P. Pierson & T. Skocpol (Eds.), *The transformation of American politics* (pp. 191–222). Princeton, NJ: Princeton University Press.

Myles, J. (1984). *Old age in the welfare state.* Boston: Little, Brown.

Myles, J., & Quadagno, J. (2002). Political theories of the welfare state. *Social Service Review, 76,* 34–57.

Nettl, J. P. (1968). The state as a conceptual variable. *World Politics, 20,* 559–592.

Niskanen, W. (1971). *Bureaucracy and representative government.* Chicago: Aldine.

O'Conner, J. (1973). *The fiscal crisis of the state.* New York: St. Martin's Press.

Orloff, A. S. (1988). The political origins of America's belated welfare state. In M. Weir, A. S. Orloff, & T. Skocpol (Eds.), *The politics of social policy in the United States* (pp. 37–80). Princeton, NJ: Princeton University Press.

Pampel, F., & Williamson, J. (1992). *Age, class, politics, and the welfare state.* New York: Cambridge University Press.

Parenti, M. (1970). Power and pluralism: A view from the bottom. *Journal of Politics, 32,* 501–530.

Peterson, P. G. (1999). *Gray dawn: How the coming age wave will transform America—and the world.* New York: Times Books.

Pierson, P. (1994). *Dismantling the welfare state? Reagan, Thatcher, and the politics of retrenchment.* New York: Cambridge University Press.

Pierson, P. (2007). The rise and reconfiguration of activist government. In P. Pierson & T. Skocpol (Eds.), *The transformation of American politics* (pp. 19–38). Princeton, NJ: Princeton University Press.

Piven, F. F., & Cloward, R. (1971). *Regulating the poor: The functions of public welfare.* New York: Vintage Books.

Polsby, N. (1963). *Community power and political theory.* New Haven, CT: Yale University Press.

Pratt, H. (1976). *The gray lobby.* Chicago: University of Chicago Press.

Price, M. C. (1997). *Justice between generations: The growing power of the elderly in America.* Westport, CT: Greenwood.

Putnam, R. (1995). Bowling alone: America's declining social capital. *Journal of Democracy, 6,* 65–78.

Quadagno, J. (1988). *The transformation of old age security.* Chicago: University of Chicago Press.

Quadagno, J. (2005). *One nation, uninsured.* New York: Oxford University Press.

Rimlinger, G. (1971). *Welfare policy and industrialization in Europe, America, and Russia.* New York: Wiley.

Robertson, D. B. (1993). The return to history and the new institutionalism in American political science. *Social Science History, 17,* 1–36.

Rosenberg, C. (1962). *The cholera years.* Chicago: University of Chicago Press.

Ryan, W. (1971). *Blaming the victim.* New York: Knopf.

Samuelson, R. J. (2005, November 16). AARP's America is a mirage. *Washington Post,* A19.

Schattschneider, E. E. (1935). *Politics, pressures, and the tariff.* New York: Prentice Hall.

Schattschneider, E. E. (1960). *The semi-sovereign people.* New York: Wiley.

Schneider, A., & Ingram, H. (1993). Social construction of target populations: Implications for politics and policy. *American Political Science Review, 87,* 334–347.

Skocpol, T. (1985). Bringing the state back in: Strategies of analysis and current research. In P. Evans, D. Rueschemeyer, & T. Skocpol (Eds.), *Bringing the state back in* (pp. 3–37). New York: Cambridge University Press.

Skocpol, T. (1991). State formation and social policy in the United States. *American Behavioral Scientist, 34,* 559–584.

Skocpol, T. (1992). *Protecting soldiers and mothers.* Cambridge, MA: Belknap Press.

Smeeding, T. (2006). Poor people in rich nations. *Journal of Economic Perspectives, 20,* 69–90.

Teles, S. (2007). Conservative mobilization against entrenched liberalism. In P. Pierson & T. Skocpol (Eds.), *The transformation of American politics* (pp. 160–188). Princeton, NJ: Princeton University Press.

U.S. Bureau of the Census. (2004, November). *Current population survey.* Washington, DC: U.S. Government Printing Office.

Walker, J. (1983). The origins and maintenance of interest groups in America. *American Political Science Review, 77,* 390–406.

Wilensky, H. (1975). *The welfare state and equality.* Berkeley: University of California Press.

Wilensky, H., & Lebeaux, C. (1958). *Industrial society and social welfare.* New York: Free Press.

Williamson, J. B., & Watts-Roy, D. (in press). Aging boomers, generational equity, and the framing of the debate over Social Security. In R. B. Hudson (Ed.), *Boomer bust? Economic and political issues of the graying society.* Westport, CT: Praeger.

Wilson, J. Q. (1973). *Political organizations.* New York: Basic Books.

Witte, E. E. (1963). *The development of the Social Security Act.* Madison: University of Wisconsin Press.

The Political Economy Perspective of Aging

30

Ben Lennox Kail
Jill Quadagno
Jennifer Reid Keene

The political economy of aging is concerned with the social, political, and economic processes involved in the distribution of scarce resources and the ways that the state and market economy participate in shaping the redistribution effort (Johnson, 1999). It views the market economy and redistributory public policies as interlocking systems involved in the production of economic inequality. It also emphasizes that social actors engage the market from different structural locations, creating barriers that restrict employment opportunities and force less privileged groups to engage the market according to a different set of rules.

The political economy perspective is particularly useful for exploring the ways in which economic inequalities accumulate over the life course and are transmitted across generations. It has often been used to examine differences in the ways that gender and class inform individual interactions with the market and the welfare state. Recently, the political economy perspective has been used to disentangle the challenges facing racial and ethnic minorities in market relationships and in the subsequent consequences for access to public and private benefits. Finally, a small but growing body of literature explores how marital arrangements and family structure reinforce and exacerbate inequalities produced in the market. Specifically, this perspective contends that individuals who enter into family formations that exist outside the once normative configuration of the male breadwinner and female caretaker model are disadvantaged both in labor market activities and during the economic redistribution that occurs in retirement.

In this chapter, we first trace the theoretical origins of the political economy perspective. We then discuss two contemporary applications: the theory of cumulative disadvantage and the moral economy approach. Finally, we describe the welfare state as a system of stratification and examine differences in distributional outcomes according to gender, race, and marital status.

Marx, Weber, and Political Economy

The political economy perspective is grounded in Marx's theory of class structure and Weber's conception of stratification. In Marxist theory, the class structure is based on property ownership with society bifurcated into a ruling class that owns the means of production and a propertyless working class (Marx, 1983b). This antagonistic economic relationship is the focal mechanism of social stratification. For Marx, the class structure not only determines "the distribution of economic goods" but also is the sorting mechanism for the distribution of political power (Giddens, 1971).

Marx rejected economists' conception of an economy that existed "independently of the mediation of human beings" (Giddens, 1971, p. 10). Rather, he insisted that there was a reciprocal relationship between the economy and the political and social order (Coser, 1977). Although the economy serves as the foundation for civil society, it is the social relations between actors that "constitutes the economic structure of society" (Marx, 1983a, p. 159). Within this relationship, the economic structure both shapes and grounds the formation and enactment of social relationships (Coser, 1977).

Weber's conception of stratification and of the mechanism behind it is more nuanced than that of Marx. He views social class as just one component of a multifaceted system of stratification and social organization rather than as the sole explanation (Gerth & Mills, 1946). Weber felt that Marx's unyielding focus on the way economic forces shape class structure prevented him from acknowledging other possible groupings of social organization that could lead to a stratified society.

In *Economy and Society,* Weber (1978) discusses three spheres of social stratification. He agrees with Marx that social class is broadly organized around the functions that actors serve in the process of production and that the primary class division is based on the ownership of private property (Gerth et al., 1946; Giddens, 1971). However, Weber also includes status groups and parties in his conceptual model as sources of stratification. Status groups are stratified by lifestyles on the basis of neighborhoods, occupations, or patterns of consumption and are connected by social honor. Parties are groups whose explicit goal is the attainment of social power. They may take the form of "social clubs," interest groups, or organized political parties competing for state power (Gerth et al., 1946). While Weber viewed these spheres of social organization and stratification as potentially overlapping, he believed that they were not confounding and that each sphere could produce its own stratification system (Giddens, 1971).

Weber also includes race in his discussion of stratification. He argues that when profit becomes scarce, profit seekers use "externally identifiable characteristics" (Weber, 1978, p. 342) of others in order to exclude them from the competition for profits. When race is "subjectively perceived as a common trait" (p. 385), it may force those who are subjectively racialized into forming a racial group.

There is also an intergenerational component to Weber's discussion of stratification. Weber argues that, in some circumstances, parents pass the advantages and disadvantages of their class, status, and party along to their children. By including the concept of intergenerational transmission in his discussion of race, status, parties, and class, Weber arrives at a more fully specified concept of stratification than Marx with his emphasis on antagonism between dichotomous classes.

Marx and Weber are the conceptual architects of the foundation on which the political economy perspective rests. Their perspectives emphasize the structural constraints that members of different social groups face when interacting with the economy and show that groups positioned differently within the political power structure reap different levels of benefits in the redistribution of social goods (Estes, 1999). These insights provide a basis for understanding the processes that create inequality in old age.

Contemporary Theory and the Political Economy of Aging

Cumulative Advantage Theory

Grounded in research on the life course, the theory of cumulative disadvantage[1] suggests that people accrue advantages or disadvantages over the life course (DiPrete & Eirich, 2006). Unlike life course perspectives that link disadvantages to biological causes of social differentiation, this approach links the accumulated effect of disadvantage to mechanisms of social stratification (Ferraro & Kelley-Moore, 2003). It suggests that while a single occurrence of disadvantage may have little effect, aggregated occurrences of systematic disadvantage over the life course have a large and meaningful impact in later life. The cumulative disadvantage approach also suggests that disadvantages not only accrue over the life course but also have a magnifying or feedback effect (Crystal & Shea, 1990; Ferraro & Kelley-Moore, 2003). Thus, the more disadvantages individuals experience, the more likely they are to accrue subsequent and greater disadvantages.

The cumulative disadvantage approach provides a useful tool for understanding inequality in old age because it attributes later-life outcomes to a variety of preretirement circumstances. As O'Rand and Henretta (1999) point out,

> *Variations in educational achievement, labor force participation, labor market opportunities, family formation and dissolution patterns, pension and asset accumulation, and health trajectories—all of which are cumulative and interrelated over time—produce diverse life chances with unequal outcomes in middle and late life. (p. 6)*

The cumulative disadvantage approach is useful to a discussion of the political economy of aging for two reasons. First, cumulative disadvantage informs us that group membership affects how individuals experience the process of aging (Dannefer, 2003). Second, it emphasizes that disadvantages not only accumulate over the life course but are also exacerbated in the transition between work and retirement (O'Rand & Henretta, 1999). This transition triggers mechanisms that makes these disadvantages even more apparent, resulting in greater economic inequality among retirees than among active workers (Crystal & Shea, 1990; Pampel & Hardy, 1994). Thus, it provides a way to explain inequality across the life course.

When viewed through the lens of cumulative disadvantage, labor force participation is a critical mechanism in the stratification processes at play among retirees. Pension generosity is related to previous labor force participation. Individuals who have been employed in high-paying jobs and have had stable employment have a greater probability of securing more generous private pension income than individuals who have not had these advantages (Crystal, Shea, & Krishnaswami, 1992). Inasmuch as social statuses like class, race, gender, and marital status are sorting mechanisms that affect employment opportunities, these status positions influence the generosity of pension benefits or the receipt of any pension income at all.

Over the past quarter century, there has been a shifting of risk from the employer to the employee. As a result, income in old age has become less stable, even for more advantaged workers (Hacker, 2006). Until the late 1970s, employer pension plans took the form of a defined benefit (DB) that guaranteed retired workers a fixed annuity with the amount determined by prior wages and years of service. In 1978, an obscure provision, section 401k, was added to the tax code, allowing workers and employers to make contributions that would not be taxed until the worker retired. These defined contributions (DC) plans liberated employers from long-term obligations by making pension benefits a fixed payment for current employees. In subsequent years, 401ks and their sister funds, individual retirement accounts (IRAs), expanded rapidly while DB pensions declined. In the 1970s, three-quarters of workers with pension coverage had a DB plan. By 2001, that figure had declined to 33% (Even & Macpherson, 2007). Such DC pension income is less secure because it has to last employees for the duration of their retirement years. The risk always exists that individuals will spend down all their assets and outlive their resources. Further, DC pensions are also much more vulnerable to fluctuations in the economy compared to DB plans. Just as the shift from DB to DC plans has increased economic risk in later life, so too has the decline of retiree health benefits. Between 1988 and 2007, the percentage of employers that paid retiree health benefits dropped from 66% to 33% (Quadagno & McKelvey, in press).

In addition to previous labor force participation, accumulated lifetime assets also affect the economic well-being of retirees. Since a home is the single largest asset for most people in the United States, home owners fare better in retirement than renters. Because home ownership varies across ethnoracial groups, minorities are generally worse off in retirement that Whites (Oliver & Shapiro, 2006). Further, having fewer income-producing assets means both lower levels of financial security and less wealth to pass along to future generations (Hogan & Perrucci, 1998). Thus, the cumulative disadvantage framework is useful for explaining not only how advantage accrues over the life course but also how it is transmitted across generations.

Moral Economy

The concept of moral economy is another component of the political economy perspective. It focuses on how such concepts as fairness, justice, and social obligation are socially constructed and used to justify particular solutions rather than alternative solutions (Clark, 1999). In regard to the elderly, the moral economy approach helps elucidate the social constructions that cast some individuals as deserving of social benefits and others as undeserving (Minkler & Cole, 1999).

Because the elderly are generally not active labor force participants and rely heavily on public benefits, they are in a prime position to be defined as a problem (Estes, 1999). This chimera of a problem may manifest itself in several ways. It may take the form of an impending "geriatric crisis" in which the demographic trend toward population aging will create an unmanageable economic burden, pitting the elderly against the young in a battle for scarce funds (Clark, 1999). According to this generational equity scenario, an aging population will bankrupt the economy and crowd out funds for other social needs (Schulz & Binstock, 2006).

The generational equity debate is based on a carefully constructed rhetorical strategy. It consists first of the premise that the distribution of Social Security favors retirees at the expense of current workers because present levels of benefits will not be available for future generations. When the problem is defined in this way, then the only viable solution is to privatize Social Security by allowing current workers to contribute a portion of payroll taxes to private accounts (Rohlinger & Quadagno, 2006; Williamson & Watts-Roy, 1999). A second component of the generational equity frame is that the elderly are doing well at the expense of children. The problem with this claim is that there is often no relationship between levels of spending on programs for the elderly and spending on children. Rather, the concept of generational equity is little more than a smokescreen masking the market risks, particularly for single mothers, that have led to increased rates of childhood poverty (Minkler & Robertson, 1991). Evidence suggests that the increased rate of childhood poverty is more closely related to the increase in single mother households than it is to a swelling of Social Security payments (Quadagno, 1989). Moreover, when tested empirically, public support for the assumptions on which the generational equity argument is founded does not hold up (Street & Cossman, 2006).

Taken together, the analytic framework provided by the cumulative disadvantage and moral economy perspective offers a nuanced explanation for economic differentiation among the elderly. The cumulative disadvantage approach informs us that differentiation is a result of systematic inequalities that accumulate according to certain statuses over the life course. These systematic inequalities are not solely the outcome of the accrual of resources through the market economy but also are associated with the availability of public benefits for retirees. The moral economy approach specifies the ways that welfare policies designed to compensate for the effects of economic disadvantage are socially constructed according to moral discussions of deserving and undeserving recipients and that the rhetoric of the old robbing the young is an indirect way to undermine support for current distributional policies.

The Welfare State as a System of Stratification

A core assumption of the political economy approach is that public polices for income, health, long-term care, and social services are an outcome of the social struggles and dominant power relations of the era. These relationships are not merely created in the private sector but also are adjudicated within the state. To a large extent, the state organizes class, gender, race, and marital relations and influences family structure through various incentives and penalties. The welfare state consists of social programs and tax policies that determine the distribution of societal resources (Estes 1979; Harrington Meyer, Wolf, & Himes, 2005; Quadagno, 1988).

Although the welfare state may seek to lessen social inequality, it is in itself a system of stratification that contributes to the ranking of individuals in a social hierarchy (Smelser, 1988). By providing differential access to power and resources, the welfare state protects and enhances the status of some individuals while reducing the power and resources of others. Thus, welfare programs may reinforce stratification based on gender, age, race, and marital status and reproduce inequality over the life course.

As the primary site of the civil functions of the state, the welfare state has become the central research focus of the political economy perspective. A large share of government expenditures in all Western, capitalist democracies is directed toward the aged. In consequence, much of the literature has been concerned with the organization of public pension systems and the distribution of public pension income. However, recent studies include a broader array of programs targeted at reducing economic insecurities at various phases of the life course.

Principles of Distribution

Welfare states are institutions designed to harmonize the production and distribution of wealth. The welfare state is articulated by its power to tax, to distribute resources, and to regulate. Although much of the literature on the welfare state has focused on its distributional component, current policy directions cannot be understood as independent of the taxation and regulatory functions. Together, these functions involve rules and policies that redistribute resources by setting levels and forms of taxation and by establishing eligibility criteria and benefit formulas.

Cross-national comparisons have been based on two distinguishing characteristics of welfare states: the forms of provision and the bases of entitlement.

Welfare programs can be classified into three types: social assistance, social insurance, and fiscal welfare. Each has its own set of rules regarding who pays for the benefit, who is eligible to receive it, and how much beneficiaries receive. Moreover, each type of program reflects a particular set of values and attitudes toward the needy.

Social Assistance

Social assistance benefits derive from the 16th-century British system of poor relief, which was based on the principle of "less eligibility," meaning that the treatment of the poor was intended to be less desirable than the treatment of the lowest wage earners (Myles, 1989). Social assistance is intentionally designed to be unattractive in order to discourage recipients from becoming overly reliant on benefits (Esping-Andersen, 2002). The basis of entitlement is need, determined through the administration of a means test. Means tests are often considered demeaning and humiliating by applicants because they subject individuals' private lives, income, assets, and behaviors to scrutiny and judgment. In some cases, people who are poor enough to meet the eligibility criteria are still denied benefits because they are viewed as thriftless or immoral.

Social assistance recipients are viewed not as entitled to benefits but rather as recipients of charity. Because means-tested benefits are quite low and accompanied by social stigma, they compel all but the most desperate to participate in the labor market (Marmor, Mashaw, & Harvey, 1992). Thus, although social assistance offers minimal relief, it does not provide individuals with a viable alternative to the market (Esping-Andersen, 1994).

In the United States, a key to understanding moral orientations toward social policies is the widespread belief in the code of individuality (Gilens, 1999). Individualism is integral to most social aspects of U.S. culture (Bellah, Madsen, Sullivan, Swindler, & Tipton, 1985) and is at the heart of the conflict between advocates of social policy expansion and advocates of welfare retrenchment (Clark, 1999). This individualistic orientation makes it difficult for the United States to enact policies that remedy social rather than individual problems. It also helps explain why the United States favors instituting means-tested programs that target individuals rather than programs of universal coverage. As long as the causes of the problems are viewed as individually based, the solutions are likely to be viewed as individually based as well.

Social Insurance

Social insurance is based on the recognition that social risks are unevenly distributed over the life course and that people share these life course risks. When risks are pooled broadly, the costs for one family or individual are distributed across an entire population (Hacker, 2006). The objective of social insurance programs is to provide security against loss of income from such risks as unemployment, disability, widowhood, or retirement.

In social insurance programs, criteria other than need determine who receives benefits. Social insurance is distinguished from social assistance by the notion that people contribute to a common pool. Unlike social assistance programs where benefits are considered a form of charity, contributory benefits are entitlements based on the concept of earned rights. Benefits may be universal and based on citizenship, or they may be related to earnings, as is the case in the United States and many other countries (Korpi & Palme, 1998). Earning-related benefits are typically calculated on the basis of some combination of age, years of service, prior earnings, or level of contributions.

Fiscal Welfare

A third, often unrecognized form of social provision is fiscal welfare. Fiscal welfare consists of provisions in the tax code that provide preferential treatment (i.e., tax breaks) for certain expenses (Shalev, 1996). Because benefits are provided through the private sector but subsidized by the tax system, they are part of the "hidden welfare state" (Howard, 1999).

In the United States, fiscal welfare benefits are termed "tax expenditures." Among the items that qualify as tax expenditures are employee contributions to employer-provided pensions, personal savings for retirement, employer-provided health insurance, and home mortgage interest. These programs represent an indirect approach to achieving public objectives such as encouraging savings for retirement, expanding health coverage insurance, and encouraging home ownership.

Tax expenditures are inherently unequal in their impact because they allow individuals receiving the same income to pay taxes at different rates (Street, 1996). For example, workers who contribute to an employer-provided pension fund pay less in taxes than workers who do not. Similarly, individuals who receive health insurance through their employer pay lower taxes than those who have no health insurance. Home owners can deduct the interest they pay on their mortgage, whereas renters with similar incomes pay more in taxes. Thus, tax expenditures promote inequality because they disproportionately benefit the middle and upper middle class at the expense of the working class and the poor, who are more likely to rent and less likely to have jobs with benefits.

Welfare states vary in the extent to which they rely on social assistance, social insurance, or fiscal welfare as well as in how the bases of entitlement to benefits are organized. The structure of the welfare state has implications for class, gender, race, and marital equality.

Processes of Stratification

Class Stratification

Class-based theories emphasize the ways that the division of labor within the economic sphere shapes the redistributive effort (Korpi, 2000). According to class-based theories, the welfare state is the product of political struggles between workers and capitalists, that is, between the owners and nonowners of the means of production (Stephens, 1979). The result of those struggles are played out in the political sphere where workers mobilize into unions, use their numerical superiority to capture the state, and then enact programs that provide unemployment or retirement benefits as an alternate to low-wage work. Thus, the welfare state "decommodifies" workers by giving them bargaining power in the conflicts with employers, with the quality of social benefits serving as a measure of success. In this sense, then, the labor market is both the source of "distributive conflict" and the battleground on which the contentious politics of the redistributive effort are fought.

The concept of welfare state "regimes" arose as a result of observed regularities in patterns of social provision across nations, according to the level of decommodification (Gran, 1997). There are three main regime types among Western, capitalist democracies based on dominant forms of social provisions, basis of entitlement, and stratification in the market (Esping-Andersen, 1990). They include social democratic, conservative, and liberal regimes.

"Social democratic" regimes do the most to decommodify workers and liberate them from the market. Benefits are universal and bestowed on the basis of citizenship with the amount independent of time employed or prior earnings (Hicks & Kenworthy, 2003). The high quality of benefits eliminates class and status cleavages (Esping-Andersen, 1990). Although class cleavages are diminished in social democratic regimes, tensions between the genders remain with men more involved in the private market and women more involved in the welfare state, both as employees and as recipients (Svallfors, 2004). "Conservative" regimes maintain traditional status relationships by providing distinct programs for different class and status groups. Benefits are based on labor market experience, not citizenship rights, and social provision is linked to labor market participation. As a result, patterns of stratification are replicated in retirement (Gran, 1997). Finally, "liberal" regimes rely heavily on a residual welfare state strategy based on a two-tired system of benefits. The first tier consists of social insurance programs where contributions provide an earned right to benefits, and the second tier consists of means-tested social assistance, with need being the condition for eligibility. The consequence is that social assistance divides society into a self-reliant majority and a dependent core of welfare state clientele (Esping-Andersen, 1999). Noticeably absent from liberal welfare states is social provision based on citizenship claims (Gran, 1997). Public benefits in liberal welfare states are often heavily subsidized with private retirement packages, reinforcing inequalities stemming from the labor market (Esping-Andersen, 2002; Hicks & Kenworthy, 2003). Of the three regime types, liberal regimes do the least to decommodify workers. As a result, divisions remain particularly salient in retirement (Svallfors, 2004).

The United States is the archetypical liberal regime. Because welfare effort does little to decommodify workers, inequalities created during the working years become increasingly pronounced in the retirement. Considered through the lens of moral economy, the reason these patterns have persisted—and in fact increased over time—is because of a normative moral philosophy centered on a belief in meritocracy. From this vantage point, it is morally justifiable that rewards in later life reflect differences in human capital accrued over the life course. What this vision of moral justice ignores is that what is often mistaken for merit is instead the result of cumulative disadvantage and intergenerational transfer. Moreover, human capital often is not accrued on the basis of merit alone but rather is bound by structural constraints based on ascriptive statuses.

Gender Stratification Theory

While the first generation of welfare state theories focused on the ability of the welfare state to separate the economic fortunes of workers from the vicissitudes of the market, the second generation was grounded in a feminist critique of the class-based approach. Feminist theorists argue that class analyses ignore the distributional effects of welfare state structure on gender equality. Because women are primarily responsible for caring for young children and elderly parents, they spend fewer years in the paid labor force than men and subsequently accrue fewer benefits in retirement. As a result, women have less income in later life because Social Security payments, private pensions levels, and wealth accumulated from lifetime earnings are contingent on work history. Thus, a class-based theory that treats the male breadwinner model as the normative order ignores important variations that occur across gender and race (Acker, 2005).

Feminist theorists criticize class-based models for centering their assessments of welfare state adequacy on such bases of entitlement as labor market status, need, and citizenship while ignoring the quality of women's entitlements as wives, mothers, and informal caregivers to elderly or infirm parents (Herd, 2005b). They argue that a primary cause of gender inequality in old age is the structure of social insurance programs, which award benefits on the basis of labor force participation and penalize caregiving (Misra, 1998). In the United States, for example, poverty rates have been higher among elderly women than among men despite the availability of Social Security, which is the sole source of income for many older women (Herd, 2005a). Although the welfare state, through its public policies, political ideologies, and principles, may decommodify men, it may also reproduce the gendered division of labor and perpetuate male domination.

Feminist theorists are also critical of Esping-Andersen's three regime types because his model of decommodification highlights the relationship between paid employment and welfare benefits but ignores the unequal ways the welfare state rewards unpaid work (Lewis, 1997). From a feminist perspective, the question is not just the degree to which workers are decommodified but also the degree to which the welfare state liberates women from male domination and provides them with an independent source of income (O'Connor, Orloff, & Shaver, 1999). Esping-Andersen has acknowledged the validity of this argument and now recognizes that the concept of decommodification misses important gendered variations in the relationship between employment and welfare benefits, in part because most programs fail to reward unpaid labor (Esping-Andersen, 1999).

In response to these criticisms, Korpi (2000) devised an alternative regime typology based on the relationship between the market, the state, and the family. In his model, the "general family support" regime provides high levels of benefits to parents independent of their labor force status. The "dual-earner support" regime encourages both partners within a familial unit to engage in the labor market by providing such benefits as state-sponsored care for the young and the elderly and parental leave for mothers and fathers. Finally, regimes with "market-oriented polices" lack social programs and policies offering any public family support.

Racial Stratification

Theoretical debates about the distributional consequences of the welfare state have paid less attention to the effect of social provision on racial equality. Although the class-based model of welfare state provision emphasizes the amelioration of life course risk, it pays less attention to the problem of the intergenerational transmission of risk that is ascriptively determined on the basis of race or ethnic origin (Esping-Andersen, 1999). The risk of being a victim of racial discrimination, which is produced in the family and then compounded in the market, is not diminished by social programs that target life course risks but fail to redistribute life chances. In this case, the problem to be solved is the systematic reproduction of inequality that produces inherited disadvantages.

In the United States, there is a wide disparity in income and wealth in old age on the basis of race. Throughout their lives, African Americans earn less than Whites, reducing their income security in old age. Income inequality in old age is partly a consequence of racial discrimination in employment opportunities over the life course, leading in turn to lower Social Security benefits and less access to private pension income. As a result, Whites also receive more in retirement benefits than racial minorities do. On average, African Americans and Hispanics receive just 70% of the Social Security benefit and 60% of private pension benefits of Whites (Hogan, Kim, & Perrucci, 1997). In 2005, the median income of elderly White men was about $10,000 more per year than that of African American or Hispanic men, while the median income of elderly White women was about $3,000 more than that of elderly African American women and $4,500 more than elderly Hispanic women (U.S. Census Bureau, 2007a). Further, minority women face double jeopardy. Although women overall are nearly twice as likely as men to be poor in retirement, African American women are more than twice as likely as White women to be poor (Herd, 2005a).

African Americans also have fewer assets in old age than Whites. The principal asset for most people is home equity, and for multiple reasons, African Americans have less home equity than Whites. Until the 1960s, federal policies did not prohibit and indeed encouraged racial segregation in public housing and allowed racial discrimination by private lenders. Although the Fair Housing Act of 1968 made racial discrimination in housing illegal, discrimination in private lending and de facto neighborhood segregation have persisted (Myers & Chung, 1996; Oliver & Shapiro, 2006). As a result, only 54% of African Americans own their homes compared to 76% of Whites (King, Ruggles, Alexander, Leicach, & Sobek, 2004). Even when African American families do purchase homes, they are often relegated to central cities where housing values are lower than in White suburbs (Shapiro & Kenty-Drane, 2005). The consolidation of African American residents within certain neighborhoods leads to housing devaluation. According to one estimate, when more than 10% of residents are African American, housing values in that neighborhood decline by 16% (Shapiro and Kenty-Drane, 2005). Less housing equity perpetuates racial inequality across generations, for it means that Black families have significantly less wealth to transmit to their children. Thus, future generations will benefit less from "transformative assets" (Shapiro, 2004).

The feminist critique of a welfare system that fails to provide care benefits to women is especially relevant to African American families. Nearly 25% of

African American grandparents have primary caregiving responsibility for their grandchildren. Although they may receive some support from means-tested programs like Temporary Assistance to Needy Families, no social insurance program protects them from economic insecurities based on care (Crewe, 2003).

Racial inequality in old age reflects underlying processes of cumulative disadvantage over the life course, which is the product of institutional racism in the labor market and exacerbated by the legacy of racially biased federal housing policies. Within the liberal welfare regime of the United States, the welfare state fails to significantly diminish race-based inequality produced by the economic market, an outcome that is consistent with the cumulative disadvantage perspective. The political economy framework is thus useful for understanding the multiplicity of structural forces that reduce economic security in old age and that replicate gender and racial inequality across the life course and across generations.

Marriage as a System of Stratification

A second line of inquiry to emerge from the feminist perspective concerns the ways in which the welfare state exacerbates economic stratification based on marital status. The central critique from this perspective is that the welfare state in general and social insurance programs in particular have been constructed around patterns of family formation that no longer represent a large percentage of beneficiaries. As a result of this bias toward the traditional family structure, the welfare state fails to provide protection against economic uncertainly resulting from divorce or widowhood as well as to people in nontraditional families.

Social Security is a prime example. It rewards married couples who engage in the traditional gendered division of labor because benefits are calculated on the basis of the male breadwinner model (Yabiku, 2000). Families with a high-earning male and a dependent spouse receive the highest benefits in retirement (Harrington Meyer, 1996). Social Security does have a spousal benefit, which is one of the few welfare benefits that is neither linked to earnings in the paid labor force nor based on a means test. However, the amount of the spousal benefit is calculated according to length of marriage and is unrelated to time spent performing care work (Harrington Meyer, 1996; Herd, 2006). Social Security also provides spousal benefits to the previously married, but the marriage must have lasted for 10 years (Social Security Administration, 2007). An individual who engaged in unpaid care work for fewer than 10 years before becoming divorced or widowed would be ineligible for any spouse benefit. This differs from some nations where care work is included in benefit determinations.

Family status has significant implications for income security in old age by gender. Few married elderly people live in poverty; being unmarried greatly increases the likelihood of poverty in old age, particularly for women (Harrington Meyer, 1990; Herd, 2005a; Schmidt & Sevak, 2006). Compared to women, men are more likely to be married, less likely to be divorced, and much less likely to be widowers (U.S. Census Bureau, 2007b). Single women, whether widowed, never married, or divorced, receive slightly more than half the Social Security income of married couples (Hogan & Perrucci, 1998). Divorced women experience roughly a 25% decline in income following a divorce, while men experience a 15% increase in income on average (Peterson, 1996). The economic consequences of divorce have an even greater impact from an intergenerational perspective. Because divorce leads to lower assets, the children of divorcees are likely to inherit less than they would if their parents had remained married.

Income disparities between married couples and single people also result from differences in eligibility and patterns of participation in private benefit plans. Single individuals are less likely to receive any pension income, and pension income they do receive is more likely to come from a DC plan, which is less secure than a DB plan. Further exacerbating the problem is the fact that single women are more likely than married couples or single men to cash out their pension funds when they change jobs, leaving them in a more precarious economic position in retirement (O'Rand & Shuey, 2007; Shuey & O'Rand, 2006). Private pensions are less likely to pay spousal benefits than public benefits and almost always are reduced when the wage earner dies (Harrington Meyer, 1990). As a result, women are less likely to benefit from pension systems and more likely to enter into poverty following the death of a spouse.

Individuals who never marry face greater economic uncertainty in retirement than married people. Without the benefit of a spousal safety net, single people are more vulnerable to the adverse effects of economic fluctuations. They are also less likely to have pension coverage, have lower IRA balances, and frequently have to cash out their pensions earlier. These patterns are particularly significant for African Americans, who tend to be single for a greater portion of their lives (O'Rand & Shuey, 2007; Shuey & O'Rand, 2006). Elderly African Americans have rates of marriage that are nearly 20% lower than Whites, but they are 20% more likely to cohabitate (King et al., 2004; Waite, 1995). They are also more likely than Whites to experience marital dissolution (Cherlin, 1998; King et al., 2004). For these reasons, African Americans are much less likely than Whites to be able to take advantage of the spousal benefits provided by Social Security (Harrington Meyer, 1996; Quadagno, 2000; Willson & Hardy, 2002). Moreover, empirical evidence suggests that divorce has long-lasting economic effects since, even when parents remarry, children of divorce receive diminished intergenerational transfers (Pezzin & Schone, 1999). Inasmuch as marital patterns vary by race and class, this phenomena may further exacerbate the diminished economic chances of poor and minority children.

Conclusion

The political economy perspective provides a lens for understanding inequality in old age. Derived from classical social theory, it is concerned with the effect of early life opportunities, constraints and choices on income security, health, and well-being in later life. It is also concerned with the social construction of particular modes of distribution and how they perpetuate inequality. A key line of inquiry concerns the effect of welfare state programs on inequality. Although the welfare state has a buffering effect that dampens the differentiation of wealth among the elderly, in the United States the degree to which social programs ameliorate inequality depends on the status characteristics of individual recipients.

Feminist theories of the welfare state have added a gender dimension to class-based arguments about inequality. Feminists have illuminated how gender inequality in old age is a consequence of political decisions about eligibility rules. Such decisions create institutionalized mechanisms that penalize women for limited life choices and restricted labor market opportunities. Combined with the cumulative disadvantage perspective, the feminist critique provides a nuanced understanding of how women's economic situation in retirement is shaped by both market and nonmarket preretirement experiences. Variations in family status that affect women's earning potential during their prime working years also carry over into retirement (Shuey & O'Rand, 2006).

In addition to considering gendered variations, welfare state theories have begun to recognize that racial stratification is embedded into social institutions. Because racial and ethnic minorities often have fewer opportunities to accumulate income and wealth during their working lives, they are more likely to experience deprivation in old age. Furthermore, the disadvantages experienced by older generations translate into diminished transfers to younger generations, thus perpetuating inequality. Welfare state theories still need to examine more fully the ways that unequal opportunities reduce economic security across the life course and the ways in which market inequalities are compounded by welfare policies.

Note

1. We acknowledge that this has been referred to as both cumulative advantage and cumulative disadvantage, but for the sake of simplicity, we refer to it only as the latter.

References

Acker, J. (2005). *Class questions: Feminist answers.* Lanham, MD: Rowman & Littlefield.

Bellah, R., Madsen, R., Sullivan, W., Swindler, A., & Tipton, S. (1985). *Habits of the heart: Individualism and commitment in American life.* Berkeley: University of California Press.

Cherlin, A. J. (1998). Marriage and marital dissolution among Black Americans. *Journal of Comparative Family Studies, 29,* 147–158.

Clark, P. G. (1999). Moral economy and the social construction of the crisis of aging and health care: Differing Canadian and U.S. perspectives. In M. Minkler & C. L. Estes (Eds.), *Critical gerontology: Perspectives from political and moral economy.* Amityville, NY: Baywood Publishing.

Coser, L. A. (1977). *Masters of sociological thought: Ideas in historical and social context.* Fort Worth, TX: Harcourt Brace Jovanovich College Publishers.

Crewe, S. E. (2003). African-American grandparent caregivers: Eliminating double jeopardy in social policy. In T. B. Bent-Goodley (Ed.), *African-American social workers and social policy* (pp. 35–54). Binghamton, NY: Haworth Social Work Practice Press.

Crystal, S., & Shea, D. (1990). Cumulative advantage, cumulative disadvantage, and inequality among elderly people. *The Gerontologist, 30,* 437–443.

Crystal, S., Shea, D., & Krishnaswami, S. (1992). Educational-attainment, occupational history, and stratification—Determinants of later-life economic outcomes. *Journal of Gerontology, 47,* S213–S221.

Dannefer, D. (2003). Cumulative advantage/disadvantage and the life course: Cross-fertilizing age and social science theory. *Journal of Gerontology: Social Sciences, 58,* S327–S337.

DiPrete, T. A., & Eirich, G. M. (2006). Cumulative advantage as a mechanism for inequality: A review of theoretical and empirical developments. *Annual Review of Sociology, 32,* 271–297.

Esping-Andersen, G. (1990). *The three worlds of welfare capitalism.* Cambridge: Polity Press.

Esping-Andersen, G. (1994). The three political economies of the welfare state. *The State: Critical Concepts, 26,* 10–36.

Esping-Andersen, G. (1999). *Social foundations of postindustrial economies.* Oxford: Oxford University Press.
Esping-Andersen, G. (2002). *Why we need a new welfare state.* New York: Oxford University Press.
Estes, C. L. (1979). *The aging enterprise.* San Francisco: Jossey-Bass.
Estes, C. L. (1999). Critical gerontology and the new political economy of aging. In M. Minkler & C. L. Estes (Eds.), *Critical gerontology: Perspectives from political and moral economy* (pp. 17–35). Amityville, NY: Baywood Publishing.
Even, W., & Macpherson, D. (2007). Defined contribution plans and the distribution of pension wealth. *Industrial Relations, 46,* 551–581.
Ferraro, K. F., & Kelley-Moore, J. A. (2003). Cumulative disadvantage and health: Long-term consequences of obesity? *American Sociological Review, 68,* 707–729.
Gerth, H. H., & Mills, C. W. (1946). *From Max Weber: Essays in sociology.* New York: Oxford University Press.
Giddens, A. (1971). *Capitalism & modern social theory: An analysis of the writings of Marx, Durkheim and Max Weber.* Cambridge: Cambridge University Press.
Gilens, M. (1999). *Why Americans hate welfare: Race, media, and the politics of antipoverty policy.* Chicago: University of Chicago Press.
Gran, B. (1997). Three worlds of old-age decommodification? A comparative analysis of old-age support using the Luxembourg income study. *Journal of Aging Studies, 11,* 63–79.
Hacker, J. (2006). *The great risk shift: The assault on American jobs, families, health care and retirement and how you can fight back.* New York: Oxford University Press.
Harrington Meyer, M. (1990). Family status and poverty among older women—The gendered distribution of retirement income in the United States. *Social Problems, 37,* 551–563.
Harrington Meyer, M. (1996). Making claims as workers or wives: The distribution of Social Security benefits. *American Sociological Review, 61,* 449–465.
Harrington Meyer, M., Wolf, D. A., & Himes, C. L. (2005). Linking benefits to marital status: Race and Social Security in the US. *Feminist Economics, 11,* 145–162.
Herd, P. (2005a). Ensuring a minimum: Social Security reform and women. *The Gerontologist, 45,* 12–25.
Herd, P. (2005b). Reforming a breadwinner welfare state. *Social Forces, 83,* 1365–1393.
Herd, P. (2006). Crediting care or marriage? Reforming social security family benefits. *Journal of Gerontology: Social Sciences, 61,* S24–S34.
Hicks, A., & Kenworthy, L. (2003). Varieties of welfare capitalism. *Socio-Economic Review, 1,* 27–61.
Hogan, R., Kim, M., & Perrucci, C. C. (1997). Racial inequality in men's employment and retirement earnings. *Sociological Quarterly, 38,* 431–438.
Hogan, R., & Perrucci, C. C. (1998). Producing and reproducing class and status differences: Racial and gender gaps in US employment and retirement income. *Social Problems, 45,* 528–549.
Howard, C. (1999). *The hidden welfare state: Tax expenditures and social policy in the United States.* Princeton, NJ: Princeton University Press.
Johnson, M. L. (1999). Interdependency and the generational compact. In M. Minkler & C. L. Estes (Eds.), *Critical gerontology: Perspectives from political and moral economy* (pp. 55–74). Amityville, NY: Baywood Publishing.
King, M., Ruggles, S., Alexander, T., Leicach, D., & Sobek, M. (2004). *Integrated public use microdata series, current population survey: Version 2.0.* [Machine-readable database]. Minnesota Population Center [producer and distributor].
Korpi, W. (2000). Faces of inequality: Gender, class, and patterns of inequalities in different types of welfare states. *Social Politics, 7,* 127–191.
Korpi, W., & Palme, J. (1998). The paradox of redistribution and strategies of equality: Welfare state institutions, inequality, and poverty in the Western countries. *American Sociological Review, 63,* 661–687.
Lewis, J. (1997). Gender and welfare regimes: Further thoughts. *State & Society, 4,*160–177.
Marmor, T. R., Mashaw, J. L., & Harvey, P. L. (1992). *America's misunderstood welfare state: Persistent myths, enduring realities.* New York: Basic Books.
Marx, K. (1983a). A contribution to the critique of political economy. In E. Kamenka (Ed.), *The portable Karl Marx.* New York: Penguin.
Marx, K. (1983b). Economico-philosophical manuscripts of 1844. In E. Kamenka (Ed.), *The portable Karl Marx.* New York: Penguin.

Minkler, M., & Cole, T. R. (1999). Political and moral economy: Getting to know one another. In M. Minkler & C. L. Estes (Eds.), *Critical gerontology: Perspectives from political and moral economy* (pp. 37–53). Amityville, NY: Baywood Publishing.

Minkler, M., & Robertson, A. (1991). Generational equity and public health policy: A critique of "age/race war" thinking. *Journal of Public Health Policy, 12,* 324–344.

Misra, J. (1998). Mothers or workers? The value of women's labor: Women and the emergence of family allowance policy. *Gender & Society, 12,* 376–399.

Myers, S. L., & Chung, C. (1996). Racial differences in home ownership and home equity among preretirement-aged households. *The Gerontologist, 36,* 350–360.

Myles, J. (1989). *Old age in the welfare state: The political economy of public pensions.* Lawrence: University Press of Kansas.

O'Connor, J. S., Orloff, A. S., & Shaver, S. (1999). *States, markets, families.* New York: Cambridge University Press.

Oliver, M. L., & Shapiro, T. M. (2006). *Black wealth/white wealth: A new perspective on racial inequality.* New York: Routledge.

O'Rand, A. M., & Henretta, J. C. (1999). *Age and inequality: Diverse pathways through later life.* Boulder, CO: Westview Press.

O'Rand, A. M., & Shuey, K. M. (2007). Gender and the devolution of pension risks in the US. *Current Sociology, 55,* 287–304.

Pampel, F. C., & Hardy, M. (1994). Status maintenance and change during old age. *Social Forces, 73,* 289–314.

Peterson, R. R. (1996). A re-evaluation of the economic consequences of divorce. *American Sociological Review, 61,* 528–536.

Pezzin, L. E., & Schone, B. S. (1999). Parental marital disruption and intergenerational transfers: An analysis of lone elderly parents and their children. *Demography, 36,* 287–297.

Quadagno, J. (1988). *The transformation of old age security: Class and politics in the American welfare state.* Chicago: University of Chicago Press.

Quadagno, J. (1989). Generational equity and the politics of the welfare-state. *Politics & Society, 17,* 353–376.

Quadagno, J. (2000). Another face of inequality: Racial and ethnic exclusion in the welfare state. *Social Politics, 7,* 229–237.

Quadagno, J., & McKelvey, J. B. (2008). The transformation of American health insurance. In J. Hacker (Ed.), *Health care at risk: Expert perspectives on America's ailing health system—and how to heal it.* New York: Columbia University Press.

Rohlinger, D., & Quadagno, J. (2006). Framing the Social Security debate. In J. R. Blau & K. Iyall-Smith (Eds.), *Public sociologies reader* (pp. 123–136). Lanham, MD: Rowman & Littlefield.

Schmidt, L., & Sevak, P. (2006). Gender, marriage, and asset accumulation in the United States. *Feminist Economics, 12,* 139–166.

Schulz, J. H., & Binstock, R. H. (2006). *Aging nation: The economics and politics of growing older in America.* New York: Praeger.

Shalev, M. (1996). *The privatization of social policy? Occupational welfare and the welfare state in America, Scandinavia and Japan.* New York: St. Martin's Press.

Shapiro, T. M. (2004). *The hidden cost of being African American: How wealth perpetuates inequality.* New York: Oxford University Press.

Shapiro, T. M., & Kenty-Drane, J. L. (2005). The racial wealth gap. In C. Conrad, J. Whitehead, P. Mason, & J. Stewart (Eds.), *African Americans in the US economy* (pp. 175–184). NY: Roman and Littlefield.

Shuey, K. M., & O'Rand, A. M. (2006). Changing demographics and new pension risks. *Research on Aging, 28,* 317–340.

Smelser, N. J. (1988). *Handbook of sociology.* Newbury Park, CA: Sage.

Social Security Administration. (2007). *How does a divorced spouse qualify for benefits?* Retrieved December 15, 2007, from http://ssa-custhelp.ssa.gov/cgi-bin/ssa.cfg/php/enduser/std_adp.php?p_faqid=299&p_created=959268213&p_sid=scIYryRi&p_accessibility=0&p_redirect=&p_lva=&p_sp=cF9zcmNoPTEmcF9zb3J0X2J5PSZwX2dyaWRzb3J0PSZwX3Jvd19jbnQ9MTUsMTUmcF9wcm9kcz0mcF9jYXRzPTMsNjImcF9wdj0mcF9jdj0yLjYyJnBfc2VhcmNoX3R5cGU9YW5zd2Vycy5zZWFyY2hfbmwmcF9wYWdlPTE*&p_li=&p_topview=1

Stephens, J. D. (1979). *The transition from capitalism to socialism.* London: Macmillan.

Street, D. (1996). *The politics of pensions in Canada, Great Britain and the United States: 1975–1995.* Tallahassee: Florida State University.

Street, D., & Cossman, J. S. (2006). Greatest generation or greedy geezers? Social spending preferences and the elderly. *Social Problems, 53,* 75–96.

Svallfors, S. (2004). Class, attitudes and the welfare state: Sweden in comparative perspective. *Social Policy and Administration, 38,* 119–138.

U.S. Census Bureau. (2007a). *Current population survey, annual social and economic supplements, historical income tables.* Retrieved December 15, 2007, from http://www.census.gov/hhes/www/income/histinc/incpertoc.html

U.S. Census Bureau. (2007b). *Statistical abstract of the United States: 2008.* Retrieved December 15, 2007, from http://www.census.gov/statab

Waite, L. J. (1995). Does marriage matter? *Demography, 32,* 483–507.

Weber, M. (1978). *Economy and society* (G. Roth & C. Wittich, Ed. and Trans.). Berkeley: University of California Press. (Original work published 1922)

Williamson, J. B., & Watts-Roy, D. M. (1999). Framing the generational equity debate. In J. B. Williamson, D. M. Wats-Roy, & E. R. Kingson (Eds.), *The generational equity debate* (pp. 3–38). New York: Columbia University Press.

Willson, A. E., & Hardy, M. A. (2002). Racial disparities in income security for a cohort of aging American women. *Social Forces, 80,* 1283–1306.

Yabiku, S. T. (2000). Family history and pensions: The relationships between marriage, divorce, children, and private pension coverage. *Journal of Aging Studies, 14,* 293–312.

Theory Informing Public Policy: The Life Course Perspective as a Policy Tool

31

Victor W. Marshall

A theoretical perspective is useful for science, in which it directs attention of the investigator to specific aspects of the phenomena under investigation, suggesting what is problematic about those phenomena and what should be examined if the phenomena are to be understood. Put simply, to invoke a theoretical perspective is to say, "look at it this way." But a perspective can be useful not only for science but also for policy, as I argue in this chapter.

The life course perspective has been developing explicitly in the social sciences for more than 40 years, and its antecedents go back well before that,

Note: This chapter draws extensively on previous work: a paper coauthored with Margaret Mueller for Canadian Policy Research Networks and a paper prepared under contract from Social Development Canada, February 2006. I am grateful to Paul Bernard, University of Montreal, and Peter Stein, UNC Institute on Aging, for helpful comments.

usually focusing on the unfolding lives of individuals over time (Elder, 1992; Marshall & Mueller, 2003). However, in the past 20 years or so, scholars have enriched the perspective by suggesting that social institutions by their very nature provide a structural basis for ordering people's lives, thus allowing us to refer to the social structure of the life course. In this perspective, individuals are seen as born into a society that features a structured set of positions to be occupied over the course of their lives and a set of mechanisms that set constraints or opportunities for mobility through this structured field. People can modify the social structure of the life course, particularly through concerted social action, but in turn, the socially structured life course is confronted as a material fact; it is something that needs to be navigated.[1]

The life course perspective has become widely adopted by aging researchers, as witnessed by creation of the Section on Aging and the Life Course of the American Sociological Association, but a great deal of research and theorizing in the perspective has dealt with earlier life. Placing the aging individual in the context of the entire life course has been a major contribution of those advocating this perspective to the development of sound social theories of aging, in effect radically changing the very nature and definition of social gerontology.[2]

The relatively small amount of life course research dealing with social structure and the social institutions that shape people's life courses has focused on the *effects of public policy in shaping the life course*. However, the life course perspective has only recently begun to be actively and explicitly applied in the service of public policy development, that is, *in developing policy* rather than in examining it. I focus on this neglected topic in this chapter. To my knowledge, the Policy Research Initiative, a Canadian exercise, is the single most important such attempt anywhere, and I draw extensively on that example. This initiative deserves attention not only because it is a unique entrée of an explicit social science perspective to public policy formation but also because it places the aging individual in the much broader context of the entire life course, and it explicitly suggests that policy to enhance the lives of older people must be directed to people earlier in their life course and not, for example, just after they reach the age of 65.

Theorizing the Life Course: Social Psychological and Structural Approaches

At issue here is not a theory—there is not a "life course theory" per se—but rather a theoretical perspective. A theory is a formally stated set of linked propositions purporting to explain something. The work of Ferraro, Shippee, and Schafer (see chapter 22 in this volume), which is developing theory within one component of the life course perspective, gives promise that the perspective might become a theory or, more likely, come to undergird some theoretical development in specific life course domains. In contrast to formal theory, a theoretical perspective is a set of principles that recommend a way of looking.[3]

The life course perspective began to crystallize in the 1960s, when Leonard Cain Jr. (1964) published an essay, "Life Course and Social Structure," in which he aimed "to identify, isolate, and systematize a life course, or age status, frame of reference", as well as to "contribute to the advancement of a sociology of age status" (p. 273). Grounding this frame of reference in a wide range of scholarship from sociology, anthropology, demography, history, developmental psychology, and biology, he suggested that terms such as "life cycle," "life span," "career," "stages of life," and even "aging" itself are approximate synonyms for the concept "life course." Cain used the term "life course" "to refer primarily to those successive statuses individuals are called upon to occupy in various cultures and walks of life as a result of aging," and he saw "age status" as referring to "the system developed by a culture to give order and predictability to the course followed by individuals" (p. 278).[4] As Cain argued,

> *Every member of a society is called upon to move through a succession of age statuses. Every society, therefore, has the tasks of preparing individual members for subsequent age statuses, of absorbing them into the successive statuses along with removing them from formerly occupied status, and of proclaiming to, or providing other means of communicating to, the society that the transfers have been accomplished. (p. 287)*

The key concepts of Cain's approach include (a) differentiation of status on the basis of age: an *age stratification system;* (b) *socialization* for passage into and out of age statuses; (c) formalized means to affect such changes in status, such as *rites of passage;* (d) *age grading* of people of similar ages into age statuses; and (e) establishment of interaction patterns among those of different age sets, or *generational phenomena* (Cain, 1964).

Fifteen years later, Matilda White Riley (1982) crystallized what she called the "emerging" life course perspective in four "central premises": (a) *aging is a lifelong process* of growing up and growing old that starts with birth (or with conception) and ends in death; (b) aging consists of biological, psychological, and social processes that are systematically interactive with one another over the life course; (c) the life course pattern of any particular person (or cohort of persons all born at the same time) is affected by social and environmental change (or *history*); and (d) *new patterns of aging can cause social change.* That is, not only does social change mold the course of individual lives, but, when many persons in the same cohort are affected in similar ways, the change in their collective lives can in turn also produce social change (Riley, 1982).

The third premise will be seen to be crucial in terms of policy implications. This premise emphasizes that biographies are profoundly influenced by the social, political, and economic contexts, as Mills (1959) had observed, and thus the aging experience is different for different birth cohorts, as Mannheim (1952) had argued. It also implies that the experiences of one cohort in a given age category cannot be reliably generalized to other cohorts, whose encounter with history will have been distinct.

The fourth premise reacts against strict social or demographic determinism to argue that individuals or cohort members can act to change social structure (again, consistent with Mannheim's [1952] position on generations). As Riley (1982) has noted, it is the intersection of individual and cohort aging (cohort flow) with age structure that defines the territory of the life course.

Glen Elder, widely recognized as the preeminent scholar in the field, defines the life course as "a sequence of socially defined events and roles that the individual enacts over time" (Giele & Elder, 1998, p. 22). Whereas many life course theorists use the term "career" to capture this notion, he uses a terminological distinction between trajectories and transitions:

> Trajectories *provide a long view by linking social or psychological states over a substantial part of the life span.* Transitions *depict a short view, a change in state or stages, such as when children leave home or a mood change from depressed feelings to happiness. Since transitions are always elements of trajectories, a substantial change in direction during a transition may represent a* turning point *as well. (Elder, 1998, p. 955)*

This frames the life course in terms of the individual rather than social structure, but the individual life course is "structured by age norms and other constraints, biological and social" (Elder, 1998, p. 955). Elder has done more than anyone to formalize the life course perspective, which especially in North America has this social psychological cast, establishing five "principles of the life course" (Elder, 1994, 1998; Elder & Johnson, 2003):[5]

1. Human development and aging are lifelong processes.

As this principle has come to be widely adopted, there has been a shift away from "age-specific" studies to research that reaches across the life course, reflecting the truism that "life is longitudinal" (Bernard, 2007, p. 14). We know that early experiences and their meanings are brought to new situations and that this context of personal biography influences how new events and transitions are experienced (Elder & Johnson, 2003). Research following children into adolescence, adulthood, and through later life allows linkages to be made between earlier and later life course experiences.

2. Historical time and place: the life course of individuals is embedded in and shaped by the historical times and places they experience over their lifetime.

Historical change can have two kinds of effects. *Cohort effects* differentiate the lives of men and women in successive birth cohorts. For example, an expanding economy can lead to expansion of educational opportunities, which in turn might benefit more recently born cohorts, such that a few decades later there will be a greater percentage of cohort members highly educated than in previously born (and now older) cohorts. On the other hand, *history* is said to have a "period effect" when the impact of a major social event, such as a war, or a social policy change, such as welfare reform, is relatively uniform across the population. Both types of effects are conditioned by place. For example, World War II stimulated tremendous economic growth in Canada and the United States while devastating the economic infrastructure of much of Europe, with attendant consequences for people (Elder & Johnson, 2003).

3. Timing: the antecedents and consequences of life transitions and events vary according to their timing in a person's life.

Three types of timing phenomena are relevant here. The first has to do with cohorts in relation to historical events, as mentioned under the second principle. Cohort effects are determined by the *timing* of historical events in relation to people's lives and are based on the fact that historical events usually have different effects on people of different ages (and therefore of different birth cohorts). Elder's (1999) book *Children of the Great Depression* showed that cohorts born a decade apart had different economic lives over time. One experienced childhood during the 1920s, a period of prosperity. The other experienced childhood during the Depression era of the 1930s. The former cohort experienced less family disruption and economic hardship as children. Elder attends to within-cohort differences, particularly family economic status and gender, but nonetheless finds lasting effects of this experienced hardship, which for some gave them greater resilience but for others presaged difficulties in their occupational careers and subsequent health status.

A second form in which timing is important is in relation to life transitions. An example is Harley and Mortimer's (2000) finding that individuals who make very early transitions to adult statuses, such as by leaving the parental home, commencing work, marrying, and having children, are more likely to experience adverse consequences for mental health (cited in Elder, Johnson, & Crosnoe, 2003). Both the timing (*when* they occur) and sequencing patterns (in what *order* they occur) of life events can condition the effects they have on the subsequent life course.

The third way in which timing is important is in terms of expectations, viewed at either the individual or the social level. Despite great ambiguity about age norms, the phrase "act your age!" is still meaningful, referencing generalized expectations for when certain events *should* occur and normative or even legal sanctions for not following the socially prescribed timetable. Events such as giving birth to a child, job loss, or widowhood are especially difficult and potentially disruptive when they happen "off time," particularly when they occur too early in a person's life (Neugarten, Moore, & Lowe, 1965).[6]

4. Linked lives: lives are lived interdependently, and social-historical influences are expressed through this network of relationships.

Lives are not lived in isolation but are experienced interdependently. Events in the life of one person can set the course of another person on a trajectory that may not have been anticipated or desired. For example, when an older widow remarries, this may relieve her children of financial and personal care burdens. When a woman has a child, her mother is suddenly placed into the role of "grandmother," an event over which the mother herself had little control. This principle was key in Elder's (1999) now-classic analysis *Children of the Great Depression*, in which he examined how economic difficulties experienced by parents had consequences for the lives of their children (see discussion in Elder [1998] and in Elder & Caspi [1988]).

In the occupational realm, the linked-lives principle is found in the research of scholars such as Angela O'Rand (O'Rand, Henretta, & Krecker, 1992) and Phyllis Moen (Han & Moen, 1999; Moen & Han, 2001), who have drawn attention to "coupled careers" and the ways in which couples synchronize their work and retirement plans. While family provides obvious examples of linked lives, colleagues, friends, neighbors, and numerous others make up the network of ties within which individuals are embedded, giving each experience a distinct orienting context. Toni Antonucci (1990; see also chapter 14 in this volume) has illustrated how kin, friends, and other social ties supplement and complement each other at various stages of life and in different contexts, creating a "convoy" of social support over the life course.[7]

5. Human agency: individuals construct their own life course through the choices and actions they take within the opportunities and constraints of history and social circumstances.

This principle, which is consistent with Riley's (1982) premise that new patterns of aging can cause social change, has been used in many different ways in the life course literature. However, it is most useful simply as a reminder that human lives are not fully shaped or determined by social circumstances (or for that matter by biology) (Marshall, 2005; Marshall & Clarke, in press). The principle also directs attention to planful change both at the individual and the collective level, such as at the political level, and will therefore be germane to the use of the life course perspective for public policy that might be directed to modify the structure of the life course.[8]

American approaches to the life course generally focus on the individual biography or types of biographies. In contrast, European and some Canadian academic approaches focus either on the social institutions that shape and constitute a structure of the life courses or on the relationship of that structure to individual lives.

For many years, a strong research program on the life course at the University of Bremen linked American-inspired social psychological foci on the individual with a greater attention to structural issues that in general is more characteristic of European social science. The first element in the Bremen model is the *cohort approach,* focusing on social change and the timing, duration, and sequences of life course transitions from generation to generation. A second element is the *constructionist* approach to agency, which focuses on personal narratives about individual action and social contexts as they interact in the construction of biographies over time. These two elements are also important in American life course research. But a third, *institutional* approach, emphasizes the interplay of policy and individuals in the regulation, timing, and sequencing of life course transitions in states.

An important example of this approach is the analysis of German welfare state policy by Leisering and Leibfried (1999; see also Leisering, 2003). Based on empirical data from the former West Germany and the former East Germany, these authors "describe policies that form and secure the life course against social risks through education, social security and old-age pensions" (Leisering & Leibfried, 1999, p. xiii). Poverty is viewed as a risk in the context of the German welfare state. Their research "combines quantitative investigations of poverty careers with qualitative biographical analyses of Social Assistance claimants" (Leisering & Leibfried, 1999, p. 6). Their emphasis on how poverty is framed by both institutional arrangements and biographical factors and on how these produce the "temporal structure of the entire life span" has a great deal to offer to those who would understand the relationship of policy to the life course. For example, the emphasis on temporalization emphasizes that poverty is not usually a permanent state but that people move in and out of poverty—something that is true in North America as it is in Germany.

Key Life Course Concepts for Policy

An understanding of the life course perspective requires us to go beyond the somewhat abstract premises and principles outlined here to a number of more specific concepts. Together with the principles described previously, these constitute a perspective that directs the attention of the life course researcher and can similarly direct the attention of the policymaker or policy analyst to certain phenomena that might otherwise be neglected (Marshall & Mueller, 2002).

Time and Context

Two fundamental characteristics of a life course perspective are its emphasis on time and context. Temporality includes issues such as *historical time* as well as the *timing* of an event within a single person's own life course. Social policies that are in place over a person's lifetime and at critical points in his or her life course, such as policies on health care, retirement planning, and social security, characterize one aspect of the historical setting or context for life course experiences. *Social time* refers to "the ordering of life-course events, and the taking on of social roles, in accordance with age-linked expectations, sanctions and options" (Gee, 1987, p. 266, drawing on Elder, 1978).

The Life Course as Social Structure

The *social structure of the life course* is defined in terms of social time and includes shared beliefs about age-appropriate behavior but also, critically, the administrative and legal apparatus in a society that formally enables and facilitates age-graded behavior and that sanctions departures from the socially structured patterns. A related construct is the behavioral structuring of the life course, which has been studied by examining the mean ages at which different cohorts experience important life course transitions in education, work, and the family (Gee, 1987; Ravanera, Rajulton, & Burch, 2004) or the age by which a specified percentage, such as a quintile, have passed through a given life course transition (Hogan 1980, 1982).

Biography as Transitions and Trajectory

Individual or cohort biographies can be described in terms of transitions and trajectories. *Transition* refers to a change in state or states, such as from work to retirement, triggered by an event but also characterized by duration. For example, retirement is both an event and a transition process. *Trajectory* refers to the life pathway resulting from a series of states, encompassing interlacing transitions over a substantial period of time. Among some life course researchers, the term "career" is used instead of "trajectory."[9]

Differentiation and the Principle of Cumulative Advantage and Disadvantage

Life course analysis focuses on the relationship between individual or cohort trajectories and social structure or, in other words, the intersection of biography and history (Mills, 1959). While there is always variability between and within cohorts, intracohort differences are generally far greater at the end of life than at the beginning. By the end of their lives, initially disadvantaged cohort members are generally doing far worse relative to their advantaged counterparts than they were at the beginning of life. As the upper and lower strata move even farther apart and differentials in various indicators of well-being increase over time, we see a process of *intracohort differentiation* with age. The net effect of this *cumulative advantage and disadvantage* (Dannefer, 1987, 1988; Ferraro & Kelley-Moore, 2003; O'Rand, 1995) or cumulative inequality (see chapter 22 in this volume) is that cohorts become increasingly heterogeneous over time. This principle applies not only to economic but also to other resources, such as health and social capital.

Flexibility and the Risk Society

The trend toward individualization in modern society has tremendous policy implications in terms of social security, the social welfare safety net, and social cohesion. "Secondary" institutions in modern society control individual behavior less directly than the older, collectivist institutions (Beck, 1994; Giddens, 1991). In the advanced societies of late modernity, many factors that threaten individual lives have come under greater control by social institutions (e.g., the threats of famine and epidemics), but new threats have arisen, and security against risk is frequently being devolved from major social institutions of the welfare state to individuals. In these cases, individuals may more often experience insecurity, as they are required to assume more personal responsibility for managing their lives within looser institutional constraints.[10] In addition to temporal differences with the rise of late modernity, there are also intersocietal differences with respect to the extent to which major institutions control the life course. For example, Germany is widely considered to have stronger institutional controls over education and work transitions than Canada and the United States (Leisering & Leibfried, 1999). Thus, the social structure of the life course can vary historically or across societies in terms of how constraining it is on the life course trajectories of individuals and cohorts or how encouraging it is of life course flexibility.

Within the vocabulary of the life course perspective, scholars suggest that, to varying degrees, societies have culturally normative conceptions of the life course. These are institutionalized in great measure by public policy and law,[11] channel or constrain behavior, and also provide reference points against which individuals view their biographies as normal or deviant, standard or not (Hagestad & Neugarten, 1985; Neugarten et al., 1965; Settersten & Hagestad, 1996a, 1996b). In many of the highly industrialized societies, such as Germany, Canada, and the United States, much of the social safety net is predicated on the belief that the majority of citizens experience *highly standardized life courses*, described earlier in terms of the tripartite division of the life course into three major segments: preparation for work, the working years, and retirement. To the extent that this was ever true, it is less true today than when the template was set for such public policy. The concept of the standardized life course now serves as reference point to understand how it is that social policies premised on it can be archaic (Marshall & Clarke, 1998) and to understand very complex patterns of stability and change in occupational trajectories over the life course (Brückner & Mayer, 2005; Grunow & Mayer, 2007).

To summarize, the life course perspective calls attention to the ways in which people experience their lives over time, as this has been differentially structured for different cohorts and for different social-demographic configurations in society. The perspective has been used in research that attempts to understand people's lives over time and the ways in which social structure and social institutions shape life course trajectories. As a tool, the life course perspective can also be used as an analytic lens through which various barriers and potential points of intervention that might otherwise go unnoticed are revealed. I next briefly describe an explicit attempt to take this approach to its next logical step, one that attempts to use the life course perspective to inform public policy development.

The Life Course Perspective in the Policy Research Initiative

The Canadian government in recent years established and has maintained an innovative Policy Research Initiative (PRI).[12] In 2004, as one of its activities, it explicitly invoked the life course perspective. The intention was to "provide the qualitative and quantitative language that is needed to move towards integrated analysis" across three streams: "Qualitative studies of individuals, social institutions and networks—especially the lives of the people and institutions that shape our understanding of the need for, and design of, public policies that affect those lives; . . . Empirical analysis of the characteristics of people and social institutions—and of trends over time . . ."; [and] The description, design and assessment of programs and policies, the measurement of their effectiveness, and support of arrangements that hold responsible agencies to account for the way those policies are implemented" (Hicks, 2006, p. 3).

The intent to use the life course perspective to *design* new social policies is imaginative and highly innovative, and its intention to incorporate both qualitative and quantitative data and to address both individual lives and social institutions suggests the adoption of a broad range of life course ideas from a broad range of life course scholarship in both North America and Europe.[13] While many PRI documents explicitly endorse the life course perspective and academic researchers have been invited to the PRI table, none of the initial formal documents emanating from government sources provided explicit links to the academic literature that deals with the life course perspective. However, an active dialogue with academic researchers has led to an infusion from the academic sector of some social science principles of the perspective. It is the case, however, that the PRI framework is more focused on some issues and not at all focused on others that are important in the academic version of the life course perspective and that have great potential in the policy context. The time is opportune to make more explicit links of academic life course research to the PRI conceptualization to the life course perspective.

Just how is the life course perspective invoked in the PRI exercise? It comes up explicitly in one of the five PRI projects, "Population Aging and Life-Course

Flexibility," which "aims at analyzing the social and economic effects of aging populations. . . . [T]his project studies how better flexibility in organizing one's time could contribute to reducing anticipated labour shortages, while at the same time obtaining important social gains" (Voyer, 2004, p. 5). It is also clear that the PRI project is based on the assumption that the life course should be restructured so as to enable and motivate people to remain working for more years than is now the case.[14] A project report, *A Life-Course Approach to Social Policy Analysis: A Proposed Framework* (PRI Project, 2004), presents the most systematic PRI statement of the life course *framework,* defined as "a consistent way of describing individuals in their relationship to society and its institutions, including how policies affect those relationships and how policies affect individual and social outcomes" (p. 5). The life course *approach* is offered as a foundation on which to build a policy framework, but the approach in fact receives just one sentence of attention in this document. The approach "focuses on individual's trajectories through life and on how key life events and transitions affect these trajectories" (p. 5).

Another project report, *Encouraging Choice in Work and Retirement* (PRI Project, 2005) has more to say:

> *Life-course analysis is beginning to enrich public policy. It is a research and analytical framework that permits the linking of longitudinal research—understanding the life context and the complicated inter-relationships of experiences, transitions and connectedness—to more traditional cross-sectional and time-series analysis, and to coordinate the findings with other tools and models. It allows us to understand the interactions of social and economic dimensions of diverse life trajectories. We can take cognizance of the need of individuals at different stages in the life cycle to have access to different kinds of resources—money, time, information and social support. We can consider how different point-in-time experiences may play out over life courses, and how policy interventions might influence and interact with, not only the targeted event or situation, but also the continuation of life experience. (p. 1)*

Documents from the PRI say very little explicitly about the conceptual apparatus of the life course perspective or "approach." Rather, they move quickly to the articulation of a framework for policy. Some of the key aspects of the academic life course perspective are captured by PRI policy writers, but many are not. An important component of the PRI initiative on "Population Aging and Life-Course Flexibility" has been the development by Statistics Canada of a specific analytical tool, called *Life-Paths,* involving sophisticated simulations and record linkage approaches (for a description of the model and an application to health trajectory analysis, see Légaré, Busque, Vézina, & Décarie, 2007; for an overview of statistical initiatives relevant to the PRI, see Voyer, 2005). It may be that statistical methods trump social theory in the PRI exercise and foster a more individualist than institutional approach. Certainly, the focus on a synthetic data file of individuals and the complex statistical methods to develop and use it have received more attention than theoretical issues, including those of history and social structure.

The Fit Between the Academic and the PRI Approaches to the Life Course

What, then, is the relationship between the academic version of the life course perspective and the life course framework found in the PRI documentation? The PRI framework is more focused than the academic perspective, and this is especially so in its explicit attention to a policy agenda. It therefore inevitably leaves out some of the richness of the life course perspective. I describe three important things that are either overlooked or given little emphasis in the PRI framework.[15] Paying more attention to these three areas and to the academic research and theorizing that has taken place within the life course perspective can nourish the PRI's use of life course thinking in support of policy. Conversely, academic life course theorists can benefit from the PRI as a landmark and pathbreaking attempt to extend the usefulness of the life course perspective through policy development.

Inattention to History in the PRI Model

The PRI neglects Elder's second principle, which speaks to the importance of historical time and place. This principle is key if it can be agreed that we can learn something from history. For example, the years immediately following World War II were characterized by deprivation throughout much of Europe but of increasing prosperity in Canada and the United States. Mayer (1988) and his colleagues have found that the cohort of German men born between 1915 and 1925 lost as many as 9 years of their occupational careers because of the war, and many were unable to find employment afterward. This cohort of men suffered high rates of imprisonment, and at least one-quarter did not survive the war. This portrait differs greatly from the effects of World War II on occupational careers in the United States (Elder, Pavalko, & Hastings, 1991).

The government of Québec, discussing reform of the Québec Pension Plan, took history into account, arguing that the elderly should receive good pensions even if benefits exceeded contributions because they went through difficult economic times and contributed to subsequent economic benefit of later generations and also because they underwent the hardships of World War II (Québec, 1996).

Canadian policies governing benefit eligibility to veterans also recognize historical factors, although weighing these factors is frequently contested. The traditional veterans (of both world wars and the Korean War) receive a broader range of benefits than the more recent, Canadian Forces Veterans (with peacekeeping and peacemaking service). And benefits also differ within these groups depending on service theater and intensity of service (Ives, 1998; Struthers, 2004).[16]

These examples also speak to Elder's third principle, which emphasizes the importance of timing. It is the individual's intersection with history that counts—an insight voiced by C. Wright Mills (1959) in his classic book *The Sociological Imagination,* in which he writes that the sociologist must study the relationship between personal troubles and public issues and between biography and history. This intersection makes cohort analysis critical for understanding the fate of people (Ryder, 1965). Birth cohort can determine whether people are already in the workforce or trying to enter the workforce as the economy enters into a historical period of decline or of boom. Generally, entry is much more difficult than retention in periods of economic decline, such as depressions.

Similarly, change in a legal pension age will have different effects on different cohorts. There are undoubtedly strong cohort effects in relation to the changing policies concerning retirement timing that first promoted "early exit" (Kohli, Rein, Guillemard, & van Gunsteren, 1991) and then promoted a shift to extension of working life (Guillemard, 2003). Consider three cohorts. The earliest of these, now fully in retirement or deceased, entered the workforce holding expectations for employment to a standardized retirement age such as 65 and completed their careers under those conditions. A slightly younger cohort would have entered employment under the standardized life course assumption, only to be surprised by changing policies and norms encouraging early exit. The third cohort, younger than the second, would be caught by the two policy changes.

The importance of history as it influences different cohorts is raised in a recent issue brief from the Center for Retirement Research. The authors point out that, despite concerns about the baby-boom generation being too consumer oriented to save for retirement, data from the U.S. Government's Survey of Consumer Finances from 1983 through 2001 showed remarkable stability in the ratio of wealth to income. This, they say, would be comforting until history is taken into account, for during this period (a) there was a huge shift from defined benefit to defined contribution pension plans, (b) interest rates fell, (c) life expectancy increased dramatically such that a given amount of wealth has to support a longer period of retirement, and (d) health care costs rose substantially (Delorme, Munnell, & Webb, 2006). These facts illustrate that policy development has to look at the experience of cohorts in their historical context if it is to be meaningful.

The principle of life course analysis that directs attention to history and the historical context provides a valuable remedy to policy thrusts that are based on "apocalyptic" or "voodoo" demography (terms used by McDaniel [1987] and Robertson [1979]). Historical analyses, such as those by Townsend (1981) and Walker (1981, 2005) for the European situation, have been valuable in showing how pension policy changes acted to initially create the association between old age and retirement, foster negative attitudes toward the elderly, and, subsequently redefine the retirement period and lower the entry to "old age" to the point where retirement and old age became dissociated.[17]

Sheppard, Myles, and Polivka (1996) point out that "much of the 'intergenerational conflict' (or competition, or tension) discussion is characterized by a virtually total ignorance of any historical perspective. At best, there might be some reference to experiences and data going back as far as ten to twenty years" (p. 605).[18]

Lack of Attention in the PRI Model to Social Institutions That Structure the Life Course

It is somewhat paradoxical that in the PRI exercise, which is explicitly a policy exercise, so much attention focuses on individuals rather than on social institutions. The German sociologist Karl Ulrich Mayer (2000) has argued that one goal of using the life course perspective "is to understand how institutions and policies on the macro- and meso-level of societies influence and pattern individual life courses in the interrelated form of educational tracks, employment trajectories and family histories." Canadian sociologist Paul Bernard (2007) notes that social institutions "play a key role in shaping life courses, through their policies in the fields of health, education, social assistance, urban affairs, transportation, the environment and so on" (p. 15), and calls for comparative life course research, which will move work in the perspective away from individualism.

The extent to which there is in fact an age structuring of the life course has been investigated quantitatively by many demographers and other social scientists in the United States (Hogan, 1982; Winsborough, 1982) and Canada (Gee, 1987; Ravanera et al., 2004; Rodgers & Whitney, 1981). By calculating the interquartile ranges in age using life tables for cohorts of men and of women born 1916–1920 through 1966–1970, Ravenera et al. (2004) were able to trace changes in the timing of school completion, starting work, leaving home, first union, first marriage, first birth, departure of first child from the household, and departure of last child from the household. Unfortunately, retirement was not considered in this analysis. Interquartile range is calculated by subtracting the age at which the first 25% of cohort members have experienced an event from the age at which three-quarters of the cohort have done so. A smaller interquartile range thus means that the transition event was more precisely defined or "structured." They found different trends for the education and work-start transitions than for the family-related transitions and differences for men and women. The picture is complex but does show a move toward somewhat greater age standardization of the school to work transition across all cohorts but more age homogeneity in family-related transitions from the first cohort through the 1941–1945 cohort, followed by a move to less homogeneity in that area.

Turning to later in the working life course, since the 1980s we have seen a significant policy shift in many countries, from policies supporting early withdrawal from the labor force to policies designed to reverse the trend toward early retirement and promote retention of workers to later years. The early policy initiatives to promote "early exit" from the workforce were motivated primarily by a concern to create job vacancies for the large baby-boom cohort (Kohli et al., 1991; McMullin, Cooke, & Tomchick, 2008; Schmähl, 1989). The shift in policy has been motivated by a concern to reduce the years of drawdown on pensions and state health care benefits while increasing the years of tax and contribution support for such state programs, in other words, as a means to reduce the so-called pension burden. However, a second reason for this policy shift to promote longer years of working life is to meet labor force demands (Penner, Perun, & Steurle, 2002). A justification made for this shift is that life expectancy has increased greatly, creating productivity and fiscal problems as larger proportions of the population withdraw from formal production and become recipients of pensions and health care at state expense (Marshall, in press).

The current policy direction faces difficulties precisely because it runs counter to previous policies that first established age 65 as a normal retirement age in North America and then acted to promote "early retirement" in relation to that normative age. As Penner et al. (2002) state,

> *Many of the economic and institutional barriers to working longer evolved when there was reason to make room for the giant cohorts of baby boomers working their way up the career ladder. Often, pressures to downsize were much stronger than pressures to retain valuable human capital. Early retirement provided a relatively painless way to shed workers. It was also a time when mandatory retirement was legal, life expectancy was shorter, health at any age was more fragile, and many more jobs were physically demanding. (p. 6)*

The timing of withdrawal from the labor force is thus much more than simply an economic issue: its normative and institutional context make it also a sociological issue. I believe it is fair to say that most of the policy options are framed by economists preoccupied with either pension or labor force issues, but the options should be viewed in a broader social context as well. Given current retirement patterns in North America, a typical citizen can expect to spend about one-third of his or her adult life in retirement. This was certainly not the expectation when the institutions that have shaped the working life course, such as state pension systems, were first put into place. The policy issues in this area, therefore, touch in important ways the expectations, plans, and hopes of citizens.

The life courses of individuals and also of cohorts cannot be properly understood without concerted analytical attention to the restructuring of the life course in terms of work, as this discussion has stressed, and in terms of its other aspects such as the family. As Settersten (2005) has put it,

> *The welfare state is, even in America, the only "overarching agency"—to use Leisering's (2003) term—that has direct and indirect bearings on the entire life course, some effects of which may be unintended. Yet welfare states rarely address the life course as a whole, instead providing spot coverage around specific periods of vulnerability and risk or specific transitions. A policy that affects the life course is not the same as a life-course policy designed with the whole of life in mind and meant to connect and integrate different life periods. (p. 551)*

Need to Elaborate the Linked-Lives Concept in the PRI Model

The PRI discussion paper *A Life-Course Approach to Social Policy Analysis* (PRI Project, 2004) comes close to recognizing the linked lives principle and also the principle of timing as it develops the trajectory of the synthetic case, Olivia.[19] Olivia is portrayed as engaged in two-way resource flows in five domains: work (markets), family, government, community organizations, and arm's-length public agencies such as educational institutions. In the working paper, each trajectory is first developed in isolation—we find a graphical figure and a verbal depiction of Olivia's family and household trajectory, for example, and one for each of the others. Then, in a more complex figure, we see financial flows portrayed for all five domains, yet the focus is always on the individual, Olivia. The PRI conceptualization moves in the direction of linked lives when, in discussing financial flows, it recognizes "the importance of taking into account of multiple sources of support. Even when limited to financial flows, as in this example, the interacting role of jobs, markets and families can be seen in her overall income and expenditures" (PRI Project, 2004, p. 17). Moreover, the draft discussion paper illustrates other aspects of linked lives in examples of Olivia taking care of her mother when she becomes ill and so forth.

It is debatable whether the current framing of the PRI model will take the exercise as far as required. Cheal (2000), with reference to aging issues, makes a persuasive case for attention to the linked-lives concept: "It is increasingly recognized by contemporary demographers of population aging that relevant variables include not only demographic characteristics of older people, but also demographic characteristics of the members of their support networks. In other words, precise assessments of the impacts of population aging require a *multi-dimensional demography*" (p. S114). The model, as developed in the PRI, is person centered and hence very individualistic. Perhaps that is a requirement for simulations and data analysis in exercises such as those using simulation. But there is a danger that the entire exercise might be unduly limited by its focus on the individual rather than on larger units of analysis, such as whole families, neighborhood, workplace populations, and so forth.

Much of the richest life course research has used the concept of linked lives, and doing so often requires taking simultaneous account of multiple actors. Qualitative research methodologies might have a special place here. This is particularly so if we would wish to move beyond the tracking of complex contingent events to achieve an understanding of the processes. The life course contingencies that link people's biographies are not things that "just happen to individuals"; they are interactions through which people negotiate their lives. People such as Olivia do not automatically become caregivers when their mothers become ill. Rather, new roles are negotiated through complex social processes.

We can learn from national-level surveys and simulations, but we can also learn from smaller-scale studies of social groupings, such as Connidis's (2003) imaginative study of divorce and union dissolution over three generations of the same lineage, studied qualitatively in 10 three-generation families. For another example, Davies (2003) gathered life histories of heterosexual, never-married childless individuals to explore the "transition to singlehood," finding it very much a gendered experience and showing the importance of social time-tables as a structural aspect of the family life course. Such studies, combining descriptive statistics with insightful quotations from qualitative interviews, can provide insight and understanding, much of which can be transferable to our interpretation of the complex statistical patterns discovered through simulation and large-scale multivariate analyses. At the very least, qualitative studies can remind us that life is, in fact, even more complex than the logistic regression models show us.

Conclusion

My purpose has been to both celebrate an innovative application of the life course perspective—its explicit use not only in the analysis of policy but also in its development—and argue that the PRI initiative, which is engaged in this pioneering effort, can benefit greatly by enlarging its view of the life course model and more explicitly drawing on academic research in this area. I introduced the life course perspective historically, in a very cursory way, as it has been developed within the academy. The North American version of the life course perspective has been quite social psychological, whereas European life course scholars have in addition addressed social structures and social institutions, as these constitute the constraints and the opportunity structures within which individuals seek to construct their lives.

I reviewed the basic principles of the life course perspective and the additional concepts—such as the concept of cumulative advantage and disadvantage—that are most useful for policy development as well as for policy analysis. I concluded by noting three major areas in which the academic perspective on the life course can be most valuable in enriching the PRI.[20] I believe that this important work will be more successful to the extent that it is more historically nuanced, that the unit of analysis moves beyond the individual to more thoroughly deal with linked-lives issues, and that the work attends more centrally to social institutions and social structure rather than the life paths of individuals. If the full conceptual tool kit of the life course perspective can be employed to *understand* social policy, it can also be used to *fashion* social policy. If it does so, public policy will attend more to early intervention in light of its understanding of cumulative advantage and disadvantage, it will recognize the importance of viewing individuals in their family and broader social networks as these change over time, and it will recognize the importance of history in providing and in constraining options for people and the consequent necessity to frame policy in light of the ways in which different cohorts or generations experience history in different ways.

Notes

1. Life course is a metaphor. The version of this metaphor invoked here is of the individual in a boat, navigating a watercourse upstream in a complex river system. Structural features such as islands, sandbars, rocks, and tributaries offer both choices and constraints, thus influencing but not fully determining the ultimate destination.
2. Life course theorists recognize the importance of gender, race, and class in shaping life course trajectories, but considering these is beyond the scope of this chapter. See, for example, Bernard (2007), Martin-Matthews and Campbell (1995), Moen and Han (2001), and O'Rand (1995).
3. Glen Elder, the most influential academic writing about the life course, prefers the term "orientation" to perspective, but in fact he uses the two terms interchangeably: "According to Merton (1968), theoretical orientations establish a common framework to guide descriptive and explanatory research. They do so in the identification and formulation of research problems, the selection of variables and rationales for them, and strategies for designing research and analyzing data. In this regard, the life course refers to age-graded life patterns that are embedded in social structures and historical change" (Elder & Johnson, 2003, p. 54; see also Elder & O'Rand, 1995).
4. More detailed histories of development of the life course perspective are found in Elder (1992, 1998) and Marshall and Mueller (2003).
5. For an earlier systematic treatment, with just three principles, see Elder (1975).
6. Cultural expectations as to appropriate timing for life events, such as when it is appropriate to marry, also vary historically and cross-culturally.
7. Consider the convoys of the Battle of the Atlantic during World War II. To make the crossing alone would be highly perilous, but ships cross in the company of others. Accompanying naval vessels provide protection. At mid-ocean, some ships will have been lost, and the ships of the Royal Canadian Navy often turned over the escort duties to Britain's Royal Navy at

mid-ocean. The metaphor is that people go through life not alone but in the company with others, not always the same others, but with considerable continuity in support.

8. This principle also acts against strict determinism that is found in rational choice and other utilitarian models. People may try to act rationally, but they cannot act in a purely rational manner because they lack complete information or the capacity to make complex calculations of the costs and benefits of different life pathways from which they choose.
9. Notably in European research at the University of Bremen and in North American research that draws on the symbolic interactionist tradition of sociology (Marshall & Mueller, 2003).
10. For example, the move from defined benefit to defined contribution pension plans shifts the risks of ensuring the individual's financial security in retirement from the employing company to the individual (Frericks, Maier, & de Graaf, 2006).
11. At the most basic level, one could describe the "legally defined" life course in terms of laws such as those requiring people to attend school during specific ages or for a specific duration; laws governing eligibility to vote, drive, marry, and so on; legally set ages for pension eligibility; age windows of eligibility for military conscription; or ages beyond which the right to work is no longer protected. The correspondence between a "legal life course" and culturally shared or normative conceptions of the life course or the extent to which actual behavior is structured in this way is a matter of investigation but also a matter of some consequence to individuals.
12. The life course is one of several areas pursued by the PRI, the mission of which is to conduct research in support of the Canadian government's medium-term agenda, focusing on "horizontal" issues (interministerial and multi-area) and to ensure the transfer of knowledge to policymakers. Other areas include the impact of science, cultural diversity, and freshwater supply. See the PRI Web site at http://www.policyresearch.gc.ca.
13. In academic life course research, qualitative data have been used, mainly in the symbolic interactionist tradition, in both North American and European research. North American research has tended to focus more on the life courses of individuals rather than the social institutions that shape the life course, whereas European research has paid more attention to social institutions (for a review, see Marshall & Mueller, 2003).
14. The PRI initiative also deals with family life course issues. I have the space in this chapter to address only the domain of work and the life course, even though these two domains obviously interact (Hareven, 1982; Marshall, 2006; Marshall & Mueller, 2002; Martin-Matthews & Campbell, 1995).
15. It is impossible to do justice to the conceptual richness of the life course perspective within the limits of this chapter. For a broad overview in depth, see Mortimer and Shanahan (2003); for a brief overview, see Marshall and Mueller (2003); and for a more detailed discussion in terms of policy, see Marshall (2006) and Marshall and Mueller (2002).
16. In the United States, recent efforts to legislate a new GI Bill recognize the importance of history in a similar way. The amount provided for postrelease education has fallen proportionate to costs. Senators Webb and Hagel, main proponents of the bipartisan bill, consider current tuition coverage reasonable in peacetime but not for those with war service in Iraq or Afghanistan.
17. The extent that these observations apply to Canada is in itself a policy concern, and the research basis for the answer, while not as solid as it might be, suggests that the observations do apply.
18. In addition to its critique of demographic determinism and ahistorical policy formation, the life course perspectives offers a critique of individualist, "rational-choice" assumptions that frequently underlie public and corporate policy. The individualized analyses of psychological and social psychological researchers support only the most limited policy formation because it is difficult to find public policy levers at that microlevel of analysis. Individual-level rationality underlying economic models (in sociology, "rational-choice" models) can take policy analysis and formation only so far because people's choices are constrained by social structure and by the contingencies of their lived lives.
19. Olivia is a synthetic Canadian member of the baby-boom generation for whom extensive statistical data relevant to the life course have been assembled through data linkage and statistical inference from several Canadian surveys, censuses, and taxation data. She illustrates the type of data that the PRI is using in microsimulation exercises. For an extensive description, see Hicks (2006).

20. In an earlier report for the Canadian Policy Research Networks (Marshall & Mueller, 2002), I deal with these and related issues in an explicit policy context and also provide additional description of important life course perspective principles and concepts.

References

Antonucci, T. C. (1990). Social supports and social relationships. In R. H. Binstock & L. K. George (Eds.), *Handbook of aging and the social sciences* (3rd ed., pp. 205–227). New York: Academic Press.

Beck, U. (1994). The reinvention of politics: Towards a theory of reflexive modernization. In U. Beck, A. Giddens, & S. Lash (Eds.), *Reflexive modernization: Politics, tradition and aesthetics in the modern social order* (pp. 1–55). Stanford, CA: Stanford University Press.

Bernard, P. (2007). The interconnected dynamics of population change and life-course processes. *Horizons, 9*(4), 13–16.

Brückner, H., & Mayer, K. U. (2005). De-standardization of the life course: What it might mean? And if it means anything, whether it actually took place? *Advances in Life Course Research 9,* 27–53.

Cain, L. D., Jr. (1964). Life course and social structure. In R. E. L. Faris (Ed.), *Handbook of modern sociology* (pp. 272–309). Chicago: Rand McNally.

Cheal, D. (2000). Aging and demographic change. *Canadian Public Policy, 26*(Suppl. 2), S109–S122.

Connidis, I. A. (2003). Divorce and union dissolution: Reverberations over three generations. *Canadian Journal on Aging, 22,* 353–368.

Dannefer, D. (1987). Aging as intracohort differentiation: Accentuation, the Matthew Effect, and the life course. *Sociological Forum, 2,* 211–236.

Dannefer, D. (1988). Differential gerontology and the stratified life course: Conceptual and methodological issues. *Annual Review of Gerontology and Geriatrics, 8,* 3–36.

Davies, L. (2003). Singlehood: Transitions within a gendered world. *Canadian Journal on Aging, 22,* 343–352.

Delorme, L., Munnell, A. H., & Webb, A. (2006). *Empirical regularity suggests retirement risks.* Issue Brief No. 41. Boston: Center for Retirement Research at Boston College.

Elder, G. H., Jr. (1975). Age differentiation in the life course. *Annual Review of Sociology, 1,* 165–190.

Elder, G. H., Jr. (1978). Approaches to social change and the family. In J. Demos & S. S. Boocock (Eds.), *Turning points: Historical and sociological essays on the family* (pp. 1–38). (Supplement to *American Journal of Sociology, 84*)

Elder, G. H., Jr. (1992). Models of the life course. *Contemporary Sociology, 21*(5), 32–35.

Elder, G. H., Jr. (1994). Time, human agency, and social change: Perspectives on the life course. *Social Psychology Quarterly, 57,* 4–15.

Elder, G. H. Jr. (1998). The life course and human development. In R. M. Lerner (Ed.), *Handbook of child psychology* (Vol. 1, pp. 939–991). New York: Wiley.

Elder, G. H., Jr. (1999). *Children of the Great Depression: Social change in life experience* (25th anniv. ed.). Chicago: University of Chicago Press. (Original work published 1974)

Elder, G. H., Jr., & Caspi, A. (1988). Economic stress in lives: Developmental perspectives. *Journal of Social Issues, 44*(4), 25–45.

Elder, G. H., Jr., & Johnson. M. K. (2003). The life course and aging: Challenges, lessons and new directions. In R. Settersten (Ed.), *Invitation to the life course: Toward a new understanding of later life* (pp. 49–81). Amityville, NY: Baywood Publishing.

Elder, G. H., Jr., Johnson, M. K., & Crosnoe, R. (2003). The emergence and development of life course theory. In J. T. Mortimer & M. J. Shanahan (Eds.), *Handbook of the life course* (pp. 3–19). New York: Kluwer Academic/Plenum Press.

Elder, G. H., Jr., & O'Rand, A. M. (1995). Adult lives in a changing society. In K. S. Cook, G. A. Fine, & J. S. House (Eds.), *Sociological perspectives on social psychology* (pp. 452–475). Needham Heights, MA: Allyn & Bacon.

Elder, G. H., Jr., Pavalko, E. K., & Hastings, T. J. (1991). Talent, history, and the fulfillment of promise. *Psychiatry, 54,* 251–267.

Ferraro, K. F., & Kelley-Moore, J. (2003). Cumulative disadvantage and health: Long-term consequences of obesity? *American Sociological Review, 68,* 707–729.

Frericks, P., Maier, R., & de Graaf, W. (2006). Shifting the pension mix: Consequences for Dutch and Danish women. *Social Policy & Administration, 40,* 475–492.

Gee, E. M. (1987). Historical change in the family life course of Canadian men and women. In V. W. Marshall (Ed.), *Aging in Canada: Social perspectives* (2nd ed., pp. 265–287). Markham, Ontario: Fitzhenry & Whiteside.

Giddens, A. (1991). *Modernity and self-identity: Self and society in the late modern age.* Stanford, CA: Stanford University Press.

Giele, J. Z., & Elder, G. H., Jr. (1998). *Methods of life course research: Qualitative and quantitative approaches.* Thousand Oaks, CA: Sage.

Grunow, D., & Mayer, K. U. (2007). *How stable are working lives? Occupational stability and mobility in West Germany 1940s–2005.* Working Paper 2007–03. New Haven, CT: Yale University, Center for Research in Inequalities and the Life Course.

Guillemard, A-M. (2003). France: Struggling to find a way out of the early exit culture. *Geneva Papers on Risk and Insurance, 28,* 558–574.

Hagestad, G. O., & Neugarten, B. L. (1985). Age and the life course. In R. H. Binstock, E. Shanas, V. L. Bengtson, G. L. Maddox, & D. Wedderburn (Eds.), *Handbook of aging and the social sciences* (pp. 35–61). New York: Van Nostrand Reinhold.

Han, S-K., & Moen, P. (1999). Clocking out: Temporal patterning of retirement. *American Journal of Sociology, 105,* 191–236.

Hareven, T. K. (1982). *Family time and industrial time: The relationship between the family and work in a New England industrial community.* Cambridge: Cambridge University Press.

Harley, C., & Mortimer, J. (2000, March 30–April 2). *Social status and mental health in young adulthood: The mediating role of the transition to adulthood.* Paper presented at the biennial meeting of the Society for Research on Adolescence, Chicago.

Hicks, P. (2006, March 23–24). *A life-course framework for social policy analysis.* Notes for a second draft of the Olivia Story. Presentation at the Expert Roundtable on Well-Being and Participation Over the Life Course. Population, Work and Family Research Collaboration Symposium, Ottawa.

Hogan, D. P. (1980). The transition to adulthood as a career contingency. *American Sociological Review, 45,* 261–276.

Hogan, D. P. (1982). *Transitions and social change: The early lives of American men.* New York: Academic Press.

Ives, D. (1998). The Veterans Charter: The compensation principle and the principle of recognition for service. In P. Neary & J. L. Granatstein (Eds.), *The Veterans Charter and post-World War II Canada* (pp. 85–94). Montreal: McGill-Queen's University Press.

Kohli, M., Rein, M., Guillemard, A-M., & van Gunsteren, H. (Eds.). (1991). *Time for retirement: Comparative studies of early exit from the labor force.* Cambridge: Cambridge University Press.

Légaré, J., Busque, M-A., Vézina, S., & Décarie, Y. (2007). The health of tomorrow's older Canadians: An application of Statistics Canada's LifePaths microsimulation model. *Horizons, 9*(4), 51–53.

Leisering, L. (2003). Government and the life course. In J. T. Mortimer & M. J. Shanahan (Eds.), *Handbook of the life course* (pp. 205–25). New York: Kluwer Academic.

Leisering, L., & Leibfried, S. (1999). *Time and poverty in western welfare states.* Cambridge: Cambridge University Press.

Mannheim, K. (1952). The problem of generations. In D. Kecskemeti (Ed.), *Essays on the sociology of knowledge* (pp. 276–322). London: Routledge & Kegan Paul. (Original work published 1928)

Marshall, V. W. (2005). Agency, events, and structure at the end of the life course. In R. Levy, P. Ghisletta, J. Le Goff, & E. Widmer (Eds.), *Towards an interdisciplinary perspective on the life course. Advances in Life Course Research, 10,* 57–91. Amsterdam: Elsevier.

Marshall, V. W. (2006, March 23–24). *The life course perspective: An overview in relation to the Policy Research Initiative.* Presentation at the Expert Roundtable on Well-Being and Participation Over the Life Course. Population, Work and Family Research Collaboration Symposium, Ottawa.

Marshall, V. W. (in press). Global aging and families: Some policy concerns about the global aging perspective. In Merril Silverstein (Ed.), *From generation to generation: Continuity and change in aging families.* Baltimore: Johns Hopkins University Press.

Marshall, V. W., & Clarke, P. J. (1998). Facilitating the transition from employment to retirement. In *Canada Health Action: Building on the Legacy* (Vol. 2, pp. 171–211). Papers commissioned by the National Forum on Health, Determinants of Health: Adults and Seniors. Sainte-Foy Foy, QC: Editions MultiMondes.

Marshall, V. W., & Clarke, P. J. (in press). Agency and social structure in aging and life course research. In D. Dannefer & C. Phillipson (Eds.), *International handbook of social gerontology.* Thousand Oaks, CA: Sage.

Marshall, V. W., & Mueller, M. M. (2002). *Rethinking social policy for an aging workforce and society: Insights from the life course perspective.* CPRN Discussion Paper No. W/18. Ottawa: CPRN.

Marshall, V. W., & Mueller, M. M. (2003). Theoretical roots of the life-course perspective. In W. R. Heinz & V. W. Marshall (Eds.), *Social dynamics of the life course* (pp. 3–32). New York: Aldine de Gruyter.

Martin-Matthews, A., & Campbell, L. D. (1995). Gender roles, employment, and informal care. In S. Arber & J. Ginn (Eds.), *Connecting gender and aging: Sociological reflections* (pp. 129–143). Philadelphia: Open University Press.

Mayer, K. U. (1988). German survivors of World War II. The impact on the life course of the collective experience of birth cohorts. In M. W. Riley in association with B. J. Huber & B. B. Hess (Eds.), *Social change and the life course: Vol. 1. Social structures and human lives* (pp. 229–246). Newbury Park, CA: Sage.

Mayer, K. U. (2000, August 12). *Life courses in the process of transformation to post-communism: The case of East Germany.* Distinguished scholar lecture, Section on Aging and the Life Course, American Sociological Association meeting, Miami Beach, FL.

McDaniel, S. A. (1987). Demographic aging as a guiding paradigm in Canada's welfare state. *Canadian Public Policy, 13,* 330–336.

McMullin, J. A., Cooke, J. M., & Tomchick, T. (2008). Work and retirement in Canada: Policies and prospects. In P. Taylor (Ed.), *Ageing labour forces: Promises and prospects* (pp. 62–83). Camberly: Edward Elgar.

Merton, R. K. (1968). *Social theory and social structure.* New York: Free Press.

Mills, C. W. (1959). *The sociological imagination.* New York: Grove.

Moen, P., & Han, S-K. (2001). Reframing careers: Work, family and gender. In V. W. Marshall, W. R. Heinz, H. Krüger, & A. Verma (Eds.), *Restructuring work and the life course* (pp. 424–445). Toronto: University of Toronto Press.

Mortimer, J. T., & Shanahan, M. J. (Eds.). (2003). *Handbook of the life course.* New York: Kluwer Academic.

Neugarten, B. L., Moore, J. W., & Lowe, J. C. (1965). Age norms, age constraints, and adult socialization. *American Journal of Sociology, 70,* 710–717.

O'Rand, A. M. (1995). The cumulative stratification of the life course. In R. H. Binstock, L. K. George, & Associates (Eds.), *Handbook of aging and the social sciences* (4th ed., pp. 188–207). San Diego, CA: Academic Press.

O'Rand, A. M., Henretta, J. C., & Krecker, M. L. (1992). Family pathways to retirement: Early and late life family effects on couple's work exit patterns. In M. Szinovacz, D. J. Ekerdt, & B. H. Vinick (Eds.), *Families and retirement* (pp. 81–98). Beverly Hills, CA: Sage.

Penner, R. G., Perun, P., & Steurle, E. (2002, November). *Legal and institutional impediments to partial retirement and part-time work by older workers.* Washington, DC: Urban Institute.

PRI Project. (2004, August). *A life-course approach to social policy analysis.* Draft Discussion Paper. Ottawa: Author.

PRI Project. (2005, October). *Encouraging choice in work and retirement: Project report.* Ottawa: Author.

Québec. (1996). *For you and your children: Guaranteeing the future of the Québec Pension Plan.* Working Paper. Sainte-Foy, QC: Régie des rentes du Québec.

Ravanera, Z. R., Rajulton, F., & Burch, T. K. (2004). Patterns of age variability in life course transitions. *Canadian Journal of Sociology, 29,* 527–542.

Riley, M. W. (1982). Introduction: Life course perspectives. In M. W. Riley, R. P. Abeles, & M. S. Teitelbaum (Eds.), *Aging from birth to death: Sociotemporal perspectives* (pp. 3–13). Boulder, CO: Westview Press.

Robertson, A. (1979). Beyond apocalyptic demography: Towards a moral economy of interdependence. *Ageing & Society, 17,* 425–446.

Rodgers, R. H., & Witney, G. (1981). The family cycle in twentieth-century Canada. *Journal of Marriage and the Family, 43,* 727–740.

Ryder, N. B. (1965). The cohort as a concept in the study of social change. *American Sociological Review, 30,* 843–861.

Schmähl, W. (Ed.). (1989). *Redefining the process of retirement: An international perspective.* New York: Springer-Verlag.

Settersten, R. A., Jr. (2005). Social policy and the transition to adulthood. In R. A. Settersten Jr., F. F. Furstenberg Jr., & R. G. Rubmaut (Eds.), *On the frontier of adulthood: Theory, research and public policy* (pp. 534–560). Chicago: University of Chicago Press.

Settersten, R. A., & Hagestad, G. O. (1996a). What's the latest? Cultural age deadlines for family transitions. *The Gerontologist, 36,* 178–188.

Settersten, R. A., & Hagestad, G. O. (1996b). What's the latest? Cultural age deadlines for educational and work transitions. *The Gerontologist, 36,* 602–613.

Sheppard, H. L., Myles, J. F., & Polivka, L. (1996). Is America exporting another new social idea? *Ageing & Society, 16,* 603–612.

Struthers, J. (2004, December). *Comfort, security, dignity: The Veterans Independence Program, a policy history.* Report prepared for the Veterans Affairs Canada. Charlottetown, Prince Edward Island: Veterans Affairs Canada.

Townsend, P. (1981). The structured dependency of the elderly: A creation of social policy in the twentieth century. *Ageing & Society, 1,* 5–28.

Voyer, J-P. (2004). *Preface to views on life-course flexibility and Canada's aging population.* Ottawa: PRI Project in collaboration with Ekos.

Voyer, J-P. (2005). The data gaps initiative at a crossroad. *Horizons, 8*(1), 4–8.

Walker, A. (1981). Towards a political economy of old age. *Ageing & Society, 1,* 73–94.

Walker, A. (2005). Towards an international political economy of ageing. *Ageing & Society, 25,* 815–839.

Winsborough, H. H. (1982). Changes in the transition to adulthood. In M. W. Riley, R. P. Abeles, & M. S. Teitelbaum (Eds.), *Aging from birth to death: Sociotemporal perspectives* (pp. 137–152). Boulder, CO: Westview Press.

Aging and Social Policy: Theorizing the Social

32

Alan Walker

This chapter examines the relationship between aging and social policy and argues that, without an adequate conceptualization of the "social," it will not be possible either to understand its meaning and operation or to envisage a new historical form in which this relationship is not driven by economic ideology and policy. It is argued, furthermore, that a theory of the social will pave the way to a reconciliation of the purported conflict between structure and agency. This endeavor starts with an outline of the connections between aging and social policy, with a specific focus on the changing relationship between aging and the welfare state, this is followed by an outline of the two current contrasting theories of the relationship between aging and the welfare state, poststructuralism and the political economy of aging perspective, which was formulated initially

Acknowledgments: I am very grateful to Wolfgang Beck and Laurent van der Maesen for their permission to use our joint work.

to examine this relationship. Then the constitution of the social is analyzed, and finally an example of its theoretical application to later life is provided.

Aging and Social Policy

The significance of aging to social policy can hardly be exaggerated even though this realization came earlier to gerontology than it did to mainstream social policy. It is not possible to understand the origins, development, and contemporary debates concerning welfare states without an aging dimension. On the one hand, most welfare states were founded on provision for old age, with the first legislative bricks being laid in by Bismarck's Germany in 1889. The other western European countries followed soon after the turn of the next century: the Netherlands in 1901, the United Kingdom in 1908, France in 1910, Sweden in 1913, and Italy and Spain in 1919. (It was not for another decade and a half that the United States introduced its first public pension.) Because of their significance in the constitution of welfare states public pension systems tend to have a defining influence over the rest of the welfare regime (Esping-Andersen, 1990; Walker, 2003). On the other hand, today, older people are the largest beneficiaries of social spending, particularly as pension recipients and users of health care services, and pensions are the largest item of such expenditures (on average 45% in Europe). In most welfare states and, certainly, in most western European ones, pensions comprise a significant proportion of national gross domestic product (GDP)—ranging from a low of 4.7% in Ireland to a high of 14.2% in Italy, with a western European average of 10.6% (European Commission, 2006). It is the sheer scale of this public expenditure commitment that put public pensions in the spotlight when policymakers began to question the received wisdom from the formative years of welfare states that decent provision for old age was a hallmark of a civilized society.

The Changing Relationship Between Aging and the Welfare State

Old age was acknowledged collectively as a risk status from the early part of the 20th century, but it was the advent of the fully fledged Western welfare state, in the post–World War II period, that both the risk of old age and, in effect, the social definition of old age itself became institutionalized (Myles, 1984; Walker, 1980). In other words, the risks associated with later life were accepted as socially legitimate, with few sanctions attached to the welfare responses, unlike those connected with people of working age. Welfare states were built at a time of relative optimism about tackling social needs and the prospects for the future funding of benefits. Given their precarious economic situation and the capitalist drive to exclude older "unproductive" workers from the labor force, older people were regarded as a deserving cause for welfare spending, in direct contrast to the unemployed. This is not to suggest that public pension systems were established without, largely, working-class action: some of the campaigns were long ones. Nonetheless, older people were regarded positively as a needy group. This was not entirely good news, though, because it also entailed their social construction as dependent in economic terms, and this encouraged popular ageist stereotypes of old age as a period of poverty and frailty (Binstock 1991; Townsend, 1981, 1986; Walker 1980). In fact, when the welfare states were created, these stereotypes were well founded, and there was widespread poverty and destitution as older people were forced out of employment and then had to rely on their families and/or poor relief. Even after the creation of public pension systems, a significant proportion of people over 65 remained in poverty: one in five in Germany, one in four in the United States, and one in three in the United Kingdom in the late 1960s. Evidence such as this led to renewed efforts to tackle poverty in old age and the expansion of pension systems. Thus, between 1960 and 1985, total public pension spending in countries in the Organization for Economic Cooperation and Development (OECD) rose significantly faster than economic output, which contributed to a rising share of GDP being allocated to pensions. The influence of the three factors determining this growth—demography, eligibility, and benefit levels—was roughly equal, suggesting that expansive policy decisions were taken concerning eligibility and the levels of pensions and related benefits for older people (OECD, 1988). That may be seen, in retrospect, as the "golden age" of the welfare state. During this period of welfare state expansion, old age was identified as a social problem, but later, in the 1980s, it was to become an economic one (for a detailed account of this transformation, see Walker, 1999).

The welfare state tide began to ebb in the mid-1970s following the world oil price rise shock and the fiscal crisis it precipitated (O'Connor, 1977). The previous consensus that had underpinned welfare state expansion, including the status of older people as the deserving poor, was rejected in some countries and replaced with increasingly critical questions about the cost of population aging. These questions were amplified in the second wave of attacks on the welfare state in which a neoliberal agenda began to take shape. Again, because pensions are the largest item of social expenditure, they were the main target. The fact that many of the public pension schemes that were established early in the 20th century were reaching maturity in the 1980s reinforced the urgency of the neoliberal arguments against the role of the state in welfare. Not surprisingly, it was the Anglo-Saxon countries that adopted most readily the neoliberal ideological prescriptions. In western Europe, this meant that the United Kingdom and Ireland and, elsewhere, Australia, New Zealand, and the United States followed a similar path. For example, in the United Kingdom, the early 1980s saw the shift from wage to price indexation for the basic public pension, and later in the decade, the earning-related component of the pension was cut substantially, while those in employment were offered tax incentives to opt for private prefunded pensions (Walker, 1991, 1993).

As well as this transformation in the policies of some countries toward older people, there was a parallel rhetorical sea change in which the previously sacrosanct status of deservingness on the part of this group was replaced by a discourse emphasizing, to a greater or lesser extent, the "burden" of pensions on the working population. Sometimes this discourse has been framed in terms of generational equity, and, invariably, the crude "dependency ratio" between those of working and pension ages is used to lend this case an aura of scientific legitimacy (Walker, 1990). Nowhere in Europe, however, has the generational equity discourse had the negative impact on public welfare intended by its proponents. Similarly, in the United States, the pressure group Americans for

Generational Equity failed to dent public support for social security (Marshall, Cook, & Marshall, 1993).

Similar discourses concerning the future costs of population aging followed in the wake of the third wave of neoliberalism in the 1990s. This time, partly because of the role of the European Union, its influence spread beyond the Anglo-Saxon countries to others in western Europe, and this led to changes in most of their public pension systems (Walker, 2003). Apart from the introduction of funded components in Italy and Sweden, these modifications were mainly parametric, such as adjustments to pension formulas or eligibility criteria. During this period, the core neoliberal concern about the current and future costs of public pension schemes was enlarged to include health and social care services. Here too a negative discourse about the potential "burden" of an aging population has become common. As with the case concerning pensions, such discourses are frequently accompanied by simple extrapolations of current disability and disease rates that assume implicitly that nothing can or will be done to ameliorate them. This ideologically inspired argument directly contradicts evidence, on the one hand, of increasing healthy life expectance (Robine, 2003) and, on the other, demography as a secondary element in the rising cost of health and social care (Jacobzone, 1999).

Thus, over the span of three decades, the relationship between aging and the welfare state has been transformed from the relatively positive one, albeit with benign ageist elements, that was rooted in the construction of welfare states to a generally more negative one that is focused primarily on costs rather than revenues. The critical role of international governmental organizations (IGOs)—the International Monetary Fund and the World Bank especially—in progressing and in some respects engineering this transformation is clear (Estes & Phillipson, 2002; Phillipson, 2006; Walker & Deacon, 2003). The impact of the IGOs on public pension systems has been particularly severe in central and eastern Europe and in Latin America. The new neoliberal policy consensus encouraged by the IGOs has the power to undermine long-established public pension and social protection schemes and, with them, the historical connection between aging and the welfare state. Against this rather pessimistic scenario must be set the empirical facts that not all western European countries have followed the prescriptions of the IGOs; in fact, it is only a small minority that have done so substantially. The European Union has encouraged a broad approach to pension system reform that includes a focus on adequacy (Walker, 2003), and the World Bank itself has recently modified its views (Holzmann & Hinz, 2005), although the original policy has already had a devastating effect on public pension provision in some countries.

Theorizing the Relationship Between Aging and the Welfare State

The Cultural Turn of Poststructuralism

This is not the place to dwell on the political economy of this transformation in the relationship between aging and the welfare state or its consequences (Estes, 1982, 2004; Estes & Phillipson, 2002; Myles & Quadagno, 1991; Walker &

Deacon, 2003). Underlying it is a general trend toward the "individualization of the social" (Ferge, 1997) in which, increasingly and not only in Western countries, governments are expecting individuals and families to take primary responsibility for risks that were previously guaranteed collectively. This radical change in social policy and the nature of welfare states is theorized not only in terms of political economy, which will be considered later, but also according to the cultural transition from modernity to late (or post) modernity. From this perspective, the purposeful shift in the relationship between aging and the welfare state is entirely predictable, as it demonstrates the breaking down of one of the major structures of modernity, the welfare state, in response to sociocultural changes in society, such as the destandardization of the life course. At the same time, it is argued, these changes open up new opportunities for individual agency, including new lifestyle preferences and choices, that demand new, more flexible institutional responses. Thus, it is argued, as needs become more diversely individual, the bureaucratic social institutions simply cannot respond to them sensitively enough. In contrast to the political economy of aging, therefore, the cultural thesis reinforces and, to some extent, attempts to legitimize the individualization of the social. It must be acknowledged, though, in making such a sweeping generalization that there are many variations in this school of thought, and some of them, with an interest in social policy, seek to reconstruct the welfare state itself into a more responsive form (Biggs, 2001; Giddens, 1998).

The cultural turn in social theory stems from the early 1980s with the pronouncement that social and cultural conditions were postmodern (Lyotard, 1984). In a nutshell, this meant that the "grand narratives" or "metanarratives" of the modernist Enlightenment project of the 18th century were to be abandoned in favor of a looser, fragmentary, heterogeneous and plural, poststructuralist understanding of social life (Harvey, 1989). Despite its critics, especially from the perspective of critical realism (Archer, 1995; Bhaskar, 1989; Sayer, 1992), poststructuralism has had a far-reaching influence. In particular, the idea of a postmodern or late modern condition has been developed in a number of directions, such as "high modernity" or "reflexive modernization," the most influential of which, in social policy terms, is the "risk society" thesis (Beck, 1992; Giddens, 1994). The essence of this analysis is that risks that were predictable and calculable under modern or "Fordist" societal arrangements become unpredictable and incalculable in the risk society. In a similar vein, using the concept of reflexive modernization, Beck, Bonss, and Lau (2003) posit two related modernities: the first consisting of industrialization and the nation-state, within which the welfare state was produced, and the second characterized by reflexivity in which the position of the state and its institutions is weakened along with other key aspects of modern social structure, such as the nuclear family and social class. Summarizing drastically, the social citizenship that was secured under the first modernity, including social rights to pensions and social security, is undermined by globalization, increasing individualization, destandardization of the life course, and the pursuit of diverse lifestyle preferences.

The implications for the welfare state and its major user group are massive (although the precise implications for older people are not considered): survival in a global market, in which uncertainty is manufactured and risks globalized, necessitates fundamental changes in the architecture of modernity. On the one hand, the institutional structures, such as social security and public pensions, have to be transformed, and, on the other, individuals can no longer rely on traditional state or community support systems but, instead, must accept personal responsibility for their lives (Giddens, 1998).

The risk theorists put a heavy emphasis on ecological, scientific, and technological risks. Their analysis of the welfare state rests on what is a functionalist argument that it must be reconstructed in the face of the new, globalized basis of risk. They see the welfare state as a system designed to respond to "external" risks (unemployment and retirement) or "accidents of fate" in Giddens's terms. But, the new form of "manufactured risk" makes obsolete the institutions designed to deal with external risks. According to Giddens (1994), "In an era of manufactured risk—the welfare state cannot continue on in the form in which it developed in the post 1945 settlement," and "the crisis of the welfare state is not purely fiscal, it is a crisis of risk management in a society dominated by a new type of risk" (p. 24).

There is very little evidence, however, for this contention with regard to the welfare state. It is undeniable that citizens face new technological and ecological risks and that many of these are global. But, at the same time, many of the modern risks continue, and there is plenty of evidence that welfare states are able to accommodate newly emerging ones. In fact, when the changing nature of risk in late modern societies is considered, it can be seen how important it is to ensure that collective arrangements are maintained in order to both pool risks and prevent them. Four such major contemporary risks may be highlighted within Europe (Boscoe & Chassard, 1999):

- A reduction in the financial risk associated with old age but with a new risk of becoming unemployable after 50
- The emergence of a new risk associated with longevity: the need for long-term care
- A change in the nature of the labor market and unemployment so that, for the unemployed, it is not just a matter of geographical mobility to find work but also skills mobility to remain employable
- New forms of insecure work with no or very low workers' rights to social protection

It is obvious that these new major forms of risk all have significant direct or indirect implications for old age. Equally obviously, the new risks are borne unequally according to class, gender, race and ethnicity, and so on. Thus, while some are able to make multiple lifestyle choices, others are faced with the insecurities associated with these risks. They also emphasize a fundamental flaw in the risk society analysis: the welfare state was designed to pool risks, to share the social costs of economic progress, and to support accumulation and not just to respond to "external risks." Indeed, in the European Union at least, the indications are that social protection systems are responding to the changing nature of risk, for example, by changing policies toward those over 50 and by introducing support for long-term care (e.g., the extension of social insurance in Germany). Nonetheless, the danger exists that this process of adaptation and, with it, the underlying collectivization of risk will be rejected in some countries in favor of privatization and individualization. This would be perverse, even in the risk society analyst's own terms, because individuals are already at the mercy of a wide variety of new risks and, arguably, should not be needlessly exposed to others. It would undermine the mature welfare states and relocate old age squarely back into the private risk market. It is not inevitable that this will happen, but it could do so if policymakers continue to encourage pessimism about both old age and the capacity of the welfare state to support it and if neo-liberalism remains the dominant response to economic globalization.

The Political Economy of Aging

This critique of the risk society thesis emanates from a political economy perspective that originated because of the need to explore the previously ignored relationship between aging and social policy (Estes, 1979; Guillemard, 1980; Myles, 1984; Walker, 1978). In contrast to poststructuralism, this theoretical perspective is rooted in materialist neo-Marxist sociology, although, later, a second paradigmatic source, critical theory, transformed it into critical gerontology (Baars, Dannefer, Phillipson, & Walker, 2006; Phillipson & Walker, 1987).

The main focus of the early gerontological analyses of political economy took the form of counterarguments to the dominant benign functionalist theories in social gerontology that implied that features of aging in advanced industrial societies were somehow natural or inevitable. For example, economic dependency and poverty were accepted too readily and uncritically as "facts" of old age to which older people had to adjust. The dominant liberal-pluralist framework of social gerontology had, hitherto, paid very little attention to the social construction of old age and the variable impact of aging, especially along class, gender, and ethnic lines (Phillipson, 1982; Townsend, 1981; Walker, 1980, 1981).

Not surprisingly, therefore, the thesis emphasized economic and material dependency and exclusion and argued that they are not an inevitable fact of aging but, in part, the result of conscious thought and action primarily in the form of social policies. Thus, it is not chronological age as such that is the main determinant of economic dependency but rather the socially constructed relationships between, principally, age and the labor market and age and the welfare state. This analysis had the effect of diverting some of the gerontological gaze away from the problems of old age and individual adjustment to features of the aging process toward structural constraints and sources of inclusion or exclusion, such as pension policies, retirement policies, age and sex discrimination, and so on. It emphasized structural inequalities between different groups of older people and focused on two key but then neglected aspects of the aging process: cumulative life course advantages and disadvantages between different groups and the consequences of economic dependency on the state (Dannefer, 2003; Ginn, 2003). It was seen by the scientific community as a radical departure and has provided the basis of an enormous flow of research in this field (Baars et al., 2006). Of particular note is the influential strand of gerontological research on gender and later life (Arber & Ginn, 1991, 1995; Estes, 2001, 2004).

Needless to say, the political economy thesis has been subject to criticism, and it was partly in response to some of this that a broader critical perspective was developed. Before considering one aspect of the critique of the political economy of aging, in case there is any doubt, the continuing need for it is demonstrated briefly here. In its absence, it is possible for gerontologists to accept uncritically both the burden-of-aging proposition, which dominates public policy in the aging field across the globe, and the benign role of IGOs in the development of national responses to population aging. For example, according to Higgs and Gilleard (2006), "Improvement in the standard of living of the retired, if funded by the state, always represented a drain on the resources of the economy" (p. 214). Leaving aside the use of burden-of-aging terminology, in economic terms, regardless of whether pensions are funded by the state, employers, or the individual saver, they represent a call on current consumption or what is termed deferred consumption (Barr, 2001). The key economic issue is not "state funding" but revolves around whether the pension system is pay-as-you-go (PAYG) or prefunded (or a hybrid). On this topic a great deal of inconclusive economic and political heat has been generated about whether funding improves economic performance by, for example, increasing the savings rate or by improving the efficiency of capital and labor markets (Davis & Hu, 2006). Certainly it should not be claimed that rates of return are necessarily higher under funded systems than PAYG ones (Orszag & Stiglitz, 2001). The transition in recent years of some PAYG public pension systems (e.g., Sweden, Italy, Poland, and Latvia) into more actuarially based ones further muddies the distinction (Holzmann & Hinz, 2005). The main point of this illustration is that, without a political economy perspective, it is possible to accept, apparently without critical questioning, the neoliberal economic and political assumptions and prescriptions that currently surround discussions of public pension reform. It is even possible to conclude that social insurance is a threat to the global financial regime (Higgs & Gilleard, 2006).

The same applies to the pronouncements of the global purveyors of neoliberalism: IGOs. Thus, policy prescriptions from the World Bank should not be taken at face value only because they embody a specific ideology concerning the role of the state and, in particular, the primacy of the market (Deacon, Hulse, & Stubbs, 1997; Phillipson, 2006). The idea that the World Bank was simply responding to demographic aging when it published its influential report *Averting the Old Age Crisis* in 1994 rather than attempting to set a global agenda for prefunded pensions, at the very least, should be subject to question (cf. Ervik, 2005; Higgs & Gilleard, 2006). A political economy of aging is required to undertake this critical analysis in exactly the same way as it is needed to assess the pension proposals from very different ideological perspectives, such as the International Labour Office (Gillion, 2000). The fact that much of the critical attention of the political economists of aging has been directed at the policies of neoliberalism is mainly because they represent the major challenge to socioeconomic security in old age and to the social status of older people.

The Cultural Critique of Political Economy

Political economy and the structured dependency theses were never posed in deterministic or purely utilitarian terms, which portrayed older people as helpless pawns in a capitalist conspiracy. They were intended to illuminate the structural features of the aging process—social class, gender, ethnicity, race, sexuality, and so on—and the role of social and economic policies precisely in order to counterbalance the previous overconcentration on individual adjustment and situational factors. Furthermore the focus on old age and the welfare state sought to counterbalance the gerontological tendency to emphasize two very different narratives of aging: the biomedical on the one hand and lifestyle and consumerist culture in old age on the other. Nonetheless, the main recurring criticism of the thesis is that it neglects agency (the ability of individuals to act within, engage with, and change social structures) (Archer, 2000; Barnes, 2000; Weber, 1968). This criticism is factually incorrect, and it is also rather ironic since the thesis originated as a critique of the implicit pessimism of acquiescent functionalism, in assuming that everyone over retirement age was a dependent burden, and for failing to recognize that many of the features associated with old age have their origins in social structures and processes that are beyond the individual's immediate control but that are amenable to collective political action, or social policy. The social construction of old age showed that, in important respects, the risks associated with aging differ between social groups—class/occupation, gender, race, and so on—and that these differences are determined to a large extent prior to old age, and this core message is as true today as it was nearly three decades ago. The trajectories of individual aging are determined by the interaction between social actors (who are also unique genetic and anatomical creations) and social structures but in conditions of relative power and powerlessness.

Nonetheless, the concepts of structured dependency and political economy have suggested to some gerontologists a view of action as overdetermined by external forces. This is not the way it was intended, and it is important to realize the limitations of the "structural" metaphor when structures are created by the actions and thoughts of people (Giddens, 1984; Weber, 1968). It is equally important to understand that agency may be exercised by not acting, for example, in refusing to claim a means-tested social security benefit, an issue that figured significantly in the early U.K. versions of the political economy thesis. However, this concept was said to limit the scope for individuals to construct their own meanings and destinies. This, in turn, led to interactionist and ethnographic approaches emphasizing agency in terms of the construction of social relations through everyday encounters (Gubrium & Holstein, 2002; Gubrium & Wallace, 1990; Kuypers & Bengtson, 1984). Unfortunately, microsociological gerontological perspectives have tended to ignore the constraints of structure and, therefore, have unnecessarily diverted attention from the sources of inequality in old age.

The latest addition to the gerontological literature that follows this path in overestimating agency is the "cultures-of-aging" thesis advanced by Gilleard and Higgs (2000). While this analysis is important in directing attention to aging as a cultural phenomenon and points the way to research on antiaging technologies and the "staying-young" culture, in trying to suggest that political economy insights are no longer relevant and have been replaced by a "culture of personal identity" its authors commit the very sin that they criticize the political economists for: one-sidedness. Unfortunately, in this case, there is no evidence to support the argument that old age has been transformed into one characterized by enhanced status and "agentic" power, even among those in their third age. Moreover, there is good evidence of the variations in the exercise of individual autonomy in later life both between social groups and across similar countries (Hagan Hennessy & Walker, 2004; Walker, 2005).

The cultures-of-aging argument may be criticized on numerous grounds, but that is not the purpose here (Walker, 2002). Its relevance for this discussion is that it purveys a false choice between agency and identity on the one hand and structural determination on the other (Gilleard & Higgs, 2000). Political economy (which is wrongly conflated with structured dependency) is caricatured as suggesting that aging is something that happens to people, while cultural explanations see aging as something that individuals have to engage with (Gilleard & Higgs, 2000):

> *Whatever heuristic value it once possessed, structured dependency theory and the "political economy" approach no longer provide a satisfactory understanding of ageing and old age. Post-work lives have become richer and more complex. Not only has this approach failed to acknowledge the agency that individuals exercise in retirement but it has signally failed to recognise the diversity of the social processes and structure that shape the choices available to people in later life. (Gilleard & Higgs, 2000, p. 193)*

As noted previously, the political economy thesis highlighted the neglected but critical role of policy; it did not suggest that policy explains everything. The previous quotation fails to recognize that there are two key elements in the political economy of aging. One is the structural impact of social and economic roles and statuses prior to retirement, and the other is the impact of retirement itself. This cultural critique focuses only on the second. It rightly observes growing affluence in Western society and a diminution in the impact of retirement on some groups, opening up new opportunities. However, in overemphasizing the potential for agency, the extent of the changes that have taken place and the degree of autonomy enjoyed by third agers are also overestimated—the gender fault line being a case in point (Ginn, 2003). Of course, how people respond individually to their own aging is a legitimate and vital aspect of microsociological analysis. Such research can reveal important narratives about how different older people negotiate old age to construct a life of quality and how creative they are in doing so (Kellaher, Peace, & Holland, 2004) and similarly with the variations in the exercise of agency by older people in different ethnic and cultural groups (Moriarty & Butt, 2004; Nazroo et al., 2004; Wray, 2003). Furthermore, it is an empirical question whether dependency on the state for pensions on the one hand and dependency on the agents of "gray capitalism" controlling the private pension funds on the other represent fundamentally different experiences (Blackburn, 2002). A serious problem arises, however, when it is suggested that the equally necessary structural analyses are no longer relevant because of factors such as increased "diversity." Leaving aside the fact that the political economy perspective was responsible for highlighting diversity in old age, in terms of structural inequalities, the evidence of continuing structural divisions based on class, age, gender, sexuality, disability, race, and ethnicity demand, in both scientific and moral terms, continued analyses. In practice, it is possible to combine these strands of analysis (Daatland & Biggs, 2006).

On the policy front, the optimism of the cultural thesis concerning the new aging, as shown earlier, can lead to a completely uncritical perspective. This entails the wholesale acceptance of the risk society thesis, as articulated by Giddens (1994, 1998), that the crumbling of the structures of modernity opens up new opportunities for agency and that, in a future era when everyone follows a different life course pattern, standardized social institutions cannot possibly respond sensitively to individual needs. In short, as emphasized here, such arguments reinforce the case for the individualization of risk and the privatization of the welfare state.

Theorizing the Social

The cultural critique of the political economy of aging is inadequate in terms of both evidence and theory. Moreover, it implies the detachment of scientific research from engagement with policy issues that have a huge potential impact on older people's lives, such as the choice between public and private pensions. The uncritical acceptance of the policy prescriptions of the risk society analysis unwittingly condones the neoliberal perspective on globalization that leads down a path of state residualization—in pensions and health and social care—and the individualization of the social. For more than two decades, the political-economy-of-aging perspective has provided a counterargument to neoliberalism by demonstrating over and over again the unequal impact of its policies on different groups of older people and the cumulative disadvantage that can accrue from such policies toward young and middle-aged people. But when the dominant global policy perspective focuses on the inevitability of inequality, with some even celebrating it as "diversity," this perspective is in danger of becoming sidelined as a worthy academic theory but one that is increasingly irrelevant to the "real world" of late modernity.

Of course, this marginalization is not peculiar to social gerontology; it is part of the wider struggle that the sociologically based social sciences have been losing with the economic one since the breakup of political economy and, especially over the past 50 years as the economic has become preeminent in the policy field. The core problem is that the *social,* for example, in social policy lacks the coherent theory and clear policy prescriptions claimed by the economic world (Walker, 1984). This challenge to theorize the social to both understand it and to pave the way for the creation of an authentic, independent rationale for social action and social policy has been taken up in Europe by the development of the "social quality" concept. It is employed here because it provides the foundations for a new approach to social policy and, in particular, to the relationship between aging and the welfare state and because it may have something to contribute to a better understanding of the tension between agency and structure in the field of gerontology.

The concept of social quality was created a decade ago as the starting point for a new approach to policy based on a revised relationship between economic and social development. The immediate European pressures behind this work need not concern us here, but part of the practical case for a new approach was the threat posed to the European Union's welfare states by the Transatlantic Consensus on economic globalization (Beck, van der Maesen, & Walker, 1997; Beck, Van der Maesen, & Walker, 2001; Walker, 1999).

In theoretical terms, it was the disappearance from social science of a clear understanding of the social that was the main impetus. Over time, the scientific distinction between the social and the individual has become entrenched, and, as noted previously, in recent decades the latter has taken analytical precedence over the former (Ferge, 1997). There is, in the social sciences, an increasing preoccupation with individual lifestyles, preferences, choices, consumptions, well-being, and quality of life, and, as we have seen, gerontology is no less immune to this "cultural turn" than other disciplines. While this paradigm offers rich possibilities in the exploration of the new dynamics of later life (Daatland & Biggs, 2006), too often its key concepts—lifestyles, consumption, preferences, and so on—have been constructed in highly individualized terms. The challenge, therefore, for both social analysis and policy is that the social is not only normatively assumed but also indirectly defined as an external entity, detached from the process of individual decision making and, therefore, not requiring either definition or understanding. The social quality concept starts from the assumption that this dominant paradigm of social science and policy is based on a false premise that the individual and society are in contradistinction. In Elias's (2000) words,

> *To understand the obstruction which the predominant modes of thinking and feeling pose to the investigation of longer-term changes of social structure and personality structure . . . it is not enough to trace the development of the image of people as societies, the image of society. It is also necessary to keep in mind the development of the image of people as individuals, the image of personality . . . one of the peculiarities of the traditional human self-image is that people often speak and think of individuals and societies as if these were two phenomena existing separately—of which, moreover, one is often considered "real" and the other "unreal"—instead of two different aspects of the same human being. (p. 468)*

The explicit theoretical aim, therefore, was to tackle this counterproductive duality that has bred confusion as well as preventing the formation of effective social policies. This account focuses on this theoretical endeavor rather than the other, more policy-oriented aspects of social quality (Beck et al. 1997, 2001).

At the heart of the social, it is contended, is the self-realization of individuals as social beings. Thus, the social is the outcome of constantly changing processes through which people, to a greater or lesser extent, realize themselves as interacting social beings. This assumes, first of all, that individuals are essentially social actors. Furthermore, individuality is a function of the social nature of humans. Rather than being the atomized economic agents of utilitarianism and neoliberalism, an individual's self-realization depends on social interaction and, especially, social recognition (Honneth, 1996). Second, therefore, the contexts for self-realization are social interactions or collective identities. There is, in other words, a constitutive interdependency between individual self-realization and the formation of collective identities (Bhaskar, 1993). Needless to say, these are dynamic relationships that change, in interaction with each other, over time. Third, in order to have the competence to act socially, individuals require the capacity for self-reference, which, again, is produced by the combination of self-realization and collective identities. Finally, there must be a "framing structure," the constructed or natural environment that creates opportunities, potential, and barriers or contingencies (such as social exclusion). Thus, the constitutive interdependency (between self-realization and the formation of collective identities) is the basic condition for the social, and this is constructed, in various expressions, by the relationships between competent social actors and their framing structure.

The historical starting points for the constitutive interdependency outlined here are created by the interactions of two reciprocal tensions. These may be illustrated by a two-dimensional model (Figure 32.1). The horizontal axis mirrors the tension between systems, institutions, and organizations on the one hand and communities, families, networks, and so on on the other. This corresponds to Lockwood's (1999) interpretation of the dynamics between system integration and social integration and also Habermas's (1987) distinction between the formally organized system and the communicatively structured lifeworld (although he posits to an antagonistic relationship between them). In social quality theory, the horizontal plane is a field of interactions between unequal actors with both poles being separate but dependent on each other (Beck et al., 2001). The vertical axis is the field of opportunities, whether realized or not, and represents the tension between societal and biographical development (Weyman & Heinz, 1996).

32.1

Reciprocity between two basic tensions.

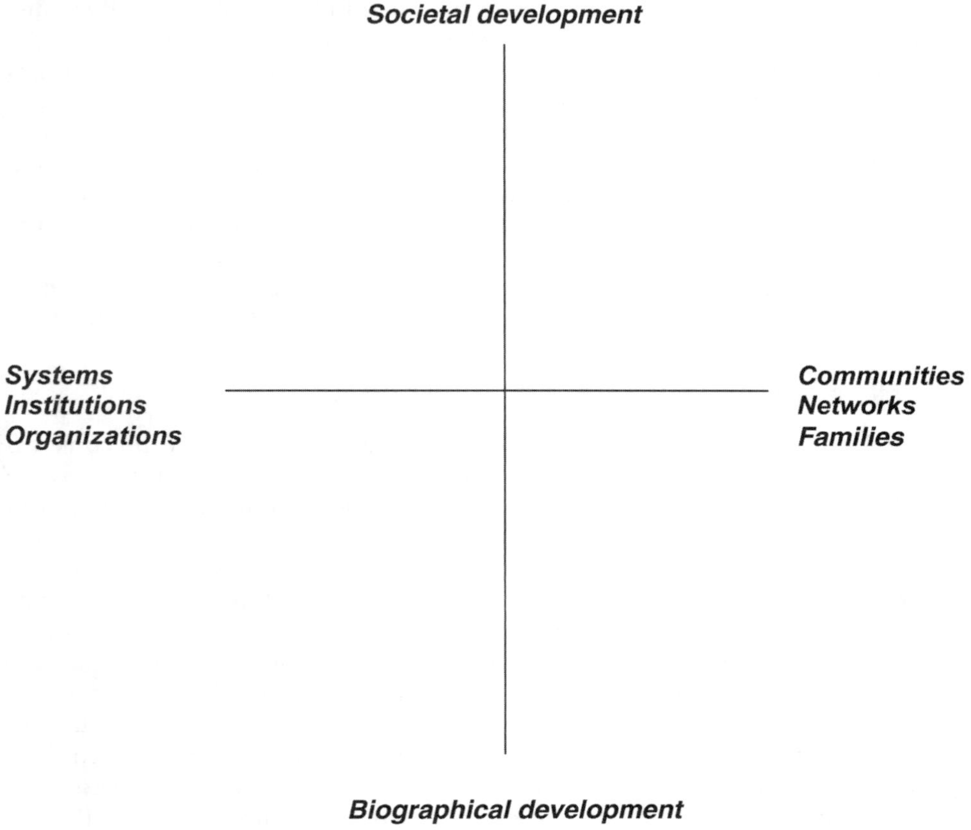

Societal development

Systems
Institutions
Organizations

Communities
Networks
Families

Biographical development

This is not a reflection of discourse theory and its individual focus but, rather, a multiperspective approach that attempts to connect symbols, meanings, constructions, values, norms, traditions, and cognition at both levels. The pursuit of opportunities for self-realization across this field occurs in both the lifeworld and the world of systems, as well as at their intersections.

This theoretical perspective is basically a critical realist one because it accepts that society does not exist independently of human activity or the product of it (Bhaskar, 1978). It has much in common with Giddens's (1981) theory of structuration but goes beyond it, with the critical realists, in arguing that all social life is embedded in a network in the sense of social relations and that social identities (here labeled collective identities) are constituted relationally (Bhaskar, 1979).

To conclude this theoretical excursion, the interaction between processes of self-realization and those concerning the construction of collective identities brings into operation four factors that seem to be essential to translate the competence of the self-referential individual into social action. In other words, if people are to take part in collective identities in order to realize themselves, these four factors are decisive in determining their scope for action in the face of opportunities or contingencies (the vertical axis) and the forms that these interactions may take (the horizontal axis). The four factors that contribute to the constitution of social actors are personal (human) security, social recognition, social responsiveness, and personal (human) capacities. As illustrated in Figure 32.2, these four factors may be located within the tensional field created by the two-dimensional model in Figure 32.1. It is not intended to imply that the influence of these factors is confined to each sector of the quadrangle, but they are located where their primary role is played.

Once reflexive social actors are constituted as such, they may participate in collective identities to experience as well as manufacture social quality. The extent to which there are opportunities to do this is determined by four conditional factors that are appropriately located in the fields of action shown in Figure 32.1: socioeconomic security (top left), social cohesion (top right), social inclusion (bottom left), and social empowerment (bottom right). Again these primary locations do not imply that there are no cross influences (Beck et al., 2001).

Structure and Agency Across the Life Course

The gerontological relevance of this theoretical understanding of the constitution of the social is, first, that it creates a platform for the conceptualization of social policy with its own distinct rationale in relation to other aspects of policy, especially the economic one. This could enable the field to move beyond the increasingly lame moral or utilitarian appeals against whatever economic ideology prevails at a particular historical moment (although there will always be a moral case for the welfare state). Certainly, without an autonomous rationale for social policy, there is little hope of a revised relationship between aging and the welfare state in which economic ideology is not dominant. Second, it offers the prospect of measuring the relative quality of the social in different countries and communities. For example, comparative studies of the extent to which older people experience socioeconomic security, social cohesion, social inclusion, and social empowerment will tell us the extent to which they are able to participate

32.2

The constitutional factors of social quality.

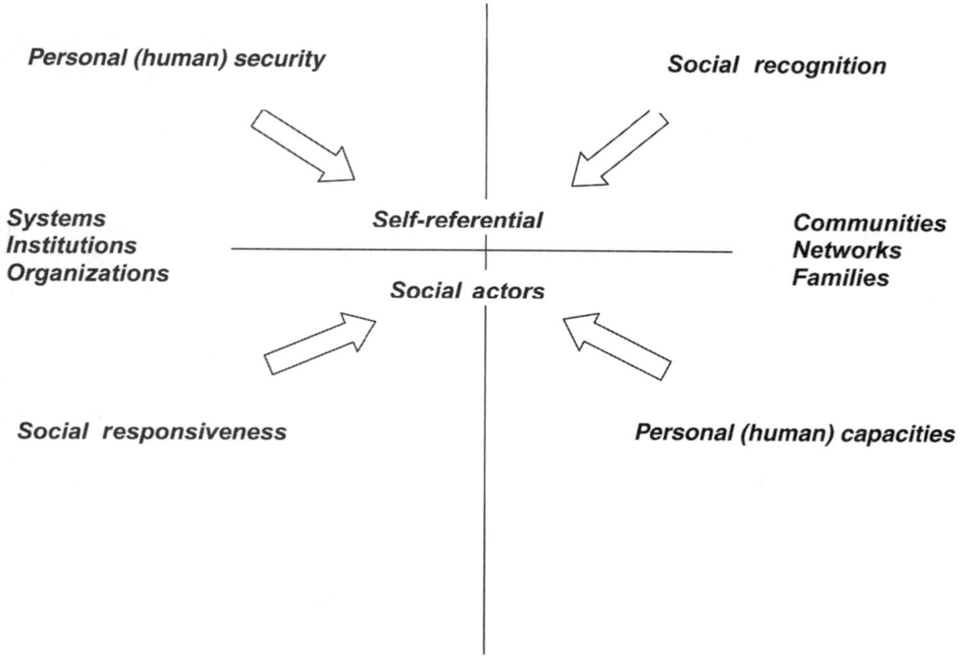

in social and economic life and how enabling are a country's welfare and other institutions. Third, by providing a methodology for understanding the constant tension between structure and agency in everyday life, including over the life course, it points the way to reconcile the critiques that political economy overemphasizes structure on the one hand (Gilleard & Higgs, 2000) while life course and some cultural perspectives overemphasize agency on the other (Dannefer & Uhlenburgh, 1999). Moreover, the conceptual approach to the social outlined here defines the relationship between social structures and human agency while retaining the distinctiveness of both of them. This contrasts with Elias's (1978) work on figuration and Giddens's (1984) theory of structuration in which the two are constitutionally enmeshed. In practice, they are not a dichotomy but rather two sides of the same coin (Layder, 1994).

Focusing on the third point, in practical terms we have the basis, if not yet a fully honed theoretical construction, to understand the interaction between agency and structure over the life course. Older people themselves are not isolated, atomized individual agents or subjects focusing only on their own identities; rather, they are interacting with and changing social structures. In fact, as Barnes (2000) has argued, social life consists of "collective agency" in which nonindependent people routinely affect each others' actions. As reflexive social subjects, older people are able to exercise the choices of agency concerning their lifestyles and approach to aging, just as when they were younger adults they decided (within constraints) on careers, housing, family formation, and so on. But these choices are always exercised within immediate and historical structural relations, and, depending on structural category, large numbers of younger and older people are not able to make any choices whatsoever about key aspects of their lives, such as about the age they retire, their level of income, and their access to health care and long-term care. Nonetheless, how they negotiate and respond to aging and the values that older people place on different aspects of their lives varies across a very broad range and is certainly not mechanically predetermined by position in the social structure. It is a matter of the continual pursuit of self-realization within collective identities that is subject to four critical conditions (as outlined previously). At earlier stages of the life course, the choice of a pension plan, for example, is not an open one; rather, it is constrained by structures such as class, gender, and race (mainly by their influence on occupation) and by factors such as income and health. Forgoing occupation and income altogether or taking part-time employment to care for an older relative or child will also have a bearing on the choices available (Evandrou & Glaser, 2003, 2004).

In other words, agency is embedded within structure. As individuals pursue identity and self-realization, they must interact with others, and in doing so they will sometimes have to compromise or simply conform to formal or informal rules, sometimes be able to exercise choice or resist constraints, and sometimes encounter good or bad luck. The ways that they exercise this agency are diverse, such as between ethnic and religious groups (Torres, 1999; Wray, 2003), as are the meanings given to autonomy and the values that they place in individual as opposed to collective action. A key question that requires further investigation is, What problems are structurally induced for older people: problems that are inevitable and must be responded to by them in their own individual or collective ways? This points to the negative aspects of social action where agency is constrained, sometimes severely, with an individual being on the receiving end with no freedom to influence another individual or an institution but only to frame their response, and in situations of abuse or extreme social exclusion, even this latter autonomy is very limited. It also reminds us of the point made earlier that the choice not to do something is a legitimate exercise of agency. A second key research question concerns the role of social policy—and the welfare state in particular—and the extent to which its institutions facilitate or obstruct the processes of self-realization engaged in by older people. Addressing this question on a comparative basis would open up a rich vein of research on the role of the social in the constitution of well-being in later life.

Conclusion

This brings us back to where we started: the welfare state and the role of social policy. Risk pooling and collective support ideally should enable people to make choices and limit the structural constraints on them. In addition, ideally welfare arrangements should promote socioeconomic security, social cohesion, social inclusion, and social empowerment. An interesting empirical question is how far the different welfare regimes do so. Thus, the roles of the welfare state should be to promote choice and flexibility and to empower people to negotiate their way through the rapidly changing life course. Public structures and constitutions should enable, not inhibit, individual and collective agency. Moreover, the welfare state should not be seen as the alternative to agency because down that route lies the individualization of the social, based on the false assumptions that the market is the only source of choice and that human beings are merely individual economic agents.

References

Arber, S., & Ginn, J. (1991). *Gender and later life.* London: Sage.

Arber, S., & Ginn, J. (Eds.). (1995). *Connecting gender and ageing,* Buckingham: Open University Press.

Archer, M. (1995). *Realist social theory: The morphogenic approach.* Cambridge: Cambridge University Press.

Archer, M. (2000). *Being human: The problem of agency.* Cambridge: Cambridge University Press.

Baars, J., Dannefer, D., Phillipson C., & Walker, A. (Eds.). (2006). *Aging, globalisation and inequality,* Amityville, NY: Baywood Publishing.

Barnes, B. (2000). *Understanding ageing: Social theory and responsible action.* Camden, NJ: Sage.

Barr, N. (2001). *The welfare state as a piggy bank.* Oxford: Oxford University Press.

Beck, U. (1992). *The risk society.* Camden, NJ: Sage.

Beck, U., Bonss, W., & Lau, C. (2003). The theory of reflexive modernisation: Problematic, hypotheses and research programme. *Theory, Culture and Society, 20,* 1–33.

Beck, W., van der Maesen, L., & Walker, A. (Eds.). (1997). *The social quality of Europe.* The Hague: Kluwer International.

Beck, W., van der Maesen, L., Thomése F., & Walker, A. (Eds.) (2001). *Social quality: A vision for Europe.* The Hague: Kluwer International.

Bhaskar, R. (1978). *A realist theory of science.* Brighton: Harvester Press.

Bhaskar, R. (1979). *The possibility of naturalism.* Brighton: Harvester Press.

Bhaskar, R. (1989). *Reclaiming reality: A critical introduction to contemporary philosophy,* London: Verso.

Bhaskar, R. (1993). *Dialectic: The pulse for freedom.* London: Verso.

Biggs, S. (2001). Towards critical narrativity: Stories of aging in contemporary social policy. *Journal of Aging Studies, 15,* 303–316.

Binstock, R. H. (1991). From the great society to the aging society—25 years of the Older Americans Act. *Generations, 15*(3), 11–18.

Blackburn, R. (2002). *Banking on death.* London: Verso.

Boscoe, A., & Chassard, Y. (1999). A shift in the paradigm: Surveying the European Union discourse on welfare and work. In M. Heikkila (Ed.), *Linking welfare and work* (pp. 43–58). Dublin: European Foundation.

Daatland, S. O., & Biggs, S. (Eds.). (2006). *Ageing and diversity.* Bristol: Policy Press.

Dannefer, D. (2003). Cumulative advantage/disadvantage and the life course. *Journal of Gerontology: Social Sciences, 58,* 5327–5337.

Dannefer, D., & Uhlenburgh, P. (1999). Paths of the life course: A typology. In V. Bengtson & W. Schaie (Eds.), *Handbook of theories of aging* (pp. 306–326). New York: Springer Publishing.

Davis, E. P., & Hu, Y-W. (2006). Funding, saving and economic growth. In G. Clark, A. Munnell, & J. M. Orszag (Eds.), *The Oxford handbook of pensions and retirement income* (pp. 201–218). Oxford: Oxford University Press.

Deacon, B., Hulse, M., & Stubbs, P. (1997). *Global social policy: International organisations and the future of welfare.* London: Sage.

Elias, N. (1978). *What is sociology?,* London: Hutchinson.

Elias, N. (2000). *The civilising process.* Oxford: Blackwell.

Ervik, R. (2005). Battle of future pensions: Global accounting tools, international organisations and pension reform. *Global Social Policy, 5,* 6–30.

Esping-Andersen, G. (1990). *The three worlds of welfare capitalism.* Oxford: Polity Press.

Estes, C. (1979). *The ageing enterprise.* San Francisco: Jossey-Bass.

Estes, C. L. (1982). Austerity and aging in the US. *International Journal of Health Services, 12,* 573–584.

Estes, C. (2001). From gender to the political economy of ageing. *European Journal of Social Quality, 2,* 28–56.

Estes, C. L. (2004). Social Security privatisation and older women: A feminist political economy perspective. *Journal of Aging Studies, 18,* 9–26.

Estes, C., & Phillipson, C. (2002). The globalisation of capital, the welfare state and old age policy. *International Journal of Health Services, 32,* 279–297.

European Commission. (2006). *Adequate and sustainable pensions,* Luxembourg: Office for Official Publications of the European Communities.

Evandrou, M., & Glaser, K. (2003). *Family work and quality of life: Changing economic and social roles* (GO Findings 5). Sheffield: Growing Older Programme, University of Sheffield.

Evandrou, M., & Glaser, K. (2004). Family, work and quality of life: Changing economic and social roles through the lifecourse. *Ageing & Society, 24,* 771–792.

Ferge, Z. (1997). A central European perspective on the social quality of Europe. In W. Beck, L. van der Maesen, & A. Walker (Eds.), *The social quality of Europe* (pp. 165–181). The Hague: Kluwer International.

Giddens, A. (1981). *A contemporary critique of historical materialism.* London: Macmillan.

Giddens, A. (1984). *The constitution of society.* Cambridge: Printing Press.

Giddens, A. (1994). *Beyond left and right.* Cambridge: Polity Press.

Giddens, A. (1998). *The third way.* Cambridge: Polity Press.

Gilleard, C., & Higgs, P. (2000). *Cultures of ageing.* Harlow: Prentice Hall.

Gillion, C. (Ed.). (2000). *Social Security pensions: Development and reform.* Geneva: International Labour Organization.

Ginn, J. (2003). *Gender pensions and the lifecourse.* Bristol: Policy Press.

Gubrium, J., & Holstein, J. (2002). Going concerns and their bodies. *Cultural Gerontology, 11,* 191–206.

Gubrium, J., & Wallace, J. (1990). Who theorises age? *Ageing & Society, 10,* 131–149.

Guillemard, A. M. (1980). *La vieillesse et l'etat.* Paris: Presses Universitaires de France.

Habermas, J. (1987). *The theory of communicative action.* Cambridge: Polity Press.

Hagan Hennessy, C., & Walker, A. (2004). *Growing older: Quality of life in old age.* Hemel Hempstead: McGraw-Hill.

Harvey, D. (1989). *The condition of post-modernity.* Oxford: Blackwell.

Higgs, P., & Gilleard, C. (2006). Class, power and inequality in later life. In S. V. Daatland & S. Biggs (Eds.), *Ageing and diversity* (pp. 207–221). Bristol: Policy Press.

Holzmann, R., & Hinz, R. (2005). *Old age income support in the 21st century.* Washington, DC: World Bank.

Honneth, A. (1996). *The struggle for recognition—The moral grammar of social conflicts.* Cambridge: Polity Press.

Jacobzone, S. (2003). *Healthy ageing and the challenges of new technologies.* The Geneva Papers, *28*(2), 254–274.

Kellaher, L., Peace, S., & Holland, C. (2004). Environment, identity and old age—Quality of life or a life of quality? In A. Walker & C. Hagan Hennessy (Eds.), *Growing older: Quality of life in old age.* (pp. 60–80). Maidenhead: Oxford University Press.

Kuypers, J., & Bengtson, V. (1984). Perspectives on the older family. In W. Quinn & G. Houghston (Eds.), *Independent aging, family and social systems perspectives* (pp. 3–19). Rockville, MD: Aspen Systems.

Layder, D. (1994). *Understanding social theory.* London: Sage.

Lockwood, D. (1999). Civic integration and social cohesion. In I. Gough & G. Olofsson (Eds.), *Capitalism and social cohesion: Essays on exclusion and integration* (pp. 63–85). London: Macmillan.

Lyotand, J. (1984). *The postmodern condition.* Manchester: Manchester University.

Marshall, V., Cook, F., & Marshall, J. (1993). Conflict over generational equity: Rhetoric and reality in a comparative context. In V. Bengtson & W. A. Achenbaum (Eds.), *The changing contract across generations* (pp. 119–140). New York: Aldine de Gruyter.

Moriarty, J., & Butt, J. (2004). Inequalities in quality of life among older people from different ethnic groups. *Ageing & Society, 24,* 729–754.

Myles, J. (1984). *Old age in the welfare state.* Bosten: Little Brown.

Myles, J., & Quadagno, J. (Eds.). (1991). *States, labor markets and the future of old age policy.* Philadelphia: Temple University Press.

Nazroo, J., Bajekal, M. Blane, D., & Grewal, I. (2004). Ethnic inequalities. In A. Walker & C. Hagan Hennessy (Eds.), *Growing older* (pp. 35–59). Maidenhead, England: McGraw Hill.

O'Connor, J. (1977). *The fiscal crisis of the state.* London: St. Martin's Press.

Organization for Economic Cooperation and Development. (1988). *Reforming public pensions.* Paris: Author.

Orszag, P., & Stiglitz, J. (2001). Rethinking pension reform: Ten myths about social security systems. In R. Holzmann & J. Stiglitz (Eds.), *New ideas about old age security* (pp. 17–56). Washington, DC: World Bank.

Phillipson, C. (1982). *Capitalism and the construction of old age.* London: Macmillan.

Phillipson, C. (2006). Aging and globalisation: Issues for critical gerontology and political economy. In J. Baars, D. Dannefer, C. Phillipson, & A. Walker (Eds.), *Aging, globalisation and inequality* (pp. 43–58). Amityville, NY: Baywood Publishing.

Phillipson, C., & Walker, A. (1987). The case for a critical gerontology. In S. de Gregario (Ed.), *Social gerontology: New directions* (pp. 1–19), London: Gower.

Robine, J. M. (2003). The relevance of population health indicators. *Journal of Epidemiology Community Health, 57,* 318.

Sayer, A. (1992). *Method in social science: A realist approach.* London: Routledge.

Torres, S. (1999). A culturally relevant theoretical framework for the study of successful ageing. *Ageing and Society, 19,* 33–51.

Townsend, P. (1981). The structured dependency of the elderly: The creation of social policy in the twentieth century. *Ageing & Society, 1,* 5–28.

Townsend, P. (1986). Ageism and social policy. In C. Phillipson & A. Walker (Eds.), *Ageing and social policy* (pp. 15–44). Aldershot: Gower.

Walker, A. (1978, July). *The social construction of old age.* Paper presented to the World Congress of Sociology, Uppsala, Sweden.

Walker A. (1980). The social creation of poverty and dependency in old age. *Journal of Social Policy, 9,* 49–75.

Walker, A. (1981). Towards a political economy of old age. *Ageing & Society, 1,* 73–94.

Walker, A. (1984). *Social planning.* Oxford: Blackwell.

Walker, A. (1990). The economic "burden" of ageing and the prospect of intergenerational conflict. *Ageing & Society, 10,* 377–396.

Walker, A. (1991). Thatcherism and the new politics of old age. In J. Myles & J. Quadagno (Eds.), *States, labor markets and the future of old age policy* (pp. 19–36). Philadelphia: Temple University Press.

Walker, A. (1993). Poverty and inequality in old age. In J. Bond, P. Coleman, & S. Peace (Eds.), *Ageing in society* (2nd ed., pp. 280–303). London: Sage.

Walker, A. (1999). Public policy and theories of ageing: Constructing and reconstructing old age. In V. Bengtson & K. Schaie (Eds.), *Handbook of theories of ageing* (pp. 361–378). New York: Springer Publishing.

Walker, A. (2002, September). *Cultures of ageing—A critique.* Paper presented to the British Society of Gerontology Annual Conference, Birmingham.

Walker, A. (2003). Securing the future of old age in Europe. *Journal of Societal and Social Policy, 2,* 13–32.

Walker, A. (Ed.). (2005). *Growing older in Europe.* Hemel Hempstead, UK: McGraw-Hill.

Walker, A., & Deacon, B. (2003). Economic globalisation and policies on ageing. *Journal of Societal and Social Policy, 2,* 1–18.

Weber, M. (1968). *Economy and society.* New York: Bedminster Press.

Weyman, A., & Heinz, W. (Eds.). (1996). *Society and biography: Interrelationships between social structure, institutions and the life course.* Weiheim: Deutscher Studien Verlag.

Wray, S. (2003). Women growing older: Agency, ethnicity and culture. *Sociology, 37,* 511–527.

33 Reconstructing Theories of Aging: The Impact of Globalization on Critical Gerontology

Chris Phillipson

The aim of this chapter is to explore a range of issues raised by the relationship between globalization and the acceleration of population aging. Debates around the theme of globalization remain influential in many areas of the social sciences, notably in sociology, economics, and political science (Held & McGrew, 2007a; Ritzer, 2007). Social gerontology has also joined the debate about the influence of globalization, for example, through work in the field of critical gerontology and political economy (Baars, Dannefer, Phillipson, & Walker, 2006; Estes & Phillipson, 2002; Vincent, 2003; Walker & Deacon, 2003). Such attention might be said to be consistent with the need to investigate what Bengtson, Putney, and Johnson (2005) refer to as the "structural contexts of aging," and the effect of these on "processes of aging independent of individual action" (p. 17). This work might also be seen as reflecting the call to bring macrosociological questions back into focus in gerontology, providing a correction to what Hagestad and Dannefer (2001) refer to as the "persistent tendency towards microfication in social science approaches to ageing" (p. 4).

The main argument developed in this chapter is that the phenomenon of globalization raises important new issues for the development of theory in social gerontology. In general, globalization confirms the importance of locating individuals within the orbit of social and economic structures, these increasingly subject to forces lying beyond the boundaries of the nation-state. At the same time, globalization has also been linked to the abandonment of those routines and institutions established in what Giddens (1991) refers to as "the first phase of modernity." Giddens (1991) and Ulrich Beck (1992, 2000) argue that we are now living in a "posttraditional society" where in comparison with the past there is greater emphasis on developing new lifestyles and making fresh choices about the conduct of daily life. This transformed cultural, economic, and social context will, it is argued, provide important challenges for the application of social theory in gerontology.

The chapter is divided into five main sections. The first section reviews the development of critical perspectives within the field of aging. The second section considers the relationship between gerontology and the impact of globalization. The third section reviews more broadly the potential influence of globalizing processes on population aging. The fourth and fifth sections draw out some specific examples of how globalization is affecting social theory in gerontology, examining issues relating to social structure, social identity, and citizenship.

Social Theory and Critical Gerontology

Social theory in gerontology brings together a variety of intellectual streams, reflecting in large measure shifts in sociological perspectives over the past 50 years (Phillipson & Baars, 2007). Over the past 10 years, one particular strand—critical gerontology—has been especially prominent, although this approach itself follows a number of paths, building on perspectives from feminism, the humanities, and political economy (Baars, 2006; Minkler & Estes, 1999; see also chapter 32 in this volume). Central to the approach taken by critical gerontology is the idea of aging as a socially constructed experience and process (Walker, 1981). In respect of political economy, this is seen to reflect the role of elements such as the state and economy in the social construction of old age (Estes, 1979, 1999). The interaction between these areas is viewed as creating significant inequalities in the experience of growing old, especially in relation to living standards, life expectancy, and expectations of daily living. The task thus becomes that of developing a critical analysis of processes that lead to empowerment and control for some older people while creating dependency and powerlessness for others (Hendricks & Leedham, 1991).

The first phase of critical gerontology, stretching over the period from 1980 to the late 1990s, was built around the application of a range of disciplinary perspectives (e.g., Marxist approaches, conflict theory, psychoanalytic perspectives, and the Frankfurt school) to problems of inequality and exploitation affecting older people within individual nation-states (Estes, Biggs, & Phillipson, 2003). Problems associated with what Townsend (1981) defined as "structured dependency," to take one example, were linked to forms of welfare organization, these viewed as contributing to the experience of alienation and poverty in old age (Phillipson, 1982; Walker, 1981). The strength of this approach, as well as that from historical and sociological work outside critical gerontology, in part arose from its linkage to clearly defined national settings, this contributing to a narrative that combined a nation's history with that of the emergence of older people as a social group (Fischer, 1977; Thane, 2000).

This research was complemented by work exploring the nature of citizenship, with particular emphasis on the influence of T. H. Marshall (1964). The main focus of Marshall's work concerned exploring links between the nation-state on the one hand and citizenship on the other (see further discussion later). In this tradition, as Delanty (2000) notes, citizenship was viewed as "the internal or domestic face of nationality" (p. 51). In the case of old age, the provision of care and support was viewed as an example of the way in which the state sought to modify class-based inequalities operating within national borders. Critical gerontology was in part a response to the perceived limitations of these policies and in particular their construction of older people as a "passive" social group (Estes, 1979). In the case of political economy, an important element in this work was exploring the role of the state in regulating and distributing life chances through the life course, with the social production of inequalities in old age a significant outcome of this process (Estes & Associates, 2001).

By the end of the 1990s, the need to extend approaches beyond the nation-state had become apparent. Pressures on welfare states were increasingly global rather than national in scope (Dannefer, 2003). The *globalization* of capital itself had a destabilizing effect in many spheres, most notably on the organization of work and welfare (Beck, 2000; Sennett, 2006). Anthony Giddens (1999) describes two views on globalization: those of the "skeptics," who view globalization as a myth, not altogether different from earlier transformational changes in society, and those of the "radicals," who view globalization as real and with consequences that are largely indifferent to national borders (see further discussion later). Giddens (1999) himself takes the view of the "radicals," noting that globalization is revolutionary on multiple economic, political, cultural, and societal levels. He argues that globalization is characterized by a complex set of forces, embodied by contradictory, oppositional processes that pull away power and influence from the local and nation-state levels while also creating new pressures for local autonomy and cultural identity.

To explore the previous argument in more detail, the next section of this chapter examines the impact of globalization on key institutions affecting the lives of older people and the institutions with which they are associated.

Social Theory, Gerontology, and Globalization

In general terms, globalization has produced a distinctive stage in the history of aging, with tensions between nation-state–based policies concerning demographic change as compared with those formulated by global actors and institutions. To fully appreciate the impact of globalization requires going back to the development of social gerontology, in particular the time from the late 1940s to the early 1970s. Lash and Urry (1987) define this period as dominated by "organized capitalism," reflected in the intensification of mass production techniques (or "Fordism"), a context of full employment, and the development of public sector services (with older people major beneficiaries). This period produce a distinctive framework for regulating and managing policies relating to aging. The outcome was what has been referred to as the "modernization of aging" (Gilleard & Higgs, 2005; Phillipson, 1998), created through the rapid expansion of biomedicine, the emergence of retirement, and the growth of the welfare state (Conrad, 1992; Graebner, 1980).

The steady growth in the proportion of elderly people in the population was, at least until the 1970s, managed in Western societies through the institution of retirement on the one side and the construction of the welfare state on the other. These elements created the social, economic, and moral space within which growing numbers of people were supported. At the same time, these institutions started the process of developing a *narrative* (in the context of a work-focused society) for *being* an older person, on the one hand, acceptance of retirement from work but maintaining activity for as long as possible—articulated in role theory and related perspectives—and, on the other, the idea of support from the state as a "reward" for a lifetime of labor. These elements became the institutional pathways through which old age was developed and around which theories of social aging were built (Estes, 2003).

From the 1970s, however, a new set of "pathways" emerged influencing the construction of old age. In narrow terms, the changes here were driven by declines in male economic activity—this occurring in most industrial countries (Künemund & Kolland, 2007). From a broader perspective, however, this period marked a reversal in the fortunes of "organized capitalism," with the decline of traditional working-class occupations, the emergence of a new service class (built around the employment of women and other social groups), and the collapse of many of the old, manufacturing-based urban areas. Initially, this was theorized as the advent of a new "disorganized capitalism," one bringing a profound instability to social relations and undermining with it the secure institutional pathways supporting old age. Lash and Urry (1987) express this development as follows:

> *The world of "disorganized capitalism" is one in which the "fixed, fast-frozen relations" of organized capitalist relations have been swept away. Societies are being transformed from above, from below, and from within. All that is solid about organized capitalism, class, industry, cities, collectivity, nation state, even the world, melts into air. (pp. 312–313)*

The instability associated with "disorganized capitalism" has subsequently been linked to the changes associated with globalization, the latter defined as the mechanisms, actors, and institutions that link together individuals and groups across different nation-states. Held, McGrew, Goldblatt, and Perraton (1999) elaborate on this as follows:

> *Today, virtually all nation-states have gradually become enmeshed in and functionally part of a larger pattern of global transformations and global flows. . . . Transnational networks and relations have developed across virtually all areas of human activity. Goods, capital, people, knowledge, communications and weapons, as well as crime, pollutants, fashions and beliefs, rapidly move*

> *across territorial boundaries. . . . Far from this being a world of "discrete civilisations" or simply an international order of states, it has become a fundamentally interconnected global order, marked by intense patterns of exchange as well as by clear patterns of power, hierarchy and unevenness.* (p. 49)

Certain aspects of globalization remain highly contested within the social sciences, with an important division between those doubting the reality of globalization and those who view it as *the* major feature of contemporary society. Critiques of globalization theory suggest that, as a social and economic trend, the evidence points as much to the continuing power of nation-states and the continuing influence of regional and localized identities (Gilpin, 2002). Moreover, some research suggests that globalization processes may be on the retreat, a product of the economic downturn affecting many countries in the period from 2000 on (Rosenberg, 2005).

Other researchers, by way of contrast, point to the continued significance of globalization, suggesting that it has proved more resilient than many expected to be the case. Held and McGrew (2007b) argue that the reasons for this are that underpinning contemporary globalization may be found a number of "deep drivers" that are likely to be around for the foreseeable future. Among these they list the changing infrastructure of global communications, the development of global markets in goods and services, the new global division of labor driven by multinational corporations, and the diffusion of consumer values across many of the world's regions.

This chapter supports the view of what has been termed "global radicals" (Giddens, 1999), who consider globalization to be challenging many of the organizing principles of modern social science. Held and McGrew (2007b) suggest that "recursive patterns of worldwide interconnectedness challenge the very principle of the bounded society and the presumption that its dynamics and development can be comprehended principally by reference to endogenous social forces. By eroding the distinctions between the domestic and the international, endogenous and exogenous, internal and external, the idea of globalization directly challenges the 'methodological nationalism' which finds its most acute expression in classical social theory'" (p. 5; see also Urry, 2000).

The following sections of this chapter take the previous statement as providing a framework for applying perspectives from globalization theory to aging societies. The next section starts this process by reviewing some general influences of globalization on demographic change.

Globalization and Aging Societies

The implications of globalization have been acknowledged in social gerontology in a variety of ways. First, it has been implicated in what has been termed the "crisis construction and crisis management" of policies for older people (Estes & Associates, 2001), notably around provision for pensions and social security. Yeates (2001) has noted that in the case of policies around provision for pensions, "both the World Bank and [International Monetary Fund] have been at the forefront of attempts to foster a political climate conducive to the residualization of state welfare and the promotion of private and voluntary initiatives" (p. 122). Deacon (2000) refers to a global discourse about pensions and retirement age that takes for granted a minimal role for the public sector and the promotion of market-based solutions.

Second, there is evidence for widening inequalities within and between different countries, produced as a consequence of global forces. Rather than leading inexorably to minimum levels of social protection (Mosley, 2007), globalization has been implicated in the rise in income inequality produced as a consequence of falling relative demand for unskilled labor and the weakened power of labor organizations (Glyn, 2007). The increase in incomes at the very top of the income distribution has been a feature of advanced industrial societies throughout the 1990s and 2000s. For those less fortunate, however, there has been the growth of what Sennett (2006) refers to as "underemployment" (affecting around 20% of men in their 50s in many advanced industrial societies), this coming alongside constraints on wages and salaries, both these elements reflecting the contraction of jobs arising from economic globalization (see also Blossfeld, Mills, & Bernandi, 2006).

Third, debates in gerontology have implicated globalization processes in the move from defining aging as a *collective* to an *individual* responsibility. On the one hand, growing older seems to have become *more* secure, with longer life expectancy, rising levels of economic well-being (Disney & Whitehouse, 2002), and enhanced lifestyles in old age (Gilleard & Higgs, 2005). Set against this, the pressures associated with the *achievement* of security are themselves generating fresh anxieties across all generations. Risks once carried by social institutions have now been displaced onto the shoulders of individuals and/or their families (Bauman, 2000; O'Rand, 2000). Dannefer (2000) summarizes this process in the following way: "Corporate and state uncertainties are transferred to citizens—protecting large institutions while exposing individuals to possible catastrophe in the domains of health care and personal finances, justified to the public by the claim that the pensioner can do better on his or her own, and that Social Security can do better diversified into equity markets" (p. 270). More generally, Stiglitz (2003) argues that risk has been turned into "a way of life" through a combination of changes in the labor market (with the erosion of jobs for life) and reliance on private pension arrangements—these subject to the volatility of the global stock market (Blackburn, 2006; Minns, 2007).

Finally, globalization—both through the spread of worldwide communications and through the power of global organizations—has elevated aging to an issue that transcends individual societies or states. Gerontology, for much of the 20th century, was preoccupied with issues affecting older people in advanced capitalist societies (Dannefer, 2003). Indeed, theories such as disengagement and modernization theory took the view that the Western model of aging would ultimately be diffused across all cultures of the world (Fennell, Phillipson, & Evers, 1988). Globalization has provided a fundamental challenge to vestiges of this approach. Global interests may indeed continue to be subject to U.S. hegemony and/or Western imperialism in various guises, but globalization also illustrates the emergence of new social and political forms at international, national, regional, and local levels (Held & McGrew, 2007a). Cerny and Evans (2004) make this point in the following way:

> *The central paradox of globalization, the displacement of a crucial range of economic, social and political activities from the national arena to a cross-cutting*

global/transnational/domestic structured field of action, is that rather than creating one economy or one polity, it also divides, fragments and polarises. Convergence and divergence are two sides of the same process. Globalization remains a discourse of contestation that reflects national and regional antagonisms and struggles. (p. 63)

But the globalization of communications has introduced a further dimension into the understanding of demographic change. Thompson (2000) has explored the processes involved in the appropriation of globalized media products as follows:

The appropriation of globalized symbolic materials involves what [may be described] as the accentuation of symbolic distancing from the spatial-temporal contexts of everyday life *[emphasis added]. The appropriation of symbolic materials enables individuals to take some distance from the conditions of their day-to-day lives—not literally but symbolically, imaginatively, vicariously. Individuals are able to gain some conception, however partial, of ways of life and life conditions that differ significantly from their own. They are able to gain some conception of regions of the world which are far removed from their own locales. (p. 212)*

The process described by Thompson is transforming aging at various levels. Global communications sharpened awareness in the 1990s of the suffering of older people in zones of conflict, notably in the former Eastern bloc countries and in sub-Saharan Africa. But from another perspective, it also generated ideas about lifestyles that might be possible to develop in middle and older age. Older people in developed countries became aware of the possibilities of travel and migration and the potential benefits of global tourism. Bauman (1998) observes that "spiritually at least we are all travellers" (p. 78). During the past 10 years, this been put into practice by a minority of wealthier retirees, even though many of their contemporaries remained tied to localities experiencing the costs associated with global change (Phillipson, 2007). Such examples confirm the way in which globalization has been radical in its transformation of aging—with, to paraphrase Beck (1992), few social groups or societies immune to its effects.

In addition to the previously mentioned factors, globalization has further implications for theory in gerontology, reflecting additional areas affected by global, social, and economic change. Understanding current pressures on older people requires acknowledgment of what has been termed the "emerging condition of globality—the growing awareness of the world as a shared social space" (Held & McGrew, 2007b, p. 5). In line with this, the next sections of this chapter discuss two major areas for developing social theory and globalization as applied to the study of aging: first, issues relating to the redefinition of the "social" and changes to personal identity, and, second, redefinitions of citizenship in old age.

Globalization and Aging: Redefining the "Social"

The influence of globalization on older people is well understood at an economic and political level, for example, in areas such pensions and policies around health care provision (George & Wilding, 2002; Yeates, 2001). In this section, however, it is argued that globalization provides additional challenges to theorizing about later life. The point has already been made regarding the extent to which old age was (re)constructed through the pathways of organized capitalism, in particular, those associated with the institutions of retirement and the welfare state. Aging, in this regard, can be viewed as a product of modernity and its associated social and cultural transformations (Conrad, 1992). Modernity created the conditions, through reforms in public health and related areas, for the development of "old age"; equally, it developed the public institutions through which older people could be supported. Underpinning both aspects was the idea of the "social" that went alongside the project of modernity. Delanty (1999) elaborates on this as follows:

> *The discourses of modernity emerged in the context of the rise of the social as a reality sui generis. The distinctive feature of the social was the mediating domain of institutions which separated subjectivity from nature. . . . [In contrast at the present time] . . . we are witnessing the decline of the social, not its rise. Just as modernity arose out of the collapse of the institutions of the Middle Ages, so too is a new historical experience arising out of the decline of the institutions of modernity. Processes of globalization have undermined the project of modernity as one of institution building. . . . Instead . . . we have the spectre of a world out of control, or at least one that is not controlled by any one social agent. (p. 49)*

This type of argument is reflected in the work of theorists such as Beck and Giddens, who point to the uncertainty and insecurity affecting daily life: a bewildering range of personal choice at one level and anxiety and awareness of risk at another. Such elements are further illustrated by the move from the prescribed roles characteristic of mass or industrial society to the mobile and indeterminate positions characteristic of the present day. Elliott and Lemert (2006) summarize this aspect in terms of an emerging conflict between globalization and personal identity, reflected in changes in the workplace, the "detraditionalization" of everyday life, and the "hollowing out" of public sector institutions.

The impact of globalization in redefining the social has considerable implications for theory in gerontology. Population aging has now to be "managed" within what has been described as a fluid and deregulated social order (Elliott & Lemert, 2006). Turner (2000) argues that ideas about instability and risk contrast with traditional assumptions in sociology that emphasize stability and regulation. He highlights concepts such as Weber's notion of rationalization and Elias's concept of the civilizing process, both of which imply that "society [over time] will become more regulated, more normal, more routine, and more administered" (p. 14). In fact, Turner makes the point that the tension is really between a macroenvironment that has become more uncertain and irregular and a microenvironment that is subject to processes of standardization and regularization. In other words, the contrast for older people is between a macroworld the dominant institutions of which offer unpredictable levels of support and a microworld constructed around ideas of planning and life scheduling (Best, 1980; Ekerdt & Clark, 2001).

This divergence between macro- and microlevels, driven by globalization, largely explains the complex and increasingly fluid transitions associated with later life, these creating elements of choice for some groups but insecurity and anxiety for many others (Elliott & Lemert, 2006; Gilleard & Higgs, 2005; Phillipson, 2002). Accepting the influence of globalization, as a factor influencing personal identity, needs further exploration within gerontology. Increasingly, older people (in common with other age-groups) experience the world as though they were riding (as Giddens [1991] expresses it in his description of high modernity) a "juggernaut": "It is not just that more or less continuous and profound changes occur; rather, change does not consistently conform either to human expectation, or to human control" (Giddens, 1991, p. 28). But what has to be theorized from the standpoint of gerontology is how older people maintain a sense of security and identity in what Beck (2000) describes as a "runaway world" or what Delanty (1999) views as a shift from the social integration offered by modernity to the fragmentation of identity characteristic of capitalism in its "disorganized phase" (Lash & Urry, 1987).

The unraveling of traditional institutions has exposed once again the cultural uncertainties surrounding old age (Cole, 1992). Western society is beset, as in the period of the 1930s and 1940s, with anxieties about the most appropriate way to respond to an aging population (Phillipson, 1998). But these uncertainties are given particular emphasis by the pressures and insecurities associated with a late modern age. Arguably, older people have had most to lose from the breakup of the relationships associated with "organized capitalism." For older people, the extension of individualization in the period of "disorganized capitalism" poses a significant threat to identity itself. As Biggs (1993) notes, modern life raises at least two possibilities: the promise of a multiplicity of identities on the one side and the danger of psychological disintegration on the other. Biggs suggests that in response to these circumstances, individual actors will attempt to find socially constructed spaces that lend some form of predictability to everyday relationships. Yet in a world of late or high modernity, spaces such as these may be difficult to locate. Bauman (1996) makes this point as follows:

> *In our postmodern times . . . the boundaries which tend to be simultaneously most strongly desired and most acutely missed are those of a rightful and secure place in society, of a space unquestionably one's own, where one can plan one's life with the minimum of interference, play one's role in a game in which the rules do not change overnight and without notice, and reasonably hope for the better. . . . It is the widespread characteristic of men and women in our type of society that they live perpetually with the "identity problem" unresolved. They suffer, one might say, from a chronic absence of resources with which they could build a truly solid and lasting identity, anchor and stop it from drifting. (p. 26)*

The type of argument advanced by Bauman points to some of the major issues that social theory applied to aging will need to tackle. Where do older people stand in a society in which priorities and values are constantly open to revision and change? What is the moral and existential space to which they are entitled in a world where social integration is achieved through the marketplace (Elliott & Lemert, 2006)? What are the costs and benefits of what Beck (2000) refers to as the "compulsion" to lead your own life? How does this "compulsion" play in a world where illness and loss of key relationships threaten? One starting point for addressing such questions may lie in considering the changing basis of citizenship in old age and the implications of this for supporting and empowering older people. The next section gives some consideration to this issue.

Globalization and Aging: Redefining Citizenship

Arguably the most radical implications of globalization for older people have emerged through the questioning of traditional forms of nationality and citizenship. Citizenship has, Turner (1993) suggests, been profoundly challenged by global developments in the organization of modern societies. This is reflected, as noted earlier, in the power of international bodies operating outside national governments, in accelerated rates of migration and mobility across different societies, and in the importance of global capital and its influence on the daily lives of individual citizens. Modern debates on citizenship have been built around the legacy of T. H. Marshall (1964), who viewed human rights as having evolved along three main dimensions: first, civil or legal rights, associated with the right to a fair trial; second, political rights, reflected in the right to vote; and, third, social rights, reflected in rights associated with the organization of the welfare state.

The framework presented by Marshall has been severely tested, however, by the loosening of rights (notably in the social sphere) accompanying globalization (Kuper, 2007). The idea of citizenship is now operating in a very different economic and social context to that understood by Marshall in the 1940s. Identity in old age, as noted in the preceding section, is increasingly subject to forces beyond both the individual's control and in some cases that of his or her nation-state. Indeed, precisely what is the individual's nation-state, for the purpose of providing resources and support, is likely to be an increasingly open and/or contested issue moving through the 21st century.

In this context, if what might be called the "first phase of aging" (which lasted for much of the 20th century) was about growing old as a reinforcement of national identity and citizenship, the second phase will involve to a much greater extent the development of what may be termed "hybrid identities" (Werbner & Modood, 1997). Growing old in the first phase was deeply rooted within particular communities and the political framework of nation-states. In the second phase, however, under the pressure of globalization, identity becomes progressively detached from particular places (and potentially even nations). Beck (2000) argues that "people are expected to live their lives with the most diverse and contradictory transnational and personal identities and risks" (p. 169). And Albrow (1996) makes the point that "under globalized conditions it becomes less easy for individuals to affirm their identity within the strict confines of nation, gender, age or any other categorical distinctions" (p. 151).

Following this, Soysal (1994) argues the case for a "postnational" model of citizenship that recognizes the variety of attachments which characterize modern nation-states. She sees the implications of this as follows:

> *In the postnational model, universal personhood replaces nationhood; and universal human rights replace national rights. . . . The rights and claims of*

> *individuals are legitimated by ideologies grounded in a transnational community, through international codes, conventions and laws on human rights, independent of their citizenship in a nation-state. Hence the individual transcends the citizen. (p. 142)*

Debates about the changing nature of citizenship raise important issues for social theory in gerontology. In the first place, the human rights focus may be a more productive field for challenging discrimination and inequality than that associated with ideas around citizenship. Some of the implications of this approach have been developed by Turner (1993, 2001), who argues that a rights-based approach is necessary precisely because individuals are ontologically frail rather than autonomous beings, this arising partly through the effects of aging but also because life is inherently risky. Turner (1993) concludes,

> *To be precise, the argument is that, from sociological presuppositions about the frailty of the body and the precarious or risky character of social institutions, it is possible to offer a sociologically plausible account of human rights as a supplement to citizenship or as an institution which goes beyond citizenship because human rights are not necessarily tied to the nation-state. (p. 180)*

Another approach to "postnational citizenship" is to view older people as a group likely to benefit from what Delanty (2000) refers to as "cosmopolitan citizenship." Cosmopolitanism is an important philosophical idea to consider in that it offers the basis for promoting new social roles for older people (see also Achenbaum, 2005; Weiss & Bass, 2002). Linklater (1998) cites Beitz's view that the essence of cosmopolitanism lies in the belief that all human beings possess equal moral standing. Linklater goes on to argue that the implications of this is that political communities should widen their ethical horizons until the point is reached where no individual or group interest is systematically excluded from moral consideration. Such an approach would challenge many of the ageist stereotypes implicated in processes leading to forms of "structured dependency" in old age. It would also consider the basis for older people to embrace active social roles (or "civic engagement" in Achenbaum's [2005] terms) as a consequence of the duties and obligations associated with membership of a multiplicity of communities.

Developing a cosmopolitan view of aging may be significant as well in challenging linkages between aging and economic and cultural decline. For cosmopolitan citizens, age is of secondary importance behind their responsibilities within civic society. This contrasts with national citizenship, where chronological age may continue to determine access to a range of resources and responsibilities. Assessing the basis of new forms of citizenship in old age will be an important task for social theory in gerontology, reflecting the changing contexts and institutions created through globalization.

Conclusion

Globalization will undoubtedly be a major factor in shaping the lives of older people in the 21st century. The types of changes it will bring are easy to predict in some respects, much less so in others. Older people will certainly be living in a culturally and socially diverse world, increasingly aware not only of the aging of their own society but also of the impact of growing old on different communities across the globe. An additional change will be the influence of supranational bodies in determining policies in areas such as social security and health care, these creating the framework for debates about resources and support for old age. Globalization—as one constituent of the "risk society"—may also generate new forms of insecurity of which anxieties and fears about aging may represent a significant dimension.

But other aspects are less easy to predict. Will a new cohort of older people (e.g., the post–World War II baby-boom generation) give a different voice and meaning to the nature of growing old? If they do, to what extent will this be determined by social networks that embrace global as much national contexts? To what extent will globalization undermine the social, economic, and cultural threads (tenuous at best given the role of class, gender, and ethnicity) linking together people with a common chronological age? Will globalization create new forms of inclusion and exclusion in later life, with greater prosperity for some groups of older people coming at the expense of marginalization for others? How will complex issues relating to pensions and health care—difficult enough to resolve at a national level—fare as they become more closely incorporated into debates around global social policy?

Globalization has certainly transformed the world, but it is changing growing old as well—and in equally radical ways. Further study of this important phenomenon will be a major task for gerontologists in the years ahead. It will almost certainly transform the nature of social theorizing about later life, creating new agendas and questions for researchers to consider. Globalization, to return to the theme identified at the beginning of this chapter, highlights the importance of a macrolevel focus within the study of aging. New opportunities are provided for understanding the way structural factors influence the organization of daily life. Analyzing the implications of this for social theory is now an urgent task for gerontologists to incorporate into their research.

References

Achenbaum, W. A. (2005). *Older Americans: Vital communities.* Baltimore: Johns Hopkins University Press.

Albrow, M. (1996). *The global age.* Cambridge: Polity Press.

Baars, J. (2006). Beyond neomodernism, antimodernism, and postmodernism: Basic categories for contemporary critical gerontology. In J. Baars, D. Dannefer, C. Phillipson, & A. Walker (Eds.), *Aging, globalization and inequality* (pp. 17–42). Amityville, NY: Baywood Publishing.

Baars, J., Dannefer, D., Phillipson, C., & Walker, A. (Eds.). (2006). *Aging, globalization and the new inequality.* Amityville, NY: Baywood Publishing.

Bauman, Z. (1996). *Postmodernity and its discontents.* Oxford: Blackwell.

Bauman, Z. (1998). *Globalization.* Oxford: Polity Press.

Bauman, Z. (2000). *Liquid modernity.* Oxford: Polity Press.

Beck, U. (1992). *The risk society.* London: Sage.

Beck, U. (2000). Living your own life in a runaway world: Individualism, globalisation and politics. In W. Hutton & A. Giddens (Eds.), *On the edge: Living with global capitalism* (pp. 164–175). London: Jonathan Cape.

Bengtson, V. L., Putney, N., & Johnson, M. (2005). The problem of theory in gerontology today. In M. Johnson, in association with V. L. Bengtson, P. Coleman, & T. Kirkwood (Eds.), *The Cambridge handbook of age and ageing* (pp. 3–20). Cambridge: Cambridge University Press.

Best, F. (1980). *Flexible life scheduling.* New York: Praeger.
Biggs, S. (1993). *Understanding aging.* Maidenhead: Open University Press.
Blackburn, R. (2006). *Age shock.* London: Verso.
Blossfeld, H-P., Mills, M., & Bernandi, F. (Eds.). (2006). *Globalization, uncertainty and late careers in society.* London: Routledge.
Cerny, P. G., & Evans, M. (2004). Globalization and public policy under new labour. *Policy Studies, 25,* 51–65.
Cole, T. (1992). *The journey of life.* Cambridge: Cambridge University Press.
Conrad, C. (1992). Old age in the modern and postmodern world. In T. Cole, D. Van Tassels, & R. Kastenbaum (Eds.), *Handbook of the humanities & ageing* (pp. 62–95). New York: Springer Publishing.
Dannefer, D. (2000). Bringing risk back in: The regulation of the self in the postmodern state. In K. W. Schaie & J. Hendricks (Eds.), *The evolution of the aging self: The social impact on the aging process* (pp. 269–280). New York: Springer Publishing.
Dannefer, D. (2003). Toward a global geography of the life course. In J. Mortimer & M. Shanahan (Eds.), *Handbook of the life course* (pp. 647–659). New York: Kluwer Academic/Plenum Press.
Deacon, B. (2000). *Globalization and social policy: The threat to equitable welfare.* Occasional Paper No. 5. Retrieved January 5, 2008, from http://www.org.unrisd
Delanty, G. (1999). *Social theory in a changing world.* Oxford: Polity Press.
Delanty, G. (2000). *Citizenship in a global age.* Buckingham: Open University Press.
Disney, R., & Whitehouse, E. (2002). The economic well-being of older people in international perspective: A critical review. In S. Crystal & D. Shea (Eds.), *Economic outcomes in later life: Public policy, health and cumulative advantage* (pp. 59–94). New York: Springer Publishing.
Ekerdt, D., & Clark, E. (2001). Selling retirement in financial planning advertisements. *Journal of Aging Studies, 15,* 55–68.
Elliott, A., & Lemert, C. (2006). *The new individualism: The emotional costs of globalization.* London: Routledge.
Estes, C. (1979). *The aging enterprise.* San Francisco: Jossey-Bass.
Estes, C. (1999). Critical gerontology and the new political economy of aging. In M. Minkler & C. Estes (Eds.), *Critical gerontology: Perspectives from political and moral economy* (pp. 17–36). Amityville, NY: Baywood Publishing.
Estes, C. (2003). Theoretical perspectives on old age policy: A critique and proposal. In S. Biggs, A. Lowenstein, & J. Hendricks (Eds.), *The need for theory: Critical approaches to social gerontology* (pp. 219–243). Amityville, NY: Baywood Publishing.
Estes, C., & Associates (2001). *Social policy and aging.* Thousand Oaks, CA: Sage.
Estes, C., Biggs, S., & Phillipson, C. (2003). *Social theory, social policy and ageing: A critical introduction.* Maidenhead: Open University Press.
Estes, C., & Phillipson, C. (2002). The globalization of capital, the welfare state and old age policy. *International Journal of Health Services, 32,* 279–297.
Fennell, G., Phillipson, C., & Evers, H. (1988). *The sociology of old age.* Milton Keynes: Open University Press.
Fischer, D. J. (1977). *Growing old in America.* New York: Oxford University Press.
George, V., & Wilding, P. (2002). *Globalization and human welfare.* London: Palgrave.
Giddens, A. (1991). *Modernity and self-identity.* Cambridge: Polity Press.
Giddens, A. (1999). *Globalization.* Reith Lecture No. 1. BBC Online Network. Retrieved January 12, 2008, from http://www.lse.ac.uk/giddens/lectures.htm
Gilleard, C., & Higgs, P. (2005). *Contexts of ageing: Class, cohort and community.* Cambridge: Polity Press.
Gilpin, R. (2002). *The challenge of global capitalism.* Princeton, NJ: Princeton University Press.
Glyn, A. (2007). *Capitalism unleashed.* Oxford: Oxford University Press.
Graebner, W. (1980). *A history of retirement.* New Haven, CT: Yale University Press.
Hagestad, G., & Dannefer, D. (2001). Concepts and theories of aging: Beyond microfication in social science approaches. In R. Binstock & L. George (Eds.), *The handbook of aging* (pp. 3–16). San Diego, CA: Academic Press.
Held, D., & McGrew, A. (Eds.). (2007a). *Governing globalization: Power, authority and global governance.* Cambridge: Polity Press.
Held, D., & McGrew, A. (2007b). Introduction: Globalization at risk. In D. Held & A. McGrew (Eds.), *Governing globalization: Power, authority and global governance* (pp. 1–11). Cambridge: Polity Press.

Held, D., McGrew, A., Goldblatt, D., & Perraton, J. (1999). *Global transformations.* Oxford: Polity Press.
Hendricks, J., & Leedham, C. A. (1991). Dependency or empowerment? Toward a moral and political economy. In M. Minkler & C. Estes (Eds.), *Critical perspectives on aging: The perspectives on aging: The political and moral economy of growing old* (pp. 51–64). Amityville, NY: Baywood Publishing.
Künemund, H., & Kolland, F. (2007). Work and retirement. In J. Bond, S. Peace, F. Dittman-Kohli, & G. Westerhoff (Eds.), *Ageing in society* (pp. 167–185). London: Sage.
Kuper, A. (2007) Reconstructing global governance: Eight innovations. In D. Held & A. McGrew (Eds.), *Governing globalization: Power, authority and global governance* (pp. 225–239). Cambridge: Polity Press.
Lash, S., & Urry, J. (1987). *The end of organized capitalism.* Cambridge: Polity Press.
Linklater, A. (1998). *The transformation of political community.* Cambridge: Cambridge University Press.
Marshall, T. H. (1964). Citizenship and social class. Reprinted in *Class, citizenship and social development.* Chicago: University of Chicago Press. (Original work published 1949)
Minkler, M., & Estes, C. (Eds.). (1999). *Critical gerontology: Perspectives from political and moral economy* (2nd ed.). Amityville, NY: Baywood Publishing.
Minns, R. (2007). The future of stock market pensions. In J. Vincent, C. Phillipson, & M. Downs (Eds.), *The futures of old age* (pp. 98–106). London: Sage.
Mosley, L. (2007). The political economy of globalization. In D. Held & A. McGrew (Eds.), *Globalization theory* (pp. 106–125). Cambridge: Polity Press.
O'Rand, A. M. (2000). Risk, rationality, and modernity: Social policy and the ageing self. In K. W. Schaie (Ed.), *Social structures and aging* (pp. 225–249). New York: Springer Publishing.
Phillipson, C. (1982). *Capitalism and the construction of old age.* London: Macmillan.
Phillipson, C. (1998). *Reconstructing old age.* London: Sage.
Phillipson, C. (2002). *Transitions from work to retirement.* Bristol: Policy Press.
Phillipson, C. (2007). The "elected" and the "excluded": Sociological perspectives on the experience of place and community in old age. *Ageing & Society, 27,* 321–342.
Phillipson, C., & Baars, J. (2007). Social theory and social ageing. In J. Bond, S. Peace, F. Dittman-Kohli, & G. Westerhoff (Eds.), *Ageing in society* (pp. 68–84). London: Sage.
Ritzer, G. (2007). *The Blackwell companion to globalization.* Oxford: Blackwell.
Rosenberg, J. (2005). Globalization theory: A post mortem. *International Politics, 42,* 2–74.
Sennett, R. (2006). *Cultures of capitalism.* New Haven, CT: Yale University Press.
Soysal, Y. (1994). *Limits of citizenship: Migrants and postnational membership in Europe.* Chicago: University of Chicago Press.
Stiglitz, J. (2003). *The roaring nineties.* London: Penguin.
Thane, P. (2000). *Old age in English history: Past experiences, present issues.* Oxford: Oxford University Press.
Thompson, J. B. (2000). The globalization of communication. In D. Held & A. McGrew (Eds.), *The global transformations reader.* Cambridge: Polity Press.
Townsend, P. (1981). The structured dependency of the elderly: The creation of policy in the twentieth century. *Ageing & Society, 1,* 5–28.
Turner, B. (1993). Contemporary problems in the theory of citizenship. In B. Turner (Ed.), *Citizenship and social theory* (pp. 1–18). London: Sage.
Turner, B. (2000). Introduction. In B. Turner (Ed.), *The Blackwell companion to social theory* (pp. 1–18). Oxford: Blackwell.
Turner, B. (2001). The erosion of citizenship. *British Journal of Sociology, 52,* 189–209.
Urry, J. (2000). *Sociology beyond societies.* London: Routledge.
Vincent, J. (2003). *Old age.* London: Routledge.
Walker, A. (1981). Towards a political economy of old age. *Ageing & Society, 1,* 73–94.
Walker, A., & Deacon, B. (2003). Economic globalization and policies on aging. *Journal of Societal and Social Policy, 2,* 1–18.
Weiss, R. S., & Bass, S. A. (Eds.). (2002). *Challenges of the third age.* Oxford: Oxford University Press.
Werbner, P., & Modood, T. (Eds.). (1997). *Debating cultural hybridity.* London: Zed Books.
Yeates, N. (2001). *Globalisation and social policy.* London: Sage.

Care for Older Adults in the Welfare State: Theories, Policies, and Realities

34

Mats Thorslund
Merril Silverstein

Population aging is often identified as one of the greatest societal challenges of the next 50 years (Kallache, Barreto, & Keller, 2005). In both the developed and the developing world, nations are anxious over this demographic transition and concerned about their ability to sustain the relatively large number of older people that are soon to be in their midst. Meanwhile, economic stagnation and growing budget deficits are prompting a reconsideration of the role of the state in the lives of individuals and families. In most Western nations, there has been a retrenchment of social welfare programs as governments seek to reduce their commitments to the elderly population and shift risk to individuals and families (O'Rand, 2006). Under pressures of globalization, the efforts of government to provide for its most vulnerable citizens have weakened (Phillipson, 2003).

Nations with the most universal, generous, and egalitarian systems of care and support to their older citizen—those labeled as *welfare states*—are said to be at the greatest risk of crisis. In this chapter, we explore the welfare state as both a sociocultural ideal and an institution tied historically to the material conditions that gave rise to it and sustains it. We maintain that the welfare state, as it is currently constituted, is being reevaluated largely because the economic, political, and social conditions that seeded its growth have changed. External constraints on the welfare state resulting from global market integration and reduced public budgets have opened up an internal contradiction between the political and moral economies that underlie the welfare state. Nowhere does this contradiction come into sharper relief than in policies toward the older population in the Scandinavian nations. Therefore, we ask how far the reality of the welfare state has strayed from its ideal form, considering the Scandinavian model as the apotheosis of welfare state development with regard to old-age support and care.

Paradigmatic Representations of the Welfare State

The allocation of formal services to dependent older persons in the community varies substantially across nations. At the macrolevel, welfare state structures differ depending on the way in which welfare production is allocated among state, market, and households. Esping-Andersen (1990, 1999) provides a succinct set of state groupings: (a) *social democratic welfare states,* in which all citizens are incorporated under a single universal insurance system (such as those found in the Scandinavian countries); (b) *liberal welfare states,* where assistance is means tested and modest social insurance plans dominate (such as those found in Australia, Canada, and the United States); and (c) the *conservative welfare states,* where the state will only intervene when the family's resources are exhausted (such as Austria, France, and Germany). The welfare state is commonly associated with the Scandinavian model, which in many instances is considered a pure, or an ideal, manifestation of social democratic principles.

Theories locate the welfare state as an evolutionary end product of societal development and modernization. Indeed, most Western nations have followed a similar historical arc in collectivizing old-age benefits, though their manifestations differ. The development of the welfare state can be divided into three distinct historical phases, each corresponding to a particular institutional response to aging populations (Phillipson, 2003). The welfare state originated in the 1950s and rapidly expanded through the mid-1970s. In terms of benefits for the aged, this first phase was marked by growth in state-supported pensions and development of readily available home help services and residential care. Fueled by economic expansion, close to full employment rates, and the near sanctification of the intergenerational contract, this period is often referred to as the "golden age" of the welfare state. The second phase, roughly from the late 1970s through the 1990s, was characterized by skepticism and even hostility toward the welfare state fueled by growing economic instability, declining real wages, and loss of faith in the viability of institutions supporting older people. The first decade of the new millennium has emerged as the third phase. This period is being shaped by the expansion of global trade, the near worship of free markets, and the perceived competitive advantage of having a smaller public sector. In this new economic environment, population aging—specifically the demands that an aging population places on the public sector—has become increasingly considered an obstacle to global competitiveness. One of the gloomiest scenarios is painted by economists Razin and Sadka (2005), who project that population aging will increase the old-age dependency ratio in European Union nations in the range of 35% to 66% between 2000 and 2050, requiring either tax increases of up 33% or debt financing to pay for obligations owed older citizens. Both solutions, in their estimation, will substantially slow economic growth of European states.

There are substantial differences in the challenges that confront nation-states with regard to population aging. For the developed welfare states of Scandinavia, the challenge is to ensure that existing systems for long-term care and pensions can withstand the demands exerted by increasing needs and numbers (both in absolute terms but especially in relative terms) of elderly persons in the population. In the less developed welfare states (e.g., Italy, Spain, and Greece), the challenge will more be to develop new systems and finding the resources necessary to fund them.

Sweden in Comparative Context

The allocation of formal services to dependent older persons in the community varies substantially across nations. This variation ranges from the universalist policies of social democratic states (such as those found in Scandinavian countries) to liberal market policies that reflect government partnerships with the private sector and the family (such as those found in Germany, Great Britain, and the United States) and residualist policies that leave the majority of care responsibility to family members (such as those found in most developing nations). In contrast to the universalist policies of Sweden, for example, U.S. policies are needs based and presume that families have central responsibility for care of the elderly. Swedish policies, on the other hand, are designed to reduce the burden placed on families, especially women, by their elder care responsibilities. Recent evidence demonstrates that the Swedish model is effective in meeting the needs of elders. Impaired elders in the United States are more likely to have unmet needs compared to similarly impaired elders in Sweden, and this disparity is almost completely explained by the lower use of formal services in the United States (Shea et al., 2003). Further, research suggests that compared to the United States the formal service sector of Sweden better targets institutional care at more vulnerable elders, suggesting that both greater coverage *and* greater efficiencies are achieved by the welfare state (Davey et al., 2005).

Comparative statistics show that in the early 1990s more than 10% of the older population received home help in Denmark, Finland, Norway, and Sweden, a rate larger than that found in other European nations and more than twice that of the United States (Organization for Economic Cooperation and Development, 1996). Contrary to other Scandinavian countries, Sweden reduced the coverage of home help during the 1990s among the Scandinavian countries (8%) but delivered the greatest intensity of care at 6.6 hours per week (Szebehely, 2003). This strategy highlights an intentional strategy to target those most in need and deliver sufficient care to keep frail elders in their homes as long as possible, but the cost is ignoring those with more moderate but still significant needs. There are clear differences among the western European states in the degree to which they prefer state and/or family support for older frail adults. At the margins, Norway and Spain represent distinctive sets of preferences, with the former overwhelming choosing public over family-provided care and the latter more likely to prefer a mix of public family care for its older citizens (Daatland & Herlofson, 2003).

Development of the Swedish Model of Old-Age Care

The Swedish welfare state is mainly a post–World War II phenomenon. Old-age care was synonymous with institutional care until the 1950s, when the municipalities gradually also began to offer in-home support to dependent elderly persons. Notably, the legal obligation of children to care for their parents was abolished in 1956, explicitly making the principles of remaining at home and receiving public help a public goal for old-age care at a relatively early date. Municipal home help was at that time given mainly to people who needed help with domestic services, such as cooking, cleaning, and doing the laundry. Persons needing more help were referred to institutional care. No particular training of home helpers was required (Larsson, Thorslund, & Silverstein 2005).

The newly offered services soon became very popular, and their use increased rapidly after the introduction of state subsidies to the municipalities in the mid-1960s. Home help was highly subsidized, and the recipients paid only a fraction of the actual costs of the services. The needs assessments focused on whether the elderly person could manage daily tasks regardless of the existence or state of health of a spouse or the availability proximate family members. Rates of home help reached a peak at the end of the 1970s, when nearly a quarter of the retired elderly population in Sweden received some services in the course of a year. Most recipients received only a few hours of weekly or monthly help, in most cases with shopping, house cleaning, or laundry. The introduction of state subsidies paved the way for the expansion of home help. It gave older people with ordinary incomes a choice. They were no longer forced to move to institutions or to be dependent on their children but could stay in their own homes and receive assistance from the municipal home help services. This period of establishing a generous (from an international perspective) public system of in-home care of the elderly coincided with the establishment of the general welfare state in Sweden. The 1960s and the 1970s were decades during which the expanding Swedish economy allowed both a wide expansion of public welfare services and room for an increasing rate of private consumption (Bergmark, Thorslund, & Lindberg, 2000).

During the 1960s and 1970s, an increasing number of women entered the labor market. The expansion of home help enabled many middle-aged women to maintain gainful employment rather than stay home and care for dependent parents. It is also argued that the expansion of public in-home care granted family members (in most cases daughters or daughters-in-law) the choice of whether to provide care to elderly relatives. By the mid-1980s, the continued expansion of home help services generated demand far in excess of what the public eldercare system could provide, leading to stricter needs assessments. Older adults with less extensive needs and those who were deemed capable of receiving help from informal sources fell outside the realm of public concern. As a consequence, the average home help recipient had more extensive health problems, placing new demands on staff and elder care organizations serving a higher proportion of highly frail elderly persons.

Under the pressure of growing population of the oldest-old (by this measure, Sweden—together with Italy—currently has the highest population in the world with more than 5% of its population 80 years of age and older [United Nations, 2007]), the demands on health and social service providers increased substantially. Criticism was directed at the organization of care for the elderly, particularly at the unclear demarcation between providers of health care (the county councils) and providers of eldercare (the municipalities). The Swedish Parliament therefore decided on a new elder care policy in 1992. This policy gave the municipalities responsibility for nursing homes for patients who still needed care after discharge from hospital in addition to the responsibility for ordinary home help services.

The reform took place at the same time as budgetary reductions due to weakening economic growth in the 1990s and resulted in a dramatic restructuring of the long-term care system. This development, however, increased the pressure on the municipal elder care organization in terms of resources and competence. Among elderly persons living at home, home help services were targeted to the most frail and dependent elderly with extended personal care needs. In the mid-1990s, every third person with home help received help during weekends, and every fourth received help during evenings or at night (Daatland, 1997). Among married persons, the spouse (usually the wife) was frequently the only caregiver, often having little or no support from formal elder care services (Larsson & Thorslund, 2002). Consequently, spouses, as well as persons with less extensive needs, had to rely on family, friends, or commercial alternatives for domestic services.

During this phase, municipalities, mainly in urban areas, began contracting services to nonpublic providers, although still publicly financed and under public control. Still, commercial and volunteer alternatives to medical or personal care, paid out of pocket, continue to be almost nonexistent. Competition among providers of care has been seen as one method of stretching the public budget and in some cases allowed elderly persons to select among different providers of care, although this trend is criticized as being a departure from the Swedish model (Szebehely, 2005).

What accounted for Swedish welfare state exceptionalism in the first place? We suggest that the Swedish welfare state came to fruition at the confluence of four conditions occurring within a small temporal window following World War II. These included (a) rapid economic growth enabled by a relatively intact infrastructure and male labor force after the war and access to rich natural resources, (b) high levels of public trust in state institutions and their representatives earned by a government with little corruption and a good degree of transparency, (c) a small and homogeneous population that minimized internal conflict over resource allocation, and (d) a strong state church that could provide institutional leverage for welfare state policies.

Several of these conditions have changed. Since 2000, Sweden no longer has a state-sanctioned church—reflecting increasing secularization as well as growing ethnic and religious heterogeneity due to a fairly generous immigration policy. However, the most important precondition for establishing a social democratic welfare state is having an economy that is sufficiently strong to fund it. Without the proper economic conditions, any political ambitions to establish a generous welfare state would be difficult to implement. The booming economy in the 1950s allowed the Social Democrats to form much of the country's social policy in a centralized, controlled, and uniform manner (Parker, 2000). With the economy flourishing, political decisions often concerned matters as in what sector of the society it might be expedient to support expansion. Some decades later, the situation is quite different. Difficult priorities must constantly be made between service sectors in terms of slashing budgets and of what services must be discontinued (Bergmark et al., 2000).

Even though the economic situation in Sweden has recovered from the recession in the 1990s, a simple thought experiment would lead to the conclusion that if Sweden had not chosen as it did in the 1950s and 1960s to develop its welfare state regime, it would unlikely have done so today. What this means for more conservative welfare states is that the establishment of a Scandinavian-style welfare state is highly unlikely. If the Scandinavian ideal is out of step with the current trend toward smaller and more conservative governments in Europe and North America (and most recently in Sweden itself), what, then, is the future of the welfare state in the very nations that brought it into being as a third way between communism and capitalism?

Tension Between Moral and Political Economies

The system of old-age support and care in Sweden embodies principles of universalism and egalitarianism in allocating benefits and services to the elderly, with the goal that socioeconomic differentials should be minimized and collectivization of risk maximized (Daatland, 1997; Thorslund, 1991). In general, Scandinavian social welfare systems provide cradle-to-grave protection against economic and social needs caused by unemployment, poor health, retirement, and family formation with every citizen in principle having equal access to benefits. To simplify a bit, the welfare state rests on two pillars: a political economy in which economic growth and relatively high taxes allowed its establishment, expansion, and sustenance and a moral economy that legitimates the universalistic and redistributive principles under which it sets policies.

As a result of the imperatives of the global economy, policymakers are under increasing pressure to apply market principles—that is, privatization—in the design of social policies while placing restrictions on public welfare programs. This is particularly evident with regard to provisions for old-age support and long-term care, raising fundamental questions about society's collective obligation to the elderly and the rights of older citizens to health and supportive services (Phillipson, 2003). In the United States, the issue of public and private risk is now central to policy debates over income security and acute and chronic health care in old age. Macroeconomic restructuring and trends toward the individualization of risk (O'Rand, 2006) have permeated all social institutions, exacerbating tensions between public and private spheres for dependent populations.

The moral economy reflects the underlying values and preferences in each national population of the "good" society—what is desirable even if not achievable. These valuations include the relationship between private and public responsibility for older adults, the role of women in the labor market and in family roles, the amount of autonomy and residential independence that care systems provide older persons, and the role of the private and voluntary sector in the care mix. When actions taken in the political economy to reduce state spending and promote private market solutions come into conflict with ideologies of the moral economy, a crisis may ensue. Whereas pensions are formulaic in balancing revenues against benefits, long-term care options are more ambiguous because many different models of care are possible and their costs are more difficult to estimate and, therefore, more difficult to control. In addition, long-term care is an area where the moral economy more obviously bumps up against the political economy because policy changes have immediate and direct consequences for the care provided by families.

Discussions among policymakers in developed welfare states tend to follow narrow technocratic lines such as how to get the most efficiency out of existing systems. The welfare state is entrenched bureaucratically and politically, making change difficult, but it is also ideologically ingrained in the public mind. The welfare state remains popular in Nordic countries, even though confidence in it is waning. Institutional inertia guarantees that change when it comes will be incremental. In addition, the welfare state has raised expectations in the population based on what an earlier generation of older adults received, making severe cutbacks politically unpopular in many circles. Given the global and demographic forces at work, modifications to the welfare state are inevitable. Acceptance of the policy changes in the offing may hinge on whether citizens perceive them as retrenchment or reconstruction of the social welfare enterprise (Quadagno & Street, 2006).

Gender Egalitarianism

The welfare state is built on the supposition that women should be released from the responsibility of caring for elderly parents (and for taking care of the children) so that they might have the opportunity to participate in the labor force. Notably, in Sweden the legal obligation of children to care for their parents was abolished in 1956, a policy that affected women more than men. Yet scholars have been uneasy about the incorporation of gender into theories of the welfare state. Anttonen and Sipilä (1996) criticize the dominant theoretical paradigms of the welfare state for ignoring this and instead grounding the welfare state on its social insurance provisions for wage earners (mostly men)—what is referred to as the "decommodification of labor power" (Esping-Andersen, 1990). Often ignored in this framework are the benefits that the welfare state has provided women by giving them the means to be economically independent of their families and spouses and free of the financial risks associated with childbearing and mothering—what is referred to as "defamilialization" of women (Sipilä, Anttonen, & Baldock, 2003). In this view, the welfare state reduces the advantages of more privileged groups in the population and specifically operates as a counterweight to gender inequality and male dominance. With regard to pensions, the welfare state compensates for wage differentials during their working lives. Liberally allocated home help services allow women to resist providing care to their older parents, a role that a traditional division of labor would have assigned to them.

The welfare state also benefits older women directly. Because women outlive men, tend more than men to be widowed, and suffer from more chronic disabilities, home help and other long-term care services are disproportionately beneficial to older women. The establishment of a publicly financed and controlled system for long-term care also creates a demand for (middle-aged) women without formal education and without paid work experience to work as home help aides.

Social Versus Family Solidarity

Social solidarity—the linking of disparate and unequal social groups through state mediation—is viewed as a virtue of the Scandinavian model of social welfare. In the United States, the age disparity between immigrant and minority populations and native-born Whites necessarily results in a working-age population that is disproportionately composed of people "of color" who transfer Social Security taxes for the benefits of a predominantly White older population.

The 1992 financial crisis in Sweden introduced a set of restrictions that narrowed eligibility for home care benefits (Thorslund, Bergmark, & Parker, 2001). These changes occurred with no legislative change and no announcement of a revision of the state's social policy goals. Evidence suggests an increase in the number of moderately impaired elders served by families over the same historical period that formal services were targeted at the more severely impaired (Larsson, 2006; Sundstrom, Johansson, & Hassing, 2002). Reliance on individual and family resources is viewed in the moral economy of the welfare state as a violation of the principle of egalitarianism in service allocation, as those older adults without sufficient resources are likely to have unmet needs.

The "Third Sector"

Increasingly, scholars have rejected the zero-sum division of care into state versus family as a false dichotomy and have turned their attention to incorporating the "third sector" into their theoretical formulations (Evers & Laville, 2004; Gonzales, 2007). Third-sector organizations represent nongovernmental organizations, community organizations, and civic and religious groups that provide care services to those in need. Indeed, in some formulations, third-sector organizations are viewed as blending with the state and the family to produce an integrated system of care. Some scholars emphasize the flexibility of the tripartite welfare mix to meet needs and praise its communitarian aspects, sometimes viewing third-sector organizations as empowering individuals and communities to achieve social change and social justice (Gonzales, 2007). Retraction of state benefits globally has induced increased reliance on traditional social obligations of family and community in a mix of public and private services that has been called a "third way" of social welfare provision (Giddens, 2000).

Yet the mixed model is still rare in the Nordic welfare state (Jegermalm, 2006), perhaps because it contradicts a moral economy that puts trust in the state's ability to equitably allocate benefits and services. Services provided by religious or ethnic organizations may be viewed as circumventing the principle of equitability, both challenging and usurping the role of the state. Particularistic solutions that rely on voluntary organizations are capable of generating inequalities in outcomes based on unequal access to services and benefits.

Egalitarianism Versus Targeting

Policy decisions inherently involve setting priorities in the context of limits. This has been difficult in a long-term care sector that has a tradition of "prioritizing everything." On the other hand, targeting is antithetical to a moral economy that stresses equal access to services. Beginning in the early 1990s, Sweden began to restrict in-home support for the aged by targeting them to those most in need, resulting in an increase in denied services for older people. Strategies to target services at elders who lived alone and had the most impairments and the least family support were an expedient reaction to an unfortunate economic downturn but, in some minds, violated the egalitarian principles on which the welfare state was established (Larsson et al., 2005). As a result, elder care policy in Sweden in the 1990s has moved closer to the more targeted policies found in the United States (Parker, 2000), representing an instance where Sweden has emulated welfare strategies associated with liberal market regimes.

Aging in Place Versus Institutional Care

Emphasis on providing home care services in welfare state regimes has the goal of preserving the dignity and well-being of frail elders by keeping them out of institutions for as long as possible. Whether home help is also a pragmatic cost-saving option is open to question and depends on the service mix available and criteria for eligibility. Meeting "the needs" of the elderly population is a moral priority in the welfare state, as it is in most developed nations. However, the definition of "needs" is also part of the moral equation. According to general surveys, virtually all elderly people want to stay in their own homes for as long as possible. But what does "possible" mean? Who is to define it? And what form of public care do the elderly who have passed the "possible" boundary want and deserve? Saving costs by keeping frail individuals at home longer may be economically efficient and ethically worthwhile, but keeping them at home longer at *greater* cost may still be a worthy societal goal from the perspective of the moral economy of the state.

Conclusion

Changes to the Swedish welfare state have been made with little public discussion about the Swedish concept of the welfare state and have been generally viewed as pragmatic reactions to changing political economies at national and global levels. Missing from the discussion is an assessment of the moral economy and how to maintain its integrity in the face of reforms.

The welfare state model hinges on a moral economy that legitimates redistributive principles as a basis for policy formation as well as a political economy that enables those policies. When each complements the other, the welfare state is likely to be stable and rely on strong public support. However, when they are dissonant, their reconciliation may require policy changes that range from targeting to universal restrictions to outright restructuring. Politicians and pundits are prone to discussing the economic limits of the welfare state as justification for its retrenchment. But there are also limits to altering the moral economy. Finding the right balance between fiscal change and ideological continuity will help guide policymakers to devise practical schemes that are more likely to find favor in the general population.

It is far more likely that an aging population and competition in the world market economy will result in the refurbishing of the welfare state rather than its demise. Mitigating circumstances may help avert the need to dramatically bend the moral economy to fit fiscal realities. Older adults in European nations with relatively generous pension programs, including Sweden, tend to provide economic transfers to needy children, suggesting a social welfare function for their surplus economic resources (Fritzell & Lennartsson, 2005; Künemund, Motel-Klingebiel, & Kohli, 2005; Spilerman, 2004). Sweden has been able to ease the acceleration of its old-age dependency ratio by immigration policies that "young" the society as well as institute policies such as providing generous child care benefits that encourage fertility. In the end, demography is not destiny for the welfare state but may require a detour that is compatible with the national character on which it is based.

References

Anttonen, A., & Sipilä, J. (1996). European social care services: Is it possible to identify models? *Journal of European Social Policy, 6,* 87–100.

Bergmark, A., Thorslund, M., & Lindberg, E. (2000). Beyond benevolence—Solidarity and welfare state transition in Sweden. *International Journal of Social Welfare, 9,* 238–249.

Daatland, S. O. (1997). Welfare policies for older people in transition? Emerging trends and comparative perspectives. *Scandinavian Journal of Social Welfare, 6,* 153–161.

Daatland, S. O., & Herlofson, K. (2003). "Lost solidarity" or "changed solidarity": A comparative European view of normative family solidarity. *Ageing & Society, 23,* 537–560.

Davey, A., Femia, E. E., Zarit, S. H., Shea, D. G., Sundstroem, G., Berg, S., et al. (2005). Life on the edge: Patterns of formal and informal help to older adults in the United States and Sweden. *Journal of Gerontology: Social Sciences, 6,* S281–S288.

Esping-Anderson, G. (1990). *The three worlds of welfare capitalism.* Princeton, NJ: Princeton University Press.

Esping-Anderson, G. (1999). *Social foundations of postindustrial economies.* London: Oxford University Press.

Evers, A., & Laville, J.-L. (Eds.). (2004). *The third sector in Europe.* Northampton MA: Edward Elgar Publishing Limited.

Fritzell, J., & Lennartsson, C. (2005). Financial transfers between generations in Sweden. *Ageing & Society, 25,* 1–18.

Giddens, A. (2000). *The third way and its critics.* Cambridge: Polity Press.

Gonzales, V. (2007). Globalization, welfare reform and the social economy: Developing an alternative approach to analyzing social welfare systems in the post-industrial era. *Journal of Sociology and Social Welfare, 34,* 187–211.

Jegermalm, M. (2006). Informal care in Sweden: A typology of care and caregivers. *International Journal of Social Welfare, 15,* 332–343.

Kallache, A., Barreto, S. M., & Keller, I. (2005). Global ageing: The demographic revolution in all cultures and societies. In M. Johnson (Ed.), *Cambridge handbook of aging* (pp. 30–46). Cambridge: Cambridge University Press.

Künemund, H., Motel-Klingebiel, A., & Kohli, M. (2005). Do intergenerational transfers from elderly parents increase social inequality among their middle-aged children? Evidence from the German Aging Survey. *Journal of Gerontology: Social Sciences, 60,* S30–S36.

Larsson, K. (2006). Care needs and home-help services for older people in Sweden: Does improved functioning account for the reduction in public care? *Ageing & Society, 26,* 413–429.

Larsson, K., & Thorslund, M. (2002). Does gender matter? Differences in patterns of informal support and formal services in a Swedish urban elderly population. *Research on Aging, 24,* 308–337.

Larsson, K., Thorslund, M., & Silverstein, M. (2005). Delivering care to older people at home. In M. Johnson (Ed.), *Cambridge handbook of aging* (pp. 630–637). Cambridge: Cambridge University Press.

O'Rand, A. M. (2006). Stratification and the life course: Life-course capital, life course risks, and social inequality. In R. L. Binstock & L. K. George (Eds.), *Handbook of aging and the social sciences* (6th ed., pp. 145–162). San Diego, CA: Academic Press.

Organization for Economic Cooperation and Development. (1996). *Caring for frail elderly people: Policies in evolution.* Social Policy Studies, no. 19. Paris: Author.

Parker, M. G. (2000). Sweden and the United States: Is the challenge of an aging society leading to a convergence of policy? *Journal of Aging Social Policy, 12,* 73–90.

Phillipson, C. (2003). Globalization and the reconstruction of old age: New challenges for critical gerontology. In S. Biggs, A. Lowenstein, & J. Hendricks (Eds.), *The need for theory: Critical approaches to social gerontology* (pp. 163–179). Amityville, NY: Baywood Publishing.

Quadagno, J., & Street, D. (2006). Recent trends in U.S. social welfare policy: Minor retrenchment or major transformation? *Research on Aging, 28,* 303–316.

Razin, A., & Sadka, E. (2005). *The decline of the welfare state: Demography and globalization.* Cambridge, MA: MIT Press.

Shea, D., Davey, A., Femia, E. E., Zarit, S. H., Sundstrom, G., Berg, S., et al. (2003). Exploring assistance in Sweden and the United States. *The Gerontologist, 43,* 712–721.

Sipilä, J., Anttonen, A., & Baldock, J. (2003). The importance of social care. In A. Anttonen, J. Baldock, & J. Sipilä (Eds.), *The young, the old and the state: Social care systems in five industrial nations* (pp. 1–23). Cheltenham: Edward Elgar Publishing Limited.

Spilerman, S. (2004). The impact of parental wealth on early living standards in Israel. *American Journal of Sociology, 110,* 92–122.

Sundstrom, G., Johansson, L., & Hassing, L. B. (2002). The shifting balance of long-term care in Sweden. *The Gerontologist, 42,* 350–355.

Szebehely, M. (2003). *Hemhjälp i Norden—Illustrationer och reflektioner* [Home help in the Nordic countries—Illustrations and reflections]. Lund: Studentlitteratur.

Szebehely, M. (2005). Care as employment and welfare provision—Child care and elder care in Sweden at the dawn of the 21st century. In H. M. Dahl & T. R. Eriksen (Eds.), *Dilemmas of care in the Nordic welfare state: Continuity and change* (pp. 80–97). Aldershot: Ashgate.

Thorslund, M. (1991). The increasing number of very old people will change the Swedish model of the welfare state. *Social Science and Medicine, 32,* 455–464.

Thorslund, M., Bergmark, Å., & Parker, M. G. (2001). Care for elderly people in Sweden. In D. N. Weisstub, D. C. Thomasma, S. Gauthier, & G. F. Tomossy (Eds.), *Aging: Caring for our elders* (pp. 49–63). Dordrecht: Kluwer Academic.

United Nations. (2007). *World population prospects: The 2006 revision.* New York: United Nations, Population Division.

Translating Theories of Aging

Jurisprudential Gerontology: Theorizing the Relationships Between Law and Aging

35

Israel Doron

Thirty years ago, in one of the first direct references to the field of law and aging made by a gerontologist, Elias S. Cohen (1978), the editor in chief of *The Gerontologist,* wrote the following words:

> *There is a growing recognition among lawyers, and more recently among gerontologists, that there are serious areas of inquiry and research in aging and law which address critical areas of social significance. . . .*
>
> *. . . But law and aging is too important to leave to the lawyers. And the research, language and analysis of lawyers are too important to be ignored by gerontologists. (p. 229)*

Unfortunately, except for very few exceptions (e.g., Levine, 1982), Cohen's call for cooperation and research and for the integration of law into the science of aging was unheard or mostly ignored. While the field of "elder law" continued to flourish and grow in the legal discipline (Frolik, 1993), the social gerontology mainstream continued to pay relatively little attention to legal developments in the field of aging. Yet the need to develop the field of "jurisprudential gerontology" (or "geriatric jurisprudence") still exists, as shown by the calls for the field's development that have appeared repeatedly in recent years (Doron, 2006b; Doron & Hoffman, 2005; Kapp, 2003).

It is my belief that the stereotypical construction of the field of law and aging was at least partly responsible for the fact that Cohen's call in 1978 failed to make a difference in reality. In its infancy, the field of law and aging was viewed using a legal-positivist approach. As will be described in this chapter, the field was seen as just another application of law, without any unique theoretical perspective, thus making it relevant mostly to lawyers working with older clients. Such a positivist construction made it very easy for social and political gerontologists to leave law outside their scope of research or interest. Moreover, as can be seen in the popular portrayal of old age in films, the legal background to important social phenomena was often simply ignored (Doron, 2006a).

However, as will be described in this chapter, the theoretical approaches that exist today have long abandoned the narrow positivist approach. Various new theoretical approaches to law and aging have been introduced in recent years. These have opened up the field of law and aging to new opportunities and avenues for integrating law and gerontology in what I think should be called "jurisprudential gerontology." I consider here the traditional positivist approaches to law and aging as well as the new approaches, both monist and pluralist.

The Positivist-Professional Approach

Lawyers have been dealing with older clients since the birth of the profession. However, the term "elder law" is relatively new and received formal recognition by the American bar only in the 1970s (Brazen, 1996; Frolik, 1993). The traditional, professional approach (i.e., that adopted by practicing lawyers in the field of elder law and the bar) defined the field of "elder law" from two different perspectives. One was a definition based on the client to be served. According to this approach, an elder law attorney was one who was concerned with the needs of the elderly client (Pohl, 1995). This kind of conceptual approach was adopted, at least in name, by what used to be called "the ABA [American Bar Association] Commission on the Legal Problems of the Elderly" (currently known as "the ABA Commission on Law and Aging"). Formed in 1978, this bar commission viewed its role as one that entailed working to involve the private bar in assisting older persons in need of legal services (Abrams & Russo, 1991). This kind of approach was also adopted by Goodstein (1993) in his essay "The Essence of Elder Law." According to his definition,

> *"Elder Law" is the entire body of law employed for the resolution of the legal problems encountered by the elderly, but with special application of the law to meet the needs and concerns of the client and family. . . . [I]t is defined by reference (1) to the client to be served, and (2) to the professional skill and understanding of the lawyer. (p. 11)*

The second professional perspective defined elder law by listing or detailing contents/topics that are unique or relevant to the field. For example, in response to the legal needs of older clients, estate planning or Medicaid planning became a legal field of expertise. Moreover, creative new legal tools, such as the "trust accounts," were invented exclusively in order to allow older persons to receive government benefits (such as Medicaid or supplemental security income), even when their income was above the minimum required for eligibility (Pohl, 1995).

This "content-specific" approach was adopted, for example, by the National Academy of Elder Law Attorneys (NAELA). Through its National Academy of Elder Law Foundation (an organization created by the board of directors of NAELA), NAELA offers "certification" in the field of elder law on successfully completing an examination covering the following topics: (1) health and personal care planning (e.g., advance directives); (b) premortem legal planning (e.g., wills); (c) fiduciary representation (e.g., guardianship); (d) legal capacity counseling; (e) individual representation (for those subject to guardianship/conservatorship procedures); (f) public benefits advice (e.g., Medicare); (g) advice on insurance (e.g., long-term care insurance); (h) resident rights advocacy; (i) housing counseling (e.g., home equity conversion); (j) employment and retirement advice (e.g., pension rights); (k) income, estate, and gift tax advice; (l) tort claims against nursing homes; (m) age and/or disability discrimination; and (n) litigation and administrative advocacy (e.g., elder abuse) (Pohl, 1995). Other scholars, such as Abrams and Russo (1991), have listed 21 content areas within elder law.

On both "client" and "content" perspectives, there was no need to develop "new" legal theories or to conceptualize the theoretical grounds for the field of law and aging. In both cases, elder law was standing, jurisprudentially speaking, on existing ground. Hence, the professional approach to the field of law and aging was well summarized by Abrams and Russo (1991) as follows:

> *Elder law embodies the diverse areas of law employed for the resolution of legal problems for the senior citizens. It is not a separate corpus of legal rules as may be applicable to subjects such as real property, torts, corporations and trusts. Rather, the elder law practitioner must be prepared to advise the client(s) and his/her family on a variety of legal and quasi-legal issues. (p. 33)*

Monist Jurisprudential Approaches to Law and Aging

The positivist-professional perspective provided sufficient grounds for excellent professional bodies such as NAELA or the ABA Commission on the Legal Problems of the Elderly to flourish. However, the perspective did not provide any new theoretical understanding of the unique ways in which the law interacts with and affects the lives of the older population. It was not surprising, then, that various elder law scholars started to look at existing and new jurisprudential approaches in order to provide a conceptual framework for the professional definition. This endeavor resulted in a rich and diverse body of scholarly writings that attempted to provide elder law with a single (or "monist"), coherent jurisprudence. Four such approaches are hereby described in short:

the later life planning approach, the law and economics approach, the therapeutic jurisprudence approach, and the feminist approach.

The Later Life Planning Approach

Lawrence Frolik has been following the development of the field of elder law since its early days (Frolik, 1993). In his article "The Developing Field of Elder Law Redux: Ten Years After" (2002), he summarizes his analysis of the development of this field as follows:

> *I believe that elder law has deviated from its original path, and is evolving into a field that is best termed later life planning. In doing so, elder law is reacting to the needs of clients, but also to the needs of attorneys who find it economically wise to expand the scope of their practice. (p. 2)*

What is later life planning? Traditionally, Medicaid planning (as also mentioned in the previous section on the professional approach) was considered to be the central issue of late life planning (Frolik, 2002). However, as Frolik describes later in his article, later life planning has expanded dramatically to include much broader and diverse legal issues that concern the elderly and the nonelderly. Health care decision-making issues are today a major legal issue for planning in old age. Included in this are not just end-of-life decisions or the appointment of a surrogate decision maker: planning also involves careful consideration of how the individual wants to be treated in old age and where and by whom. Within this field, "dementia planning" is practically a subspecialty in itself. As described by Frolik (2002), this requires property management planning, long-term care arrangements and planning for surrogate decision making, as well as final estate planning arrangements.

Traditional legal fields, such as those concerned with wills and estates, are changing in response to the reality of aging populations and the breakdown of traditional family structures. As noted by Frolik (2002), one motivation for late-life estate planning is often the behavior of the children, grandchildren, and other potential heirs of the client. Even older clients who do not have estates large enough to be subject to the federal estate tax may need a complicated estate plan that reflects the reality of families in the 21st century (Frolik 2002). These "new" families are the result of familiar dynamics that include divorce, remarriage, second families, late-life children, alternative lifestyles, and even drug and alcohol abuse.

When it comes to the older-old population, later life planning is less about planning for future contingencies and more about dealing with present realities. Moreover, as Frolik (2002) correctly points out, such planning must be undertaken with a client who is in many cases physically frail, perhaps mentally less acute than in the past, and possibly very confused as to what is "proper" behavior by the possible heirs and who is therefore looking for moral support and intellectual guidance from his or her lawyer. Therefore, there is no doubt that conceptualizing elder law as a legal planning tool for older people will lead to the continued development of creative legal solutions in light of a diverse and an ever-changing older population.

The Law and Economics Approach

While later-life planning is elder law specific, law and economics is a broad jurisprudential approach that is not elder specific. Nevertheless, as some scholars have proved, adopting this approach as an analytical framework is very useful in understanding the unique legal dimension of elder law (Kaplan, 2005). One leading scholar, famous for his law and economics analysis, is Richard Posner. A former chief judge of the U.S. Court of Appeals and senior lecturer at the University of Chicago Law School, Posner is one of the leading voices in the economic analysis of law. Posner (1995) has taken on himself the task of providing a comprehensive economic analysis of the field of law and aging in his book *Aging and Old Age*. His goal was "to show, in fact, that economics can provide a unifying perspective in which to view the whole range of social problems concerning the elderly" (p. 1).

To showcase one example of his many analyses, I present here Posner's economic analysis of age discrimination legislation in the United States. While this is considered to be an important piece of legislation that advances the rights of older workers and breaks down ageist stereotypes against them, Posner (1995), using his economic analysis, argues that

> *age discrimination law is largely ineffectual, but to the extent it is effective it has a perverse impact both on the welfare of the elderly and on the equality of income and wealth across the entire population. The age discrimination law is at once inefficient, regressive, and harmful to the elderly. (p. 319)*

To prove his point, Posner (1995) provides ample evidence from various empirical researches in this field. An example of one piece of supporting evidence is the very small number of lawsuits concerning age discrimination in the hiring process. In practice, employers are reluctant to hire older persons. The cost of training compared to the expected return on the investment in training is usually lower than for younger workers because the older worker has a shorter working life expectancy. The law, which pertains to eradicating such discriminating behavior, actually fails to achieve its goal. Posner presents empirical data that shows that, when considering cases of age discrimination litigation, only a small proportion of them concern hiring issues (10.5% of all cases). Moreover, within these hiring cases, the success rate (i.e., where the plaintiff won) was relatively low (4.4%). These figures are easily explained by the extreme difficulty of proving substantial damages in such cases and by the fact that disappointed applicants are unlikely to be satisfied with an order requiring the employer to hire them, as they would then have to enter a most inauspicious employment environment. Thus, adopting such a theoretical perspective can provide a much better understanding of the actual relationships between law and the elderly.

The Therapeutic Jurisprudence Approach

Another important conceptual lens or prism that allows us to better examine and understand the extent to which laws intended to benefit older persons actually end up accomplishing that mission is the therapeutic jurisprudence (TJ) approach. Law professor David Wexler (1990), who along with Bruce Winick

(1997) was one of the original developers of TJ, has defined this concept as follows:

> *The therapeutic jurisprudence perspective suggests that the law itself can be seen to function as a kind of therapist or therapeutic agent. Legal rules, legal procedures, and the roles of legal actors . . . constitute social forces that, like it or not, often produce therapeutic or antitherapeutic consequences. Therapeutic jurisprudence proposes that we be sensitive to those consequences, rather than ignore them, and that we ask whether the law's antitherapeutic consequences can be reduced, and its therapeutic consequences enhanced. (Wexler, 1996, pp. 453–455)*

The leading legal scholar who adopted and applied the TJ approach to the field of law and aging was Marshall Kapp. In his book *The Law and Older Persons: Is Geriatric Jurisprudence Therapeutic?,* Kapp (2003) applies the TJ approach to a whole range of legal issues regarding older persons, from legal guardianship over older adults to the legal reply to elder abuse and neglect. Kapp shows in his analysis how critically examining current legal policies toward the aged under the TJ approach reveals how law fails to achieve its intended or declared goals.

One example Kapp uses in his book is the legal regulation of nursing homes. Nursing homes, or institutional long-term care settings for the aged, are important and central players in the field of long-term care services for the dependent older population. As described by Kapp, on average, nursing home residents are older and more disabled than persons using home- and community-based long-term care services. These characteristics make this population more susceptible to neglect or abuse, and hence they require more stringent legal protection.

When describing the legal regulation of the nursing homes industry in the United States, Kapp (2003) uses the "octopus" metaphor:

> *The regulatory octopus entangling nursing homes possesses multiple tentacles. . . . The centerpiece of the regulatory puzzle is a set of mandatory conditions contained in the Nursing Home Quality Reform Act, enacted as a portion of the Omnibus Budget Reconciliation Act (OBRA) of 1987. . . .*
>
> *To implement OBRA '87, DHHS over the past two decades has promulgated regulations—Requirements and Participation—that set forth very specific mandates on which nursing homes will be surveyed for compliance. These federal survey requirements are classified into 17 major categories. (pp. 32–33)*

However, after describing the complex legal system of rules, regulations, and case law that surrounds the nursing homes industry in the United States, his TJ analysis brings Kapp to argue a quite unusual point in the world of elder advocacy and elderly rights:

> *Rather than admitting the often countertherapeutic limits and shortcomings of the current regulatory and litigation approaches in the nursing home context, the majority of public policy makers are stuck in the analytical "box" that says, "If regulation and litigation have failed, the answer is to make more of*

> *the same." Thus we continue to see a proliferation of legislative and regulatory proposals to "toughen up" on command and control supervision of nursing home process. (p. 66)*

It is through the unique TJ analysis that Kapp reaches his conclusion that what is needed in the realm of nursing home regulation is not more "new laws to solve current bad laws." Instead, he posits that the solution is to think creatively and to carefully allow the loosening of the existing regulatory reins and discard the habit of solving problems within the context of regulation. Therefore, the TJ approach toward nursing home regulation supports more consumer choice within a competitive marketplace. This consumer choice avenue is based on the autonomy model, which respects older individuals by allowing and encouraging them to make their own voluntary and informed choices about the terms of their health care coverage as well as the financing and delivery arrangements. From this TJ perspective, "consumers can and should manage their own care instead of relying on agencies or professional case management" (Kapp, 2003, pp. 102–103).

The Feminist Ethic of Care Approach

The feminist approach to law and aging, especially a feminist ethic of care approach (Gilligan, 1982), begins with the argument that any discussion of the field must consider gender issues (Korzec, 1997). Feminist legal theory tries to provide an alternative basis to the dominant male-based jurisprudence (e.g., the law and economics jurisprudence or the professional approach) (Olsen, 1990). Under this dominant male-based approach, dispute resolution is based on a rational, rights-based system that emphasizes the use of generalized principles and rules. Furthermore, under this traditional approach, "the justice-oriented 'neutral' problem-solver/decision-maker embodies a heightened moral development" (Korzec, 1997, p. 550).

The feminist ethics of care, by contrast, is totally different. It focuses on the unique factual context as well as on the parties' interdependencies and interpersonal responsibilities and rights (Gilligan, 1982; Korzec, 1997). It rejects adversarial disputes in favor of preserving ongoing relationships and forging cooperative solutions grounded in the specific facts of the problem at hand (Korzec, 1997). Applying the feminist ethic of care jurisprudence to the current field of law and aging not only exposes its sexist grounds but also broadens its insights and produces a more responsive elder law jurisprudence (Korzec, 1997).

One example of using a feminist jurisprudence to critically examine a law and aging issue is in the field of legislation, which addresses the rights of informal carers for older parents or other older family members. Empirical data in this field show again and again not only that most care for the elderly is provided by informal caregivers but also that it is usually women, either partners or daughters, who carry most of the burden of care.

When examining existing legislation (which pretends to address the needs of informal caregiving by family members) through a feminist lens, some critical insights appear. For example, critically analyzing the U.S. Family and Medical Leave Act of 1993 reveals that it "fails to adequately address the many problems facing the 'sandwich generation' of middle-aged women responsible for caretaking their own children as well as their elderly parents" (Korzec, 1997, p. 556; see also Rector [1995], who makes a similar point). The act gives unpaid workers leave to care for a seriously ill son, daughter, or parent. However, the act provides only 12 weeks of job-protected leave and thus cannot meet the long-term needs of elderly parents and their adult children. Moreover, coverage limitations mean that only about half of all workers and less than one-third of steadily employed new mothers receive this leave (since the act covers only employees who have worked for their employer for 12 months and for 1,250 hours in the previous year and whose employer has 50 or more employees working within 75 miles of the work site) (Ruhm, 1997).

Feminist jurisprudence, however, goes beyond examining specific pieces of elder rights legislation and use of a gender-based lens (Olsen, 1990). Examining law and aging through a feminist jurisprudence analysis compels us to reexamine the existing, positivist elder law approach, which stresses principles of autonomy and independence in old age. It allows us to expose how elder law is another social construct of patriarchy, especially within the social reality of an expanding older population and the growing need for informal care and support.

A Pluralist Approach

Unlike all the monist approaches described previously, which try to provide a conceptual framework of the field using a single conceptual lens, the multidimensional approach to law and aging proposes a different approach—a pluralistic one. This approach does not require us to believe that the uniqueness of the legal perspectives on aging can be fully conceptualized using a single theoretical framework. The pluralistic model was developed in response to the argument that the only way to fully grasp the richness and diversity of elder law is through a multidimensional model that connects the different functions and targets that law wishes to achieve.

The multidimensional model presented here is an ongoing developmental process. The first version of the model was published in Doron (2003a). The model has been further developed, and an updated version was published in Doron (2003b). The multidimensional model is described graphically in Figure 35.1.

The Legal Principles Dimension

The center of the multidimensional model is embedded in general and universal legal principles. Every legal system has a core composed of the system's underlying principles: the general, constitutional, and administrative norms that apply to any legal event in the given society. Such a core naturally includes the teachings of the constitution of the legal system as well as the basic principles and values underlying the various legal areas (Raz, 1972). The legal core protects the human and civil rights of the country's citizens on a universal basis. Historically, the existence of such a juristic core has supported the argument that there is no need to create a separate legal branch to deal with the legal issues of the elderly. Legislators and the courts thought it unnecessary to create specialized norms for the elderly on the assumption that these issues could be

35.1

The elder law multidimensional model (Doron, 2003b).

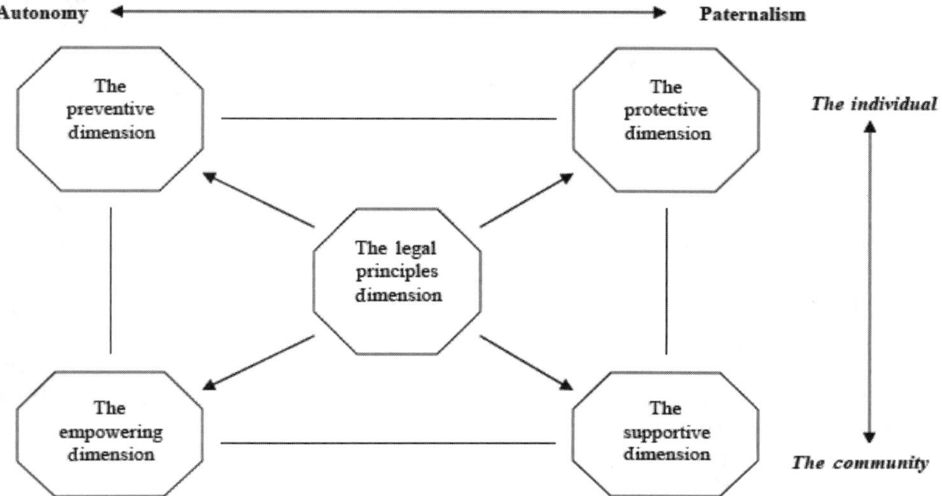

dealt with by means of the general legal principles that pertain to the entire population (Bonfield, 1989). Thus, for example, a case concerned with the financial exploitation of an older person would be handled through the general directives and rulings pertinent to contract law that forbid deception, exploitation, and coercion.

The juristic core of the justice system has its advantages and its disadvantages. The advantage is twofold: its breadth transcends the boundaries of issues, while its expanse is universal and pertains to all periods and to all areas of the law. In fact, this core provides legal protection to older persons in the same way as it does to the entire population, regardless of the content of the case or its circumstances. The second advantageous aspect of this universal core is its implicit notion of normalization: the older population is perceived as an integral and equal part of society. The law treats the aged as it does other parts of the population, and the rights of the aged are an integral part of civil rights as a whole.

However, this same claim of normalization also constitutes a disadvantage: the egalitarian principle cannot adequately contend with some of the particular issues that pertain concretely and specifically to the aged. Unique social phenomena that have a distinct effect on the older population cannot be dealt with by means of this universal core. Thus, despite its advantages, this legal core is not a fully adequate tool, as it is incapable of providing adequate legal responses to the needs of older persons.

The Protective Dimension

The point of departure for this second dimension is the need to address the unique and particular legal problems with which the older population must cope. The legal system responded by introducing point-specific legislation, intended for the most part to protect the aged (among other especially weak groups) against negligence, poverty, and exploitation.

There are many legal examples of the protective dimensions of elder law. One is the legal regime that ensures quality of care in nursing facilities. As described by Frolik and Barnes (2003), nursing home care presents special problems of quality assurance. Although the industry is increasingly professionalized, it is also subject to recurring incidents of notoriously poor care tied to high profit taking. Family members may have little power to ensure quality and good value. Thus, both federal and state laws attempt to ensure quality care and fairness in financial dealings with nursing homes, thus providing another legal layer of protection to institutionalized older persons. Such laws include diverse statutory measures, such as licensing, periodical surveys and certification, minimum staff numbers, ongoing training, and more.

The advantage of the protective dimension is that, used wisely, it provides protection to those among the elderly who need protection. It is worth noting that findings indicate that the problem of elder abuse is a serious social problem of an apparently broad scope (Decalmer & Glendenning, 1997). With these findings in mind, the establishment of this legislative dimension was a necessary response to a real social problem.

However, there is criticism over the protective dimension. First, there are those who question the effectiveness of "protective" policies (e.g., criminal justice or "command-and-control" regulations) in actually making a difference in reality and in providing real protection (Kapp, 2003). Moreover, despite the phenomenon of elder abuse, it should also be noted that not all elderly individuals are weak, vulnerable, or subject to abuse. This state of affairs makes this legal dimension a double-edged sword: by treating the elderly paternalistically and by making it possible to detract from their autonomy—based on the ethical claim that the state has the right and obligation to intervene in people's lives in order to protect them either from others or from themselves—the law substantiates the negative stereotype of the elderly population.

The Familial and Informal Supportive Dimension

The third legal dimension relating to the protection and promotion of older people's rights is actually directed at a population other than the elderly themselves. This dimension reflects an awareness and an understanding that, for a society that wishes to respect the rights of its elderly, attending to their legal status is not enough. Attention to the social context or setting is also warranted, particularly to the immediate circle of people who actually care for the needs of the older population. This conviction was based on research findings that identified a correlation between quality of life, health, and the ability to age in a respectful manner and the involvement of informal, social support networks. Older persons who had a strong supportive network, such as that of nearby family members who felt obligated to provide for and support them, were less likely to be ill, placed in institutions, or have a guardian appointed to ensure their proper care (Kane & Penrod, 1995).

To continue to help and assist social support networks for older persons, a variety of legal tools have been developed. First, laws were passed to enable relatives who act as ongoing informal caregivers of elderly family members to minimize the conflict between their obligations to the workplace and their burden of care. Second, statutory frameworks were created to provide monetary support for relatives who act as informal caregivers of elderly individuals to help compensate them for the expenses and financial losses incurred as a result of this role. Finally, formal networks were established to provide temporary or continuous nursing or palliative care in an attempt to complement or facilitate (but not be a substitute for) the informal care (Gerald, 1993).

The advantage of legally protecting older persons' rights by supporting those who care for them is derived from the link between the legal tool and the findings of other, extralegal, scientific disciplines, such as gerontology, sociology, and psychology. Thus, the nonlegal disciplines are instructive, as they demonstrate the significant role played by the social support networks in ensuring the rights of the older population and creating a more positive image of the elderly. Nevertheless, here too the moral and social strength of this legal dimension is not without limitations and apprehensions for those involved. First, there are doubts regarding the ability of such legal tools to influence the existence of informal support networks. Second, there are also political and moral reservations as to the justification of legal involvement in this regard: does this dimension enable the state to relinquish its obligation to take care of its older citizens, or, conversely, aren't the issues addressed in this dimension part of a personal moral obligation to the older generation that should not involve the law?

The Preventive and Planning Dimension

The fourth legal dimension that relates to the status of the older population concerns legal ways of preventing unnecessary intervention in the lives of the older population—by means of creating legal planning tools. This dimension was discussed in length within the monistic framework of elder law as "later-life planning" (described previously). Certainly, the greatest advantages of this dimension are its individualistic and autonomous perspective as well as its preventive dimension. This acknowledges the significance of older persons' independence and self-respect and the value of maintaining their personal autonomy. Moreover, these legal planning tools make it possible to avoid the need—on a social scale—to resort to the formal judicial system and its drawn-out adversarial procedures.

However, it seems that the main weakness of this preventive dimension is the gap between its theoretical rigor and its actual implementation, as experienced by many elders. The application and use of these planning tools requires a combination of awareness of and familiarity with the tools as well as financial and intellectual know-how. Thus, in fact, these tools remain unused by large portions of the older population. Even if it were possible to overcome the issues of awareness and faulty implementation, the moral and social basis of this dimension may be questionable. Some will argue that promoting individualistic tools may entail the risk of isolating the older person if it ignores the desires, interests, and worries of family members, professionals, and others involved in caring for the older individual (King, 1996).

The Empowerment Dimension

The final legal dimension in the multidimensional model was formed once legal systems came to realize that guarding the physical and financial welfare of older persons was insufficient, as were the individual planning tools, which remained, for the most part, unused. Research in all the previously mentioned dimensions found a lack of awareness, a lack of knowledge, or little use of existing rights (Doron & Gal, 2006; Doron & Werner, in press). Without legal means that could initiate a movement toward change, progress, and realization, the previously described dimensions of legal tools would not accomplish their intended goals.

This understanding was based on an observation of the current reality, which revealed that adding new legislation to the law books did not influence the real-life, daily experiences of many older persons. The older population would be not be able to realize their legal rights as long as they remained unaware of them, uninformed about their purpose, and unassisted in implementing them. This perspective led to the recognition that legal support for the empowerment of the older population was the step necessary to initiate a change in the older population's social and political status and that this would help attain the goals of all the prior legislative dimensions (Thursz, 1995).

Empowerment as a theoretical term is complex and implies various definitions and approaches, the scope of which exceeds the limits of this chapter. However, it is worth noting that, for our purposes, empowerment of the older population attempts to address the political asymmetry in power distribution and particularly the weak social status of the elderly by both increasing their power and changing the social environment in which they function (Handler, 1995).

The legal dimension of empowerment is well accepted by those interested in promoting older people's rights. However, it is also the focus of criticism that is far from insignificant. The first claim against this dimension is that its point of departure defines the older population once again as a powerless group in contrast to the powerful group that is either willing or forced to "grant" or "transfer" some of its powers (Sykes, 1995). The second critical claim casts doubt on the efficacy of empowerment tools as a means of changing the social status of the elderly or of any weak social group in general (Weissberg, 1999). Finally, it is claimed that the empowerment of the elderly usually comes at the expense of another social group that becomes disempowered. This dynamic may lead to a result that is contrary to the original intention: instead of empowering the elderly, it places them in conflict with other social groups vying for power in society. Often these competing groups are in fact stronger than the elderly, and thus instead of improving the social status of the elderly, this approach results in further detriment to their legal status (Lightman & Aviram, 2000).

The Broad Picture of the Pluralist Approach

The multidimensional model introduced here affords a clear presentation of the diversity and variability that characterize the field of elder law. Elder law, so the multidimensional model suggests, includes distinct types of legal tools, a range of political and philosophic approaches, and multiple perspectives on the concept of "elder rights." In other words, this field is by no means directed by a single conceptual or theoretical viewpoint: it cannot be considered either "individualistic" or "paternalistic," nor can it be portrayed as promoting "negative" as opposed to "positive" rights or as favoring the individual over the family or the private over the public. Elder law covers the range of possible approaches and perspectives, and it can be fully appreciated only by understanding the internal balance between all its components.

The model also encompasses two central dichotomies that are key to many discussions within the field of elder law. The "paternalism" versus "autonomy" dichotomy is represented on the one hand by the protective and family support dimensions, both of which represent society's willingness to provide care for the older population while sometimes paying the price of limiting autonomy or freedom of choice. On the other hand, the preventive and empowering dimensions stress the value of personal autonomy and willingness to assign legal power in line with the older person's personal preferences, even if such preferences are against his or her "best interests," family members' preferences, or society's moral views. Another important dichotomy is the "individual versus society" dichotomy: while both the protective and the preventive dimension work mostly on the individual levels, the family support and empowerment dimensions work mostly or more strongly at the broader community and social levels.

Conclusions

The diverse theoretical approaches presented in this chapter reveal the richness of this field. This should not be surprising: Martin Levine (1982) concluded his seminal article on the frame of nature, gerontology, and law in the following words:

> *How significant is aging to law? The problems of gerontology touch deep concerns of the individual, the society, even the race. Gerontology may not be a discipline in itself, but its important problems include the aging of the body, the individual, and society, as well as ageism. The received wisdom is no longer a satisfactory guide to these problems . . .*
>
> *How significant is law to the elderly? The law has a great deal to do with many of the basic problems of gerontology. The law is a major part of the context within which the individual grows old . . .*
>
> *Legal scholarship in this era will be one of many forums through which our society works out responses to the changing frame of nature. (p. 288)*

More than 24 years later, the author of this chapter wrote in an article regarding current issues and future frontiers of elder law (Doron, 2006b, p. 66) that

> *elder law should not limit itself to being a specialized field of law, but rather should become an integral part of gerontological science, or transform into "jurisprudential gerontology." In light of the interdisciplinary and multidisciplinary nature of gerontology, it is only natural for legal knowledge, methodology and philosophy to contribute its own unique perspective to the gerontological imagination.*

One can then conclude with the hope that further awareness, knowledge, and the development of theories on law and aging will enrich our understanding of the phenomenon of aging in its social and political context.

References

Abrams, R., & Russo, V. J. (1991). The phenomenon, scope and practice of elder law. *New York State Bar Journal, 63,* 32–39.

Bonfield, L. (1989). Was there a "third age" in the pre-industrial English past? Some evidence from the law. In J. Eekelaar & D. Pearl (Eds.), *An aging world—Dilemmas and challenges for law and social policy* (pp. 37–53). Oxford: Clarendon Press.

Brazen, L. (1996). A brief history of elder law. *Illinois Bar Journal, 84,* 16–18.

Cohen, E. S. (1978). Editorial: Law and aging, lawyers and gerontologists. *The Gerontologist, 18,* 229.

Decalmer, P., & Glendenning, F. (Eds.). (1997). *The mistreatment of elderly people.* London: Sage.

Doron, I. (2003a). Law and geriatrics: An Israeli perspective on future challenges. *Medicine & Law, 22,* 285–300.

Doron, I. (2003b). A multi-dimensional model of elder law: An Israeli example. *Ageing International, 28,* 242–259.

Doron, I. (2006a). Bringing law to the gerontological stage. *International Journal of Ageing and Human Development, 62,* 237–254.

Doron, I. (2006b). Elder law: Current issues and future frontiers. *European Journal on Ageing, 3,* 60–66.

Doron, I., & Gal, I. (2006). The emergence of preventive elder law: An Israeli example. *Journal of Cross-Cultural Gerontology, 21,* 41–53.

Doron, I., & Hoffman, A. (2005). Time for law: Legal literacy and gerontological education. *Journal of Gerontological Education, 31,* 627–642.

Doron, I., & Werner, P. (in press). Facts on law and aging quiz. *Ageing & Society.*

Frolik, L. A. (1993). The developing field of elder law: A historical perspective. *Elder Law Journal, 1,* 1–18.

Frolik, L. A. (2002). The developing field of elder law redux: Ten years after. *Elder Law Journal, 10,* 1–14.

Frolik, L. A., & Barnes, A. M. (2003). *Elder law: Cases and materials* (3rd ed.). New York, LexisNexis.

Gerald, L. B. (1993). Paid family caregiving: A review of progress and policies. *Journal of Aging & Social Policy, 5,* 73–89.

Gilligan, C. (1982). *In a different voice: Psychological theory and women's development.* Cambridge, MA: Harvard University Press.

Goodstein, M. J. (1993). The essence of elder law. *New York State Bar Journal, 65,* 10–12.

Handler, J. F. (1995). Community care for the frail elderly: A theory of empowerment. *Ohio State Law Journal, 50,* 541–593.

Kane, R. A., & Penrod, J. D. (Eds.). (1995). *Family caregiving in an aging society—Policy perspectives.* Newbury Park, CA: Sage.

Kaplan, R. L. (2005). Who's afraid of personal responsibility? Health savings accounts and the future of American health care. *McGeorge Law Review, 36,* 535.

Kapp, B. M. (2003). *The law and older persons: Is geriatric jurisprudence therapeutic?* Durham, NC: Carolina Academic Press.

King, N. P. (1996). *Making sense of advance directives,* Washington, DC: Georgetown University Press.

Korzec, R. (1997). A feminist view of American elder law. *University of Toledo Law Review, 28,* 547–561.

Levine, M. L. (1982). Introduction: The frame of nature, gerontology, and law. *Southern California Law Review, 56,* 261–288.

Lightman, E. S., & Aviram, U. (2000). Too much, too late: The Advocacy Act in Ontario. *Journal of Law and Social Policy, 22,* 25–48.

Olsen, F. (1990). Feminism and critical legal theory: An American perspective. *International Journal of the Sociology of Law, 18,* 199–215.

Pohl, A. E. (1995). Introduction: What is elder law anyway? *Nova Law Review, 19,* 459–464.

Posner, R. A. (1995). *Aging and old age.* Chicago: University of Chicago Press.

Raz, J. (1972). Legal principles and the limits of law. *Yale Law Journal, 81,* 823–854.

Rector, J. M. (1995). Family and Medical Leave Act of 1993. *The Journal of the Kansas Bar Association, 64*(4), 22–46.

Ruhm, C. J. (1997). Policy watch: The Family and Medical Leave Act. *Journal of Economic Perspectives, 11,* 175–186.

Sykes, J. T. (1995). A second opinion. In D. Thursz, C. Nusberg, & J. Prather (Eds.), *Empowering older people: An international approach* (pp. 47–59). London: Cassell.
Thursz, D. (1995). Introduction. In D. Thursz, C. Nusberg, & J. Prather (Eds.), *Empowering older people: An international approach* (pp. xi–xiv). London: Cassell.
Weissberg, R. (1999). *The politics of empowerment.* New York: Praeger.
Wexler, D. B. (1990). *Therapeutic jurisprudence: The law as a therapeutic agent.* Durham, NC: Carolina Academic Press.
Wexler, D. B. (1996). Therapeutic jurisprudence in clinical practice. *American Journal of Psychiatry, 153,* 453–455.
Winick, B. J. (1997). The jurisprudence of therapeutic jurisprudence. *Psychology, Public Policy and Law,* 184–206.

Spirituality, Finitude, and Theories of the Life Span

36

Malcolm L. Johnson

Perhaps gerontologists are not very spiritual or are like so many others captured by the "death taboo" identified by Aries (1981) or its "sequestration" as Giddens (1991) chose to describe it. Whatever the reasons, there is a marked aversion to addressing end-of-life issues among researchers and writers on aging. While we may describe our field of study as "the study of aging and the life span," comparatively little attention is given in the literature to the far end of the life span—death—or psychosocial aspects of the endings of lives. There is a body of work, of course. But in volume, it is massively outranked by social gerontological inquiries into families, generational relations, long-term care, pensions, ethnicity, gender, work, and retirement.

Opening with this observation is not simply special pleading or any sense of grievance that some areas of the experiences of aging get more attention than others. Nor is there cause to make a case for diverting attention (and research funds) to a new and emergent theme, such as might be made for, say, the social impact of nanotechnology on older people. Death and dying have been central issues in world literature, theology, history, philosophy, drama, and jurisprudence for as long as the written word has been available. Some literary critics argue that there are only three themes in the history of the novel: sex, death, and money. So it is not unreasonable to speculate why students of aging and old age have largely avoided the very end of the living process.

Until the middle of the 20th century, even in economically developed nations death occurred throughout the life span. Infant and perinatal mortality, maternal deaths in childbirth, children of infectious diseases, and adults in hazardous workplaces died of industrial accidents, while work environments, polluted air, and poor domestic dwellings gave rise to premature deaths in middle adulthood and later. By the commencement of the 21st century, 80% of all deaths in western Europe are of people over 65 years of age.

In a similar way, we may observe the now vast corpus of research on aging and see as Achenbaum (1995) did in his benchmark history of gerontology that the past 50 years has seen a growing focus on the "problems" of aging, the characteristics of successful aging, and the sociomedical correlates of old age. In more recent times, the shift from basic patterns of ill health associated with advancing years has been toward the psychological aspects of well-being and life satisfaction. The dispositions of gerontological researchers and theorists continue to display a curious avoidance of the inner lives of their subjects (unless they are in the turmoil we call mental illness or the particular old-age variant, dementia).

Typically, textbooks in the field will include a short chapter at the end (or none) on death and dying. Classic works of social investigation on the experiences of very old age, such as Gubrium's (1975) *Living and Dying in Murray Manor,* an insightful revelation of the underlife of a nursing home, devotes only 11 pages to death and dying and provides no analysis of the spiritual and death work that is the very stuff of long-term care. Even the benchmark sixth edition of the 2006 *Handbook of Aging and the Social Sciences* is so blind to these matters that neither the word "death" nor the word "spirituality" appear in the index.

Such observations could well be seen as selective and unrepresentative, and this cannot be denied. But they serve to make a serious point about the peculiarities of the gerontological research gaze—a topic I have addressed at a little more length previously (Johnson, 2005). Without providing an extensive and documented critique, the point to be made is clear; the key words in the title of this chapter represent underdeveloped areas of study. But they surely belong in any full assessment of the human life course—and theories about it.

Theories of the Life Course

There is some consensus among the principal commentators and contributors to life course studies and those who have tried to provide theoretical formulations that its development has been most evident from around 1980. There were, of course, many who adopted what is now termed the life course perspective before it was labeled and designated—but then there were structural functionalists before Talcott Parsons and symbolic interactionists before the American explosion of the 1950s and practitioners of grounded theory before Glaser and Strauss.

It is not the purpose of this chapter to provide a detailed account of theories of the life span. My objective is to reveal a sketch map of the burgeoning literature, to supply an overview of its main preoccupations, and, most particularly, to draw attention to the continued reserve among social scientists to seeing the end of the life span as intrinsically interesting or worthy of social investigation. This observation sits in some contrast to Erikson's (1950, 1982) willingness to include the final stages of life as aspects of his theory of generativity. However, he depicted the eighth stage as one of old age and despair, while some who are able to achieve ego integrity gain final life satisfaction—a marked difference in orientation to the prevalent school of "successful aging" and one of the principal reasons that end of life has been all but excluded from theories of the life course.

The shift in sociological thinking from consideration of the life path as a circular journey, embodied in the paradigm the "life cycle" to a recognition that human experience should be characterized not as proceeding from childhood dependency through independent adulthood and back to a second childhood of dependency in old age but as a trajectory that may result in many different experiences of later life, was fundamental. Not only did it release the idea of progression through human existence from its established place within the sociology of family; it could then become a framework for social scientists who were engaged in gerontology to explore the multiple and interacting life careers that make up personal and collective life histories. So while Glick (1977) was still promulgating his "life cycle of the family" thesis, the Committee on Human Development in Chicago, spearheaded by Neugarten and her colleagues (see Neugarten & Hagestad, 1976) and Elder (1974), then at Berkeley, were taking psychological and sociological studies of aging down parallel pathways.

Glen Elder's seminal contribution in his *Children of the Great Depression* (1974) was to go beyond the age- and stage-focused developmental theories by providing a methodology that explicated the ways in which historical change impacts on the lives of individuals. His sophisticated analyses of data sets already collected over several decades revealed how the experiences of childhood directly shaped the rest of the life course but in remarkably different ways. By following the dynamics of a cohort of children into adulthood, he avoided the limitations of cross-sectional, point-of-time studies. Through this perspective, he observed the differential and often serendipitous influence of social origins, societal and personal crises, family and socialization processes, and the opportunities that presented themselves. Elder remarks, "Such comparisons rest on the assumption that social change has differential consequences for persons of unlike age, which suggests that age variations in the meaning of a situation, in adaptive potential or options, and thus in linkages between the event and the life course" (p. 8).

As Dannefer and Uhlenberg (1999) point out, the received wisdom that derived from a large body of cross-sectional studies was severely challenged by the increasing evidence of more authentic analyses of life experiences. The trajectories of individuals with common origins that early post–World War II studies had laid in the public mind were of a somewhat rigid and predictable forward path. Based on the developmental biology of the times, both psychological and sociological research had conformed to a social determinism that depicted lives as being bounded by what we would now refer to as the social capital inherited by each child located in its historical and cultural environment.

With the erosion of confidence in generalizations about the predictability of developments contained within the shared constraints of the accepted understanding of life stages, a period of new conceptualizing emerged to reflect the expansion of longitudinal studies. In addition to Elder's work, Baltes established the Berlin Ageing Studies in Germany, and his collaborations with Schaie (Baltes & Schaie, 1968) produced valuable methodological developments. Riley and Foner (1968) commenced their sociologically significant aging society program of studies, while Bengtson initiated his Longitudinal Study of Generations, which has continued to explore the complexity of intergenerational relations to the present day (Bengtson, Biblarz, & Roberts, 2002; Bengtson & Kuypers, 1971).

A number of excellent reviews of the patterns of development in life course studies and the conceptual discourses that have emerged from the nature of longitudinal research as it affects older people and gerontology as a field have been published in recent years. Among the most persuasive is Settersten (2006), who provides, in addition to the intellectual story and notes on the key players, a perceptive assessment of the impact that this body of research has had on gerontology as a special area of study and on the distinctiveness of old age as a research focus and as a human experience. Earlier I noted a view of aging that was almost predetermined by structural variables. But current discourse represents the diversity of postretirement life as its signal characteristic. Life span studies have served to highlight difference rather than the commonalities arising from being in a postemployment phase. The question is posited: is there so little distinctiveness about old age that gerontology itself as an age related enterprise is approaching its own demise?

Intellectual fashions and the periodic salience of moral or socially sanctioned views of human groups can and do distort theories and research. Cumming and Henry's (1961) valuable study of disengagement in old age was initially hailed as a truly important revelation. It gave gerontology a clear set of observations of human beings in late life, withdrawing from various arenas of social endeavor, apparently because of decrements of physical and psychological functioning, associated with failing physical health and reduced economic status. Nearly 50 years later, that proposition looks to be a likely description of many people in the fourth age (if not of the expanding legions of healthy third agers) who may well have been out of the central economic and employment arena for two decades or more. But by the early 1960s, the structural functionalist perspective (associated with Talcott Parsons) had been toppled from its sociological ascendancy. So "disengagement theory" (it never was a theory) was discredited and has been in the academic doghouse ever since.

From the mid-1960s, it was seen as necessary for age researchers to challenge the prevailing negative stereotypes of old age. We became evangelists for a better old age. Gerontologists carried their positive old-age credentials as a badge of identity and honor—despite the empirical evidence that for all but the fortunate few, retirement was a time of restricted opportunity, ageism, and ill health resulting from occupational hazards, smoking, and poor housing. While critical gerontology gained its respected status from the work of Carroll Estes (1979), Alan Walker (1981), Chris Phillipson (1982), Martin Kohli (Kohli, Rosenow, & Wolf, 1983), Jill Quadagno (1988), Tim Diamond (1992), Ann Robertson (1997), and others who exposed the structural disadvantages imposed on older people in developed societies, the general disposition was to argue that later life was getting better and better.

The later decades of the 20th century saw a genuine increase in the well-being of older people. They were living healthier and longer. Pension provision and social security was improved (except in the United States during Reagan's smiling gerontocratic presidency). Representative organizations and pressure groups, like the American Association of Retired Persons (AARP) in the United States and Age Concern in the United Kingdom, raised the political profile. Indeed, by the early 1990s, there was the beginning of a backlash. Americans for Generational Equity (AGE) began a well-funded lobby of state legislatures to redress what they saw as a generational imbalance. AGE spoke of "greedy geezers" depriving their children of federal and state dollars that should have been going into education and youth services (Fairlie, 1988). AGE closed down in 1990, marking a failure to ignite generational conflict but leaving a greater awareness. As the baby-boomer generation moves into retirement and the third age, the topic could reappear on the political agenda.

However, the subject of generational equity was under active scholarly scrutiny long before it became a public issue. Eisenstadt's (1956) essay "From Generation to Generation" marked out an early mainstream sociological interest, while Rawls's (1971) *A Theory of Social Justice* galvanized contemporary philosophers to return to a discourse reaching back through Hobbes, Locke, and Rousseau to Aristotle. Gerontologists found themselves drawn into interdisciplinary collaborations that began to map the theoretical and the empirical realities of aging societies and distributive justice. Among them was Callaghan's (1987) profoundly controversial *Setting the Limits,* which argued that the health care of older people should take a lower priority than that of younger people. John Myles's (1983) command of the complexities of social security provided a database for the wider debate that drew in important contributions from Jill Quadagno (1988), a challenging volume from the United Kingdom (Johnson, Conrad, & Thompson, 1989) *Workers Versus Pensioners: Intergenerational Conflict in an Ageing World,* and influential collections from Bengtson and Achenbaum (1993) and Alan Walker (1996), among others, that grounded this core set of issues in the literature of aging studies.

Once the debate regarding justice across age-group entered the public policy arena, it became evident that there were ethical dilemmas at the microlevel as well: family responsibilities to old and young, economic transfers, inheritance, wills and advance directives, care and nursing home costs, and the proper treatment of the vulnerable old. Harry Moody became gerontology's most reliable and lucid guide, and his *Ethics in an Aging Society* (1992) has become a key sourcebook.

In all the fertile discussions that were stimulated by the reconceptualization of gerontology brought about by the life course perspective (Bengtson, Elder, & Putney, 2005), few have served to bring the subjects of death and spirituality into the central arena. Instead, it has reinforced the focus on the beguiling prospects of healthy immortality, sponsored by the more optimistic biologists of aging and the emergence of more and more data about "the oldest-old." With the fastest-growing sector of the populations of western Europe being those over age 85—a situation masked in North America by the youth of its immigrant population and their fecundity—there is a pervasive belief in the continuing increase in life expectation.

Not all that expectation is attributable to possibilities arising from mapping of the human genome. On the other hand, analysis of European demographic data since 1840, by Oeppen and Vauppel (2002), revealed the astonishing fact that female life expectancy (and for men equally consistently) in the lead nation, Sweden, has risen for 160 years at a steady pace of 3 months per year—and shows no sign of relenting. Their claim is that there are no known limits to the extension of life.

Yet the undeniable reality is that we all die. What is often overlooked is the dramatic movement of death along the life path. In the world's richer societies where premature death has been vastly reduced and dying in childhood or adulthood up to retirement has become rare, the very nature of death has been transformed.

Death in the Province of Old Age

I have already noted that the systematic reductions in premature death that took place across the developed world during the 20th century have made death in childhood, youth, or adulthood prior to retirement a comparative rarity. When such deaths occur, they create a sense of shock. Where the person is under 50, the reactions tend to focus on the unfairness of a life tragically ended long before time. Child deaths arouse the strongest emotions and produce the most elaborate well-attended funerals. The culturally accepted stretched life span has incorporated the marked extension of life expectancy. So there is a new norm for death, which is embedded in the collective psyche, though the normative framework has yet to permeate into any socially recognizable patterns that signify the importance and meaning of dying in later life.

A range of social scripts exists for premature deaths. "His life has been cut off in its prime." "She still had so much to give." "How tragic he has left a growing family—how will they manage?" "Her whole life was ahead of her, and now it will never happen." Underpinning these ready responses is an implicit theory of the life span. It is based on a demographic assumption that our cohort can expect to live beyond pensionable age and well into retirement. Even deaths of individuals in their late 60s produce indications of a too-early demise. "He was still quite young—could have lived for years yet."

This taken-for-granted calibration of the life span is realistic. Modern societies now experience a historically unprecedented longevity, meaning that four out of every five deaths are of people aged 65 or over. For the first time, death is in the province of old age. But where are the signs of recognition beyond the extended mental maps of the members of society and the observations of obituary writers? In a market-driven world, we might expect to see those in the death industry marketing special bespoke funerals for the mature citizen. Here is a market for new trends in memorialization to match the European fashion for family vaults and sculpted angels in the 19th century. There are memorial Web sites, interesting wicker and ecocoffins, and caskets emblazoned with pictures, images, or photographs that reflect the life and interests of the deceased person. Why are they not advertised in the lifestyle magazines, in the Sunday papers, and on television? The market is large and growing and in part well resourced.

It took some time for the older persons market to grow out of its ageism. The very existence of AARP is due to the unwillingness of travel companies to offer insurance to retired teachers. Now, 40 years after its founding, AARP is reputed to be the largest membership organization in the world and has transformed the consumer markets and public policy forums in favor of older people. To its credit, there is a good deal on its Web site that deals openly and well with death, dying, funerals, bereavement, advance directives, wills, and so on.

But the products and the services that relate to these issues have still to make it into the wider commercial arena. Perhaps the United States will have to wait for that group of attention grabbers, the boomers, to bring death back out of the closet? As for western Europe and Australasia, the signs of market recognition are few. A survey by the U.K. Office of Fair Trading (OFT) in 2001 revealed that 95% of funerals were "a distress purchase" made within 2 days of the death, where the selected funeral director was chosen from the Yellow Pages and almost all first contacts were confirmed. A study my colleagues and I undertook for the OFT review (Johnson, Cullen, Heatley, & Hockey, 2001) demonstrated that because the great majority of deaths were of old people, the person who made the arrangements for the funeral did not feel that their normal commercial judgments were affected by grief. Despite this, there was almost no reported "shopping around." This was explained by a reluctance to "haggle over a funeral" and a concern about peer pressure from siblings over any insinuations about being mean over mother's/father's funeral. This in turn highlights the low level of death and funeral planning by British older people, completing the circle of reluctance to deal with end-of-life matters.

Finitude: The Anticipation of Endings

Thoughts about the imminence of death and the effect they have on how individuals live the remaining portion of their lives is an age-old topic. From the last words of the great and the good to the sage pronouncements of the remarkably old to contemporary preoccupations with the psychological adaptations of people with life-threatening illnesses, the contemplation of expected death is a heightened feature of modern considerations of life expectancy.

Against a backdrop of apocalyptic changes in demography that has seen the average life span in developed societies almost double in a century, there is a new set of paradoxes that focus attention on lives truncated by diseases that have still eluded biomedical controls. While a century ago the common causes of death among adults included infectious diseases such as influenza, tuberculosis, and polio, the contemporary causes of premature death include cancers and HIV/AIDS.

With the aid of sophisticated diagnostic techniques and drug therapies that inhibit symptoms, there are legions of people who know they will die in the near future and have time to contemplate how to use what imagination and capacity they have to reflect on their pasts and to consider what death means to them.

Such opportunities for engaging with finitude are not new. Many great writers of the past have written about facing imminent death. Leo Tolstoy (1899) wrote movingly and sanely about his increasing illness and the struggles he had with maintaining reason and faith. "My situation was a terrible one. I knew that I should not find anything on the path of rational knowledge but the negation of life, and there, nothing but the negation of reason, which was still more impossible than the negation of life." The perceptive but cantankerous Cicero, who enjoyed his ill health (though no one else was allowed to), wrote extensively about it. At times his prognostications of death were fearful and deeply depressive, like Tolstoy's. At other times, he was charmed by the notion that death is only a transitive state, "as an inn in which to stay, but not to dwell."

Such thoughts are widely in currency today as testified by the extensive use at funerals of the poem "Death Is Nothing at All" by Henry Scott Holland (1847–1918), in which he consoles, "Death is nothing at all; I have only slipped into the next room," and concludes, "Nothing is past, nothing is lost; one brief moment and all will be as it was before" (for more accounts of predeath reflections, see Dickenson & Johnson, 1993). Indeed, the essential character of pressing finitude has not changed over time. It inevitably relies on recollection of the life lived and personal evaluations of the worth of that time of existence. Throughout history, these life reviews have used the moral and religious frameworks of the time as benchmarks of personal goodness.

Faced with a life almost at its end and now beyond reconstruction has been a source of dismay, depression, self-loathing, guilt, and anger for many. In my own work, I have termed the most distressing and intractable version of this state *biographical pain* (Johnson, 2002). I found that the term "spiritual pain," which the hospice movement had turned into a portmanteau description for all nonphysical pain, was not comprehensible to nonspecialists and implied levels of spiritual awareness that are simply not present in contemporary societies. Yet my own research has constantly encountered deeply anguished older people facing finitude whose fears are derived from life review and biographical reflection.

The Dutch psychologist Joep Munnichs (1966), an early postwar gerontologist, observed the social and psychological importance of finitude as a feature of old age, drawing attention to the psychological demands placed on the individual who faces death. His interest in the significance of the concept remained isolated. Shortly after his book was published, Kubler-Ross's *On Death and Dying* (1969) was published and drew sustained attention to the "stages" conception of the pathway to death and beyond for several decades. In turn, parallels were made between Kubler-Ross's fifth stage of "acceptance" and Cumming and Henry's (1961) "disengagement," and the discussions filled the space for some time. The notion, nonetheless, found its way into the studies of other psychologists as evidenced by the Kalish's (1976) excellent and comprehensive chapter. There he considers many of the issues that form the map of end-of-life studies today.

Kalish (1976) notes without reservation that death in old age is emotionally and qualitatively different from death earlier in life. One key feature of that is the way declining health is likely to affect the sense of finitude. He goes on to argue that finitude presents the older person with a requirement to detach from physical possessions, all experiences, and everything that is transient. Second, he notes that the imminence of death alters the meaning of the way we use time. On this topic, Kastenbaum's (1966) research showed that those dying in old age felt unable to make radical changes to their use of time, feeling that there was little they could do to change things that troubled them. This contrasted starkly with the responses of people aged 20 to 29 and 40 to 59 (Kalish & Reynolds, 1976), for whom finitude presented a need to use the heightened awareness in very active ways (a situation widely observed by the patterns adopted by younger HIV/AIDS sufferers). At that time, three decades ago, this study revealed that older people would change little with the prospect of only 30 days to live. "Nearly three times as many older persons as younger would spend their remaining time in prayer, reading, contemplation or other activities that reflect inner life, spiritual needs, or withdrawal" (p. 478).

More recent studies offer broad confirmation of these age-related patterns of response to the approach of death, but the intervening years have experienced significant cultural changes at the societal level and in the values of age cohorts as they pass along the life path (what Peter Laslett engagingly called the procession of the generations). What contemporary studies show is the same kind of dispersion of behaviors that were observed by Elder (1974) that challenged the prevailing age stereotypes. It should be a feature of revisions of life span theories that cohorts differ from one another—and it is—but also that individuals and cohorts change over time. Clearly, such inquiries have been conducted and some gained audiences well beyond the academy (e.g., Levinson, 1978; Sheehy, 1976), but they focused on young and middle-aged people.

More recently, the major multicohort studies, such as the Bengtson Longitudinal Study of the Generations, have seen their first cohorts enter retirement and even great grandparentdom. From the point of view of this chapter, it is good news that the latest study to be conducted by the University of Southern California team is on the transmission of religion across the generations—a sign perhaps that beliefs and spiritual values are being encompassed in the moving tide of life span studies.

Current cohorts of older people in the third and fourth ages represent significant differences in life experiences, not least in their religious affiliations and practices. Furthermore, there are distinctive patterns across societies (especially throughout Europe) where secularization has emerged in idiosyncratic sociocultural ways. Such divergences of experience in the nations said to be in late modernity are important for our understanding of the social, moral, and spiritual underpinnings of those whose lives are pressing close to finitude. The life span researchers' preoccupations with successful aging, well-being, and life satisfaction will need to take much more account of the spiritual dimension.

Spirituality in Later Life

All discussions of spirituality commence with acknowledgments that the term has no single definition or meaning. There is insufficient space in this chapter for a proper review. But some consideration is required. First, it must be conceded that present-day uses of the term have served to add complexity to an already difficult definitional task. Definitions conventionally begin with the spiritualities set within world religions, where the relationship with God and immersion in prayer generates both a sense of otherness that may become transcendent and a deepening of selfhood. The religious spiritual life may include adherence to specified practices often repeated (such as the Muslim daily prayer schedule or the Roman Catholic regular attendance at Mass and confession), where the rituals provide a devotional schedule of engagement with God, priest, and the community of the faithful.

Other, nonreligious models are less easy to specify because there are so many and their form and purposes are extremely diverse. A recognized starting point, when looking for an anchor, is the work of Viktor Frankl (1987), an Austrian psychiatrist who created the definition "the search for meaning." As Walter (2002) points out, Frankl himself termed this as an existential rather than a spiritual search. "It is primarily the English who have replaced the term 'existential' with 'spiritual'" (p. 133). Nonetheless, the many new and refurbished secular spiritualities are ready to shelter under this canopy definition, even if their practices, rituals, and orthodoxies are distinct.

Contemporary commentators appear to agree that the leading proponents of the search-for-meaning approach are to be found in the health professions, particularly nurses. In their paper on the links between spirituality and successful aging, Sadler and Biggs (2006), drawing on a review of the nursing literature by Oritz and Langer (2002) report a series of elements in the nursing spiritual repertoire: a transcendent belief in a higher power, experiencing a sense of connection, and drawing on inner resources, such as strength and peace.

Other features, such as "meaning making" and "manifest expressions," are to be found in the literature. Extensive debates about the descriptive and heuristic value of these statements can be found in the health professional press and most notably in writings within and about palliative care (see the following discussion). Rumbold (2000) provides some clarification by treating spirituality as a worldview, a way of looking at the meaning and purpose of life. A more comprehensive taxonomy of meanings within health care is provided by Kellehear (2000), who classifies the key "needs" domains in which spirituality operates or is perceived to be present in the lives of people experiencing serious or life-threatening illness. He identifies situational, moral, biographical, and religious needs and suggests that practitioners seeking to assess spiritual needs first clarify which category is being explored.

The debates about meaning will continue. If researchers and practitioners are trying to reveal, assess, measure, and interpret what we call the spiritual, further distillation will be required. Yet without this desired exactness, there is more than sufficient evidence that human beings desire to understand themselves, the world they live in, and the forces that guide it. Their understandings provide them with a moral compass, an external source of reference, and a way of measuring themselves against higher standards than those of the society. This is clearly evident in the world religions and often in the revered writings which accompany other belief systems.

Within the study of aging, there is ample evidence that as people age and get closer to the expected end of their lives, the spiritual dimension gains in prominence. In recent years, there have been more systematic studies that attempt to make the measurement of spirituality more possible. MacKinlay (2001) set out to map the spiritual dimension of a number of independently living adults and to design a tool for measuring the spiritual needs of older people. She was truly honest in recognizing that she was more successful with the former than the latter. Nonetheless, her well-documented journey has provided valuable advances in measurement potential.

More boldly and in a more macropiece of theorizing, Tornstam (2005) produced his theory of *gerotranscendence*. As a mainstream gerontologist, his explorations of this explanatory framework for positive aging have appeared in the literature since the term was first brought to prominence in 1990 (Tornstam, 1989) as a reformulation of disengagement theory. His purposes have been to shift gerontological thinking from the despairing old age of Erikson and Cumming and Henry into a paradigm that sponsors old age as a period of living worth achieving because of its own true benefits. Tornstam (2005) questions the underlying assumptions of the "successful aging" concept "with the typical emphasis on activity, productivity, independence, efficiency, wealth, health and sociability" (p. 3). Having observed the normative expectation that good aging is the continuation of the midlife patterns indefinitely, Tornstam asserts that there is continuous development into old age.

His theory of the gerotranscendent individual depicts him or her as someone who experiences a redefinition of the self and of relationships to others and a new understanding of fundamental, existential questions.

In this stage of transcendence (a term selected from the core lexicon of spirituality), the individual becomes less self-occupied, becomes more selective about social activities, has a greater affinity with past generations, and takes less interest in superfluous social interaction, even exhibiting a decreasing interest in material things and developing a need for solitary meditation. After a thorough critique of the negative ascriptions made to old age by society and gerontologists alike and the false optimism of the "successful aging" movement, Tornstam (2005) takes his readers into a set of complex empirical analyses that indicate the characteristics of gerotranscendence.

In addition to the substantive body of research employed and the theoretical rigor of his argument, Tornstam's work marks a transition point in the gerontological discourse. He engages with both the theory and the knowledge base in order to reformulate received notions of aging. This radical redefinition places spiritual transformation in the central arena of late life. By challenging the functionalist assumptions not only of the early formulations but also of the life course theorists, he marks out a serious challenge to the existing paradigm and notions of the life span that has no end.

In the world of care for these very same individuals at the far end of life is another kind of discourse that has its own powerful orthodoxies, incorporating entrenched presumptions about who should be the societal managers of dying, death, and bereavement. Palliative care and its sponsor, the hospice movement, have articulated their own rules about the appropriate ways to die and how pain should be palliated through a religiomedical model. Here concepts of spirituality and finitude are formulated in very specific ways and in line with the life span theorists and the "successful aging" proponents with a focus on "living to the end" while avoiding the distasteful reality of death and its aftermath.

Well-Managed Death: The Ageist Hospice and Palliative Care Paradigm

Hospices as places of respite, physical care, and spiritual concern for the dying have existed across Europe since the Middle Ages. Religious foundations (mainly Christian) provided such care as part of their ministry of healing to the poor and sick. But the commencement of the modern hospice movement is widely attributed to Cicely Saunders. Originally trained as a hospital almoner (social worker), then as a nurse, and finally as a medical doctor, she observed that dying patients in London hospitals, particularly those with cancers, received less-than-good attention to relieve the pain they experienced and to their deepest personal needs as their lives came to a close. Her dream of building a place for the terminally ill that would be "a combination of deeply rooted spirituality with the very best care that medicine can provide" (Du Boulay, 1984, p. 88) was realized in the opening of St. Christopher's Hospice in South London in 1967.

From the outset, the modern hospice was conceived of as a fusion of medical and religious ideals. It proved to be a powerful and refreshing mix that made it possible to talk about dying (but not death) openly and in a positive manner. Not only was a problem revealed to wider society, but an attractive and wholesome solution was presented by its highly persuasive advocate. Out of the hospice idea emerged the new medical specialty of palliative medicine, based on the development of pain-relieving drug therapies and the titration of this medication up the analgesic ladder. Yet for Saunders, the control of physical pain was based not simply on the administration of opioids but rather on their combination with spiritual care.

Configured in this way, we were presented not simply with an innovation in end-of-life care but also an ideology and praxis that were grounded in two other conceptual and moral domains—religion and medicine. Such a syncretization of Christian and secular spirituality and the medical model of physical pain management delivered with vigor and honesty rapidly spread. This model has proved attractive and effective for centuries, so its manifestation in a new context only reinforced the acceptability. Saunders's insistence on hospices being outside the established National Health Service and run by charitable bodies from public subscription, with services free to patients, touched a deeply socialist/communitarian susceptibility. On the basis of this moral and healing package, the hospice model was admired and reproduced around the world.

Four decades later, health care systems internationally speak the rhetoric of end-of-life care but still deliver death in hospitals to 55% of those who die annually and have learned little. But they accord high esteem to the hospices, which they do not pay for and which ration their services largely to people dying of cancers. Even in the United Kingdom, where the movement began, only 4% of annual deaths take place there. The standard hospice script is about living life to the end, of all pain being manageable, and with little talk of death itself. Palliative care has similarly attained respected status while being starved of resources yet is being used by the medical establishment to remedicalize death. So, not for the first time, a spectacular innovation has from its own well-meaning efforts created a new set of problems. They relate to the restrictions that exist on extending good end-of-life care to the many who need it and the dominance of one legitimate but not (socially) comprehensive concept of spirituality.

In his *A Social History of Dying,* Kellehear (2007) uses the term "the well managed death" as a descriptor of the hospice model. It aims to deliver "a good death," where clinical staff view dying in terms of the ease or otherwise of the patient's passing. Staff categorize deaths as "good," "bad," or "good enough." While this model might satisfy many westerners, it bears only tangential relationship to the "good death" prescribed for Hindus, Muslims, Jews, or those of many faiths in West Africa, where dying communally with family in loud presence is desired. It is a medicocultural construct, one that has angered Sinclair (2007) and mobilized him to systematize his critique on the basis of the experience of witnessing the lives and deaths of people with learning disabilities. He is perplexed as to why people were admitted to hospices not for clinical reasons but for social ones "yet palliative care activities and programmes and almost all palliative care research were about symptom control, pain management and clinical issues" (p. 2). His extended participant observations (in Australia) prompted him to disassemble the entire palliative care system by looking through the lens of the *social valorization theory* devised by Wolfensberger (1972) to understand and value people with learning disabilities and create normalization with and for them. As a result, he wants to normalize death and deinstitutionalize hospice care.

A feature of the rise of hospice care is the adoption by the caring professions, notably palliative care nurses, of a mélange of multicultural/individualistic/secular "care for the inner person," which extends their repertoire and domain while remaining loyal to the medical models. Walter (2002) depicts this as a product of the concurrent movements of secularization, globalization, and multiculturalism.

To this I would add a curious professional ageism that severely restricts the availability of palliative care to older people. A spin-off from the hospice focus on cancer among children and adults of working age, this ageism fails to recognize the equal needs of long-lived people to die with dignity and without avoidable pain.

Conclusions

If "finitude" is a proxy word for the awareness of the imminence of one's own death—and it is—and if "spirituality" is a term that embraces transcendental, religious, and self-explorations, then this chapter has attempted to demonstrate the scholarly and citizen avoidance of their meaning in considering the life path. We have acknowledged serious academic inquiries that address the end of life and have observed the unspectacular emergence of wider societal engagement with death matters. Yet this is in profound contradistinction to the studies that have uncovered extensive concerns of older people with life review, personal accounting, and spiritual reflexiveness, both satisfying and deeply troublesome.

Theories of the life span and the empirical studies that have prompted and elucidated them have added a considerable and authentic dimension to the conceptualization of human progression through the life path. This stream of work has released frameworks for considering the social and psychological *dynamics* of aging. This has, in turn, enabled a theoretical space for empirical work as diverse as intergenerational relations, work and retirement, generational equity, and the interaction of parallel life careers. The "story" of this development, so ably analyzed by Marshall (1999), reveals a steady conceptual progression of ideas and constructs that marks out the single most influential theoretical innovation in gerontology.

Over a similar time span, social and behavioral scientists, philosophers, and theologians who identify themselves as gerontologists have created an impressive body of work about dying, death, and end-of-life issues. From Kastenbaum's now-classic *The Psychology of Death* (2000) and the leading work of scholars like Neimeyer (1994) and de Vries (1999) has grown up a group of gerontologists interested in illuminating the experiences of older people at the end of life. They include research scientists and practitioners, so the menu is a strong mix of the practical and the conceptual. Yet it seems reasonable to suggest that this area of work is largely separate from mainstream gerontology—an academic subculture.

Whether this observation is acceptable or not, it is clear that there is too little integration of end-of-life work and ideas with that of the overwhelming output of age-related investigation and theorizing. If our field of study is to be described as aging and the life span, it is logical and intellectually coherent to advocate the incorporation of death and dying into theories of the life span. Howarth (2007), in reviewing sociological commentaries, has convincingly argued that death in modern society has been removed from the public realm and placed within the private sphere of the family and the individual. This chapter has agued there is a parallel in the academy. Like Giddens (1991), she argues that this sequestration removes the problem of mortality from an overtly public or social context. And with Bauman (1992), I wish to argue that it is the very fact of our mortality that produces the cultures we live in. Without death, there would be no culture (Walter, 1991).

References

Achenbaum, W. A. (1995). *Crossing frontiers: Gerontology emerges as a science.* Cambridge: Cambridge University Press.

Aries, P. (1981). *The hour of our death.* Harmondsworth: Allen Lane.

Baltes, P. B., & Schaie, K. W. (1968). Longitudinal and cross sectional sequences in the study of age and generation effects. *Human Development, 11,* 145–171.

Bauman, Z. (1992). *Mortality, immortality and other life strategies.* Cambridge: Polity Press.

Bengtson, V. L., & Achenbaum, W. A. (Eds.). (1993). *The changing contract across the generations.* New York: Aldine de Gruyter.

Bengtson, V. L., Biblarz, T. J., & Roberts, R. E. L. (2002). *How families still matter: A longitudinal study of youth in two generations.* Cambridge: Cambridge University Press.

Bengtson, V. L., Elder, G. H., Jr., & Putney, N. M. (2005). The lifecourse perspective on aging. In M. L. Johnson, with V. L. Bengtson, P. G. Coleman, & T. B. L. Kirkwood (Eds.), *The Cambridge handbook of age and ageing* (pp. 493–501). Cambridge: Cambridge University Press.

Bengtson, V. L., & Kuypers, J. A. (1971). Generational differences and the generational stake. *Aging and Human Development, 2,* 249–260.

Callaghan, D. (1987). *Setting the limits: Medical goals in an aging society.* New York: Simon & Schuster.

Cumming, E., & Henry, W. (1961). *Growing old: The process of disengagement.* New York: Basic Books.

Dannefer, D., & Uhlenberg, P. (1999). Paths of the lifecourse: A typology. In V. L. Bengtson & K. W. Schaie (Eds.), *Handbook of theories of aging* (pp. 306–326). New York: Springer Publishing.

de Vries, B. (Ed.). (1999). *End of life issue: Multidisciplinary perspectives.* New York: Springer Publishing.

Diamond, T. (1992). *Making gray gold: Narratives of nursing home care.* Chicago: University of Chicago Press.

Dickenson, D., & Johnson, M. L. (Eds.). (1993). *Death, dying and bereavement.* London: Sage.

Du Boulay, S. (1984). *Cicely Saunders: Founder of the modern hospice movement.* Sevenoaks, UK: Hodder and Stoughton.

Eisenstadt, S. N. (1956). *From generation to generation.* New York: The Free Press.

Elder, G. H., Jr. (1974). *Children of the Great Depression: Social change in life experience.* Chicago: University of Chicago Press.

Erikson, E. H. (1950). *Childhood and society.* New York: Norton.

Erikson, E. H. (1982). *The life cycle completed: A review.* New York: Norton.

Estes, C. (1979). *The aging enterprise.* San Francisco: Jossey-Bass.

Fairlie, H. (1988, March 28). Greedy geezers: Talkin 'bout my generation. *New Republic,* 19.

Frankel, V. (1987). *Man's search for meaning.* London: Hodder and Stoughton.

Giddens, A. (1991). *Modernity and self-identity: Self and society in the late modern age.* Cambridge: Polity Press.

Glick, P. (1977). Updating the life cycle of the family. *Journal of Marriage and the Family, 39,* 5–13.

Gubrium, J. (1975). *Living and dying in Murray Manor.* New York: St. Martin's Press.

Howarth, G. (2007). *Death and dying: A sociological introduction.* Cambridge: Polity Press.

Johnson, M. L. (2002). *Committed to the asylum: The long term care of older people.* Leveson Paper No. 3. Temple Balsall: Leveson Centre for Ageing and Spirituality.

Johnson, M. L. (2005). Ageing in the modern world. In M. L. Johnson, with V. L. Bengtson, P. G Coleman, & T. B. L. Kirkwood (Eds.), *The Cambridge handbook of age and ageing* (pp. xxi–xxvi). Cambridge: Cambridge University Press.

Johnson, M. L., Cullen, L., Heatley, R., & Hockey, J. (2001). *The psychology of death: An exploration of the impact of bereavement on purchases of "at need" funerals.* London: Office of Fair Trading.

Johnson, P., Conrad, C., & Thomson, D. (1989). *Workers versus pensioners: Intergenerational conflict in an ageing world.* Manchester: Manchester University Press.

Kalish, R. A. (1976). Death and dying in social context. In R. H. Binstock & E. Shanas (Eds.), *Handbook of aging and the social sciences* (pp. 483–507). New York: Van Nostrand Reinhold.

Kalish, R. A., & Reynolds, D. K. (1976). *Death and ethnicity: A psychosocial study.* Los Angeles: University of Southern California Press.

Kastenbaum, R. (1966). As the clock runs out. *Mental Hygiene, 50,* 332–336.

Kastenbaum, R. (2000). *The psychology of death* (3rd ed.). New York: Springer Publishing.

Kellehear, A. (2000). Spirituality and palliative care: A model of needs. *Palliative Medicine, 14,* 149–155.

Kellehear, A. (2007). *A social history of dying.* Cambridge: Cambridge University Press.

Kohli, M., Rosenow, J., & Wolf, J. (1983). The social construction of ageing through work: Economic structure and life-world. *Ageing & Society, 3,* 23–42.

Kubler-Ross, E. (1969). *On death and dying.* New York: Macmillan Publishing.

Levinson, D. (1978). *The seasons of a man's life.* New York: Knopf.

MacKinlay, E. (2001). *The spiritual dimension of aging.* London: Jessica Kingsley.

Marshall, V. W. (1999). Analysing social theories of aging. In V. L. Bengtson & K. W. Shaie (Eds.), *Handbook of theories of aging* (pp. 434–458). New York: Springer Publishing.

Moody, H. (1992). *Ethics in an aging society.* Baltimore: Johns Hopkins University Press.

Munnichs, J. M. A. (1966). *Old age and finitude.* Basel: Karger.

Myles, J. (1983). Conflict, crisis and the future of old age security. *Milbank Memorial Fund Quarterly, 61,* 462–472.

Neimeyer, R. A. (1994). *Death anxiety handbook.* Philadelphia: Taylor & Francis.

Neugarten, B. L., & Hagestad, G. O. (1976). Age and the lifecourse. In R. H. Binstock & E. Shanas (Eds.), *Handbook of aging and the social sciences* (pp. 35–56). New York: Van Nostrand Reinhold.

Oeppen, J., & Vaupel, J. W. (2002). Enhanced demography: Broken limits to life expectancy. *Science, 296,* 1029–1031.

Ortiz, L. P. A., & Langer, N. (2002). Assessment of spirituality and religion in later life: Acknowledging clients' needs and personal resources. *Journal of Gerontological Social Work, 37,* 5–21.

Phillipson, C. (1982). *Capitalism and the construction of old age.* London: Macmillan.

Quadagno, J. (1988). *The transformation of old age security.* Chicago: University of Chicago Press.

Rawls, J. (1971). *A theory of social justice.* Oxford: Oxford University Press.

Riley, M. W., & Foner, A. (1968). *Aging and society: Vol. 1. An inventory of research findings.* New York: Russell Sage Foundation.

Robertson, A. (1997) Beyond apocalyptic demography: Towards a moral economy. *Ageing & Society, 17,* 425–446.

Rumbold, B. (Ed.). (2000). *Spirituality and palliative care.* Melbourne: Oxford University Press.

Sadler, E., & Biggs, S. (2006). Exploring the links between spirituality and "successful ageing." *Journal of Social Work Practice, 20,* 267–280.

Settersten, R. A., Jr. (2006). Aging and the lifecourse. In R. H. Binstock & L. K. George (Eds.), *Handbook of aging and the social sciences* (6th ed., pp. 3–19). Amsterdam: Elsevier.

Sheehy, G. (1976). *Passages: The predictable crises of adult life.* New York: Dutton.

Sinclair, P. (2007). *Rethinking palliative care: A social valorisation approach.* Bristol: Policy Press.

Tolstoy, L. (1899). *A confession* (Leo Werner, Trans.). New York: Thomas Y. Crowell.

Tornstam, L. (1989). Gerotranscendence: A metatheoretical reformulation of the disengagement theory. *Ageing: Clinical and Experimental Research, 1,* 55–63.

Tornstam, L. (2005). *Gerotranscendence: A developmental theory of positive aging.* New York: Springer Publishing.

Walker, A. (1981). Towards a political economy of old age. *Ageing & Society, 1,* 73–94.

Walker, A. (1996). *The new generational contract: Intergenerational relations in old age and welfare.* London: Taylor & Francis.

Walter, T. (1991). Modern death: Taboo or not taboo. *Sociology, 25,* 293–310.

Walter, T. (2002). Spirituality in palliative care: Opportunity or burden. *Palliative Care, 16,* 133–140.

Wolfensberger, W. (1972). *The principle of normalization in human services.* Toronto: National Institute for Mental Retardation.

37 A Good Old Age: Theories of Mental Health and Aging

Steven H. Zarit

Old age is widely regarded as a time of illness, loss, and disability. Despite the best efforts of gerontologists to dispel stereotypes and myths about aging, it remains the case that older people face significant challenges that can undermine emotional and physical well-being and compromise quality of life. Paradoxically, however, older people appear, on average, to be remarkably resilient. Apart from dementia, the risk of which increases with age, older people have lower rates of mental disorders than other adult age-groups and generally report higher emotional well-being. Indeed, given all the possible losses and challenges in later life, one might ask why older people are so happy.

In this chapter, I examine briefly the evidence on well-being and mental health in later life and then consider possible factors that might account for this apparent paradox. I begin by examining methodological and conceptual problems in the available research that might account for these findings and then turn to developmental theories that suggest why older people may be able to maintain high levels of well-being.

Mental Health and Well-Being Among the Older Population

Let me begin with some definitions. When I write about mental health and mental health problems, I am referring to clinically significant problems that interfere with daily functioning and quality of life. I use the term "disorder" to reflect a pattern of symptoms that meets established criteria for a particular psychiatric diagnosis and the term "symptoms" to indicate people who have specific complaints, such as depressive feelings that may or may not meet diagnostic criteria for a depressive disorder. I use the term "well-being" to encompass a person's typical emotional state. Well-being is often defined in a more comprehensive way to include health, but I limit my focus in this chapter to emotion, that is, how people feel on a day-to-day basis.

Older people have long been characterized in the media and among the general public as lonely, sad, and depressed and as increasingly rigid and neurotic. These qualities have been considered the outcomes of the aging process and/or the result of illness or loss. Many older people do, in fact, suffer from mental health problems, primarily depression and anxiety but also schizophrenia, bipolar disorders, and personality disorders. But the vulnerability of older people to mental disorders is tempered in two ways (for a review, see Zarit & Zarit, 2007).

First, older people have a lower prevalence of mental disorders than do young and middle aged adults. This is a finding supported by virtually every epidemiological survey that has been conducted (e.g., Blazer, George, & Hughes, 1991; Kessler et al., 2003; Regier et al., 1988; Ritchie et al., 2004; Weissman et al., 1988). Let me illustrate with three problems: depression, anxiety, and personality disorders. Estimates of the prevalence among older people of the most serious form of depression, major depressive disorder (MDD), have varied between 1% and 5% of the population, depending on the method used for determining diagnosis (Kessler et al., 2003; Ritchie et al., 2004; Weissman et al., 1988). Although a considerable amount, these prevalence estimates are lower than for young and middle-aged adults. About 9% of older people have been found to suffer from significant levels of anxiety. Again, this is a substantial amount though lower than for younger age-groups (Blazer et al., 1991; Regier et al., 1988). Estimates of the prevalence of personality disorders such as borderline, narcissistic, and paranoid schizoid patterns vary widely because of disagreement over diagnostic criteria, but as many as 10%–15% of the older population may have a personality disorder (Girolamo & Reich, 1993; Grant et al., 2004; Samuels, Nestadt, Romanoski, Folstein, & McHugh, 1994). This is a considerable burden, especially because personality disorders are quite distressing both to the affected person and to family and friends, but, again, rates are lower than for younger adults (Ames & Molinari, 1994; Cohen et al., 1994; Engels, Duijsens, Haringsma, & van Putten, 2003; Grant et al., 2004).

Second, an abundance of evidence suggests that serious mental illness in later life is usually a problem that originated at a younger age and has continued or recurred in old age. It is less common for a mental disorder other than dementia to have its first onset in late life. MDD, for example, is likely to occur for the first time in adolescence or young adulthood (Andrade et al., 2003; Burke, Burke, Regier, & Rae, 1990). Incidence of new cases declines steadily after age 30, with a small increase after 75. The story for anxiety disorders is similar. First onset typically occurs during adolescence or young adulthood (Blazer et al., 1991; Kessler, Walters, & Wittchen, 2004), though new cases have been reported in later life (Lenze et al., 2005; Stanley & Beck, 2000). As for personality disorders, onset in adolescence and young adulthood is considered an essential feature of diagnosis, and late life forms have not been reported.

This pattern is found for every serious disorder; that is, most people have their first onset of a problem earlier in life, though new cases can emerge in old age. In other words, the mental health problems experienced by many older people are not problems of aging but are chronic and recurrent difficulties that they have experienced since earlier in life. Biomedical, social, and psychological processes in later life can trigger a new episode or lead to worsening of symptoms, but the basic vulnerability emerged at an earlier point in the life span. As Abraham (1977) observed many years ago, it is essential to differentiate the age of the person from the age of the problem.

By drawing a picture of mental disorders as generally part of a lifelong pattern, I do not mean to diminish the extent to which older people do, in fact, suffer from serious problems and should receive adequate treatment for those problems. The point that I want to make is that mental health problems *are* a serious concern in later life, but the prevalence is lower than at earlier ages, and most but not all cases are recurrent episodes of an earlier problem. In other words, for many older people the etiology of their mental health problems may have to do with risk factors that have been present for a long time and not to the aging process.

There are two caveats to these conclusions. First, we need to keep in mind that with only a few exceptions such as personality disorders, there are both early-onset and late-onset cases of major mental disorders. It is not known whether the late-onset form of a disorder shares the same etiology as early onset cases. Considerable attention has been given in recent years to the question of whether late-onset depression represents a different form of the disorder than earlier in life. Late-onset cases have been found to be associated with cognitive problems, especially in executive functions (Alexopoulos et al., 2000) and white matter hyperintensities in the brain (Alexopoulos, Kiosses, Choi, Murphy, & Lim, 2002). The possibility that depression and other mental disorders have different origins in late life has implications for treatment and prevention.

Second, older people who have serious medical illnesses and/or who live in nursing homes and other institutional settings have a high prevalence of mental health problems, particularly depressive and anxiety symptoms. Between 10% and 30% of older patients seen in outpatient clinics have clinically significant levels of depression (Lyness, King, Cox, Yoediono, & Caine, 1999; Robison et al., 2003), while rates of MDD among hospital inpatients have been found to range between 6% and 44%, depending on the type of medical problem studied. In nursing homes, 16% of people have been found to meet diagnostic criteria for MDD, and another 16% have clinically significant depressive symptoms (Parmalee, Katz, & Lawton, 1992). Rates of anxiety symptoms in these populations are similarly elevated.

The picture that emerges for emotional well-being is similar. Older people may, in fact, be somewhat better off—happier, less depressed, and even less lonely than other adult age-groups. Studies of emotions have found that negative affect is stable or declines over the adult years, at least until age 60, rising slightly after that point (Carstensen, Pasupathi, Mayr, & Nesselroade, 2000; Charles, Reynolds, & Gatz, 2001; Filipp, 1996; Gross, Carstensen, Pasupathi, Tsai, Skorpen, & Hsu, 1997; Lawton, Kleban, Rajagopal, & Dean, 1992; Mroczek & Kolarz, 1998). Positive emotions have also been found to be stable, again at least until 60, and then decline a small amount.

These effects can be found both for typical retrospective measures of well-being where people are asked to report about their feelings during the past week and for newer approaches where people report emotions on a daily basis. Daily measures are less prone to recall biases, for example, glossing over negative feelings that may have been experienced 3 or 4 days earlier but are now resolved. Using this type of approach, Carstensen and colleagues (2000) found that reports of negative daily emotions occurred less often with age. Young adults aged 18 to 34 had the highest rates of daily negative emotions, and people in midlife, aged 35 to 64, had the lowest. People over 65 were slightly higher in reports of negative emotions that the middle aged but still much lower than the youngest group. Other researchers (e.g., Birditt, Fingerman, & Almeida, 2005; Cichy, Fingerman, & Lefkowitz, 2007; Mroczek & Almeida, 2004) have reported similar findings that older people experience less distress on average than younger people in their reaction to daily stressors.

In sum, older people are somewhat better off, on the whole, than younger age-groups in these various markers of mental health—incidence and prevalence of disorders and well-being. I now turn to methodological and conceptual issues that might account for these findings.

Methodological and Conceptual Issues in Findings on Mental Health and Aging

It is possible that older people appear to be better off than younger individuals because of systematic biases in the available data and problems in how mental health and well-being are defined and estimated. I explore three possibilities—selective attrition, definitions of mental illness, and reliance on cross-sectional data.

The lower rates of disorders among the old may be the result of selective attrition. Simply put, people with serious mental disorders earlier in life are less likely to live to old age. They have a shorter life expectancy due to higher rates of suicide (e.g., Barak, Knobler, & Aizenberg, 2004), high comorbidities of alcohol and drug problems, and lifestyles that create vulnerabilities to illness (Parks, Svendsen, Singer, & Foti, 2006). Another consideration is that people with severe, chronic mental health disorders may be less likely to respond to community surveys or may underreport symptoms, leading to the impression that disorders are less common in later life. There may also be a more positive type of attrition.

Some people who experienced one or more episodes of a serious mental disorder earlier in life recover or improve substantially with treatment or time (e.g., Ciompi, 1987; Huber, 1997). All three of these factors would contribute to reduced prevalence of mental health disorders in the older population compared to younger adults.

A second possible explanation of the differences in mental health problems and well-being between young and old is that the form that disorders take in later life or how people report symptoms may change with aging. In studies of the incidence and prevalence of mental disorders, diagnosis is made using structured interviews that yield information for determining if an individual meets explicit criteria for diagnosis of a particular disorder. Criteria for diagnosis have been developed largely using younger samples. If a disorder, such as MDD, presents in later life in a somewhat different way, it is possible that some people may not meet the diagnostic criteria. It has been suggested, for example, that some older adults will report somatic symptoms when experiencing emotional disturbances (Beck & Averill, 2004; Sadavoy & Fogel, 1992).

One way of evaluating this possibility is to focus on rates of symptoms rather than diagnosis. Taking depression as an example, the prevalence of clinically significant depressive symptoms has been estimated as between 10% and 25% of older people (Blazer, 2002; Gurland et al., 1983; Lindesay, Briggs, & Murphy, 1989; Livingston, Hawkins, Graham, Blizard, & Mann, 1990). Most of these people do not meet the diagnostic criteria for MDD but experience symptoms that are severe enough to interfere with everyday functioning. These findings on prevalence of symptoms suggest that depression is a more extensive problem in later life than when typical diagnostic categories are used. On the other hand, both cross-sectional and longitudinal studies indicate that symptoms of depression decline with age, at least until 75 years (Haynie, Zarit, Berg & Gatz, 2000; Heikkinen & Kauppinen, 2004; Zarit, Femia, Johansson, & Gatz, 1999). These findings of declining levels of symptoms thus mirror results for prevalence of disorders. After age 75, some studies have found rates of symptoms are as high as in young populations (Lewinsohn, Rohde, Fischer, & Seeley, 1991), though other research reports low rates even past age 80 (Haynie et al., 2000). Looking at types of depressive symptoms, Gatz and Hurwicz (1991) found that people over age 70 were less likely to report depressive symptoms compared to younger adults but more likely to indicate a lack of well-being. In one of the few longitudinal analyses, Fiske, Gatz, and Pedersen (2003) followed a sample of adults originally aged 20 to 93 over a 9-year period. Depressive symptoms increased a small amount on average over time. Increases were somewhat more pronounced among older adults and were associated with negative life events and poorer health status. Other longitudinal studies of the oldest-old have reported no (Haynie et al., 2000) or small (Zarit et al., 1999) increases in depressive symptoms.

Finally, we need to consider the possibility that the findings on differences in rates of mental disorders between younger and older adults, as well as on symptoms and well-being, may be affected by reliance on cross-sectional research designs. As noted, some longitudinal data are available, but most of these studies are relatively short term, and the overwhelming predominance of studies are cross-sectional.

Three factors need to be considered as affecting the results of cross-sectional studies. First, as noted in many areas of gerontological research, the differences that emerge from a cross-sectional comparison may be the result of the effects of cohort rather than aging. Older cohorts may be less likely to report symptoms like depression than younger, more psychologically sophisticated generations (Kessler et al., 2003).

Second, cross-sectional findings do not inform us about the severity of recurrent episodes. The available data suggest some lessening of symptoms, although it is possible that selected individuals experience increasingly severe symptoms as they grow older. A study by Mroczek and Almeida (2004) suggests that changes in well-being reflect an interaction of personality and age. Looking at response to daily stressors, they found that older people, on average, reported less distress than did younger people. Older people who scored high on the dimension of neuroticism, however, reported high distress. In other words, there may be some truth to the observation that one's quirky or neurotic relatives become more eccentric with age.

A third factor is that cross-sectional studies, which look at people at only one point in time, may not adequately identify the actual risk in later life. Although prevalence at any point in time might be lower among older people, the probability of developing a significant disorder at some point in later life may be as high or higher than during comparable periods earlier in life. This kind of argument that "sooner or later" something bad will happen describes patterns found with dementia. Prevalence of dementia rises with age to rates of about 30% to 35% by the decade of the 80s. If lifetime risk is taken into account, however, more than 50% of the oldest-old will suffer from symptoms of dementia for some period of time before their deaths (Johansson & Zarit, 1995). The reason for this discrepancy of prevalence and lifetime risk is that incidence rises with age and people with dementia have a shortened life expectancy compared to older persons without dementia. A similar analysis of anxiety or depression might indicate a high lifetime risk, even though prevalence at any point in time is low.

There are several factors, then, that may influence the estimates of prevalence of disorders and symptoms and reports of well-being in the older population. It is important to take into account that many older people do suffer from severe mental illness and that others experience frequent feelings of sadness, loneliness, and worry. At the same time, there may be protective factors that make it possible for older people to adapt better to major life challenges as well as daily hassles. I turn next to theories that identify potential protective factors that make it possible for older people to regulate their daily lives and emotions in a positive manner.

Developmental Theories of Mental Health and Aging

The work of Rowe and Kahn (1987, 1997, 1998) on successful aging serves as a starting point for examining the question of how older people might make a positive adaptation in later life. In their landmark paper "Human Aging: Usual and Successful," Rowe and Kahn (1987) observed that much of the research on aging contrasts people with illnesses and other losses to people who are considered "normal," that is, who do not have serious illnesses. Rowe and Kahn point out that normal aging includes people who may differ widely from one another on key medical and psychological indicators. Some people may be very active, and others may fatigue easily and have little activity besides taking care of basic needs. Normal aging encompasses people with excellent cognitive functioning as well as those who have slowed down or have more difficulties with learning and remembering new information. In other words, the broad term "normal" aging includes two groups. The first group is people who are productive and engaged in their lives and excited about what they are doing. Rowe and Kahn call this pattern "successful aging." The second group is just getting by. They do not have major limitations, but they may have minor difficulties in functioning, mild health problems or symptoms of depression, and so on. The challenge that Rowe and Kahn propose to the gerontology field is to identify the factors that promote successful and vital old age and not just usual aging.

Drawing on findings from the MacArthur study of successful aging, as well as other literature, Rowe and Kahn (1987, 1997) suggest three factors that contribute to successful aging. The first factor concerns health. To be successful in old age, people need to avoid disease and disability. Rowe and Kahn stress that a healthy lifestyle can help delay or avoid many of the major illnesses of later life. The second factor is maximizing cognitive and physical functioning. Physical and cognitive exercise will contribute to continued high performance in these domains. To maintain cognitive functioning, people can learn new things or exercise their mental capacity with puzzles, games, and other challenges. The third is engagement with life. Rowe and Kahn argue that people who age successfully will maintain good relationships with family and friends and will engage in activities in their life that they care deeply about and that give life a sense of purpose.

Rowe and Kahn have made an important contribution by calling attention to the distinction between usual and successful aging. A major limitation in their theory is the emphasis they place on maintaining health. Although good health habits, such as getting regular exercise and eating healthy foods, can be useful in preventing disease and disability, people with good health habits can get sick, too. There is a risk that placing too much emphasis on our ability to prevent illness may lead to a "blaming of the victim," that is, where we hold older people responsible for their poor health. Many of the preventive measures that are generally advocated remain supported only by correlational data that may or may not provide an accurate map of how to promote health or prevent disease. I am not advocating that we abandon a healthy lifestyle but rather that we recognize that it is only one part of the determinants of health in later life.

A more basic issue in Rowe and Kahn's approach is the assumption that health is a necessary component of successful aging. Many people who suffer from chronic illness and disabilities can be productive members of their families and communities. Indeed, by the time people are 80, almost everyone has one or more chronic disease (Femia, Zarit, & Johansson, 2001). The real challenge for successful aging may be how to create the conditions so that people can have a good quality of life, even if they have an illness or other significant age-related changes.

Paul Baltes (1987, 1997) took a different approach to successful aging based on a dynamic model of development as a continuous process of specialization and loss. According to Baltes, successful aging takes place through a process called "selective optimization with compensation" (SOC). He used the example of the famous pianist Artur Rubenstein to illustrate this process. Rubenstein continued to perform concerts when he was in his 80s despite vision loss and other health problems. When asked in an interview how he managed, he replied as follows:

- He practiced and played fewer musical pieces. That helped him remember the music and play it at a higher level. In Baltes's terms, he "selected" fewer pieces.
- He practiced more often; in other words, he "optimized" his performance.
- Knowing that he could not play the piano as fast as when he was young, Rubenstein would deliberately slow down before he reached a fast portion of a musical piece. Then, when he reached the fast portion, it would seem to the audience that he was now playing fast. Slowing of reaction time is a prominent change with aging. In Baltes's terms, Rubenstein "compensated" for slowing by playing especially slow before he reached a fast part of a musical piece (cited in Baltes, 1997).

This model of selective optimization with compensation can be used to explain some of the paradoxes found in research on older people. One paradox is how older people are able to maintain high performance in areas of expertise, such as music, chess, or other activities (Charness, 2000; Salthouse, 1990). Salthouse's (1984) study of older, expert typists provides an example of this process. Despite slowing in their reaction time, these older typists were as fast and accurate in their work as younger typists. They were able to maintain their speed in typing because they could better anticipate the next words in the text than less experienced typists. In others words, they used their experience to compensate for age-related losses.

One implication of these findings is that the effect of aging on a particular ability may depend on the person's prior level of achievement in that domain. Those activities in which people have achieved a high degree of competence may be more stable in later life because of the ability to compensate, while less practiced abilities may be at greater risk of decline. That is not to say that all people will be able to compensate in the face of decline. The limited empirical literature suggests that engaging in SOC has both general effects, including on well-being, as well as an impact on specific domains such as work (Riediger, Li, & Lindenberger, 2006).

The concepts of expertise and SOC help us understand the central question posed in this chapter—why older people report high levels of well-being and have low rates of depression. The available data suggest that young people are emotional and become easily upset by setbacks in their lives. By contrast, many, though not all, older people have learned through experience to become experts at managing their lives and emotions. They do not let everyday events bother them, or they avoid the people or activities that upset them. Not all older people can manage their emotions well, and some become depressed or fearful. But some learn to select their experiences so that they can optimize feelings of well-being even when they encounter stress and disappointment in their lives. The difference noted earlier in response to daily hassles by people high and low in neuroticism (Mroczek & Almeida, 2004) may reflect to a large extent learned ability to regulate emotion.

Laura Carstensen (1992) and her colleagues (Carstensen, Fung, & Charles, 2003; Carstensen, Isaacowitz, & Charles, 1999) have extended the model of selective optimization with compensation to social relationships and emotions. Calling this process "socioemotional selectivity," Carstensen proposes that people become increasingly aware as they age that they have a limited amount of time left in their lives. As a consequence, they regulate their social activities so that they interact more with those individuals with whom they have positive interactions and decrease or avoid contact with people with whom they have conflict. In this manner, they can optimize feelings of well-being.

Building on Carstensen's (1992) work (see also Carstensen et al., 1999), Fingerman and her colleagues (Birditt & Fingerman, 2003; Birditt et al., 2005; Fingerman, 1995, 2000; Lefkowitz & Fingerman, 2003) have examined close personal relationships and emotions in later life. They found that older adults generally report fewer interpersonal conflicts in their daily interactions, perceive conflicts as less stressful, are less likely to respond in an angry or confronting way, and experience less emotional distress than younger adults. Conflicts are more likely to occur with a spouse but less likely to involve children (Birditt et al., 2005).

Looking specifically at mother–daughter relationships, which are a key source of support in later life, Fingerman (1995, 2000) found that daughters are more likely to report complaints about their mothers, while mothers underestimate daughters' negative feelings and behaviors. These tendencies were confirmed in an observational study of mother–daughter interactions. Mothers acted in more positive ways toward their daughters and experienced fewer negative emotions (Lefkowitz & Fingerman, 2003). Fingerman (1995, 2000) suggests that mothers may have a greater investment in this relationship than their daughters and are therefore less likely to admit to negative emotions or conflict. Again, I do not want to suggest that all close interpersonal relationships are harmonious. Some mother–daughter relationships are characterized by chronic tension and conflict that does not abate with age. But on average, these studies suggest that older people regulate conflict and emotions in relationships better, and this may contribute to their well-being.

These findings on greater emotional regulation in later life are consistent with developmental theories of personal control and emotion regulation. Schulz and colleagues (Schulz & Heckhausen, 1996; Schulz, Wrosch, & Heckhausen, 2003) have proposed that the type of control strategies that people use shifts with aging. Young people are more likely to employ primary control strategies, in which they take direct approaches to modify the events or challenging situations in their lives. In contrast, older people are more likely to employ secondary control mechanisms, which involve management of thoughts and feelings. People adjust their own beliefs, expectations, and motivations rather than trying to change the situation. They will, in other words, make the best of a bad situation. From a somewhat different perspective, Labouvie-Vief and colleagues (Labouvie-Vief, Hakim-Larson, DeVoe, & Schoeberlein, 1989) have reported that older people use more sophisticated strategies than younger individuals in regulating negative emotions.

Another dimension of control is the beliefs people hold about the extent to which they can influence the events in their lives. Although often viewed as the same, beliefs about control and control strategies or behaviors are different dimensions, correlating only modestly with each other (Wrosch, Heckhausen, & Lachman, 2000). Both Rowe and Kahn (1987, 1997) and Baltes (1987, 1997) suggest that control beliefs, including mastery and self-efficacy, are related to positive outcomes in later life. Blazer (2002) has proposed that self-efficacy is a key protective factor for depressive feelings in later life. Specifically, older people who believe that their actions can make a difference are more likely to take steps that will improve their lives. My colleagues and I have found evidence for the role of control beliefs in preventing the onset of disabilities in the oldest-old (Fauth, Zarit, Malmberg, & Johansson, 2007; Femia, Zarit, & Johansson, 1997). In samples of people in their late 80s and early 90s, we found those individuals with higher mastery beliefs were less likely to develop disabilities over time. Even after taking into account the effects of illness and physical limitations, mastery remained a strong predictor of continued independence. Focusing on health-related goals, Wrosch and colleagues (Wrosch et al., 2000) found that both control strategies and control beliefs contribute to well-being.

The increased control over emotions that is found in later life suggests another paradox. Emotional control is part of a set of cognitive abilities referred to as executive functioning that also includes problem solving, flexibility in thinking, abstract thinking, and planning. Changes in executive functioning, however, are considered one of the vulnerabilities of normal aging and a precursor of some types of dementia (e.g., Alexopoulos et al., 2000; Bäckman & Small, 2007). Yet, as discussed, emotional control appears better, on average, in later life. Consistent with SOC, people can draw on experience to compensate for mild changes in executive functioning. Of course, the more dramatic decline that unfolds in cases of dementia eventually overwhelms compensatory strategies and leads to poorer emotional regulation.

One other cognitive-emotional process that should be considered in examination of a good old age is wisdom. We know that aging is associated with decline in intellectual abilities, but there is a long-standing belief in many cultures that some older people have a special intellectual quality called wisdom. Baltes and his colleagues (Baltes & Smith, 1990; Baltes & Staudinger, 2000; Kunzmann & Baltes, 2003) conducted a series of studies that defined and examined wisdom across the life span. They view wisdom as a special type of expertise about the meaning of life and the pragmatics of how things work in a particular situation. According to Baltes and Smith (1990), older people can give wise advice in the areas where they have expertise. Another aspect of wisdom is something Baltes calls "virtue." Virtue includes openness to a range of ideas as well as putting aside one's own needs and instead understanding how the other person is thinking and feeling.

Using this framework, Baltes and his colleagues have examined age differences in wisdom (Baltes, Staudinger, Maercker, & Smith, 1995). First, they asked people to nominate individuals they considered to be wise. Interestingly, it was not just older people who were nominated as wise. In fact, people often identified as wise someone who was close to their own age (Baltes et al., 1995). Second, Baltes and his colleagues (Baltes, 1997; Smith, Staudinger, & Baltes, 1994) developed scenarios of common life problems and asked people of different ages to suggest how the protagonist in the scenario might handle the problem. The responses were rated using a scheme that identified the qualities of wisdom. Again, "wise" people were found all across adulthood and not just in old age. It also appeared that people were more likely to give better-quality suggestions for scenarios about which they had some knowledge. In other words, in a scenario about a college student with roommate problems, the best advice might come from a current or recent college student, while older people would give better advice about situations that were more familiar to them. Rather than being a universal quality of aging, then, wisdom can be identified in adults of varied ages. But those older people who have a combination of expertise and virtue can give wise advice and become valued by their family and community.

I want to talk about one more model of a good life. The work of Erik Erikson (1950; Erikson, Erikson, & Kivnick, 1986) has long been prominent in the gerontological field. In the light of contemporary approaches, Erikson's proposals for adaptation in middle and late life are both similar and different. Both Rowe and Kahn (1987, 1997) and Baltes (1987, 1997) suggest that a good life involves actively engaging the world to the extent possible. This premise is consistent with Erikson's notion that the psychological challenge of middle age is "generativity or stagnation." People who are successful in middle age become mentors of younger individuals, nurture their own maturing children in positive ways, and contribute to their communities. Erikson's theory, however, diverges from these other perspectives in its approach to old age. According to Erikson, the unique challenge of later life is "integrity or despair." The psychological task for older people is finding meaning and purpose in the whole of their life. They do so by turning inward and reflecting back over the events and accomplishments of their life. If they fail to do so, they will experience the despair of having lived a life with little meaning or purpose.

Drawing on Erikson's theory, many people have been interested in finding ways to promote a sense of integrity in old age. One widely used method is that of life review (Butler, 1963, 1974). In this approach, older people are encouraged to review the events of their lives. The goal is for them to draw comfort from their successes, resolve past conflicts, and become reconciled to their disappointments. Life review and a related process called reminiscence therapy can be conducted individually or in groups. Another variant of life review is the guided autobiography (Birren & Deutchman, 1991). Although the evidence is limited, these approaches appear useful for reducing depressive feelings in older adults (Gatz et al., 1998).

Finally, we should not overlook a quite straightforward explanation of well-being among older people. Today's elders are better off financially than in the past, have more education, and notably have universal health insurance (Smith, 2003). About 10% of elders currently live under the federal poverty line compared to historic levels of 20% or more. These improvements in the conditions of life should not be underestimated for their contributions to quality of life.

A Call for Prevention

This chapter began by reviewing the evidence that a good old age is possible and, indeed, fairly common. Blazer (2002) has made a powerful case that we have the knowledge to move beyond treatment of mental health problems in old age to programs that emphasize prevention. Based on the evidence of factors that contribute to quality of life in old age, what might prevention programs look like?

1. Develop good health habits. This factor currently receives the most attention in both the research literature and the media. Good nutrition, regular exercise, not smoking, and other health habits have a positive influence on life expectancy and well-being and may delay the onset of some diseases. People need, however, to approach health habits in a balanced way, doing sensible things and avoiding fads that are supported by little or no evidence. The downside of all the attention to health habits is that some people become so preoccupied with extreme diet or exercise regimens that they lose sight of what factors might contribute to the quality of their lives.
2. Develop skills for managing chronic illness. As noted, it is easy to recommend that people stay healthy, but the key to a good old age may be in knowing how to manage chronic illness and disability. Medical care has become increasingly complex and fragmented, and patients often have to make a series of choices for themselves that they are unprepared for. Even the manner in which they present their symptoms to a busy physician can affect whether they get appropriate treatment. People need to learn strategies for communication with physicians and how to access good-quality information about medical problems and their treatment (Zarit & Zarit, 2007). They also need to develop a particular type of self-efficacy, the belief that when a medical condition cannot be reversed, there may still be rehabilitation strategies that lead to improved functioning. Prosthetic devices such as hearing aids can be important for maintaining activities and social relationships. A key part of managing chronic illness may be learning how to select and compensate to maintain valued activities.
3. Develop good social skills. Social relationships are central to well-being throughout life. Maintaining good relationships with family and friends and knowing when to withdraw from a relationship that is one sided, noxious, or abusive is critical. People need skills for developing and maintaining good relationships and ending bad ones. The assumption that everyone knows how to relate to family or friends is belied by all the conflicted relationships in people's lives. A core set of skills that includes active listening, empathy, and assertion can go a long way toward improving relationships.
4. Develop skills for managing emotions. The findings reviewed earlier suggest that emotional regulation can lead to better relationships and well-being. We have emerged from an era where people were encouraged to express their feelings no matter what the consequences. Focusing solely on expressing emotions has largely disappeared from contemporary psychotherapy, replaced by learning behavioral and cognitive approaches that allow people to decrease their experience and expression of negative emotions (e.g., Beck, Rush, Shaw, & Emery, 1979). This shift is not a return to an earlier era where emotions were largely suppressed. Rather, it reflects the recognition that strong emotions often emerge from a faulty understanding of one's own experience and of the meaning and intention of other people's behavior. Good functioning depends on expressing emotions based on accurate appraisals of events and experiences and on learning skills to identify interpretations of events that are overly pessimistic or otherwise distorted.

5. Develop good cognitive skills. Although the benefit of cognitive enhancement for preventing dementia has probably been exaggerated, a lot of research shows that people who remain intellectually active and who continually learn new skills will have more resources for responding to the challenges in their lives. By remaining current with new ideas and technologies, older people will be better able to build bridges across generations.
6. Develop interests. Most people can expect to live many years after they retire, and they need interests and activities that give purpose to their lives. Often viewed as a burden to society, older people could be a valuable resource for helping with community needs. More opportunities for meaningful involvement would benefit everyone.
7. Develop good economic skills. Much of the current well-being of older people may be due to their relatively good economic status. The prospects for the future, however, may not be as rosy. A higher proportion of retirees in society compared to working-aged persons and continued erosion of support for guaranteed pensions such as Social Security may undermine the financial status of older adults. In this context, being competent at management of finances may become increasingly important for personal economic success and for overall well-being.
8. Develop a sense of self-efficacy for the ability to change one's life. With self-efficacy, people will believe that they can make a difference in their lives and so will be more likely to take the steps necessary to improve personal habits. As noted, self-efficacy may be particularly important for preventing depression and in managing chronic illness.

The timing of prevention is also critical. Although programs that address life skills could be implemented in old age, a better approach is to make these types of skills part of a program of lifelong learning. In that way, people will be prepared for the challenges and hazards that lie ahead.

In conclusion, economic, social, and political development has provided us with the gift of years. The challenge is to make those years meaningful and productive. A good old age is possible, and the means for helping older people discover meaning and direction in their lives may be within our reach. We cannot abolish disease and other hardships that are associated with later life, but we can establish the conditions that allow people to continue, despite age and its limitations, to contribute to their families and community and, in turn, to feel valued for their contributions.

References

Abraham, K. (1977). The applicability of psychoanalytic treatment to patients of advanced age. In S. Steury & M. L. Blank (Eds.), *Readings in psychotherapy with older people* (pp. 18–20). Rockville, MD. National Institute of Mental Health. (Original work published 1953)

Alexopoulos, G. S., Kiosses, D. N., Choi, S. J., Murphy, C. F., & Lim, K. O. (2002). Frontal white matter microstructure and treatment response of late-life depression: A preliminary study. *American Journal of Psychiatry, 159,* 1929–1932.

Alexopoulos, G. S., Meyers, B. S., Young, R. C., Kalayam, B., Kakuma, T., Gabrielle, M., et al. (2000). Executive dysfunction and long-term outcomes of geriatric depression. *Archives of General Psychiatry, 57,* 285–290.

Ames, A., & Molinari, V. (1994). Prevalence of personality disorders in community-living elderly. *Journal of Geriatric Psychiatry and Neurology, 7,* 189–194.

Andrade, L., Caraveo-Anduga, J. J., Berglund, P., Biji, R. V., DeGraff, R., Volebergh, W., et al. (2003). The epidemiology of major depressive episodes: Results from the International Consortium of Psychiatric Epidemiology (ICPE) Surveys. *International Journal of Methods in Psychiatric Research, 12,* 3–21.

Bäckman, L., & Small, B. (2007). Cognitive deficits in preclinical Alzheimer's disease and vascular dementia: Patterns of findings from the Kungsholmen Project. *Physiology and Behavior, 10,* 80–86.

Baltes, P. B. (1987). Theoretical propositions of life-span developmental psychology: On the dynamics between growth and decline. *Developmental Psychology, 23,* 611–626.

Baltes, P. B. (1997). On the incomplete architecture of human ontogeny: Selection, optimization, and compensation as foundation of developmental theory. *American Psychologist, 52,* 366–380.

Baltes, P. B., & Smith, J. (1990). Toward a psychology of wisdom and its ontogenesis. In R. J. Sternberg (Ed.), *Wisdom: Its nature, origins, and development* (pp. 87–120). New York: Cambridge University Press.

Baltes, P. B., & Staudinger, U. M. (2000). Wisdom: A metaheuristic (pragmatic) to orchestrate mind and virtue toward excellence. *American Psychologist, 55,* 122–136.

Baltes, P. B., Staudinger, U. M., Maercker, A., & Smith, J. (1995). People nominated as wise: A comparative study of wisdom-related knowledge. *Psychology and Aging, 10,* 155–166.

Barak, Y., Knobler, C. Y., & Aizenberg, D. (2004). Suicide attempts amongst elderly schizophrenia patients: A 10-year case-control study. *Schizophrenia Research, 71,* 77–81.

Beck, A. T., Rush, A. J., Shaw, B. F., & Emery, G. (1979). *Cognitive therapy of depression.* New York: Guilford.

Beck, J. G., & Averill, P. M. (2004). Older adults: Epidemiology. In R. G. Heimberg, C. L. Turk, & D. S. Mennin (Eds.), *Generalized anxiety disorder: Advances in research and practice* (pp. 409–433). New York: Guilford.

Birditt, K. S., & Fingerman, K. L. (2003). Do we get better at picking our battles? Age group differences in descriptions of behavioral reactions to interpersonal tensions. *Journal of Gerontology: Social Sciences, 60,* P121–P128.

Birditt, K. S., Fingerman, K. L., & Almeida, D. M. (2005). Age differences in exposure and reactions to interpersonal tensions: A daily diary study. *Psychology and Aging, 20,* 330–340.

Birren, J. E., & Deutchman, D. E. (1991). *Guiding autobiography groups for older adults.* Baltimore: Johns Hopkins University Press.

Blazer, D. G. (2002). Self-efficacy and depression in late life: A primary prevention proposal. *Aging & Mental Health, 6,* 315–324.

Blazer, D., George, L. K., & Hughes, D. (1991). The epidemiology of anxiety disorders: An age comparison. In C. Salzman & B. Lebowitz (Eds.), *Anxiety in the elderly* (pp. 17–30). New York: Springer Publishing.

Burke, K. C., Burke, J. D., Jr., Regier, D. A., & Rae, D. S. (1990). Age at onset of selected metal disorders in five community populations. *Archives of General Psychiatry, 47,* 511–518.

Butler, R. N. (1963). The life review: An interpretation of reminiscence in the aged. *Psychiatry, 26,* 65–76.

Butler, R. N. (1974). Successful aging and the role of life review. *Journal of the American Geriatrics Society, 22,* 529–535.

Carstensen, L. L. (1992). Social and emotional patterns in adulthood: Support for socioemotional selectivity theory. *Psychology and Aging, 7,* 331–338.

Carstensen, L. L., Fung, H. H., & Charles, S. T. (2003). Socioemotional selectivity theory and the regulation of emotion in the second half of life. *Motivation and Emotion, 27,* 103–123.

Carstensen, L. L., Isaacowitz, D. M., & Charles, S. T. (1999). Taking time seriously: A theory of socioemotional selectivity. *American Psychologist, 54,* 165–181.

Carstensen, L. L., Pasupathi, M., Mayr, U., & Nesselroade, J. R. (2000). Emotional experience in everyday life across the adult life span. *Journal of Personality and Social Psychology, 79,* 1–12.

Charles, S. T., Reynolds, C. A., & Gatz, M. (2001). Age-related differences and change in positive and negative affect over 23 years. *Journal of Personality and Social Psychology, 80,* 136–150.

Charness, N. (2000). Can acquired knowledge compensate for age-related declines in cognitive efficiency? In S. H. Qualls & N. Abeles (Eds.), *Psychology and the aging revolution: How we adapt to a longer life* (pp. 99–117). Washington, DC: American Psychological Association.

Cichy, K. E., Fingerman, K. L., & Lefkowitz, E. S. (2007). Age differences in types of interpersonal tensions. *International Journal of Aging and Human Development, 64,* 171–193.

Ciompi, L. (1987). Review of follow-up studies on long-term evolution and aging in schizophrenia. In N. E. Miller & G. D. Cohen (Eds.), *Schizophrenia and aging: Schizophrenia, paranoia, and schizophreniform disorders in later life* (pp. 37–51). New York: Guilford.

Cohen, B. J., Nestadt, G., Samuels, J. F., Romanoski, A. J., McHugh, P. R., & Rabins, P. V. (1994). Personality disorders in later life: A community study. *British Journal of Psychiatry, 165,* 493–499.

Engels, G. I., Duijsens, I. J., Haringsma, R., & van Putten, C. M. (2003). Personality disorders in the elderly compared to four younger age groups: A cross-sectional study of community residents and mental health patients. *Journal of Personality Disorders, 17,* 447–459.

Erikson, E. H. (1950). *Childhood and society.* New York: Norton.

Erikson, E. H., Erikson, J. M., & Kivnick, H. Q. (1986). *Vital involvement in old age.* New York: Norton.

Fauth, E. B., Zarit, S. H., Malmberg, B., & Johansson, B. (2007). Physical, cognitive, and psychosocial variables from the disablement process model predict patterns of independence and the transition into disability for the oldest old. *The Gerontologist, 47,* 613–624.

Femia, E. E., Zarit, S. H., & Johansson, B. (1997). Predicting change in activities of daily living: A longitudinal study of the oldest old. *Journal of Gerontology: Social Sciences, 52,* P292–P304.

Femia, E. E., Zarit, S. H., & Johansson, B. (2001). The disablement process in very late life: A study of the oldest-old in Sweden. *Journal of Gerontology: Social Sciences, 56,* P12–P23.

Filipp, S. H. (1996). Motivation and emotion. In J. E. Birren & K. W. Schaie (Eds.), *Handbook of the psychology of aging* (4th ed., pp. 218–235). San Diego, CA: Academic Press.

Fingerman, K. L. (1995). Aging mothers' and their adult daughters' perceptions of conflict behaviors. *Psychology and Aging, 10,* 639–649.

Fingerman, K. L. (2000). "We had a nice little chat": Age and generational descriptions of enjoyable visits. *Journal of Gerontology: Social Sciences, 55,* P95–P106.

Fiske, A., Gatz, M., & Pedersen, N. (2003). Depressive symptoms and aging: The effects of illness and non-health related effects. *Journal of Gerontology: Social Sciences, 58,* P320–P328.

Gatz, M., Fiske, A., Fox, L. S., Kaskie, B., Kasl-Godley, J. E., McCallum, T. J., et al. (1998). Empirically validated psychological treatments for older adults. *Journal of Mental Health and Aging, 4,* 9–46.

Gatz, M., & Hurwicz, M. (1991). Are older people more depressed? Cross sectional data on Center for Epidemiological Studies Depression Scale factors. *Psychology and Aging, 5,* 284–290.

Girolamo, G., & Reich, J. H. (1993). *Personality disorders.* Geneva: World Health Organization.

Grant, B. F., Hasin, D. S., Stinson, F. S., Dawson, D. A., Chou, S. P., Ruan, W. J., et al. (2004). Prevalence, correlates, and disability of personality disorders in the United States: Results from the national epidemiologic survey on alcohol and related conditions. *Journal of Clinical Psychiatry, 65,* 948–958.

Gross, J. J., Carstensen, L. L., Pasupathi, M., Tsai, J., Skorpen, C. G., & Hsu, A. Y. C. (1997). Emotion and aging: Experience, expression, and control. *Psychology and Aging, 12,* 590–599.

Gurland, B. J., Copeland, J., Kuriansky, J., Kelleher, M. J., Sharpe, L., & Dean, L. (1983). *The mind and mood of aging.* New York: Haworth.

Haynie, D., Zarit, S. H., Berg, B., & Gatz, M. (2000). Depressive symptoms in the oldest old. *Journal of Gerontology: Social Sciences, 56,* P111–P118.

Heikkinen, R. L., & Kauppinen, M. (2004). Depressive symptoms in late life: A 10-year follow-up. *Archives of Gerontology and Geriatrics, 38,* 239–250.

Huber, G. (1997). The heterogeneous course of schizophrenia. *Schizophrenia Research, 28,* 177–185.

Johansson, B., & Zarit, S. H. (1995). Prevalence and incidence of dementia in the oldest old: A study of a population based sample of 84–90 year olds in Sweden. *International Journal of Geriatric Psychiatry, 10,* 359–366.

Kessler, R. C., Berglund, P., Demler, O., Jin, R., Koretz, D., Merikangas, K. R., et al. (2003). The epidemiology of major depressive disorder. *Journal of the American Medical Association, 289,* 3095–3105.

Kessler, R. C., Walters, E. E., & Wittchen, H. (2004). Epidemiology. In R. G. Heimberg, C. L. Turk, & D. S. Mennin (Eds.), *Generalized anxiety disorder: Advances in research and Practice* (pp. 29–50). New York: Guilford.

Kunzmann, U., & Baltes, P. B. (2003). Wisdom-related knowledge: Affective, motivational, and interpersonal correlates. *Personality and Social Psychology Bulletin, 29,* 1104–1119.

Labouvie-Vief, G., Hakim-Larson, J., DeVoe, M., & Schoeberlein, S. (1989). Emotions and self-regulation: A life span view. *Human Development, 32,* 279–299.

Lawton, M. P., Kleban, M. H., Rajagopal, D., & Dean, J. (1992). Dimensions of affective experience in three age groups. *Psychology and Aging, 7,* 171–184.

Lefkowitz, E. S., & Fingerman, K. L. (2003). Positive and negative emotional feelings and behaviors in mother-daughter ties in later life. *Journal of Family Psychology, 17,* 607–617.

Lenze, E. J., Mulsant, B. H., Mohlman, J., Shear, M. K., Dew, M. A., Schulz, R., et al. (2005). Generalized anxiety disorder in late life: Lifetime course and comorbidity with major depressive disorder. *American Journal of Geriatric Psychiatry, 13,* 77–80.

Lewinsohn, P. M., Rohde, P., Fischer, S. A., & Seeley, J. R. (1991). Age and depression: Unique and shared effects. *Psychology and Aging, 6,* 247–260.

Lindesay, J., Briggs, K., & Murphy, E. (1989). The Guy's/Age Concern Survey: Prevalence rates of cognitive impairment, depression and anxiety in an urban elderly community. *British Journal of Psychiatry, 155,* 317–329.

Livingston, G., Hawkins, A., Graham, N., Blizard, B., & Mann, A. (1990). The Gospel Oak Study: Prevalence rates of dementia, depression and activity limitation among elderly residents in Inner London. *Psychological Medicine, 20,* 137–146.

Lyness, J. M., King, D. A., Cox, C., Yoediono, Z., & Caine, E. D. (1999). The importance of subsyndromal depression in older primary care patients: Prevalence and associated functional disability. *Journal of American Geriatrics Society, 47,* 647–652.

Mroczek, D. K., & Almeida, D. M. (2004). The effect of daily stress, personality, and age on daily negative affect. *Journal of Personality, 72,* 355–378.

Mroczek, D. K., & Kolarz, C. M. (1998). The effect of age on positive and negative affect: A developmental perspective on happiness. *Journal of Personality and Social Psychology, 75,* 1333–1349.

Parks, J., Svendsen, D., Singer, P., & Foti, M. E. (Eds.). (2006). *Morbidity and mortality in people with serious mental illness.* Alexandria, VA: National Association of State Mental Health Program Directors.

Parmalee, P. A., Katz, I. R., & Lawton, M. P. (1992). Incidence of depression in long-term care settings. *Journal of Gerontology, 47,* M189–M196.

Regier, D. A., Boyd, J. H., Burke, J. D., Jr., Rae, D. S., Myers, J. K., Kraemer, M., et al. (1988). One-month prevalence of mental disorders in the United States. *Archives of General Psychiatry, 45,* 977–986.

Riediger, M., Li, S.-C., & Lindenberger, U. (2006). Selection, optimization, and compensation as developmental mechanisms of adaptive resource allocation: Review and preview. In J. E. Birren & K. W. Schaie (Eds.), *Handbook of the psychology of aging* (6th ed., pp. 289–313). San Diego, CA: Academic Press.

Ritchie, K., Artero, S., Beluche, I., Ancelin, M. L., Mann, A., Dupuy, A. M., et al. (2004). Prevalence of *DSM—IV* psychiatric disorder in the French elderly populations. *British Journal of Psychiatry, 184,* 147–152.

Robison, J., Curry, L., Gruman, C., Covington, T., Gaztambide, S., & Blank, K. (2003). Depression in later-life Puerto Rican primary care patients: The role of illness, stress, social integration, and religiosity. *International Psychogeriatrics, 15,* 239–251.

Rowe, J. W., & Kahn, R. L. (1987). Human aging: Usual and successful. *Science, 237,* 143–149.

Rowe, J. W., & Kahn, R. L. (1997). Successful aging. *The Gerontologist, 37,* 433–440.

Rowe, J. W., & Kahn, R. L. (1998). *Successful aging.* New York: Pantheon.

Sadavoy, J., & Fogel, B. (1992). Personality disorders in old age. In J. E. Birren, R. B. Sloane, G. D. Cohen, N. R. Hooyman, B. D. Lebowitz, M. Wykle, et al. (Eds.), *Handbook of mental health and aging* (2nd ed., pp. 433–463). New York: Academic Press.

Salthouse, T. A. (1984). Effects of age and skill in typing. *Journal of Experimental Psychology: General, 113,* 345–371.

Salthouse, T. A. (1990). Cognitive competence and expertise in aging. In J. E. Birren & K. W. Schaie (Eds.), *Handbook of the psychology of aging* (3rd ed., pp. 310–391). New York: Academic Press.

Samuels, J. F., Nestadt, G., Romanoski, A. J., Folstein, M. F., & McHugh, P. R. (1994). *DSM—III* personality disorders in the community. *American Journal of Psychiatry, 151,* 1055–1062.

Schulz, R., & Heckhausen, J. (1996). A life-span model of successful aging. *American Psychologist, 51,* 702–714.

Schulz, R., Wrosch, C., & Heckhausen, J. (2003). The life span theory of control: Issues and relevance. In S. H. Zarit, L. I. Pearlin, & K. W. Schaie (Eds.), *Personal control in social and life course contexts* (pp. 233–262). New York: Springer Publishing.

Smith, D. (2003). *The older population in the United States: March 2002.* U.S. Census Bureau Current Population Reports, P20-546. Washington, DC: U.S. Census Bureau.

Smith, J., Staudinger, U. M., & Baltes, P. B. (1994). Occupational settings facilitating wisdom-related knowledge: The sample case of clinical psychologists. *Journal of Consulting and Clinical Psychology, 65,* 989–999.

Stanley, M. A., & Beck, J. G. (2000). Anxiety disorders. *Clinical Psychology Review, 20,* 731–754.

Weissman, M. M., Leaf, P. J., Tischler, G. L., Blazer, D. G., Karno, M., Bruce, M. L., et al. (1988). Affective disorders in five United States communities. *Psychological Medicine, 18,* 141–153.

Wrosch, C., Heckhausen, J., & Lachman, M. E. (2000). Primary and secondary control strategies for managing health and financial stress across adulthood. *Psychology and Aging, 15,* 387–399.

Zarit, S. H., Femia, E. E., Johansson, B., & Gatz, M. (1999). Prevalence and incidence of depression in 80 and 90 year olds: The OCTO study. *Aging and Mental Health, 3,* 119–128.

Zarit, S. H., & Zarit, J. M. (2007). *Mental disorders in older adults* (2nd ed.). New York: Guilford.

38 Translational Theory: A Wisdom-Based Model for Psychological Interventions to Enhance Well-Being in Later Life

Bob G. Knight
Ken Laidlaw

Over the past 15 years or so, the two of us have worked independently on conceptual models designed to draw on gerontological theory and research to guide adaptations of psychological interventions for depression and other mental health disorders common in later life: Knight (1996, 2004; Knight & Lee, 2008) with what is now the contextual adult life span theory for adapting psychotherapy (CALTAP) and Laidlaw, Thompson, & Gallagher-Thompson (2004) with the comprehensive conceptualization framework (CCF). Recognizing some convergence in these approaches, we recently decided to collaborate on a broader theoretical approach to psychological interventions for older adults, with the starting assumption that it should be based on current theory and research in scientific gerontology. We also decided to take a positive approach to development across the life course and ground the new theory in what is currently known about wisdom. The starting point is the assumption that many older adults mature and grow wise across the adult life span. Rather than seeing psychological intervention only in terms of correcting psychological disorders, we pose the question of why some older adults do not mature and grow wise and what psychotherapy can do to facilitate the attainment of wisdom. The potential target of wisdom attainment in later life as a goal for psychotherapy with adults of all ages is consistent with Knight (2004), who suggested that the understanding of psychotherapy with older adults could potentially lead to prospective psychological interventions with younger adults that were aimed at the attainment of a "good old age."

Empirical evidence suggests that psychotherapy for depression and anxiety in later life is efficacious (Gatz, 2007; Pinquart, Duberstein, & Lyness, 2006; Scogin, Welsh, Hanson, Stump, & Coates, 2005). While the literature for outcome research in psychotherapy with older people is quite mature, particularly evidence for cognitive-behavioral therapy (CBT; Laidlaw, Thompson, Dick-Siskin, & Gallagher-Thompson, 2003), it is evident that research has tended to evaluate outcome with nonmodified therapies using models borrowed largely from adult mental health settings without consideration to conceptual input from life span developmental and gerontological theories (Laidlaw & Thompson, 2008). Our theory in progress can be seen as also addressing the question as to how a psychotherapy designed specifically for use with older people would look different from current interventions based on work with younger adults.

The CALTAP and CCF Models

Advocating a broad and inclusive pantheoretical approach, Knight (Knight 1996; Knight 2004) developed a contextual, cohort-based maturity/specific challenge model (CCMSC) for psychotherapy with older people. More recently, Knight developed CALTAP (Knight & Lee, 2008; Knight & Poon, 2008), which explicitly draws on gerontology and life span developmental psychology and endorses a contemporary positive portrayal of the aging process (see also Satre, Knight, & David, 2006). The CALTAP model considered the role of both age-related decrements in cognitive abilities and positive age changes as well as the influence of age-specific social context, the effects of being born and raised within a specific cohort with its unique sociohistorical context, and the influence of cultural identity on older adults. While the focus of this model was on helping the psychotherapist understand the older adult client, the same framework could arguably be used to help older adults understand their own aging process and the nondevelopmental influences that make them different from younger contemporaries. That is, understanding that differences from younger family members or friends are due to one's cohort membership or to age-based social rules rather than developmental aging often leads to both a different perception of one's self and new ideas for addressing interpersonal issues.

To address concerns that CBT may require adaptation or modification for use with older people, Laidlaw et al. (2004) developed a CCF drawing on insights from gerontology as a way of contextualizing older adults' problems within CBT while maintaining the emphasis on interventions that optimize symptom reduction. The main elements of the CCF are cohort beliefs, role transitions, intergenerational linkages, sociocultural context, and health status. More recently, Laidlaw & McAlpine (in press) have considered age-appropriate conceptual rather than procedural-level modifications to enhance treatment outcome in CBT with older people. These conceptual-level modifications to CBT include the incorporation of an age-appropriate conceptualization model, a focus on understanding life span development and the interaction with depression, and an emphasis on goal-focused-optimized coping of loss experiences.

The CALTAP and CCF models share many features with each other and with life span developmental and life course perspectives on gerontology: an emphasis on cohort membership as an important explanatory alternative to chronological age and presumed developmental influences and an emphasis on social context in addition to intraindividual development. There are some differences in emphasis with regard to potential need for adaptations in psychological interventions with older adults: CALTAP emphasizes cultural differences somewhat more and places health status effects under the heading of challenges of later life (along with grief and caregiving), whereas CCF emphasizes role transitions and intergenerational linkages more than CALTAP. In addition, CCF has been more clear in how it can be used to inform older adults' understanding of their own aging process.

Wisdom and the Adult Life Span

Commonly held implicit theories of wisdom assume a positive correlation of wisdom with advancing age (Bluck & Glück, 2005). When wisdom is studied by having judges rate the wisdom of responses to life problems, however, wisdom is not correlated with advancing age after adulthood is attained (Jordan, 2005), although there are advances in wisdom from childhood through adolescence to adulthood (Richardson & Pasupathi, 2005). We take this disjuncture between common understandings of the increase of wisdom with adult development and the existing evidence on the relationship of wisdom to age in cross-sectional studies to pose challenges for psychotherapy: why do some older adults not attain wisdom?

When translating positive theories of aging for application to psychotherapy with older people, a working definition of wisdom is needed. The first step is to agree on some working ecological definition of wisdom. This is a formidable task given the great variety of such definitions across cultures and across history (see, e.g., Birren & Svensson, 2005). Within life span developmental psychology, the Berlin wisdom model developed by Paul Baltes and associates (e.g., Scheibe, Kunzmann, & Baltes, 2007) provides an important formulation of wisdom along five criteria: a store of factual knowledge about human nature and the life course, rich procedural knowledge about handling life problems, an awareness of the many contexts of life and how they change over the life span ("life span contextualism"), an understanding of the relativism of values and resulting tolerance for others, and understanding how to handle uncertainty (Scheibe et al., 2007). In discussing contrasts between Eastern and Western views of wisdom, Takahashi and Overton (2005) note that Western conceptions place a great deal of emphasis on knowledge and intelligence as components of wisdom, whereas Eastern views delete knowledge and academic intelligence and focus more on direct experience of life and integrating emotion and thought and other aspects of life seen as dialectic opposites in Western thought. In adult developmental thought, Sternberg and Lubart's (2001) description of balance theory retains some of the Western emphasis on intelligence and knowledge but emphasizes metacognition and "knowing how" over "knowing what" while also focusing on balancing intrapersonal, interpersonal, and extrapersonal aims as well as assimilation and accommodation as styles of interacting with the environment.

For our working definition of wisdom as a goal for adult development, we would emphasize the focus on life span contextualism, understanding of the contextual relativism of individual values and increased tolerance for individual differences in values, acceptance of uncertainty in life, a greater ability to integrate and balance emotion and reason, and an accumulation of "knowing how" expertise. The growth of life span contextualism across adulthood supports the role of the gerontological worldview in CALTAP and CCF in application to psychological interventions with older adults. The other elements of wisdom are generally consistent with goals of psychotherapy in promoting better relationships with others and an improved ability to regulate one's emotional life.

Wisdom and Psychotherapy

While retrospective in time orientation and aimed at ameliorating psychological disorders rather than enhancing wisdom, the CALTAP and CCF models (Knight & Lee, 2008; Laidlaw et al., 2004) provide the beginning of a bridge between psychotherapy with older adults and conceptions of wisdom. The models provide a framework for thinking about therapy with older clients, including helping older adults understand their own development through life review, that utilizes key concepts from life span developmental psychology and scientific gerontology. A main theme of positive aspects of maturation is the development of expertise, including expertise in personal relationships and in family dynamics through experience: a focus on "knowing how," especially in relationship to others. The models emphasize understanding the role of current social context and also the role of one's cohort (generational) membership as it shaped the formation of personal identity and the opportunities to engage in social roles that change from cohort to cohort. CALTAP introduces a more explicit attention to cultural values and ethnic identity and the influence exerted on understanding oneself and others. These connections between understanding of aging in psychotherapy and wisdom suggest a potential role for psychological research and intervention in understanding and encouraging the development of wisdom. On the other hand, the focus of psychotherapy on emotional pain and life's challenges reminds us that the attainment of wisdom is neither easy nor automatic.

Barriers to Wisdom

We next describe some of the barriers to learning from life experience and developing wisdom. Three such barriers are physical aging, societal ageism, and psychological disorders.

The Stronger Emergence of the Physical in Later Life

Experiencing loss and change is a universal experience in the life span (Boerner & Jopp, 2007). People who enter what is termed the fourth age (Baltes & Smith, 2002) are more likely to have to deal with greater challenges of living longer. Likewise, therapists will likely see an increase in complexity of issues and problems with a chronicity and longevity attached to them that is rarely seen currently. Questions about the suitability of psychological treatments become especially important when working with the oldest-old section of society.

The signs that prompt awareness of one's own aging are often primarily physical. Some of these are largely symbolic and without functional implications (e.g., gray hair and wrinkles), while others have some functional impact but are minor enough to allow for correction or adaptations (e.g., the normative visual and hearing changes associated with middle age and the young-old years). Finally, there are illnesses and disabling conditions associated with the later stages of life that bring serious dysfunction. Some of these medical disorders limit life expectancy, and some are progressive with increases in disability over time. A similar distinction can be made in the cognitive domain between normative changes with aging that are mainly minor and that can be compensated for and the quite serious impairments associated with the dementias of later life.

Even the symbolic and the normative physical changes can bring on a concern with what it means to grow older. In our culture, they are often unwelcome and become the occasion for sadness over growing older and ageist humor in birthday cards. These reactions fuel the growth of the antiaging industry, much of which is oriented toward preventing the visible signs of aging. Imagine an aging-positive culture in which people would use hair dyes to color their hair gray and makeup to produce more wrinkles. The difficulty in taking such an idea seriously is an indicator of the pervasive ageism of our culture.

The reactions to normative changes in perception and cognition and to the stiffening of muscles and joints are more realistic and occasion some real changes in day-to-day activities, although they typically do not prevent the aging adult from accomplishing valued goals. They do occasion an awareness of not being able to do things that were done before and the approach of older adulthood. Finding an acceptance of these changes that supports satisfaction with one's life is one part of aging well. The acceptance of this greater intrusion of the physical into daily life is one element of wisdom, an aspect of understanding the life course and the changing context of one's own life over time.

Biological theories of aging point to the wear-and-repair model (Ricklefs & Finch, 1995), with a decline in the repair functions with aging. One aspect of living longer is the accumulation of more wear and tear in the body, combined with less ability to do effective repairs (e.g., a declining immune system response). Another class of theories points to accumulations of error over time in various physiological systems (e.g., mutations in genetic replications of cells that reproduce and replace and accumulation of free radicals produced by exposure to sunlight and background radiation). Aging and death may also be programmed into our bodies as a way to make room for younger generations. From a biological standpoint, aging and death are universal and understandable and desirable at the population level. In our sociocultural context, we find them psychologically distressing to unacceptable. Part of wisdom is coming to terms with the biological inevitability of aging and death. Indeed, clinical experience suggests that older adults are more comfortable with these topics than the young and the middle aged (Knight, 2004).

To this point as we consider symbolic and normative changes in the body, the ways in which enhanced understanding and cognitive-behavioral interventions to change internalized ageism can result in a more positive view of aging and so greater satisfaction with life are relatively straightforward. As one gets older, however, the growing sense of dread about what aging will bring can often be accompanied by an increased vigilance for the first signs of the "the slippery slope" (Laidlaw & Baikie, 2007). This may be triggered by bereavement, deterioration in loved ones, or the onset of physical illness. In these situations, the older person may reflect on his or her aging as a negative and frightening experience.

While some people die without a period of chronic disability and frailty before death, high rates of chronic illness and disability are a common part of later life. For example, Tabbarah, Mihelic, and Crimmins (2001) found that about 40% of the over-70 population in the United States had at least one disability related to activities of daily living or instrumental activities of daily living. On average, people can expect to spend about 4.3 years after age 65 with heart disease, 8 years with arthritis, and/or 1.9 years with diabetes (Crimmins, Kim, & Hagedorn, 2002). The most common chronic diseases of later life also have theoretical roots in the biology of aging: the wearing out of organs that do not replace themselves with cell division and replacement of old cells (heart and brain) or the uncontrolled cell division when the process goes wrong in the organs that do (cancer). As with normative aging, what goes wrong and when is highly idiosyncratic.

The CCMSC and CALTAP models have argued that these processes constitute specific challenges rather than generic losses of later life. In this approach, the specific illness and disability matter for understanding their impact on the individual as do their prognosis and treatment. Psychological intervention is often aimed at decreasing high levels of distress rather than achieving pre-illness levels of life satisfaction. The process includes grieving for lost abilities, learning what can be done with remaining abilities, and planning a life on the basis of the realities of these specific challenges of chronic illness and disability. The assessment of current ability level is often complex and involves trial and error, and developing a new life that incorporates the reality of the illness and related disability is an ongoing challenge of constant experimentation (Freund & Baltes, 1998; Jopp & Smith, 2006).

These challenges are even greater when the illness is one of the late-life dementias and the disabilities are cognitive. The assessment process is even more difficult for the individual, the family, and helping professionals. The adjustment to disability is even more difficult when the deficits are not due to externally visible causes. Despite these difficulties, it is possible to improve the emotional distress of persons with dementia, at least into the moderate stages of the disorders.

In summary, one theme of growing older and a challenge for achieving wisdom is the growing impact of the physical body on the lives of older persons. The degree of this greater significance of the physical for psychological well-being varies greatly, from largely symbolic changes such as gray hair through normative changes such as longer healing times due to lessened immune system response to the devastating effects of terminal cancer or Alzheimer's disease. In all cases, the acceptance of physical changes, their integration into life, and the preparation for the end of life are aspects of the search for wisdom.

Internalized Ageism as a Barrier to Wisdom

Schaie (2008) notes that it is a common assumption among psychologists that universal cognitive decline is an outcome of aging, but while a few unfortunately experience decline and dementia, many do not, and a lucky few may even go on to achieve selective gains in later life. Growing older therefore does not have to be something to dread; it can (and should) be a time of continued personal growth (see Carstensen, Isaacowitz, & Charles, 1999). Indeed, older people with positive self-perceptions of aging are more likely to have better health and may increase their life expectancy (Levy et al., 2002). As people live longer and remain healthier for longer in late life (Kinsella & Velkoff, 2001), there may be new challenges of growing older in the 21st century.

We give particular emphasis to ways in which societal and introjected ageism interfere with the development of a complete and accurate understanding of life span development. Implicit and uncritical acceptance of loss-deficit models of aging (i.e., negative age stereotypes; Levy, 2003) encourage passive acceptance of suboptimal levels of quality of life. A more realistic evaluation of the challenges and gains of aging can help remove some of the barriers to guide the individual's understanding of adult development and the resulting life span construct (cf. Whitbourne, 1985), which can be seen as an older person's elaboration of self-concepts formed in young adulthood without the perspective provided by decades of adult life experience.

Laidlaw et al. (2004) note that many older people can be quite ageist and have internalized negative social stereotypes about aging. This is neatly conceptualized by Levy (2003) as meaning that "when individuals reach old age, the aging stereotypes internalized in childhood, and then reinforced for decades, become self-stereotypes" (p. 204). The importance of aging self-stereotypes is that they operate outside of many people's awareness and influence health status. As such, it is important to ascertain an individual's self-perception of aging because challenges of aging may activate negative aging stereotypes (Levy, 2003; Levy et al., 2002). In this sense, an internalized negative age stereotype acts as a latent maladaptive belief (dysfunctional attitude) that can be activated by a challenging experience associated with aging. Thus, a stress–diathesis relationship is set up, leaving an individual vulnerable to develop emotional distress following a negative experience associated with aging. This idea is consistent with the Beck theory of cognitive therapy (Beck, Rush, Shaw, & Emery, 1979) and suggests that certain transitional experiences in aging (such as developing a chronic illness associated with aging) will result in emotional dysfunction in older people who do not reappraise growing older in light of their own experiences.

Clearly, self-perceptions of aging are important to index when considering psychotherapy with older people. There are very few reliable measures of self-perception of aging (Laidlaw, Power, Schmidt, & the WHOQOL Group, 2006). The most commonly used means of indexing attitudes to aging was the Philadelphia Geriatric Morale Scale (Lawton, 1975), which had a five-item subscale assessing attitudes. While this measure reports acceptable psychometrics, the small number of items makes it less useful. Recently, two new measures of the self-perception of aging (Aging Perceptions Questionnaire; Barker, O'Hanlon, McGee, Hickey, & Conroy, 2007) and a cross-cultural attitudes-to-aging questionnaire (AAQ) have been developed (Laidlaw et al., 2006). The AAQ has been developed to provide a profile of aging perception and reports on three broad domains of aging: physical change, psychological growth, and psychological loss. It has been developed with 5,566 participants in 16 countries and promises to permit an adequate means to characterize how an individual perceives and experiences aging. From the development of this measure, Laidlaw et al. (2006) noted that older people appear quite resilient in the face of aging and endorse mainly a high subjective appraisal of health despite evidence of a number of physical health complaints for which they were in receipt of treatment. It is also evident that depression can have an impact on the perception of aging, as Chachamovich, Fleck, Laidlaw, and Power (in press) have noted that even small increases in depression can have a negative impact on scores on the AAQ. Thus, when working with older people, therapists may wish to take account of negative attitudes to aging when assessing depression.

Psychological Disorders as Barriers to Attainment of Wisdom

In addition to these pervasive and perhaps normative barriers to the attainment of wisdom, psychological disorders can interfere with successful adult development and the attainment of a wise old age. The disorders of anxiety and depression tend to bias people to negative perceptions of life and memories of the past and also interfere with successful coping strategies. Many personality disorders begin in adolescence and young adulthood and are characterized by impaired interpersonal relationships and a reduced ability to profit from life experience. Serious mental illnesses like psychosis and the dementias of later life produce even more severe cognitive deficits and impairments in daily functioning. Psychotherapeutic interventions, guided by wisdom-oriented gerontological theories, make up one method for overcoming the effects of both the normative barriers to wisdom and these psychological disorders.

For example, we argue that the attainment of wisdom is blocked by the emotional, cognitive, and behavioral consequences of depression because perception of events are negatively biased, rigid, and nonspecific (see also Nolen-Hoeksema, 1991). In particular, in depression recall of autobiographical memory is general rather than specific (Kuyken & Dalgleish, 1995) and likely to be negative in emotional tone (Knight, Maines, & Robinson, 2002). That is, in depression, people will experience difficulty in recalling specific details of events, seeing them in more global and rigid terms of failure. The character of memory in depression is "like fuel to the fire of depressive thinking" (Kuyken, 2006, p. 280). Rumination results in a downward depressive spiral that can be very aversive as depressed individuals castigate themselves for their (perceived) failings. It results in a heightened, repetitive, and perseverative focus that contributes to emotional disturbance (Papageorgiou & Wells, 2003). The importance of depression as a potential block to wisdom attainment comes from this lower likelihood that people who are depressed will appraise problematic situations in ways that facilitate learning from experience. Thus, treatment of depression can facilitate the development of wisdom with aging.

Depressed older people often appraise their age and associated physical changes as negative attributes and assume that change is impossible since one cannot become younger again. Rather than this being a realistic evaluation of their capabilities or ability to change, it may indicate an emotionally dysfunctional response to aging. Stated simply, when asked about their experience of aging, the majority of nondepressed older people will often appraise aging as being less of a negative experience than expected (Laidlaw et al., 2006) or report high life satisfaction despite loss experiences, termed the aging paradox (for review, see Carstensen & Lockenhoff, 2003). Therefore, when an individual states that aging is a negative or depressing experience, it may be not a sign of depression but rather a realistic appraisal of aging or of associated diseases.

Translating Wisdom Theory Into Action: Facilitating Attainment of Wisdom

Wisdom enhancement can take a number of different forms. It can be developed by education or difficult life circumstances, or, as Glück & Baltes (2006) showed, it can be enhanced by a simple request, such as "try to give a wise response." This simple statement may provide a wisdom-enhancing and empowering set of self-directed action-oriented strategies. Its effect may be delivered via the process of reflection that activates a metaheuristic to activate organized sets of strategies and goals that individuals will draw on to arrive at a wise response (Baltes & Staudinger, 2000).

Stated simply, wisdom enhancement may be construed as a skill or a strategy to be developed by encouraging older people to reflect on wise responses and to put this in action as a set of behavioral experiments in order to generalize this skill outside the therapy room. Indeed, one observation about therapy with older adults is that it often takes the form of reminding the older client of longstanding coping skills and finding ways to apply them to late-life challenges (Zarit, 1980). However, to promote the effectiveness of this simple intervention, Glück and Baltes (2006) indicate that it is important to index the individual's internal resources to use this task; therefore, for some individuals, more emphasis may need to be placed on psychoeducation before wisdom enhancement activities can be encouraged.

The assumptions of societal ageism that old age inevitably means loss and decrepitude can and should be challenged in therapy using cognitive restructuring. Cognitive restructuring works by identifying rigid, unhelpful, and unrealistic appraisals and substituting these with more helpful and realistic evaluations and appraisals (Beck et al., 1979). Thus, evidence from the aging experience of an individual can be used to achieve a more realistic appraisal of the process of growing older, and erroneous assumptions associated with poor functioning attributed to age rather than depression may be corrected in psychotherapy. The use of one's own experience of aging as evidence incongruent with a negative age stereotype is consistent with the concept of wisdom enhancement in therapy.

McAdam and de St. Aubin (1992) have developed a scientific framework to study generativity and have expanded on the concept so that it extends beyond middle age as a discrete developmental stage and is linked with an individual's personal life narrative (Grossbaum & Bates, 2002). The individual seeks identity, purpose, and meaning for a life well lived: "The generativity script is an inner narration of the adult's own awareness of where efforts to be generative fit into his or her own personal history, into contemporary society and the social world he or she inhabits" (McAdams & de St. Aubin, 1992, p. 1006). In qualitative analyses, individuals who were highly generative were noted to group affective scenes so that a positive affective sequence followed a negative affective sequence. This affective sequencing is termed a redemptive sequence, where bad events are "redeemed" or reframed, a good outcome is achieved, and a coherent sense of meaning and identity can be sustained in good times and in bad. As people age and have to confront many challenges throughout life, learning this skill could be highly useful in preventing the development of distress.

Summary

We intend this chapter as a first step toward articulating a theoretical framework that can serve to link a positive view of adult development and aging as captured by psychological and gerontological theories of wisdom to psychological interventions that might be used to facilitate this process by counteracting common barriers. We take wisdom to be rooted in development of a self-concept and a coherent life narrative that incorporates life span contextualism, an understanding of others that comes from appreciation of differing contexts and points of view, accumulated life experience in "knowing how," greater tolerance of uncertainty, and a balancing of dialectics such as emotion and thinking.

Barriers to wisdom attainment cut across the areas of life studied by the component disciplines of gerontology: physical changes in the body and especially disabling chronic illnesses, societal ageism and its acceptance by the aging individual, and psychological disorders that interfere with positive adult development. As psychologists and psychotherapists, we focus discussion of intervention on psychological approaches and feel that these are possible for the individual even when the causes of the barriers to wisdom are biological or societal. We recognize that removal of barriers through biomedical advances and social changes is also possible and desirable, although perhaps even slower than individual change through psychological intervention.

References

Baltes, P. B., & Smith, J. (2002, April). *New frontiers in the future of aging: From successful ageing of the young old to the dilemmas of the fourth age.* Paper presented at the Valencia Forum, Researchers, Educators and Providers contribution to the Second World Assembly on Ageing, Valencia, Spain.

Baltes, P. B., & Staudinger, U. M. (2000). Wisdom: A metaheuristic (pragmatic) to orchestrate mind and virtue toward excellence. *American Psychologist, 55,* 122–136.

Barker, M., O'Hanlon, A., McGee, H., Hickey, A., & Conroy, R. (2007). Cross-sectional validation of the Aging Perceptions Questionnaire: A multidimensional instrument for assessing self-perceptions of aging. *BMC Geriatrics, 26,* 9–17.

Beck, A. T., Rush, A. J., Shaw, B. F., & Emery, G. (1979). *Cognitive therapy of depression.* New York: Guilford.

Birren, J. E., & Svensson, C. M. (2005). Wisdom in history. In R. J. Sternberg & J. Jordan (Eds.), *A handbook of wisdom: Psychological perspectives* (pp. 3–31). New York: Cambridge University Press.

Bluck, S., & Glück, J. (2005). From the inside out: People's implicit theories of wisdom. In R. J. Sternberg & J. Jordan (Eds.), *A handbook of wisdom: Psychological perspectives* (pp. 84–109). New York: Cambridge University Press.

Boerner, K., & Jopp, D. A. (2007). Improvement/maintenance and reorientation as central features of coping with major life change and loss: Contributions of three major life-span theories. *Human Development, 50,* 171–195.

Carstensen, L., Isaacowitz, D., & Charles, S. T. (1999). Taking time seriously: A theory of socio-emotional selectivity. *American Psychologist, 54,* 165–181

Carstensen, L., & Lockenhoff, C. A. (2003). Aging, emotion, and evolution: The bigger picture. *Annals of the New York Academy of Science, 1000,* 152–179.

Chachamovich, E., Fleck, M., Laidlaw, K., & Power, M. J. (in press). Impact of major depression and subsyndromal symptoms on quality of life and attitudes to aging in an international sample of older adults. *The Gerontologist.*

Crimmins, E. M., Kim, J. K., & Hagedorn, A. (2002). Life with and without disease: Women experience more of both. *Journal of Women & Aging, 14,* 47–59.

Freund, A. M. (2006). Age-differential motivation consequences of optimization versus compensation focus in younger and older adults. *Psychology and Aging, 21,* 240–252.

Freund, A. M., & Baltes, P. B. (1998). Selection, optimization, and compensation as strategies of life management: Correlations with subjective indicators of successful aging. *Psychology and Aging, 13,* 531–543.

Gatz, M. (2007). Commentary on evidence-based psychological treatments for older adults. *Psychology and Aging, 22,* 52–55.

Glück, J., & Baltes, P. B. (2006). Using the concept of wisdom to enhance the expression of wisdom knowledge: Not the philosopher's dream but differential effects of developmental preparedness. *Psychology and Aging, 21,* 679–690.

Grossbaum, M. F., & Bates, G. W. (2002). Correlates of psychological well-being at midlife: The role of generativity, agency, and communion, and narrative themes. *International Journal of Behavioral Development, 26,* 120–127.

Jopp, D. A., & Smith, J. (2006). Resources and life-management strategies as determinants of successful aging: On the protective effect of selection, optimization, and compensation. *Psychology and Aging, 21,* 253–265.

Jordan, J. (2005). The quest for wisdom in adulthood: A psychological perspective. In R. J. Sternberg & J. Jordan (Eds.), *A handbook of wisdom: Psychological perspectives* (pp. 160–190). New York: Cambridge University Press.

Kinsella, K., & Velkoff, V. A. (2001). *US Census Bureau, Series P95/01-1, an aging world: 2001.* Washington, DC: US Government Printing Office.

Knight, B. G. (1996). Overview of psychotherapy with the elderly: The contextual cohort-based, maturity-specific-challenge model. In S. H. Zarit & B. G. Knight (Eds.), *A guide to psychotherapy and aging: Effective clinical interventions in a life-stage context* (pp. 17–34). Washington, DC: American Psychological Association.

Knight, B. G. (2004). *Psychotherapy with older adults* (3rd ed.). Thousand Oaks, CA: Sage.

Knight, B. G., & Lee, L. O. (2008). Contextual adult life span theory for adapting psychotherapy. In K. Laidlaw & B. G. Knight (Eds.), *Handbook of emotional disorders in late life: Assessment and treatment* (pp. 59–88). Oxford: Oxford University Press.

Knight, B. G., Maines, M. L., & Robinson, G. S. (2002). The effects of mood and memory in older adults: A test of the mood congruence effect. *Psychology and Aging, 17,* 653–661.

Knight, B. G., & Poon, C. (2008). The socio-cultural context in understanding older adults: Contextual adult life span theory for adapting psychotherapy. In B. Woods & L. Clare (Eds.), *The handbook of the clinical psychology of ageing* (pp. 439–456). Chichester: Wiley.

Kuyken, W. (2006). Digging deep into depression. *The Psychologist, 19,* 278–281.
Kuyken, W., & Dalgleish, T. (1995). Autobiographical memory and depression. *British Journal of Clinical Psychology, 34,* 89–92.
Laidlaw, K., & Baikie, E. (2007). Psychotherapy and demographic change: *Nordic Journal of Psychology, 59,* 45–58.
Laidlaw, K., & McAlpine, S. (in press). Cognitive-behaviour therapy: How is it different with older people? *Journal of Rational Emotive Cognitive Behaviour Therapy, 26*(4).
Laidlaw, K., Power, M. J., Schmidt, S., & the WHOQOL Group. (2006). The attitudes to ageing questionnaire (AAQ): Development and psychometric properties. *International Journal of Geriatric Psychiatry, 21,* 1–13.
Laidlaw, K., & Thompson, L. W. (2008). Cognitive behaviour therapy with depressed older adults. In K. Laidlaw & B. G. Knight (Eds.), *The handbook of the assessment and treatment of emotional distress in later life* (pp. 91–115). Oxford: Oxford University Press.
Laidlaw, K., Thompson, L. W., Dick-Siskin, L., & Gallagher-Thompson, D. (2003). *Cognitive behaviour therapy with older people.* Chichester: Wiley.
Laidlaw, K., Thompson, L. W., & Gallagher-Thompson, D. (2004). Comprehensive conceptualization of cognitive behaviour therapy for late life depression. *Behavioural and Cognitive Psychotherapy, 32,* 389–399.
Lawton, M. P. (1975). The Philadelphia geriatric morale scale: A revision. *Journal of Gerontology, 30,* 85–89.
Levy, B. R. (2003). Mind matters: Cognitive and physical effects of aging stereotypes. *Journal of Gerontology: Social Sciences, 58,* P203–P211.
Levy, B. R., Slade, M. D., Kunkel, S. R., & Kasl, S. V. (2002). Longevity increased by positive self-perceptions of aging. *Journal of Personality and Social Psychology, 83,* 261–270.
McAdam, D., & de St. Aubin, E. (1992). A theory of generativity and its assessment through self-report, behavioral acts, and narrative themes in autobiography. *Journal of Personality and Social Psychology, 62,* 1003–1015.
Nolen-Hoeksema, S. (1991). Responses to depression and their effects on the duration of depressive episodes. *Journal of Abnormal Psychology, 100,* 569–582.
Papageorgiou, C., & Wells, A. (2003). An empirical test of a clinical metacognitive model of rumination and depression. *Cognitive Therapy and Research, 27,* 261–273.
Pinquart, M., Duberstein, P. R., & Lyness, J. M. (2006). Treatments for later-life depressive conditions: A meta-analytic comparison of pharmacotherapy and psychotherapy. *American Journal of Psychiatry, 163,* 1493–1501.
Richardson, M. J., & Pasupathi, M. (2005). Young and growing wiser: Wisdom during adolescence and young adulthood. In R. J. Sternberg & J. Jordan (Eds.), *A handbook of wisdom: Psychological perspectives* (pp. 139–159). New York: Cambridge University Press.
Ricklefs, R. E., & Finch, C. E. (1995). *Aging: A natural history.* New York: Scientific American Library.
Satre, D., Knight, B. G., & David, S. (2006). Cognitive behavioral interventions with older adults: Integrating clinical and gerontological research. *Professional Psychology: Research and Practice, 37,* 489–498.
Schaie, K. W. (2008). A lifespan developmental perspective of psychological aging. In K. Laidlaw & B. G. Knight (Eds.), *Handbook of emotional disorders in late life: Assessment and treatment* (pp. 59–88). Oxford: Oxford University Press.
Scheibe, S., Kunzmann, U., & Baltes, P. B. (2007). Wisdom, life longings, and optimal development. In J. A. Blackburn & C. N. Dulmas (Eds.), *Handbook of gerontology: Evidence-based approaches to theory, practice, and policy* (pp. 117–142). Hoboken, NJ: Wiley.
Scogin, F., Welsh, D., Hanson, A., Stump, J., & Coates, A. (2005). Evidence-based psychotherapies for depression in older adults. *Clinical Psychology: Science and Practice, 12,* 222–237.
Sternberg, R. J., & Lubart, T. I. (2001). Wisdom and creativity. In J. E. Birren & K. W. Schaie (Eds.), *Handbook of the psychology of aging* (5th ed., pp. 500–522). San Diego, CA: Academic Press.
Tabbarah, M., Mihelic, A., & Crimmins, E. M. (2001). Disability: The demographics of physical functioning and home environments of older Americans. *Journal of Architectural and Planning Research, 18,* 183–193.

Takahashi, M., & Overton, W. F. (2005). Cultural foundations of wisdom: An integrated developmental approach. In R. J. Sternberg & J. Jordan (Eds.), *A handbook of wisdom: Psychological perspectives* (pp. 32–60). New York: Cambridge University Press.
Whitbourne, S. K. (1985). The psychological construction of the life span. In J. E. Birren & K. W. Schaie (Eds.), *Handbook of the psychology of aging* (2nd ed., pp. 594–618). New York: Van Nostrand.
Zarit, S. H. (1980). *Aging and mental disorders.* New York: Free Press.

The Construction of Knowledge: A New Gerontological Education Paradigm

39

Ariela Lowenstein
Sara Carmel

Educational institutions play a major role in facilitating the necessary social adaptation to the challenge of global aging and the related changing social and health needs (Hyman, 1979). Developing knowledge and educational programs in gerontology is one of the essential means of sensitizing the public and professionals working with older people to the impact of aging societies (Peterson, 1986).

In 1981, the White House Conference on Aging recommended the development of educational and training programs in gerontology and geriatrics in order to develop highly qualified personnel in the provision of services for the aged. The rationale was based on the approach that professionals exposed to a richer training environment will acquire a wide knowledge base and will act as leaders in higher academic and administrative echelons, thereby providing better and more effective services for older adults and their families. Since then, an abundance of educational programs have been developed in the United States. Based on the accumulated experience, it becomes clear that in order to develop gerontological knowledge and construct a paradigm of gerontological education, societies have to go through three interrelated stages: a new and growing social need, recognition of the need, and acting on the need.

The demographic revolution that modern societies have undergone—dramatic increases in elderly population creating the phenomenon of global aging (Bengtson, Lowenstein, Putney, & Gans, 2003) as well as new and complex age-related social and health needs—necessitates raising academic, professional, and public awareness to the needs of older persons. This recognition should be raised through the creation of specific and unique gerontological knowledge bases.

Social policy in the developed countries has come to recognize the importance of providing quality care to the growing aged population, as manifested by the accelerated development of long-term care systems. The designation by the United Nations of the year 1999 as the "International Year of the Older Persons" and the Madrid International Plan of Action on Aging of 2002 were expressions of increasing recognition.

Gerontological knowledge and research databases have proliferated over the past few decades. This is reflected in a wide array of master's- and doctoral-level educational and training programs that have developed, especially in the United States, in response to the need to train researchers, educators, and professionals to serve the growing and diverse older populations (Haley & Zelinski, 2007).

Population aging is a global phenomenon, and most societies face the related common challenges. However, countries differ in the pace with which they go through this transition as well as in their response to it. In European countries, population aging occurred over a longer period of time than in the Unite States. Furthermore, significant differences in responding to the challenges have been reported among European countries. For example, in 2003, there were 23 gerontological programs in the United Kingdom, whereas only one program was found in Finland, Italy, and Austria (Meyer, 2003).

Gerontology Emerging as a Unique Discipline

A discipline is first and foremost a body of distinctive knowledge bases with its own terminology. The goal of this body of knowledge is to promote the understanding of specific phenomena and the implementation of this body of knowledge by developing distinct talents and expertise by means of education and training. A profession cannot develop without the existence of an accompanying discipline.

Gerontology, defined nearly a century ago as "the scientific study of old age" (Metchnikoff, 1905), has been transformed from a "protodiscipline" (Levine, 1981) into an actual discipline by compiling gerontological knowledge through research dedicated to the study of aging from the broadest perspective and expanding and integrating its knowledge bases (Bass & Ferraro, 2000). Bass and Ferraro (2000) claim that already at selected schools in the United States, the trend is moving from multidisciplinarity toward interdisciplinarity. They further suggest that if a new paradigm were to be developed, gerontology will truly turn into a new discipline. In this chapter, we propose such a paradigm.

The perception of gerontology as a discipline aimed at professionalization stems from the general consensus among researchers and professionals in this field that while a body of academic knowledge exists, gerontology by its very nature embraces, incorporates, and integrates knowledge from a variety of disciplines (Hendricks & Hendricks, 1986). Additionally, there is a consensus over the existence of a core body of knowledge (Johnson et al., 1980).

This perception is reflected in a discussion by Rosenberg (1979) on the role of professionals in promoting knowledge based on three elements that can indeed be traced in the development of gerontology as an academic discipline. The first element is the content of research and education in gerontology. Contents reflect societal dilemmas regarding old age and aging on the individual, familial, and societal levels. The second element is the structure of the discipline, which is reflected in the outcome of the intellectual tools used to disseminate and entrench knowledge, that is, who the professionals are in the various disciplines who are involved with research, teaching, and training in the area of gerontology. The third element is to understand the organization of knowledge, that is, where the knowledge is produced and to whom it is conveyed.

The case for the importance of gerontology as a separate academic discipline that requires the development of distinct curricula was made in the late 1960s in the United States by Kleemeier, Havighurst, and Tibbitts (1967). They argued that education in gerontology is the key tool for the dissemination and entrenchment of existing knowledge and the development of new knowledge and is thereby the vehicle for molding the discipline.

What would gerontology as a discipline look like? Based on previous research, Bramwell (1985) posited four criteria for an academic discipline: (a) It must have a central, all-pervading theme. In gerontology today, a predominant theme is the study of human aging from a life course perspective with emphases on time as a key element (Bengtson, Cutler, Mangen, & Marshall, 1985) and the integration of structural and contextual elements with human agency (Hagestad & Dannefer, 2001), (b) It must have its own distinctive methods of inquiry. In gerontology, these include the identification of biomarkers of age, the use of phenomenological criteria and qualitative methods, and promotion of the triangulation of data and longitudinal research (Alwin & Campbell, 2001; Maddox & Campbell, 1985). (c) Its experts should constitute a self-instructive community. Gerontological organizations such as the Gerontological Society of America (established in 1945), the International Association of Gerontology (established in 1949), and the Association of Gerontology in Higher Education (established in 1974) represent more than 1,000 academic gerontological programs today. (d) It should develop a tradition of intellectual activity—a body of fundamental knowledge bases with a distinctive philosophical perspective and its own terminology.

Lowenstein (2001) proposed an analytic framework, presented in Figure 39.1, demonstrating that gerontology has reached the stage of transformation into a distinct academic discipline. It shows the distinctive as well as integrated nature of the knowledge bases in gerontology that warrant defining it as a discipline. The elements that make up the framework define the parameters of the "knowledge infrastructure" concept. This framework was adapted for the goals of this analysis from that proposed by Sivan (1995).

The framework shows the growth of an academic research base, and the professional application of academic knowledge. The integration of these two

39.1

Analytic framework for assessing the development of gerontology as a discipline.

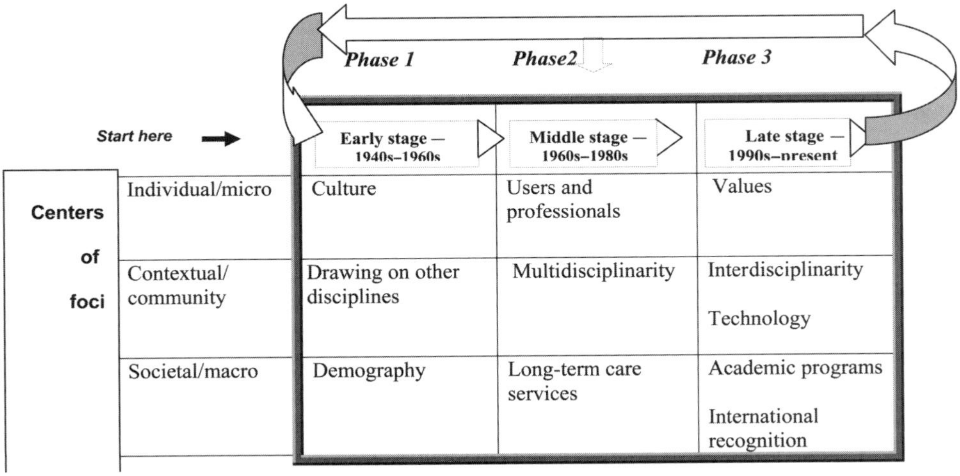

		Phase 1	Phase2	Phase 3
		Early stage — 1940s–1960s	Middle stage — 1960s–1980s	Late stage — 1990s–present
Centers of foci	Individual/micro	Culture	Users and professionals	Values
	Contextual/ community	Drawing on other disciplines	Multidisciplinarity	Interdisciplinarity Technology
	Societal/macro	Demography	Long-term care services	Academic programs International recognition

Start here →

dimensions of gerontology has become more pronounced with the passage of time. Thus, one can say that gerontology today comprises of "a range of biological, behavioral, and social sciences that are brought to focus upon aging and the aged. The interpenetration of these at this focus provides the gerontologist with his unique point of view, and to this extent, he is entitled to call the subject of his study a discipline" (Bramwell, 1985, p. 202).

Notably, the field of gerontology had matured considerably over the past several decades, as evidenced by accumulating knowledge bases, an increasing number of academic programs offering graduate and doctoral degrees, the publication of a growing number of professional journals as well as several encyclopedias on aging, and a growing number of scholars in the field. However, as is frequently true of emerging fields of scholarship, what is missing is a bridge between three elements: theoretical development, the proliferation of educational programs, and the institutionalization of the discipline.

A Proposal: The Gerontological Education Paradigm

Today, the multiple and complex needs of older people are understood to require interdisciplinary collaboration, and programs and learning experiences must be developed to facilitate a better understanding of the various roles and expertise required (Deveau, Blumberg, & Joshi, 1997). We posit that before proposing a paradigm for knowledge construction, or what we call the gerontological education paradigm, in gerontology, there is a necessity to consider the standards for knowledge development and dissemination. As Toffler (1990) points out, the struggle to develop standards, whether in the academic, political, economic, or technological realms, will determine the promotion of distinct bodies of knowledge in disciplines and professions. Conceivably, it will alter accepted gerontology perceptions and propel them toward further disciplinary developments.

How are we to assess the adequacy of a gerontological educational paradigm? Sivan (1995) provides a useful multidimensional approach in the area of education by proposing four factors that should be considered: (a) *Level of development and promotion of knowledge*—Should it be from the individual level through the organizational and supraorganizational to the national and international or vice versa? (b) *Goal*—Does it aim to simplify complex processes and facilitate their understanding, enhance communication and create a common language and/or unity among various professionals in order to achieve harmony and protect users of the knowledge, or influence the value system regarding the fixing of goals? (c) *Influence*—Does the knowledge development and dissemination exert a constructive, positive influence on the field, or is its influence unknown? (d) *Patronage*—Is there a patron, and, if so, does it consist of a single body or several, and is there an existing mandate for the field?

We argue that there is a need today to promote excellence and develop knowledge bases and research on processes of aging on the micro- and macrolevels from an interdisciplinary standpoint, adhering to the previously outlined standards. Such knowledge bases should be theory driven and reflective of an understanding of the special and dynamic nature of age and aging in different cultural and national contexts on the micro-, mezzo-, and macrolevels. Additionally, there should be closer and more harmonious integration between research and practice, emphasizing the interdisciplinarity nature of studies; the response to unique needs of heterogeneous aging populations by strongly incorporating issues of ethnicity, migration, and comparative cross-cultural and cross-national research; and the needed practice skills to work with the aged such as case management.

A new gerontological educational paradigm is guided by theoretical precepts drawn from the political economy of aging, a perspective that attends to the macrolevel structures and related processes of the demographic revolution, an evolving aging enterprise, and the technological and information changes that characterize advanced industrialized societies today. This outlook is illuminated in the model presented in Figures 39.2a and 39.2b. The model in Figure 39.2a shows the relationships between the demographic revolution, the aging enterprise (Estes, 1979), and the technological information revolutions that modern societies underwent. We discuss their significance for the development of educational standards and educational knowledge in gerontology here. Figure 39.2b shows a six-foci model with different links and impacts (processes) between the three structural components. Some of the processes are mutual, and some components are directly or indirectly impacting the others.

The bases for the demographic developments and, as a result, the growing aging enterprise serve as foundations in modern society for the need to construct *a paradigm of gerontological education.* Given the scope of service delivery—the developing markets of the aging enterprise—where a very large number of social and health care professionals are employed, many of them without or with very little knowledge base or training in gerontology and geriatrics, the time is ripe to develop innovative academic programs and to upgrade the level and prestige of those working in the field of aging. Furthermore, in the era of technological and information revolutions, a new culture is created—the information culture—which becomes yet another important element in modern society, especially today in the 21st century.

The model in Figure 39.2b shows the linkages between these three areas or structural components—the major "revolutions" that took place in 20th-century

39.2a

Relationships between the demographic revolution, the aging enterprise, and the technological and information revolutions.

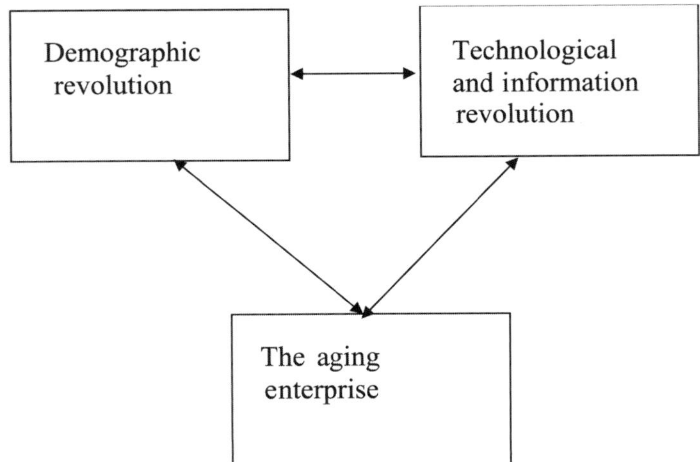

39.2b

A six-foci model: The links between the components. The three components represent structural aspects, whereas the vectors represent process aspects.

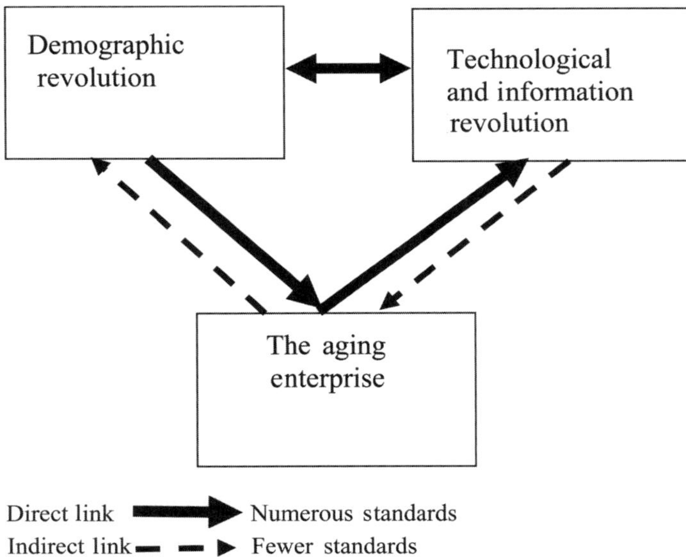

society and that are still relevant to aging societies: the demographic and the growing aging enterprise combined with the technological and information revolutions. These linkages are not equal in intensity or impact. The linkages between the demographic developments and the aging enterprise are more intensive than those between the other components. However, as these three areas represent structural components, there are also process components that affect the relationships between the areas.

These processes include (a) the pace of change in the area of the demographic revolution, (b) the markets and professional developments for the aging enterprise, and (c) the pace of development of the technological and information revolutions. In order to reinforce the mutuality between these three areas—or strengthen the direct impact that might *determine standards* for the development and dissemination of bodies of knowledge in gerontology—distinctive curricula must be developed that will stimulate research and theory advancements.

Implications for Developing Interdisciplinary Curricula

The complexity this model allows for is evident when linkages between the constructs are considered. A direction for trying to implement the model in a distinct interdisciplinary curricula is to understand the linkages between these foci. As shown in Table 39.1, the six-foci model affords the development of

39.1 Linkages Between the Structural Components of the Demographic Revolution, the Aging Enterprise, and the Technological and Information Revolutions and Their Interrelated Processes: Examples of Future Directions for the Discipline of Gerontology

	Structures		
Processes	Demographic revolution (DR)	The aging enterprise (AE)	Technological and information revolution (TIR)
Pace of change	Immigration, life expectancy, fertility rates DL	How does the DR impact the AE? IDL	Uses of TIR DL
Markets and professional development	Do they "catch" up with DR? IDL	How to answer needs of expansion of AE—using the gerontological paradigm DL	Using TRI toward improving level of professionalization IDL
Pace of development	What impact does it have on DR? IDL	Upgrading level of services—exposure to interdisciplinary programs DL	Improving tools for development of educational programs DL

future directions that is illustrated in the bivariate relationships shown in the cells by crossing structures with processes.

The construction of such a paradigm aims to develop and promote knowledge mainly for three target populations in gerontology: academic and research personnel, educators, and professional leaders and service providers. Such a conceptualization prompts the development of distinctive curricula with an interdisciplinary thrust and that at the same time attempt to achieve harmonization, create a common language between professionals working in the area, and stimulate teamwork. These developments will influence the field and will need to strengthen leaders to work and "invade" as many institutions of higher learning as possible.

Implementing a Gerontological Educational Paradigm

Goals

The *gerontological paradigm* should be formulated to achieve the following three goals. The first goal is to establish truly interdisciplinary research-oriented graduate and doctoral programs in gerontology with an emphasis on excellence. The aim should be to enhance the scientific study of aging and develop new and innovative knowledge bases unique to the needs of aging societies, thereby educating a new cadre of academic and practice-oriented leadership. In order to achieve interdisciplinarity, programs should draw and collaborate with other scholars from departments and schools, such as schools of law and business administration.

The second goal should be to upgrade the level of different professionals, planners, and administrators working in the health and social services for the aged. This could be achieved by providing academic expertise and training clinical practitioners in various research techniques while paying special attention to the unique population groups they are working with, like ethnic minorities, immigrant groups, or the chronically disabled.

The third goal should be to achieve closer and more harmonious integration between research and practice at all levels. This could be accomplished by the close collaboration of gerontology programs with centers for research on aging as well as working closely with the major ministries of health, welfare, education and others relevant in each country and with local and national service organizations. Students should be exposed to an integrative interdisciplinary seminar that would be geared to build a common professional language among the different professionals.

Program Premises

Programs should be based on the following premises. First is the multidimensionality of education, research, and training in gerontology. A flexible modular program must be developed geared to the individual needs of students. The second premise is the importance of educating and training professionals and potential academic and research cadre to answer the growing and complex needs of a heterogeneous and diverse aging population based on a holistic approach. Thus, a strong emphasis on research, policy, and management is imperative in order to promote understanding of issues like autonomy of elders and quality of life.

Examples of Paradigm-Based Curricula

The potential curricula stemming from such a paradigm should be as modular as possible, depending on the target populations but building a knowledge base for all that incorporates skills in research, theories of aging, and policy. There are several examples of various programs that utilized such an approach. One example is the European Masters of Gerontology (van Rijsselt, Parkatti, & Troisi, 2007). In another case, this approach guided the development of the two master's programs in Israel during the past decade that were described and analyzed by Carmel and Lowenstein (2007). The aim was to be on the forefront of international cutting-edge gerontological educational initiatives. The establishment of the graduate Department of Gerontology at the University of Haifa, as well as the graduate Program at Ben-Gurion University, constitutes another milestone in the road toward gerontology becoming a distinct discipline in Israel (Lowenstein, 2001, 2004).

Challenges in Implementing a Gerontological Educational Paradigm

There are several challenges when we aim to construct such a paradigm and adhere to the standards outlined previously.

Level of Development and Promotion of Knowledge

In the United States, for example, the field has been organizationally institutionalized since the 1970s with the establishment of the Association for Gerontology in Higher Education. This development was also reflected in a workshop on the topic "graduate education in gerontology worldwide: exploring options for cross-national articulation, student exchanges and more" organized by the International Association of Gerontology and Geriatrics in 2004 (Gutman, 2007). It aimed to contribute to achieving the goals related to education and training expressed in the Second United Nations World Assembly on Ageing and articulated in the Madrid International Plan of Action on Ageing (United Nations, 2003).

Yet this effort remains problematic, as aptly expressed by Robert Kastenbaum (1992) several years ago and still relevant today: "Gerontology remains a kind of shadow land today, despite all the studies, courses, conferences, publications and service programs. . . . Gerontology is still highly dependent on the whims of the academic/governmental complex" (p. 135).

Goals

The development of gerontological topics and their establishment in the curricula are influenced by societal values regarding aging, and those of various professionals. The goal is to train a potential cadre of researchers, lecturers, care professionals for the aged in various fields (especially in social and health care services), and qualified top management administrators; to develop interdisciplinary research; and to assume leadership roles in the field of aging, still lacking in many countries.

Determining the Main Topics and Study Areas

Should the focus be, for example, on management or research or on practice and interventions? Should policymakers and the array of services be recognized as "agents of change" and a practicum experience started? An educational program should be flexible enough to understand the need to develop, for example, new practice skills in management.

Influence and Impact

For an educational program to be effective, it must exert a positive influence in training top professionals and impacting the prestige of the professionals as well as preparing a potential academic cadre. This could be reflected in the number of graduates who will hold key positions in health and welfare services after graduation. Additionally, the number of new programs established by graduates and the number of those who did not work in the field previously and after graduation are absorbed in the labor market.

Integrating Research and Practice

An important issue has been the integration of two historic trends in the development of gerontological knowledge: the growth of an academic research base and the professional application of academic knowledge. The integration of the two trends has become more pronounced with the passage of time and will impact and produce social change. It should address critical issues of scientific, intellectual, social, economic, and/or cultural significance in the area of gerontology.

Such integration will also allow for more theory development, which has lagged in gerontology. The main reasons for such a lag were an unwillingness by researchers to integrate data with theory, insufficient synthesis of theoretical insights with existing knowledge, the "problem-solving" focus of gerontology that may detract from "basic research" where theory is so important, and ongoing epistemological debates (e.g., "positivism" versus "antipositivism"; Bengtson, Burgess, & Parrott, 1997). Developing curricula based on the previously mentioned model should be evaluated by the two criteria: (a) enhancement of the excellence of the research program and (b) development of highly qualified personnel.

Advantages of a Gerontological Education Paradigm

The proposed gerontological paradigm is innovative, as it offers an opportunity to develop programs with a rich and diversified range of courses in the social, behavioral, psychological, medical, legal, economic, and physiological aspects of aging, policy planning, organization, and management of service provision. It should pose a challenging experience for participants and should be tailored to individual and small groups' needs. It should be innovative by being flexible and continuously changing, based on feedback from the academic community, service networks, and students. It should be innovative in the sense of aiming for all students not only to generate, evaluate, and effectively disseminate new and existing knowledge and best practices but also to train others to identify priority gaps in knowledge needed for practice and policy development.

Three strategies might be suggested to further the advancement of the paradigm. The first strategy is to build as broad an interdisciplinary faculty as possible within the various programs developed—assembling a committed staff of social gerontologists, social workers, sociologists, psychologists, geriatricians, biologists, psycho biologists, policy planners, philosophers, architects, and lawyers.

Second, there should be a strengthening of the university–community links through consultation with top management and policymakers and actively involving the major service organizations. A third strategy is to build a strong research base through close collaboration with centers or institutes for research on aging and centers of excellence. Such collaboration will allow students to work on their research theses and become involved in studies conducted by faculty members. The aim here should be on the advancement of students' research skills, supporting their theses and other research projects, and disseminating this knowledge through active involvement of faculty and students in conferences and publications.

Conclusion

The proposed paradigm of the gerontological education constitutes a framework for looking at the linkages between the "three revolutions"—the demographic revolution, the growing aging enterprise, and the technological and information revolution—and the evolution of gerontology from a field of study into a distinct scientific discipline (outlined in Table 39.1). The approach can contribute to an analysis of the current state of knowledge in the field as well as to an analysis of a particular knowledge system or the design of new knowledge initiatives. Such varied uses of the proposed framework point to its potentially generative capacity.

As with every framework, the gerontological education paradigm has inherent limitations. Essentially, certain parts of it may look quite different in the real world because translating the actual meaning of each component of the proposed paradigm into educational programs is difficult. Certainly, the proposed analytic model is not a definitive framework. It can be modified and refined to support evolving demands, different paces of change, and new circumstances. If it stimulates new ideas about the components of a knowledge infrastructure in gerontology, it will have contributed to enhancing the establishment of gerontology as a distinct scientific discipline with an emphasis on interdisciplinarity. This will override questions about the multidisciplinarity versus the interdisciplinarity of new curricula and new programs. Today, the multiple and complex needs of the elderly are understood to require interdisciplinary collaboration, and programs and learning experiences must be developed to facilitate a better understanding of the various roles and expertise required (Deveau et al., 1997).

The goal of the paradigm is to make available knowledge usable. A logical means to accomplish this is to ensure that the educational programs that are developed are responsive to changing needs. In this context, definitive educational standards must be established for the ongoing development, evaluation, and dissemination of future gerontological knowledge bases.

In summary, one can conclude that gerontology is on its way to becoming an academic discipline, moving from multidisciplinarity to interdisciplinarity. As Kunkel (2001) observes in reviewing the fifth edition of Binstock and George's *Handbook of Aging and the Social Sciences,* "The book portrays a field characterized by a reflective maturity in theory, sophistication in methods, a high degree of breadth and depth in topical areas, and scholars able to offer historical and analytical reviews of those areas" (p. 130).

The proposed gerontological educational paradigm attempts to emphasize the relationships between the three societal age-related revolutions, containing two basic elements: time-related changes at the micro-, mezzo-, and macrolevels and their interrelations and interactions (Morgan & Kunkel, 1998)—what Ferraro (1997) calls the "gerontological imagination."

References

Alwin, D. F., & Campbell, R. T. (2001). Longitudinal methods in the study of human development and aging. In R. H. Binstock & L. K. George (Eds.), *Handbook of aging and the social sciences* (5th ed., pp. 22–43). San Diego, CA: Academic Press.

Bass, S. A., & Ferraro, K. F. (2000). Gerontology education in transition: Considering disciplinary and paradigmatic evolution. *The Gerontologist, 40,* 97–106.

Bengtson, V. C., Burgess, E. O., & Parrott, T. M. (1997). Theory, explanation, and a third generation of theoretical development in social gerontology. *Journal of Gerontology: Social Sciences, 52,* S72–S88.

Bengtson, V. L., Cutler, N. E., Mangen, D. J., & Marshall, V. W. (1985). Generations, cohorts, and relations between age groups. In R. H. Binstock & E. Shanas (Eds.), *Handbook of aging and the social sciences* (2nd ed). New York: Van Nostrand Reinhold.

Bengtson, V. L., Lowenstein, A., Putney, N. M., & Gans, D. (2003). Global aging and the challenges to families. In V. L. Bengtson & A. Lowenstein (Eds.), *Global aging and challenges to families* (pp. 1–26). New York and Berlin: Aldine De Gruyter.

Bramwell, R. D. (1985). Gerontology as a discipline. *Educational Gerontology, 11,* 201–211.

Carmel, S., & Lowenstein, A. (2007). Addressing a nation's challenge: Graduate programs in gerontology in Israel. *Gerontology and Geriatrics Education, 27,* 49–64.

Deveau, E. J., Blumberg, P., & Joshi, A. (1997). Charting the outcomes of an interdisciplinary summer institute on gerontology. *Educational Gerontology, 23,* 707–723.

Estes, C. L. (1979). *The aging enterprise.* San Francisco: Jossey-Bass.

Ferraro, K. F. (1997). The gerontological imagination. In K. F. Ferraro (Ed.), *Gerontology: Perspectives and issues* (pp. 3–18). New York: Springer Publishing.

Gutman, G. M. (2007). IAGG's role in graduate education in gerontology. *Gerontology and Geriatrics Education, 27,* 1–10.

Hagestad, G. O., & Dannefer, D. (2001). Concepts and theories of aging: Beyond microfication in social science approaches. In R. H. Binstock & L. K. George (Eds.), *Handbook of aging and the social sciences* (5th ed., pp. 3– 21). New York: Academic Press.

Haley, W. E., & Zelinski, E. (2007). Progress and challenges in graduate education in gerontology: The U.S. experience. *Gerontology and Geriatrics Education, 27,* 11–26.

Hendricks, J., & Hendricks, D. C. (1986). *Aging in mass society* (3rd ed.). Boston: Little, Brown.

Hyman, H. (1979). *Education's lasting influence on values.* Chicago: University of Chicago Press.

Johnson, H. R., Britton, J. H., Lang, C. A., Seltzer, M. M., Stanford, E. P., Yanick, R., et al. (1980). Foundations for gerontological education. *The Gerontologist, 20*(Pt. 2), 1–61.

Kastenbaum, R. (1992). Visiting hours in shadowland. *The Gerontologist, 20,* 1–60.

Kleemeier, R. W., Havighurst, R. J., & Tibbitts, C. (1967). Social gerontology. In R. E. Kushner & M. E. Bunch (Eds.), *Graduate education in aging within the social sciences* (pp. 67–90). Ann Arbor, MI; Division of Gerontology.

Kunkel, S. R. (2001). Mapping the field: Shifting contours of social gerontology. A review essay of the Handbook of Aging and the Social Sciences. *The Gerontologist, 43,* 128–131.

Levine, M. (1981). Does gerontology exist? *The Gerontologist, 21,* 2–3.

Lowenstein, A. (2001). The multidimensionality of gerontological education—The experience of Israel. *Educational Gerontology, 27,* 493–506.

Lowenstein, A. (2004). Gerontology coming of age. *Educational Gerontology, 30,* 129–142.

Maddox, G. L., & Campbell, R. T. (1985). Scope, concepts, and methods in the study of aging. In R. H. Binstock & E. Shanas (Eds.), *Handbook of aging and the social sciences* (2nd ed., pp. 3–28). New York: Van Nostrand Reinhold.

Metchnikoff, E. (1905). *The nature of man: Studies in optimistic philosophy.* New York: G. P. Putman's Sons.

Meyer, M. (2003). The current state and developments in gerontology in European higher education. *Educational Gerontology, 29,* 55–70.

Morgan, L., & Kunkel, S. (1998). *Aging: The social context.* Thousand Oaks, CA: Pine Forge Press.

Peterson, D. (1986). Extent of gerontology instruction in American institutions of higher education. *Educational Gerontology, 12,* 519–529.

Rosenberg, C. (1979). Towards an ecology of knowledge: On discipline, context and history. In A. Oleson & J. Voss (Eds.), *The organization of knowledge in modern America, 1890–1920* (pp. 449–455). Baltimore: Johns Hopkins University Press.

Sivan, Y. Y. (1995). *Setting standards in the age of knowledge.* Bloomington, IN: Technos Press.

Toffler, A. (1990). *Powershift: Knowledge, wealth and violence at the edge of the 21st century.* New York: Bantam.

United Nations, Economic and Social Council. (2003). *Madrid plus 5.* New York: United Nations.

Van Rijsselt, R. J., Parkatti, T., & Troisi, J. (2007). European initiatives in postgraduate education in gerontology. *Gerontology and Geriatrics Education, 27,* 79–98.

The Future of Theories of Aging

The Future of Theories of Aging

40

Daphna Gans
Norella M. Putney
Vern L. Bengtson
Merril Silverstein

This handbook brings together the theoretical insights of some of the most prominent researchers in the filed of aging. Their chapters present a diverse array of current inter- and intradisciplinary theorizing about the phenomena of aging. The authors come from a variety of disciplines and are guided by different theoretical perspectives. These intellectual differences are reflected in the conceptual contrasts and theoretical tensions in the field of aging research today. However, across most of the chapters in this handbook, a novel trend can be recognized: an integration of theoretical perspectives both within and across disciplines. There is agreement among authors concerning the interrelatedness of aging phenomena. It is not enough to understand specific aspects of the aging process. Rather, given the interconnectedness among the various dimensions of aging, there is a growing recognition that understanding the whole is greater than just the sum of its parts. Scientific progress in the field of aging requires a stance and a discourse that crosses theoretical and disciplinary boundaries. To understand the processes of aging requires an intellectually inclusive approach.

The contributors to this handbook have devoted an astonishing amount of intellectual effort to developing innovative explanations that advance knowledge in their fields. Their chapters present important innovations in theory and highlight important new questions for future theorizing. These innovations and questions will shape the future of aging research.

Our goal in this chapter is to summarize current theoretical trends in the field of aging and to suggest future directions for theory development. We begin by discussing four kinds of contrast or tension that differentiate theories presented in this volume: (a) differences in theoretical scope—for example, general theory or middle-range and single-aspect theories; (b) uncertainty *versus* predictability as a theme in theorizing; (c) emphasis on resilience and health or decline and disease; and (d) a focus on individual agency or on structural constraints. We then turn to discuss four main themes that appear to be common across the theories and disciplines represented in this handbook: (a) aging as a lifelong process, (b) cumulative advantages and disadvantages at both individual and population levels, (c) the interrelationships between context or environment and aging individuals, and (d) the focus on variability over universality in aging. We consider how these areas of communality can guide the development of future theory building and end our chapter with a discussion of cross-disciplinarity and its prospects for continued development in the future.

Contrasts in Theories of Aging

In chapter 2, Achenbaum discusses the usefulness of a dialectic approach in advancing a historical understanding of theories of aging. He proposes that it is through such an approach that a new and better explanation is eventually created, one that acknowledges both "sides" yet creates a deeper and more meaningful explanation. The chapters in this handbook reflect four sets of dualisms, or what we term theoretical contrasts, in the study of aging.

General Theory or Single-Aspect Theories?

In providing a panoramic view of the history of general theories of aging, Achenbaum (chapter 2) observes that some fields (for example, the sociology of aging) had in the past worked toward developing a grand theory—an *all-inclusive* theory, such as disengagement or activity theories, that attempted to explain basic principles of aging and well-being—but such efforts were subsequently abandoned after being severely criticized for reductionism. With growing recognition of the complexities of aging, researchers opted to develop middle-range or single-aspect theories, reducing the theoretical scope to focus on smaller parts of the larger set of aging phenomena (Bengtson, Putney, & Johnson, 2005). Those supporting middle-range or single-aspect theorizing feel that all-inclusive theories are too reductionistic. Middle-range or single-aspect theories are usually treated as complementing rather than competing with each other. Vasunilashorn and Crimmins (chapter 4), for example, discuss a number of theories in biodemography and typologize them into two main types: those that explain the "why" versus those explaining the "who." These theories coexist and complement each other as each attempts to explain different parts of the aging phenomena.

Several authors have asserted recently that gerontology is becoming an *integrative* discipline (Bass, chapter 19; Alkema & Alley, 2006), one that incorporates and organizes the various research and theoretical efforts across various disciplines. Such an integrative model, according to these authors, does not only acknowledge the complementary nature of the various middle-range or single-aspect theories but also embraces the multiplicity of theories of aging. This would seem to be fertile ground for the development of a grand theory in aging.

The search for a grand theory is highly appealing to some gerontologists. Fry (chapter 27) argues that a grand theory of aging is the ideal or the "Holy Grail"; it is the complexity of reality that may prevent us from achieving it. Perhaps the strongest view supporting grand theory in this handbook is that of Austad (chapter 8). A theory in Austad's view is a comprehensive all-encompassing explanation that is universal but parsimonious. He argues that a good theory will explain a variety of phenomena, providing explanations not only of the rule but also the exceptions to the rule. He further suggests that theories, unlike hypotheses, are mutually *exclusive, and therefore cannot* coexist. If one is demonstrated to be supported by empirical evidence, the other is debunked by default.

Reviewing the chapters in this handbook raises the question: Are we going to see more attempts of grand theory building in the future, or will other theoretical strategies, such as integrating across middle-range theories, take its place? We feel that the pursuit of an all-inclusive general explanation for aging phenomena (a grand theory) will likely prevail, at least in biology and (in some cases) psychology. We feel there is renewed interest in developing an all-encompassing theory of aging in the social sciences. While it is clear that such explanation cannot be unidisciplinary, we think that the growing trend toward interdisciplinarity may indeed reflect an implicit pursuit of a general, all-encompassing theory.

Uncertainty or Predictability?

A number of authors in this handbook highlight the increase of uncertainty in the lives of older individuals and theorize its likely ramifications. Perhaps the most urgent concern is the future of old-age policy. Faced by financial constraints, many countries (see chapter 29 for the United States and chapter 34 for Sweden) may be required to make changes to their old-age welfare programs, including possibly decreasing benefits or changing eligibility age. While the well-being of the aged population as a group in the United States has improved since the introduction of Social Security, uncertainty about the future of public programs is increasing. A decline in the level of benefits can undo the progress that these programs achieved in improving the situation of the elderly in the United States. As Hudson (chapter 29) notes, such changes may have more than just practical or financial consequences. In fact, an arbitrary age of eligibility to this program defines who is "old" in our society. Uncertainty about age of eligibility, therefore, means that we cannot even define who is old.

Uncertainty about aging is accelerated in an era of globalization. Walker (chapter 32) and Phillipson (chapter 33) discuss the effects that globalization will continue to have on the lives of the elderly. When national borders are replaced with a postnational reality, the lives of aging individuals in one country will necessarily be affected by economic and social forces in all other countries, and thus lead to increased insecurity. Settersten and Trauten (chapter 24) further express concerns that in a reality governed by such uncertainty, the ability of researchers to make predictions about the lives of older adults becomes more problematic.

Thematic contrasts between uncertainty and predictability take form in other areas of study as well. A good example is the debate between the two general theories in the biology of aging: programmed senescence (structured genetic expressions in old age) versus stochastic processes (such as random genetic mutation and oxidative stress). Several scholars suggest ways to bridge these ostensibly opposing explanations of biological aging. For example, Martin (chapter 10) suggests that stochastic processes in genes *and* exposures to random elements in the environment are inseparable in evolutionary theory, thereby bridging the two sides of the debate.

While Martin offers a bridge between these divergent biological explanations of aging, how will the theoretical tension between uncertainty or predictability be addressed in other disciplines? In social gerontology and the sociology of aging, there is a growing movement toward deemphasizing prediction. Proponents of critical gerontology and feminist theories, for example, call for considering multiple perspectives in an attempt to discover the experience of aging. Allen and Walker (chapter 28) suggest that such approaches allow researchers to be more comfortable with the challenges of uncertainty. As opposed to positivistic approaches, where the researcher is expected to know, critical approaches emphasize ambivalence and focus on diversity. As a result, Allen and Walker suggest, researchers guided by such approaches may be better equipped to conduct research on aging in the future, an era of growing uncertainty.

Resilience or Decline?

Many psychological theorists in aging emphasize the positive aspects of aging. Several authors in this handbook focus on resilience to change in old age, or the ability of older adults to compensate for possible declines and losses; some emphasize positive changes in old age. For example, Blanchard-Fields and Stange (chapter 15) suggest that emotional processing, social expertise, and emotion regulation may in fact improve in old age. Zarit (chapter 37) and Kryla-Lighthall and Mather (chapter 18) discuss the robustness of emotional well-being in old age, noting that older adults as a group enjoy a higher level of emotional well-being than their younger counterparts. Kryla-Lighthall and Mather suggest that older adults are "uniquely suited to live healthy emotional lives." They emphasize the importance of emotional well-being as it is interrelated with cognitive functioning and physical health.

Three chapters in the handbook (Blanchard-Fields & Stange, chapter 15; Kryla-Lighthall & Mather, chapter 18; Willis, Schaie & Martin, chapter 17) expand on the socioemotional selectivity theory proposed by Carstensen (Carstensen, 1995).

Three other chapters (Knight & Laidlaw, chapter 38; Labouvie-Vief, chapter 16; Zarit, chapter 37) base their discussions on the selective optimization with compensation model, proposed by Baltes (Baltes, 1997). Both these theoretical models emphasize how older adults can adapt to changes, losses, and declines that may accompany old age. Acknowledging the role of both biological factors and social structures, Zarit (chapter 37) and Knight and Laidlaw (chapter 38) suggest that individuals can prepare for their old age and, with the right preparation, can achieve better results in dealing with possible losses and decline.

While many psychological theories in aging emphasize resilience, most biological theories focus on decline and senescence in old age. Proponents of the antagonistic pleiotropy theory, for example, would argue that the very mechanisms or systems that support and promote adaptation earlier in life can have devastating effects in late life. The immune system is suggested as an example (Effros, chapter 9). Other biological theories consistent with the wear-and-tear approach (such as Shringarpure & Davies, chapter 13) focus on inevitable damage caused to the various systems in the body with age.

What will be the focus in the future? It is likely that theorizing on both resilience and decline with age will involve examination of the interaction between biological factors, individual choices, and environmental factors. Willis, Schaie, and Martin (chapter 17) present a theory explaining plasticity in cognitive functioning across the life span as a function of the interplay between three levels: brain, behavior, and society or culture. Labouvie-Vief (chapter 16) points out that emotional resilience in later life depends on factors such as the level of activation (older individuals respond more negatively to stress) and the level of already established vulnerability (levels of anxiety and depression). Future theories will likely focus on unveiling the ways in which this interaction changes over the life span for different individuals. Biologists of aging may continue to focus on decline, whereas psychologists may continue to focus on resilience. Either way, we believe that the focus will shift toward understanding interindividual variation across the life span and will center around why and how some individuals show more resilience and others more decline at the same chronological age. Such theoretical efforts will set in motion a trend toward understanding mechanisms of adaptability and plasticity over the life course.

Individual Agency or Structural Constraints?

Concepts of successful aging or productive aging focus on the individual's role in shaping his or her aging experience. They emphasize the importance of making healthy choices by staying physically active, socially engaged, and cognitively involved. Applications of successful aging in psychotherapy (e.g., Knight and Laidlaw, chapter 38; Zarit, chapter 37) are based on the premise that older individuals can be guided to make changes in their lives. While these theories recognize the role of social and biological constraints, they focus on individuals' agency in making positive changes toward a positive aging experience.

On the other hand, some theorists in the social sciences section suggest that greater theoretical weight should be given to societal constraints in contrast to individual agency. Guided by political economy theory (Kail, Quadagno, & Keene, chapter 30; Walker, chapter 32) and critical perspectives such as feminist theories (Allen & Walker, chapter 28; Calasanti, chapter 25), these authors emphasize the role of social structures in shaping individuals' behaviors. Individuals have differential access to various opportunities and constraints based on various characteristics, including gender, race, ethnicity, socioeconomic status, age, marital status, and sexual orientation. These differentials translate into structural inequalities that are beyond the individual's control. Earlier discussions focused on risk factors across the life course note that individuals may be placed in more than one at-risk group, signified by such concepts as "double jeopardy" or "triple jeopardy" (Bengtson & Dowd, 1978; Estes, 2001). More recent theoretical development reflects advancement in critical theories, and feminist theories introduced the concept of intersectionality (Allen & Walker, chapter 28; Calasanti, chapter 25) to denote the complexity and interconnectedness of myriad structures of inequality. These authors further suggest that these inequalities have cumulative disadvantageous effects over the life course; thus, differences across various population groups accelerate with age and grow more pronounced in old age. Focusing on *structural* opportunities and constraints suggests that change in the lives of individuals cannot be achieved by the individuals themselves but can occur only through larger structural societal change such as policy initiatives.

The theme of choice *versus* structural constraints can be extended beyond theories of aging in the social and psychological sciences to theorizing in biology and epidemiology. While it is clear that individuals' choices in health behavior, including healthy nutrition, exercise, and smoking cessation, play a significant role in one's longevity and healthy life expectancy, the effect of such health behaviors are limited by biological predispositions on the one hand and by social conditions, such as damaging factors in the environment, on the other.

Will future theories of aging focus more on individual agency or on structural constraints? Or will future theories of aging be successful in linking individual agency and structural constraints, long considered a central theoretical challenge? One way this might occur is through application of the concept of intersectionality (see Calasanti, chapter 25, and Dilworth-Anderson & Cohen, chapter 26). Hendricks and Hatch (chapter 23) offer a theory specifically addressing this issue. It is likely that new theories will be developed to explain trajectories of individuals in various intersections across inequalities of gender, race, ethnicity, class, age, marital status, and sexual orientation. The concept of cumulative advantage or disadvantage (see more detailed discussion in the next section) adds another dimension to this discussion, addressing the cumulative effects of these interacting factors over the life course. Furthermore, in many chapters, an underlying theme of balance between agency and structure is apparent. It is clear that most authors would agree that agency is embedded within structure. We discuss this notion of the individual as nested with the multiple social and other macrocontexts or environments in the next section.

Beyond Disciplinary Boundaries: Common Themes Guiding Future Theory Development

Despite some obvious theoretical contrasts or tensions within and across the various disciplinary approaches, there are striking similarities that can be noted among contemporary theorists of aging. We believe that these commonalities will become even more evident in the future. We suggest four themes or common areas of focus in theorizing about aging that cut across disciplinary boundaries in the field of aging. Much like the areas of theoretical contrasts discussed earlier, there is considerable overlap and interconnectedness among these areas of similarity. By recognizing common themes, researchers can identify future areas of theory building and research that will benefit from cross-disciplinary collaboration. Additionally, by finding common threads that cut across the various disciplines, we can not only summarize what is already known but also decide on new research initiatives that should be pursued in the future. We can begin to raise new questions about aging phenomena and theorize about possible explanations.

Aging as a Lifelong Process: Understanding the Mechanisms

Referred to as life span development in psychological and biological theories of aging (Shringarpure & Davies, chapter 13; Willis, Schaie, & Martin, chapter 17), life course in sociological theories of aging (Dannefer & Kelley-Moore, chapter 21; Marshall, chapter 31), or life cycle models in economy of aging (Hurd, Smith, & Zissimopoulos, 2007; Yaari, 1965), the idea of aging as a lifelong process appears to be universal across all disciplines. Aging does not start at some arbitrary point in life but rather is a gradual, lifelong process. As a result, explaining aging phenomena is dependent on the understanding of processes occurring earlier in the lifetime. The recognition that aging is a lifelong process is closely linked to another common theoretical theme—the process of cumulative advantage and disadvantage, which we will discuss separately.

The concept of life span development is inherent to most biological theories of aging. For example, the free radical theory of aging (see review in Shringarpure & Davies, chapter 13) and other wear-and-tear theories suggest that aging is the result of an accumulation of harmful changes and a diminishing adequacy of self-repair mechanisms over time. Classical psychological life span development models (Erikson, 1959) view aging as a stage in the life span and focus on transitions from one state to the next over the life span. Successful attainment of goals in later stages in life is dependent on successful achievement of goals in earlier stages of the life span.

Marshall (chapter 31) tracks the development of the life course theoretical perspective in the sociology of aging. What is different about the sociological use of the life course perspective is that it goes beyond consideration of time as a factor in aging or change with age. Time is viewed as a contextual factor within which aging occurs (Baars, chapter 5). In fact, the perspective guides the researcher to consider multiple contextual factors, including historical time or change, cohort effects, geographic location, and other contexts at the macrolevel (Dannefer & Kelley-Moore, chapter 21).

The life course perspective is typically considered a theoretical perspective, representing a set of lenses, or a framework, rather than explanation—a theory. The question of whether the life course perspective will become an explanatory theory in the future is raised by Marshall (chapter 31). This question is closely related to the first area of contrast suggested in this chapter, the desirability of one all-encompassing theoretical explanation of aging.

Perhaps the more pressing question to ask is not whether the life course perspective will become a theory but rather whether future theories of aging will attempt to explain how time and aging phenomena interact. There is much empirical evidence in all disciplines that the passing of time is related to aging phenomena. We know from biological theories of aging that self-repair mechanisms decline in efficiency over the life span; we know from sociological theories that inequality increases over time and that in old age differences across various population groups amplify. What is missing, however, is the understanding of the *why* and *how,* or, in other words, how these processes occur and what are the *mechanisms* that govern interrelationships between the various factors that are associated with aging over time. Biological theorists have long been focused on understanding mechanisms and pathways; now such interest is emerging in other disciplines as well. For example, Willis, Schaie, and Martin (chapter 17), in their theory of cognitive plasticity, discuss the need to understand mechanisms that explain change in the interplay between the three components of cognitive plasticity (brain, behavior, and society) over the life span. Another example is the theory of cumulative inequality proposed by Ferraro, Shippee, and Schafer (chapter 22).

Previous psychological and social theories of aging focused more on describing cognitive changes over the passage of time or on accumulation of advantages or disadvantages over time. For the most part, they remained at the description stage and did not pursue understanding of mechanisms and change in mechanisms over time. Future theorists should focus on the mechanisms of aging: How do factors associated with aging phenomena interact over the life course? Do factors associated with aging interact in the same fashion throughout the life course, or does the nature of the interplay between the various factors change over time? If it changes, what might *explain* such change? How do individuals' trajectories over the life course differ? Are there different mechanisms throughout the life course for different individuals, and, if they change, what explains change for one compared to another? It is only through answering such questions that we can advance in our efforts to explain aging as a lifelong process.

Cumulative Advantages and Disadvantages at the Individual and Population Levels

The concept of accumulation of benefits or liabilities over time and with aging is common to most theories of aging and is closely related to the view of aging as a lifelong process. However, it is important to note that the various disciplines discuss the accumulation of these characteristics at different levels of observation and analyses. In most biological theories of aging the focus is on intraindividual change over time at the level of the molecule, cell, system, or organism. Wear-and-tear theories of aging view aging as the accelerated accumulation of harmful events and the progressive weakening of self-repair mechanisms over time. Psychological theories have traditionally viewed the decline in mental capacity with age from an intraindividual perspective. The relatively new field of positive psychology maintains that some skills strengthen or resist decline with aging, particularly the ability to integrate knowledge (i.e., wisdom) and use an emotional focus in addressing practical problems. Psychological theories have increasingly taken into account individual differences in rates of cognitive decline, regulation of emotion, and reactivity to various stimuli based on intrinsic and extrinsic factors.

In contrast, most social theories discuss accumulation of characteristics from a population perspective, focusing on interindividual divergences in health and financial resources with the passage of time. Further, differentiation leading to inequalities that magnify over time "is a not a property of individuals but of populations or other collectivities (such as cohorts)" (Dannefer, 2003, p. S327). Political economy and critical theories of aging attribute individual differences in old age to social structures in a society that systematically denies powerless groups access to various resources and opportunities. Time serves to reinforce and amplify earlier disadvantages, thereby increasing inequalities between groups and individuals in later life.

Typically, these two lines of examination—those addressing intraindividual and those addressing interindividual accumulation of characteristics—have been conducted independently. But understanding the reciprocal relationship between the intra- and interaccumulation processes is closely related to the next common area of focus we discuss: interrelationships between the individual and the environment. A good example of theory that addresses the interplay of intra- and interindividual processes over time is the interdisciplinary stress theory of aging (see Finch & Seeman, 1999). Stress theories of aging suggest that age changes in various regulatory systems in the body result in declining ability to not only adapt to various environmental changes or stressors but also recover from challenges and traumas to achieve homeostatic balance. They further suggest that it is the cumulative exposure to environmental stressors that affect the rate of loss of resiliency. Thus, individuals who belong to a disadvantaged population in the society are at higher risk of exposure to stressors throughout their life and are thus more likely to suffer from steeper decline in biological resiliency.

Future theories of aging that focus on inequality can benefit from deeper examination of the interplay between intra- and interindividual changes over time. As Krause (chapter 6) notes, theories of aging must include consideration of social structure components, psychosocial and behavioral aspects, and biological and genetic processes. Some of the questions that need to be addressed are the following: Does the intersectionality of various inequality systems (gender, race, ethnicity, marital status, and sexual orientation) change over time, or does it remain constant? Is the relationship over time simply linear and additive? Or, alternatively, do certain factors weigh more than others? Additionally, does the same set of factors have the same effect on different individuals? Or, alternatively, do individuals' biological predispositions to changes over time interact with the set of inequalities? If there is interaction, we would expect that some individuals respond better to inequality factors than others. And if this is the case, further exploration is required to clarify the mechanisms and pathways of the reciprocal relationship between intra- and interindividual accumulation of factors over time.

Focusing on average rates of change due to aging in a species downplays not only variation in the aging process—deviations that can be relegated to random components of a model—but also *diversity* in the aging process due to mixed environmental exposures. In humans, such structured differentiation or inequality may be remedied by changes in public policies and institutional arrangements. To address this issue, we first need to gain a better understanding of how much of the "rate of change" due to aging is immutable and how much it is the product of resource inequalities across social groups and cohorts.

Interrelationships Between Environment and Aging Individuals

There appears to be a consensus across disciplines in gerontology that understanding the environment and the individual's place within it is crucial for understanding the aging process. The surrounding of an individual can be termed *environment* or *ecology* in biological theories (Kaplan, Gurven, & Winking, chapter 3); *context* in sociological theories of the life course (Marshall, chapter 31); *systems, social structures,* or *social locations* in theories addressing inequality (Calasanti, chapter 25); or *the social,* as proposed in a recently developed theory by Walker (chapter 32). Regardless, the message is universal: aging must be understood within the environments in which individuals are embedded.

Despite recognition of the importance of integrating personal and environmental factors in aging research (Bass, chapter 19), prior to today there have been few attempts to develop aging theory by integrating comparable concepts of individual and environment across disciplines. Instead, most previous efforts at theorizing involved holistic classification frameworks that listed various environmental concepts in one figure, typically involving a series of concentric circles whereby individuals were presented as being nested within a set of increasingly wider environments. In some cases, such as the human ecological model (Bronfenbrenner, 1979), there was a hierarchical order among the different environments, suggesting that environments closer to the individual have a stronger effect on the individual than those farther removed. While these approaches were helpful in recognizing the relationship between individuals and their surroundings, they are now replaced with more sophisticated explanations that recognize the interplay between individuals and their environments.

This handbook reflects some innovative theoretical developments that address the complex interplay of properties intrinsic and extrinsic to the individual. The concepts *mechanisms* and *pathways* are frequently used in discussing individuals and their environments. In developing their theory of biopsychosocial process of healthy aging, Ryff and Singer (chapter 7) provide specific postulates that address various pathways connecting psychosocial processes with biological ones. Effros (chapter 9) discusses the immune system as an example of the relationship between what she calls internal and external environments. As the immune system protects organisms from harmful attacks of external agents, it serves as a useful metaphor for how the effects of the environment are mediated by mechanisms internal to the organism. In another but altogether different example, Hendricks and Hatch (chapter 23) discuss how human agency in making lifestyle choices is shaped by social structural forces that lie outside the individual. While many of the chapters on biological and evolutionary theories of aging (Effros, chapter 9; Kaplan, Gurven, & Winking, chapter 3; Shringarpure & Davies, chapter 13) suggest that most mechanisms underlying the interplay between biological and environmental factors are still unknown, they specify the importance of asking and resolving such questions if we are to fully explain why and how we age. Asking these questions is already a step toward answering them.

What these chapters indicate is the need to better understand how processes *outside* individuals variously get "under the skin" *within* individuals, how these processes are structured by social characteristics and societal conditions, and how individuals and social groups act to shape the environments that affect them. Rather than rely on a static hierarchical design to organize persons within environments, new models of aging present a more complex picture of the engagement between persons and their environments—one that is more process driven, interactive, and reciprocal than before. We believe that these discussions will pave the course in which theories of aging are likely to travel. Theories that better incorporate the interplay between individuals and their environments will move the field from models that, as Krause (chapter 6) puts it, promote a "piecemeal understanding" of aging to those that provide a more inclusive and comprehensive solution to the aging puzzle.

Focusing on Variability Rather Than Universality

Most chapters in this handbook discuss variability in the aging process at several levels: within individuals, between individuals and within and across population groups, across societies, and across species. In some disciplines, the focus on variability is fundamental. Theories of biological aging focus on variability within molecules, cells, systems, or organisms. The field of genetics, for example, focuses on differences between genotypes (DNA sequences) and phenotypes (gene expressions) (Martin, chapter 10). Neuropsychological theories address individual variations such as differentials in neuron cell numbers and their relationship to outcomes of aging (Woodruff-Pak, Foy, & Thompson, chapter 11). Vasunilashorn and Crimmins (chapter 4) note that biodemography focuses on variability in the rate of aging across different species and across various human populations. Psychological theories of aging address differences by asking why older adults differ in the degree of emotional well-being, cognitive ability, emotional resilience and social engagement they experience in old age (Zarit, chapter 37; Labouvie-Vief, chapter 16). Critical theories such as feminist theories and the political economy of aging are particularly focused on structures of inequality across subgroups within populations (Allen & Walker, chapter 28; Calasanti, chapter 25; Kail, Quadagno, & Keene, chapter 30). Dilworth-Anderson and Cohen (chapter 26) discuss the importance of theorizing across cultures in attempting to understand variation and inequalities. While traditionally focused on intercohort differences, the life course perspective has been enriched by the theoretical attention paid to processes of cumulative advantage/disadvantage and is now addressing intracohort variability as well (Dannefer & Kelley-Moore, chapter 21).

Several handbook chapters indicate a growing interest in understanding interindividual variation in subjective meaning and in subjective experience of aging. A concern with meaning in aging (Baars, chapter 5; Krause, chapter 6; Longino & Powell, chapter 20) or spirituality (Johnson, chapter 36) emphasizes the role of an individual's interpretation and appraisal of the aging process. This has important implications for individuals' quality of life; research suggests that individuals with a greater sense of meaning enjoy better physical and mental health as well as higher levels of life satisfaction and happiness (Krause, chapter 6).

The concepts of meaning and experience, and specifically their variability and fluidity, also have implications for the methods scholars use in their research. Some disciplines such as anthropology have traditionally used qualitative methods to contrast and explain individual experiences situated within unique cultural settings (Fry, chapter 27). A phenomenology of aging approach can illuminate individual differences in the subtleties of meaning and interpretive evaluations of the ways aging is experienced in everyday life (Longino & Powell, chapter 20). Settersten and Trauten (chapter 24) argue that our understanding of aging may be flawed if it is not directly based on the aging individual's perspectives as appraised by a qualitative approach. But does a focus on subjective or cultural variation automatically dictate the use of qualitative approaches? Or can quantitative methods be utilized to capture such variation? While typically quantitative methods focus on means and other measures of central tendency, they are widely used to look at variance and examine divergence from means, as well as heterogeneity between individuals.

There has been a growing tendency among scholars in social theories of aging to approach the study of differential outcomes in aging using mixed methods, integrating both qualitative and quantitative analyses (Dilworth-Anderson & Cohen, chapter 26). Is the utilization of a mixed methods approach the wave of the future? Indeed a mixed method model provides a bridge between the two epistemological approaches. And, more important, such a model may indeed provide researchers with the needed tools to approach the study of aging. The chapters in this handbook indicate that contemporary focus is placed on variability rather than universality; individuals operate in diverse contexts and differ in the way they subjectively appraise extrinsic events, and in the way their intrinsic processes are affected by the extrinsic events. There is not a simple explanation to address such complexity, and any attempt to explain the processes of aging must recognize the great variability in these processes.

The Future of Interdisciplinarity: Cross-Disciplinarity as a Continuum

Grounding in a specific disciplinary orientation is generally considered a necessity for scientific research on aging. Guided by a specific set of lenses, a defined point of view, the researcher has a clear sense of where to look and what he or she is interested in uncovering. However, when studying complex phenomena such as aging, this disciplinary point of view may in fact hinder the development of knowledge. Using any unidisciplinary point of view is too narrow a framework for understanding aging. A unidisciplinary point of view on aging creates a set of blinders rather than lenses, and this may obstruct the ability to see other aspects of the aging process. Such an outlook not only limits the completeness of a theoretical understanding of the phenomenon of interest, but may also impede the scholar from asking the right questions.

The chapters in this handbook illustrate that most if not all researchers in aging have moved away from the unidisciplinary model. Most have recognized the importance of crossing over disciplinary boundaries to search for explanations of theories of aging. The cross-fertilization of different theoretical perspectives and knowledge bases is evident in almost all chapters. Authors include more than one theory in their development of innovative explanations. Several (Antonucci, Birditt, & Akiyama, chapter 14; Blanchard-Fields & Stange, chapter 15; Dannefer & Kelley-Moore, chapter 21) discuss the expansion of existing theories to account for new empirical evidence and new interdisciplinary developments in the field. Others (Ferraro, Shippee, & Schafer, chapter 22; Hendricks & Hatch, chapter 23; Knight & Laidlaw, chapter 38; Kryla-Lighthall & Mather, chapter 18; Labouvie-Vief, chapter 16; Walker, chapter 32; Willis, Schaie, & Martin, chapter 17) integrate existing theories within their discipline and across disciplines to formulate new theories of aging. Still others (Krause, chapter 6; Ryff & Singer, chapter 7; Vasunilashorn & Crimmins, chapter 4) focus explicitly on new interdisciplinary theorizing.

Based on these contributions, the movement toward cross-disciplinary theorizing can be conceptualized as a continuum. At the lower end, theorists may still operate from a paradigm that is consistent with one specific discipline but recognize the value of the work done in other disciplines. At the high end is full interdisciplinary theorizing and collaboration. The majority of the theoretical endeavors in this handbook fall somewhere along the high end of the continuum. In the first chapter, we suggested that interdisciplinarity is the wave of the future. The chapters indicate that indeed interdisciplinarity is growing in importance in theories of aging and that future explanations of aging will move more swiftly in that direction, toward more fully interdisciplinary explanations.

Conclusion

Our goal in this chapter has been to use current theoretical trends as illustrated in this handbook to suggest future directions in the development and application of theories about aging. We identified four areas of theoretical contrasts or tensions within the multidisciplinary field of aging as well as four areas of shared common foci across disciplines. These tensions will probably continue into the future, further differentiating theories of aging.

The four areas of contrast operate both within and across disciplines. The first involves differences in the scope of theory: should efforts at developing explanations be directed to general or grand theories, or should theorizing be much more limited, geared toward explaining single aspects of aging? Second is the contrast between theories targeting predictability in aging and those emphasizing uncertainty. Given that the environment within which we age is becoming more uncertain, making any scientific predictions becomes more difficult. A third contrast among theories of aging involves the focus on explaining decline and disease, on the one hand, or resilience and health, on the other. Fourth is the tension between individual agency and structural constraints. Theories of successful or productive aging, for example, focus on the individual's role in shaping his or her aging experience, emphasizing the importance of making healthy choices; political economy and critical theories, by contrast, focus on social forces (age, gender, race, social class, family status) and social institutions (the economy, the polity and civil society) that promote and reinforce structural inequalities beyond the individual's control.

At the same time, the theoretical developments discussed in this handbook reflect several important commonalities, themes that can be seen across current theories of aging. First is the importance of developing theories that reflect the lifelong process of aging. Explaining aging, from the cell to the person, is dependent on understanding processes manifest earlier in life. Second, cumulative advantage and disadvantage over the life course is an important aspect of aging at both the individual and population levels. The concept of accumulation of benefits or liabilities with aging is common to almost all current theories across all disciplines. A third common theme is the interface between context and individual in aging. There is consensus across the disciplines constituting gerontology that understanding the environment and the individual's place within it is crucial for understanding the aging process whether at the molecular or the societal level. Fourth, there appears to be a common interest in attempting to explain variability in aging—differences between individuals, across populations, between species—rather than focusing on universal characteristics. This is an interesting development; 25 years ago most theoretical work in aging attempted to identify common, or universal, predictors of age differences.

Despite ongoing theoretical contrasts or tensions discussed previously, we believe that the commonalities reflected in contemporary theorists of aging are likely to become even more evident in the future. Future theories are likely to focus on mechanisms and pathways that emphasize variation and diversity in the aging experience. There is a growing consensus across disciplines that understanding phenomena of aging must involve examination of the interplay between factors that are intrinsic and extrinsic to the individual. Individuals age within context; they are affected by the micro- and macroenvironments within which they age, and in turn, play an active role in shaping these environments to accommodate their aging.

It is important to note that theory construction is an evolving enterprise. Research provides new findings that may gradually shift theoretical perspectives within a discipline, and, in the most extreme scenario, overturn existing scientific dogma. Although paradigmatic revolutions in the field of aging are rare, we note several emergent trends since the last volume of this handbook was published. In biology, gene-selection theories from the field of evolutionary biology have gained significant traction toward becoming the dominant paradigm to explain why we age and die. In psychology, and to a lesser degree in sociology, the melding of traditional content with the biological underpinnings of aging has produced more inclusive, synthesized models that have proven to have great utility. We also note greater emphasis on purposeful, positive, and adaptive theories of aging in psychology, and greater use of social constructivism as a theoretical lens in the social sciences—with each discipline putting a greater premium on intentionality and meaning-making in the aging experience. In the policy arena, the macroforces of globalization and their effects on aging policy at the national level has become a dominant theme in the political economy of aging. Paradigmatic shifts may also be detected by what is absent in theoretical orientations today, such as the drift away from the concept of so-called normal aging in favor of diversity in the aging process.

What is still needed in our field is a deeper understanding of how processes external to the individual variously interact with internal mental and physical changes, and how aging individuals give meaning to those internal changes and society's response to them. Developing a comprehensive explanation of *how* and *why* aging-related changes occur is likely to be the goal of future theories of aging. By considering dynamic mechanisms across multiple systems and levels of analyses, and increasing the permeability of disciplinary boundaries, we will move the field toward more comprehensive solutions to the multifaceted puzzle of aging.

References

Alkema, G. E., & Alley, D. (2006). Gerontology's future: An integrative model for disciplinary achievement. *The Gerontologist, 46,* 574–582.

Baltes, P. B. (1997). On the incomplete architecture of human ontogeny: Selection, optimization, and compensation as foundation of developmental theory. *American Psychologist, 52,* 366–380.

Bengtson, V. L., & Dowd, J. J. (1978). Aging in minority populations: An examination of the double jeopardy hypothesis. *Journal of Gerontology, 33,* 427–434.

Bengtson, V. L., Putney, N. M., & Johnson, M. (2005). Are theories of aging necessary? In M. Johnson, V. L. Bengtson, P. Coleman, & T. Kirkwood, (Eds.), *The Cambridge handbook of age and ageing* (pp. 3–20). Cambridge: Cambridge University Press.

Bronfenbrenner, U. (1979). *The ecology of human development.* Cambridge, MA: Harvard University Press.

Carstensen, L. L. (1995). Evidence for a life-span theory of socioemotional selectivity. *Current Directions in Psychological Science, 4,* 151–156.

Dannefer, D. (2003). Cumulative advantage/disadvantage and the life course: Cross-fertilizing age and social science theory. *Journal of Gerontology: Social Sciences, 58,* S327–S337.

Erikson, E. H. (1959). Identity and the life cycle. *Psychological Issues Monograph I.* New York: International University Press.

Estes, C. L. (2001). *Social policy and aging.* Thousand Oaks, CA: Sage.

Finch, C. F., & Seeman, T. E. (1999). Stress theories of aging. In V. L. Bengtson & K. W. Schaie (Eds.), *Handbook of theories of aging* (pp. 81–97). New York: Springer Publishing.

Hurd, M., Smith, J. P., & Zissimopoulos, J. (2007). *Inter-vivos transfers over the lifecycle.* RAND Working Paper No. 524. Santa Monica, CA: RAND.

Yaari, M. E. (1965). Uncertain lifetime, life insurance and the theory of the consumer. *Review of Economic Studies, 32,* 137–150.

Author Index

Subject Index